Chemotherapy: Cancer Treatment

Chemotherapy: Cancer Treatment

Editor: Brielle Pittman

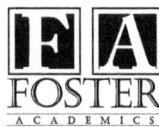

FA
FOSTER
ACADEMICS

www.fosteracademics.com

www.fosteracademics.com

FA
FOSTER
ACADEMICS

Cataloging-in-Publication Data

Chemotherapy : cancer treatment / edited by Brielle Pittman.
    p. cm.
Includes bibliographical references and index.
ISBN 978-1-63242-744-1
1. Cancer--Chemotherapy. 2. Chemotherapy. 3. Cancer--Treatment. I. Pittman, Brielle.
RC271.C5 C44 2019
616.994 06--dc23

Foster Academics,
118-35 Queens Blvd., Suite 400,
Forest Hills, NY 11375, USA

ISBN 978-1-63242-744-1 (Hardback)

Contents

Chapter 26

Chapter 27

Chapter 28

Permissions

Contributors

Index

Preface

Cancer is the condition in which there is an abnormal growth of cells that is coupled with malignant behavior relative to metastasis and invasion. Environmental factors along with genetic susceptibility contribute to genetic mutations in tumor suppressor genes and oncogenes. Such combined action gives rise to cancer. Chemotherapy is a cancer treatment, which uses chemotherapeutic agents or anti-cancer drugs for the treatment of cancer. It may also be performed for the reduction of symptoms. It comprises of intracellular poisons that inhibit cell division and extracellular signals. Some of the side effects of chemotherapy are the damage to healthy cells of the body, myelosuppression, mucositis and alopecia. This book presents the complex subject of chemotherapy in the most comprehensible language. Different approaches, evaluations, methodologies and advanced studies on cancer treatment have been included in this book. It will be a valuable resource for medical oncologists, oncological surgeons, residents and students alike.

The information contained in this book is the result of intensive hard work done by researchers in this field. All due efforts have been made to make this book serve as a complete guiding source for students and researchers. The topics in this book have been comprehensively explained to help readers understand the growing trends in the field.

I would like to thank the entire group of writers who made sincere efforts in this book and my family who supported me in my efforts of working on this book. I take this opportunity to thank all those who have been a guiding force throughout my life.

Editor

Evodiamine Synergizes with Doxorubicin in the Treatment of Chemoresistant Human Breast Cancer without Inhibiting P-Glycoprotein

Shengpeng Wang[1☺], Lu Wang[1☺], Zhi Shi[2], Zhangfeng Zhong[1], Meiwan Chen[1]*, Yitao Wang[1]*

1 State Key Laboratory of Quality Research in Chinese Medicine, Institute of Chinese Medical Sciences, University of Macau, Macau, China, 2 Department of Cell Biology & Institute of Biomedicine, College of Life Science and Technology, Jinan University, Guangzhou, Guangdong, China

Abstract

Drug resistance is one of the main hurdles for the successful treatment of breast cancer. The synchronous targeting of apoptosis resistance and survival signal transduction pathways may be a promising approach to overcome drug resistance. In this study, we determined that evodiamine (EVO), a major constituent of the Chinese herbal medicine *Evodiae Fructus*, could induce apoptosis of doxorubicin (DOX)-sensitive MCF-7 and DOX-resistant MCF-7/ADR cells in a caspase-dependent manner, as confirmed by significant increases of cleaved poly(ADP-ribose) polymerase (PARP), caspase-7/9, and caspase activities. Notably, the reversed phenomenon of apoptosis resistance by EVO might be attributed to its ability to inhibit the Ras/MEK/ERK pathway and the expression of inhibitors of apoptosis (IAPs). Furthermore, our results indicated that EVO enhanced the apoptotic action of DOX by inhibiting the Ras/MEK/ERK cascade and the expression of IAPs without inhibiting the expression and activity of P-glycoprotein (P-gp). Taken together, our data indicate that EVO, a natural product, may be useful applied alone or in combination with DOX for the treatment of resistant breast cancer.

Editor: Ming Tan, University of South Alabama, United States of America

Funding: This study was supported by the Macao Science and Technology Development Fund (102/2012/A3, 077/2011/A3) and the Research Fund of the University of Macau (MYRG 208 (Y3-L4)-ICMS11-WYT, MRG012/WYT/2013/ICMS, MRG005/CMW/2014/ICMS). The funders had no role in study design, data collection and analysis, decision to publish, or preparation of the manuscript.

Competing Interests: The authors have declared that no competing interests exist.

* E-mail: mwchen@umac.mo (MC); yo'wang@umac.mo (YW)

☺ These authors contributed equally to this work.

Introduction

One of the most serious problems responsible for the failure of cancer chemotherapy in the clinic is the occurrence of multidrug resistance (MDR). Cancer cells can exhibit resistance to multiple functionally different agents, such as vinca alkaloids, anthracyclines and taxanes, after treatment with one type or class of drugs [1]. In recent decades, the mechanisms responsible for MDR have been heavily investigated, although the available treatment options in the clinic remain limited [2]. It has been suggested that increased drug efflux by one or more energy-dependent transporters, including P-glycoprotein (P-gp), multidrug resistance associated proteins (MRPs), and breast cancer resistance protein (BCRP), and changes in the targeted enzymes, altered cell cycle checkpoints and anti-apoptotic mechanisms could all result in MDR [3].

Apoptosis resistance and increased survival signaling are the major regulators of cancer cell survival against chemotherapy, and targeting only one of these pathways may be insufficient to obtain chemotherapeutic effects [4]. The inhibitors of apoptosis (IAPs), an effective group of conserved endogenous proteins that includes X-linked inhibitor of apoptosis (XIAP), survivin and cellular inhibitor of apoptosis protein 1 and 2 (cIAP1 and cIAP2), can inhibit apoptosis by binding to caspase-9 and the downstream caspase-3 and caspase-7 in the intrinsic apoptosis pathway [5–7]. The overexpression of IAPs has been demonstrated to confer protec-

tion against apoptosis in several resistant cancers [8,9]. Targeting IAPs to release caspases and subsequently activate apoptosis has become a popular strategy in designing novel drugs to conquer MDR. Meanwhile, IAP antagonists have been shown to enhance the chemotherapeutic effect of different classes of cytotoxic drugs against various cancers [10].

Survival signals help cells to overcome stressful or deleterious stimuli by increasing the expression or activity of many survival factors [4]. The Ras/MEK/ERK cascade is one of the key signaling pathways involved in the regulation of cell cycle progression, growth and differentiation [11,12]. Activation of the Ras/MEK/ERK signaling can alter the expression, activity and subcellular localization of many proteins that play key roles in apoptosis, and has been associated with resistance to chemotherapeutic agents in many cancers [13]. Chemotherapeutic agents can activate the Ras/MEK/ERK pathway by diverse mechanisms, including ROS-induced calmodulin-dependent kinase (CaM-K) activation [14]. Chemotherapeutic drugs such as doxorubicin (DOX) can also activate p53 to increase the expression of the discoidin domain receptor (DDR), which in turn activates the Ras/MEK/ERK pathway [13]. Therefore, synchronously targeting IAPs and survival signal transduction pathways may be a promising approach to overcome drug resistance.

Evodiamine (EVO), a naturally occurring indole alkaloid, is one of the main bioactive components of the herbal medicine *Evodia rutaecarpa* (Juss.) Benth. [15]. EVO has been shown to exhibit antitumor properties by suppressing tumor growth [16], metastasis [17] and angiogenesis [18]. Furthermore, EVO can induce apoptosis by inhibiting nuclear factor kappa B (NF-κB) activation, leading to the downregulation of NF-κB-regulated gene products such as Cyclin D1, XIAP, Bcl-2, and Bcl-XL [19,20]. The PI3K/Akt and ERK signaling pathways also play important roles in cancer cell apoptosis in responses to EVO [21-23]. The objective of the present study was to determine the effects of EVO on DOX-resistant breast cancer cells when treated alone and in combination with DOX. We hypothesized that EVO would enhance DOX sensitivity in DOX-resistant breast cancer cells by synchronously inhibiting IAPs and survival signal transduction pathways. Our results indicated that EVO induced apoptosis of both DOX-sensitive and DOX-resistant cells and enhanced the apoptotic action of DOX by inhibiting both IAPs and the Ras/MEK/ERK cascade without inhibiting P-glycoprotein (P-gp).

Materials and Methods

Reagents

EVO (98% purity) was purchased by Sigma-Aldrich. DOX (98% purity) was obtained from Meilun Biology Technology Company (Dalian, China). Dulbecco's Modified Eagle Medium (DMEM), fetal bovine serum (FBS), penicillin-streptomycin (PS), phosphate-buffered saline (PBS), propidium iodide (PI) and 0.25% w/v trypsin/1 mM EDTA were purchased from Gibco Life Technologies (Grand Island, USA). The lactate dehydrogenase (LDH) release detection kit was obtained from Roche Diagnostics. Hoechst 33342 and 3-[4,5-dimethyl-2-thiazolyl]-2,5-diphenyl tetrazolium bromide (MTT) were obtained by Molecular Probes (Grand Island, USA). Primary antibodies against cleaved caspase-7, cleaved caspase-9, cleaved PARP, Ras, phosphorylated MEK, MEK, phosphorylated ERK1/2, ERK1/2, XIAP, cIAP1, survivin, P-gp and GAPDH and secondary antibodies were purchased from Cell Signaling Technology.

Cell Lines and Cell Culture

MCF-7 human breast cancer cells were obtained from the American Type Culture Collection (ATCC). The DOX-resistant MCF-7/ADR cells were obtained from stepwise exposure to increasing concentrations of DOX as originally described [24]. Cells were cultured in DMEM medium with antibiotics (100 μg/ml streptomycin, 100 U/ml penicillin) and heat-inactivated 10% (v/v) FBS at 37°C in a humidified atmosphere of 5% CO_2.

MTT Assay and LDH Assay

The colorimetric MTT assay was modified and executed to quantify cell proliferation [25]. Exponentially growing MCF-7 and MCF-7/ADR cells were seeded in 96-well plates at a final concentration of 5×10^3 cells/well. After incubation for 24 h, cells in designated wells were treated with different concentrations of EVO. After 24, 48 and 72 h incubation, cell viability was detected by with the addition of free serum DMEM medium containing 1 mg/ml MTT for 4 h and subsequently dissolving the formed formazan crystals with DMSO. The absorbance in each individual well was determined at 570 nm by microplate reader (SpectaMax M5, Molecular Devices). The proliferation rates of cancer cells were evaluated by using triplicate assays. The LDH release rates from cells were evaluated by a commercial kit according to the manufacturers' protocol (Roche).

Analysis of Nuclear Morphology

MCF-7 cells and MCF-7/ADR cells were treated with different doses of EVO for 24 h. After treatment, cells were washed twice with PBS and fixed with 4% paraformaldehyde for 20 min. After incubation with Hoechst 33342 (5 μg/ml) at room temperature for 15 min, cells were observed by Incell Analyzer 2000 (GE Healthcare Life Sciences, USA) to survey the apoptotic morphology of the cell nucleus of MCF-7 cells and MCF-7/ADR cells. Condensed, fragmented or degraded nuclei indicated apoptosis in MCF-7 and MCF-7/ADR cells, and the results were based on at least three independent experiments.

Annexin V/PI Staining Assay

Apoptotic cells were detected by an Annexin V-FITC/PI apoptosis detection kit (BioVision) according to manufacturer's instruction. MCF-7 cells and MCF-7/ADR cells were treated with different concentrations of EVO. After 48 h of incubation, cells were trypsinized and collected by centrifugation at 500 g/min for 5 min. After being washed twice with cold PBS and gently suspended in 100 μl binding buffer, cells were stained with 5 μl of Annexin-FITC and 10 μl of PI solution and incubated in the dark at room temperature for 15 min. Cell apoptosis was analyzed by a flow cytometer (BD Biosciences). All experiments were performed in triplicate.

Caspase Activity Assay

Caspase-Glo assay kits (Promega) were used to measure the caspase activities according to the manufacturer's instructions. MCF-7 cells and MCF-7/ADR cells were plated into 96-well white-walled plates (PerkinElmer). Twenty-four hours after seeding, cells were treated with different concentrations of EVO for 48 h. Subsequently, 100 μl of caspase-3/7 or caspase-9 assay reagent was added to each well, and the plate was incubated in the dark for 1 h. The luminescence was measured by using a SpectraMax M5 microplate reader (Molecular Devices). Caspase activity was expressed as a percentage of the untreated control treatment (DMSO). All samples were assayed in triplicate.

Western Blotting

MCF-7 cells and MCF-7/ADR cells were treated with different concentrations of EVO for 48 h, and the total protein was extracted with RIPA lysis buffer containing 1% phenylmethanesulfonylfluoride (PMSF) and 1% protease inhibitor cocktail. As previously reported, protein concentrations were determined with a BCA protein assay kit (Thermo Scientific) [26]. Equivalent amounts of proteins from each group were separated by SDS-PAGE and were transferred to PVDF membranes. After being blocked for 1 h with 5% non-fat dried milk, the membranes were incubated with specific primary antibodies (1: 1000) and subsequently incubated with the corresponding secondary antibodies (1: 1000). An ECL Advanced Western Blotting Detection kit (GE Healthcare) was used to visualize and detect the specific protein bands. All band densitometries were calculated using Quantity One Software (Bio-Rad).

Combination Studies of EVO and DOX

Exponentially growing MCF-7 cells and MCF-7/ADR cells (5×10^3) were seeded in 96-well plates and incubated for 24 h. Cells were pretreated with different concentrations of EVO for 12 h and incubated with the indicated concentrations of DOX for another 48 h. Cell viability was measured by MTT assay as described previously. Apoptotic cells were detected by Annexin V-FITC/PI dual staining as described previously.

Determination of Intracellular DOX

MCF-7 cells and MCF-7/ADR cells were pretreated with different concentrations of EVO. After 12 h incubation, the media were removed, and the cells were washed two times with PBS. Cells were then incubated with different concentrations of DOX for an additional 4 h. Extracellular DOX was removed, and the cells were collected and washed with PBS three times. The fluorescence of intracellular DOX was analyzed by flow cytometry (BD Biosciences). The corresponding single parameter histogram of the fluorescence signal of the collected cells (1.0×10^4) was amplified and generated by using FlowJo software.

P-gp Activity Assay

A fluorometric MDR assay kit (Abcam, Cambridge, UK) was used to determine the activity of P-gp. Following the user protocol provided in the fluorometric MDR assay kit, MCF-7 cells and MCF-7/MDR cells (1.0×10^4 cells/well) were seeded into 96-well flat clear-bottom black-wall microplates and incubated for 24 h. The cells were treated with different concentrations of EVO for 12 h. Next, 100 µl MDR dye-loading solution was added to each well and incubated at 37°C for 1 h avoiding light. Intracellular fluorescence was detected using a microplate reader (SpectraMax M5, Molecular Devices, USA) at an excitation wavelength of 490 nm and an emission wavelength of 525 nm. All experiments were performed in triplicate and compared to controls.

Statistical Analysis

All data were presented as means ± SE. Each value exhibited the mean of at least three independent experiments in each group. In all cases, Student's t-test was used for statistical comparison. P values less than 0.05 were considered significant.

Results

The Effect of EVO on Proliferation and Cytotoxicity in DOX-Sensitive and DOX-Resistant Breast Cancer Cells

We first assessed the effect of EVO on the proliferation of MCF-7 and MCF-7/ADR cells. As shown in **Figure 1A and 1B**, EVO exhibited time- and concentration-dependent inhibitory effects on both MCF-7 and MCF-7/ADR cells. The IC_{50} values of MCF-7 cells treated with EVO for 24, 48, and 72 h were 7.68 µM, 0.64 µM and 0.30 µM, respectively. The IC_{50} values of the MCF-7/ADR cells were higher than those for MCF-7, with values of 24.47 µM, 1.26 µM and 0.47 µM for 24, 48 and 72 h treatment of EVO, respectively. The cytotoxicity induced by EVO in MCF-7 and MCF-7/ADR cells was determined by LDH assay. The LDH released profiles of MCF-7 (**Figure 1C**) and MCF-7/ADR (**Figure 1D**) cells exposed to EVO for 24 h were nearly equivalent, whereas higher levels of LDH were released by MCF-7 cells after treatment with EVO for 48 h and 72 h compared with MCF-7/ADR cells, which was consistent with the results of the MTT assay.

EVO Induced Apoptosis in MCF-7 and MCF-7/ADR Cells

Hoechst staining revealed marked nuclear morphological changes in MCF-7 and MCF-7/ADR cells after EVO treatment, including the condensation of chromatin and nuclear fragmentation (**Figure 2A**). To further confirm the results, we performed Annexin V/PI double staining to quantitatively detect apoptosis. As shown in **Figure 2B**, after 48 h of treatment, EVO (1 µM) induced apoptosis in 62.7% and 50.1% of MCF-7 and MCF-7/ADR cells, respectively. PARP is a protein involved in many cellular processes as DNA repair and cell apoptosis [27], and cleaved PARP is a marker of apoptosis. EVO treatment increased the expression of cleaved PARP in the present study in a concentration-dependent manner (**Figure 2C**). Taken together, these results revealed that the inhibitory effects of EVO on the proliferation of MCF-7 and MCF-7/ADR cells were caused by the induction of apoptosis.

The Effects of EVO on Caspase Processing

As EVO induced MCF-7 and MCF-7/ADR cell apoptosis, the mechanism of apoptosis induced by EVO was further investigated. Caspases exist as inactive zymogens in normal cells and undergo proteolytic processing upon activation during apoptosis [28]. As caspases are responsible for the execution of apoptosis, we further examined caspase activation using caspase activity kits (Promega). The data confirmed that the caspase-7 activities (**Figure 3A**) of MCF-7 and MCF-7/ADR cells were increased by 1.46-fold and 2.08-fold after 48 h EVO (1 µM) treatment compared with control cells, and the caspase-9 activities (**Figure 3B**) were increased by 1.77-fold and 1.45-fold in MCF-7 and MCF-7/ADR cells, respectively. We then explored whether caspases were processed and cleaved during the course of EVO-induced apoptosis. MCF-7 cells do not express caspase-3, as described previously [29,30]; thus, we examined caspase-7 and caspase-9 as the indicators of apoptosis. As shown in **Figure 3C**, concentration-dependent proteolytic fragments of caspase-7 and caspase-9 were observed after 48 h treatment of EVO.

EVO Induced Apoptosis by Inhibiting Both the Ras/MEK/ERK Cascade and IAPs

To elucidate the potential mechanisms underlying apoptosis induction by EVO, several proteins related to apoptosis were measured by Western blotting. Treatment of the cells with 0.25 to 1 µM EVO markedly inhibited the levels of Ras, P-MEK and P-ERK1/2, whereas the levels of total MEK and ERK1/2 protein were not affected significantly in either of the tested cell lines (**Figure 4**). We further examined the effects of EVO on the expression levels of IAP family proteins, including survivin, XIAP and cIAP1. Treatment of MCF-7 cells with EVO at 1 µM completely inhibited survivin, XIAP and cIAP1 expression. Moreover, marked inhibition of the levels of survivin, XIAP, and cIAP1 was also detected in the resistant breast cancer MCF-7/ADR cells (**Figure 5**).

EVO Enhanced DOX Induced Growth Inhibition

The sensitizing cytotoxic effect of EVO in MCF-7 and MCF-7/ADR cells exposed to DOX is presented in **Figure 6**. At a concentration of 2 µM, 48 h DOX treatment inhibited MCF-7 cell viability by 60% but inhibited MCF-7/ADR cell viability by only 10%, indicating the resistance of MCF-7/ADR cells to DOX. However, when DOX was administered in combination with EVO, a significant decrease in cell viability was observed in both MCF-7 and MCF-7/ADR cells (**Figure 6A and 6C**). To characterize the interaction of these two agents, we analyzed the above results using the CalcuSyn program (Biosoft), which uses the Chou-Talalay Method, a derivation of the mass-action law principle [31]. The combination index (CI) is a quantitative measurement of the relationship between two agents, where a CI greater than 1 indicates antagonism and a CI less than one indicates synergism [32]. The CI for the interaction between DOX and EVO in MCF-7 and MCF-7/ADR cells were calculated and listed in **Figure 6B and 6D**. We observed that the sensitization effect of EVO in MCF-7/ADR cells was more significant than the sensitization effect in MCF-7 cells, as most of

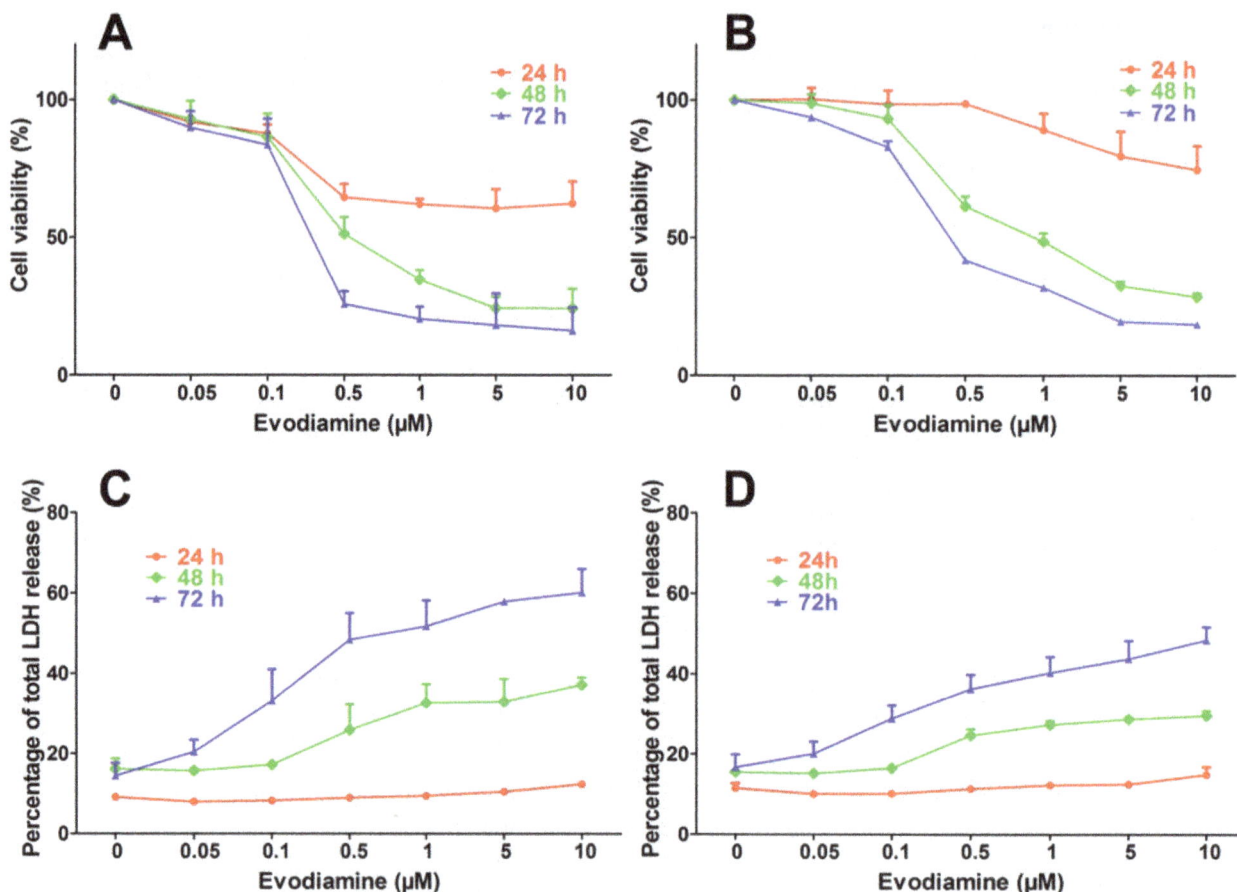

Figure 1. Effects of different concentrations of EVO on the proliferation of Dox-sensitive MCF-7 (A) and Dox-resistant MCF-7/ADR (B) cells by MTT assay. The cytotoxicity caused by different concentrations of EVO in MCF-7 (C) and MCF-7/ADR (D) cells was determined by LDH assay. Each point represents the mean ± SE.

the CI values in MCF-7/ADR cells were less than those in MCF-7 cells.

EVO Enhanced DOX-Induced Apoptosis in MCF-7/ADR Cells by Inhibiting IAPs and the Ras/MEK/ERK Cascade

The combination of DOX and EVO resulted in a significantly higher percentage of apoptosis in MCF-7/ADR cells than either drug alone (**Figure 7A**). Individual treatment with DOX (2 μM) or EVO (1 μM) induced apoptosis in 11.27% and 11.77% of the cells, respectively. In contrast, concurrent treatment with DOX and EVO increased the apoptotic cell population to 30.05%. We then examined the status of PARP and caspases. As shown in **Figure 7B**, activated PARP and caspases were slightly or moderately induced by DOX or EVO as single agents, whereas the combination of DOX and EVO caused an obvious increase in the cleaved PARP, caspase-7 and caspase-9 levels, indicating that EVO sensitized MCF-7/ADR cells to DOX by inducing cell apoptosis. To further examine the mechanisms behind the combinatorial synergism, the roles of the Ras/MEK/ERK cascade and IAPs were examined in response to concurrent treatment. In MCF-7/ADR cells, combination treatment with DOX and EVO resulted in the marked decrease of Ras expression and the phosphorylation of MEK and ERK1/2 (**Figure 7C**). Furthermore, DOX and EVO potentiated the inhibitory effect on

the expression of IAPs, including XIAP, survivin and cIAP1 (**Figure 7D**).

EVO did not Increase the Intracellular Level of DOX and Exhibited Minimal Effect on P-gp Expression and Activity

Flow cytometric analysis indicated that EVO did not augment the intracellular concentration of DOX in both MCF-7 and MCF-7/ADR cells (**Figure 8A and 8B**), unlike verapamil, a specific inhibitors of P-gp. We further investigated whether EVO could down-regulate the expression of P-gp and affect P-gp activity. As shown in **Figure 8C**, we observed that, over the 48 h treatment of EVO, the P-gp expression levels were not decreased. Furthermore, P-gp activity was examined using a fluorometric MDR assay kit in DOX-resistant cells (**Figure 8D**). No difference in the mean intracellular fluorescence value was observed between cells pretreated with EVO for 12 h compared with untreated cells, where greater numbers suggest more inhibitory effects on the P-gp activity.

Discussion

To date, in many cases, there remains no remedy to overcome drug resistance and improve clinical outcomes in resistant cancers [33]. Many attempts have been made to inhibit membrane transporters, however, most of these drug transporter inhibitors

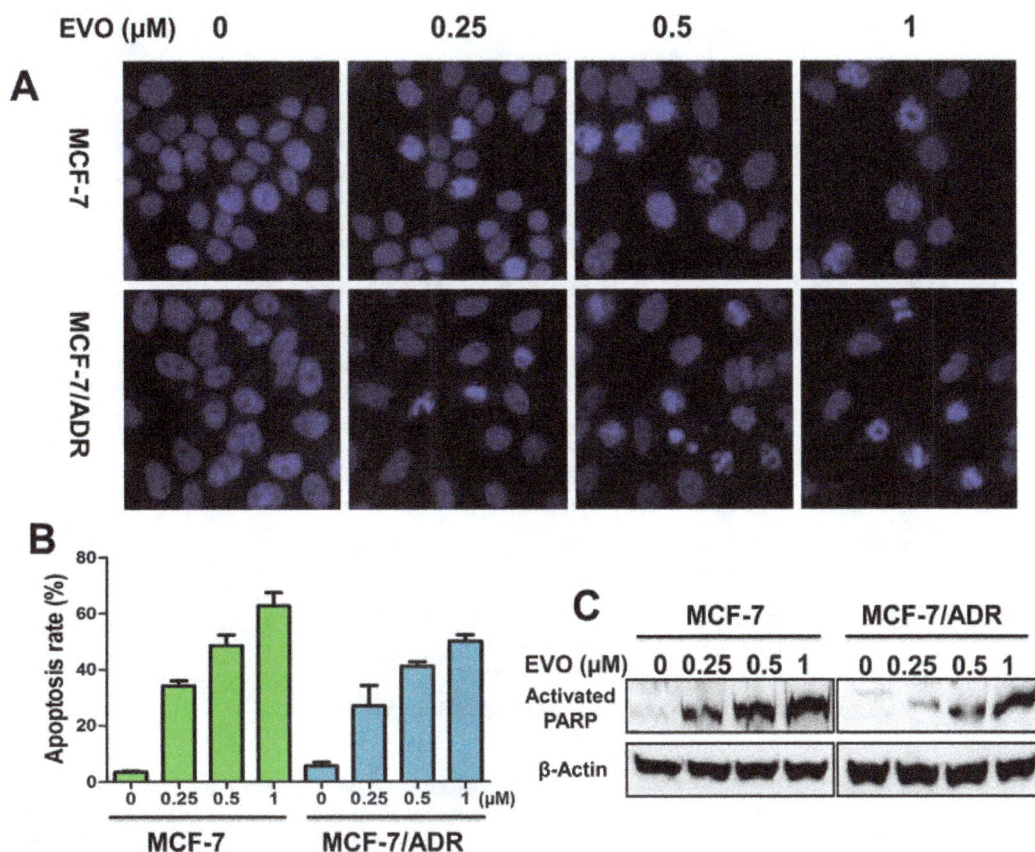

Figure 2. EVO induces apoptosis in MCF-7 and MCF-7/ADR cancer cells. (**A**) Hoechst 33342 fluorescent staining to detect apoptotic morphology of MCF-7 and MCF-7/ADR cells after treatment of different concentrations of EVO for 48 h. Apoptotic cells were recognized by condensed, fragmented and or degraded nuclei. Cells were observed of three experiments using Incell Analyzer 2000 (GE healthcare) (**B**) Quantitative apoptotic measurement by Annexin V/PI double staining in MCF-7 and MCF-7/ADR cells after treatment of different concentrations of EVO for 48 h. Data were expressed as mean $\pm$ SE of three independent experiments. * P<0.05 vs. untreated control (MCF-7), # P<0.05 vs. untreated control (MCF-7/ADR). (**C**) MCF-7 and MCF-7/ADR cells were plated on 100 mm-diameter dishes and treated with different concentrations of EVO for 48 h. The cells were used for Western blot analysis using antibodies against activated PARP and β-Actin.

have not proven to be effective in the clinic [11]. Therefore, more specific, targeted and low-toxicity therapies have attracted the interest of researchers as promising approaches to kill resistant cancer cells. The IAPs play key roles at the intersection of the mitochondria pathway and death receptor pathway and widely and potently inhibit apoptosis against multiple apoptotic stimuli, including chemotherapeutic agents and radiation [34]. Therefore, IAPs have been proven to be closely related to therapy resistance, and strategies targeting IAPs may be effective for overcoming apoptosis resistance [35]. For example, overexpression of XIAP can increase resistance to tumor necrosis factor-related apoptosis-inducing ligand (TRAIL), whereas down-regulation of XIAP restored the cell response to TRAIL [36]. Meanwhile, chemotherapeutic drugs such as DOX and docetaxel can induce the activation of the Ras/MEK/ERK pathway, and the activated cascade may regulate downstream factors that are involved in DNA repair and apoptosis, thereby contributing to drug resistance [11]. Therefore, synchronously targeting IAPs and the Ras/ MEK/ERK pathway may prevent drug resistance and the reemergence of cancer initiating cells.

Many plant-derived compounds are known to enhance the chemotherapeutic effects of anticancer agents by modulating the main ABC (ATP-binding cassette) transporters responsible for cancer drug resistance, including P-gp, MRPs and BCRP, as well as regulating both cell survival- and cell death-related signaling pathways, which makes them a promising group of low toxicity candidates for reversing MDR [37]. As EVO has been reported to inhibit the expression of IAPs, such as XIAP, survivin and cIAP1 [19], and to modulate ERK signaling [21–23], we hypothesized that EVO could reverse DOX-resistant breast cancer cells by inhibiting the Ras/MEK/ERK pathway and IAPs.

In the present study, we observed that EVO significantly inhibited the proliferation and promoted the cytotoxicity on both DOX-sensitive MCF-7 cells and DOX-resistant MCF-7/ADR cells in a time- and concentration-dependent manner, as confirmed by MTT and LDH assay. We also observed that EVO induced apoptosis in MCF-7 and MCF-7/ADR cells in a caspase-dependent manner, as confirmed by the elevated levels of PARP, caspase 7 and caspase 9 as well as a significant increase in caspase activities. Furthermore, treatment of the cells with 0.25 to 1 μM EVO markedly inhibited the levels of Ras, P-MEK and P-ERK1/2 and decreased the expression levels of IAP family proteins, including survivin, XIAP and cIAP1, in both MCF-7 and MCF-7/ADR cells.

Cancer cells can abnormally activate survival pathways and upregulate the expression of IAPs after chemotherapy agent treatment, potentially preventing the downstream apoptotic responses and decreasing the sensitivity of the cells to these agents

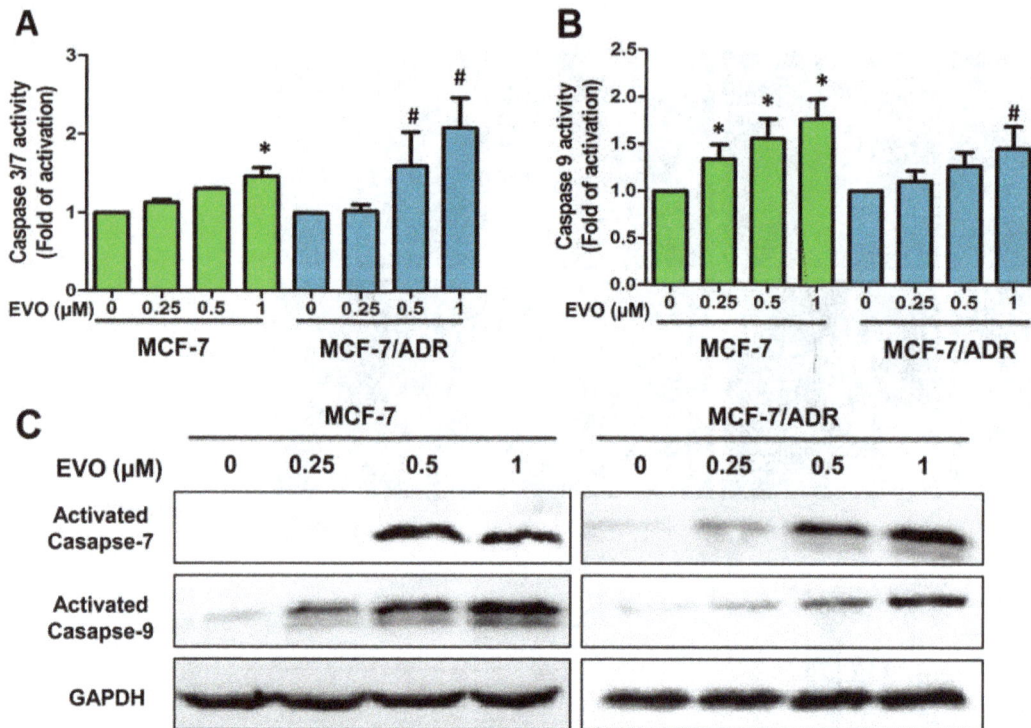

Figure 3. Involvement of caspase activation in MCF-7 and MCF-7/ADR cells after treated with EVO for 48 h. EVO increase the activities of caspase 3/7 (**A**) and caspase 9 (**B**) in MCF-7 and MCF-7/ADR cells by a dose-dependent manner. Data were expressed as mean ± SE of two or three independent experiments. * $P<0.05$ vs. untreated MCF-7 cells, # $P<0.05$ vs. untreated MCF-7/ADR cells. (**C**) MCF-7 and MCF-7/ADR cells were treated with different concentrations of EVO for 48 h. The cells were used for Western blot analysis using antibodies against activated Caspase 7, 9 and GAPDH. Similar results were obtained in two or three separate experiments.

[38]. In the present study, MCF-7 cells were more sensitive to EVO than MCF-7/ADR cells, as EVO treatment resulted in greater growth inhibition, cytotoxicity and apoptosis and inhibited the Ras/MEK/ERK pathway and IAP expression. These effects may be attributed to the activation survival pathways and apoptosis resistance induced by DOX in chemotherapy. Meanwhile, because Ras/MEK/ERK pathway is normally activated and the levels of IAPs are quite low in normal cells, EVO may

selectively induce cancer cell death, which further facilitates its application in the clinic.

The one-dimensional mechanism of action of single-drug chemotherapy often activates and heightens alternative pathways, thereby prompting the emergence of chemoresistance mutations and tumor relapse [39–42]. Synergistic combination of two or more drugs is an effective strategy for targeting both apoptosis resistance and increased survival signaling to overcome chemore-

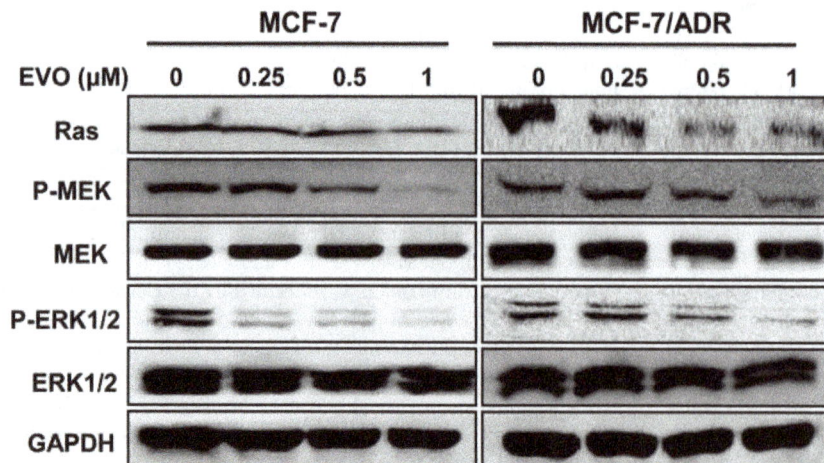

Figure 4. Inhibition of Ras/MEK/ERK signaling pathway in MCF-7 and MCF-7/ADR cells by EVO. Whole-cell lysates were generated and immunoblotted with antibodies against Ras, phosphorylated MEK (P-MEK), MEK, phosphorylated ERK (P-ERK1/2), ERK1/2 and GAPDH. Similar results were obtained in two or three separate experiments.

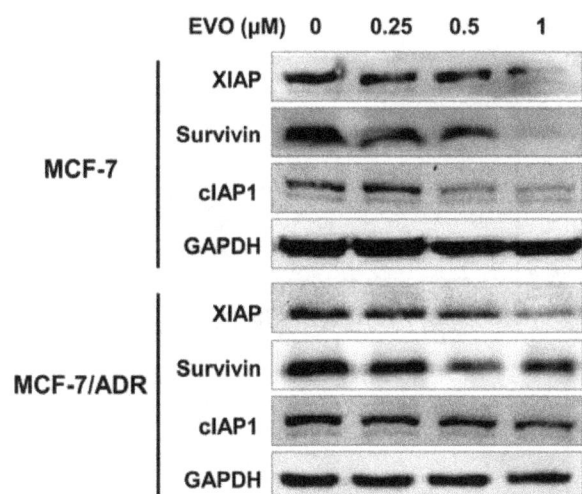

Figure 5. Inhibition of Inhibitor of Apoptosis (IAPs) in MCF-7 and MCF-7/ADR cells by EVO. Whole-cell lysates were generated and immunoblotted with antibodies against XIAP, Survivin, cIAP1 and GAPDH. Similar results were obtained in two or three separate experiments.

Therefore, increasing the sensitivity to DOX is an attractive strategy for improving the clinical management of breast cancer [44]. In this study, we observed that DOX and EVO exhibited a synergistic effect in the induction of apoptosis in MCF-7/ADR cells, which was evidenced by the presence of cleaved caspase-7, caspase-9 and PARP. The ability of EVO to block both the Ras/MEK/ERK pathway and IAP expression may sensitize human cancer cells to chemotherapy. In our experiment, we demonstrated that treatment with DOX had little effect on the Ras/MEK/ERK pathway and IAP expression, whereas the combination of DOX and EVO led to the decreased expression of Ras, P-MEK, P-ERK1/2, XIAP, survivin and cIAP1 simultaneously. We believe that EVO inhibition of the Ras/MEK/ERK pathway and IAP expression may have led to the higher levels of caspase activity observed in the resistant cancer cells after the combination treatment, thus significantly enhancing the effects of DOX.

The development of MDR is frequently associated with the overexpression of ATP-dependent membrane transporters like P-gp and MRP1, which actively pump out cytotoxic drugs from cancer cells, thus reducing their intracellular concentration and efficiency[45]. Previous studies have reported that EVO could inhibit TNF-induced expression of P-gp in KBM-5 cells [19]. However, in our present study, though obviously higher cytotoxicity was observed when DOX was combined with EVO, further studies demonstrated that EVO did not result in the down-regulation of P-gp expression or the severe impairment of its function. The effects of EVO on P-gp expression may be cell-type specific and may be related to the expression levels in targeted cancer cells. These results indicate that the sensitization mecha-

sistance. DOX is commonly used as a first-line chemotherapeutic agent for the treatment of breast cancer. DOX can incorporate into the DNA of cancer cells and prevents cell replication by suppressing protein synthesis [43]. However, unwanted side effects and the development of drug resistance limit its application.

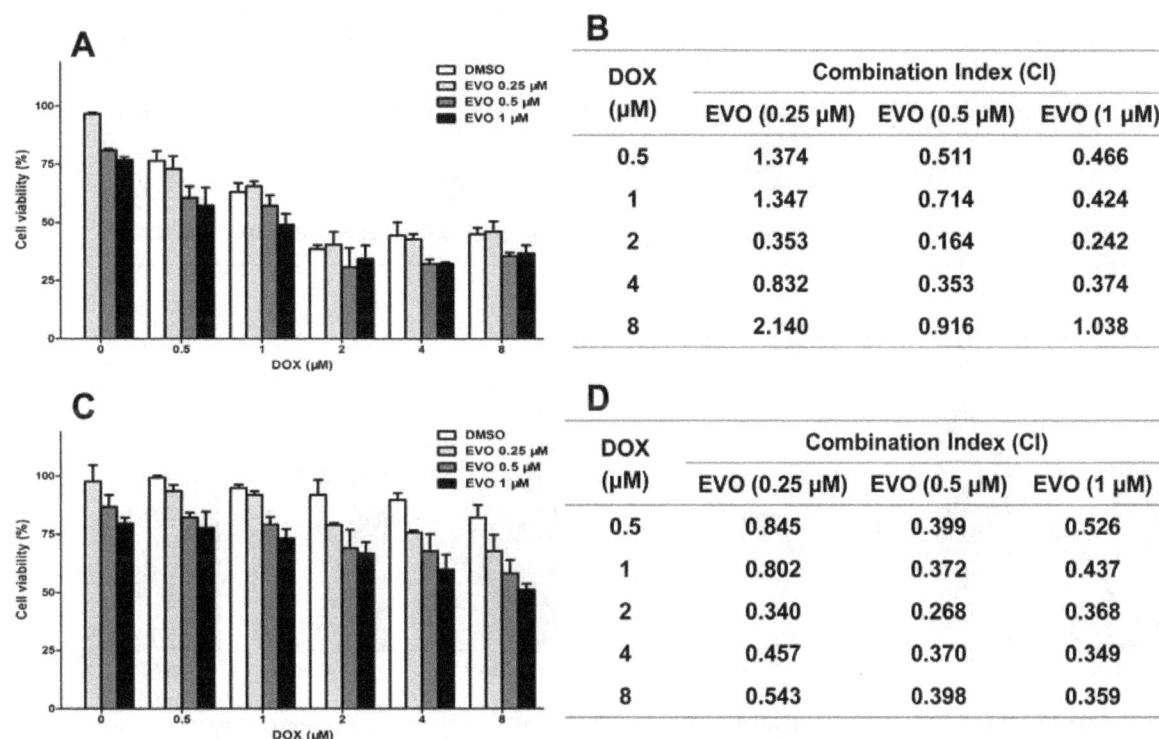

B

DOX (µM)	Combination Index (CI)		
	EVO (0.25 µM)	EVO (0.5 µM)	EVO (1 µM)
0.5	1.374	0.511	0.466
1	1.347	0.714	0.424
2	0.353	0.164	0.242
4	0.832	0.353	0.374
8	2.140	0.916	1.038

D

DOX (µM)	Combination Index (CI)		
	EVO (0.25 µM)	EVO (0.5 µM)	EVO (1 µM)
0.5	0.845	0.399	0.526
1	0.802	0.372	0.437
2	0.340	0.268	0.368
4	0.457	0.370	0.349
8	0.543	0.398	0.359

Figure 6. Combinational treatment of MCF-7 and MCF-7/ADR cells with EVO and DOX showed synergistic effect in reducing cell viability. MCF-7 and MCF-7/ADR cells were pretreated with different concentrations of EVO for 12 h, followed by treating with DOX for another 48 h. Cell viabilities of MCF-7 (**A**) and MCF-7/ADR (**C**) cells were measured by MTT assay. The combination index (CI) of EVO and DOX in MCF-7 (**B**) and MCF-7/ADR (**D**) cells were conducted using CalcuSyn software (Biosoft, Cambridge, UK), where CI<1 indicated synergistic effect. Data presented mean ± SE from three independent experiments conducted in triplicate.

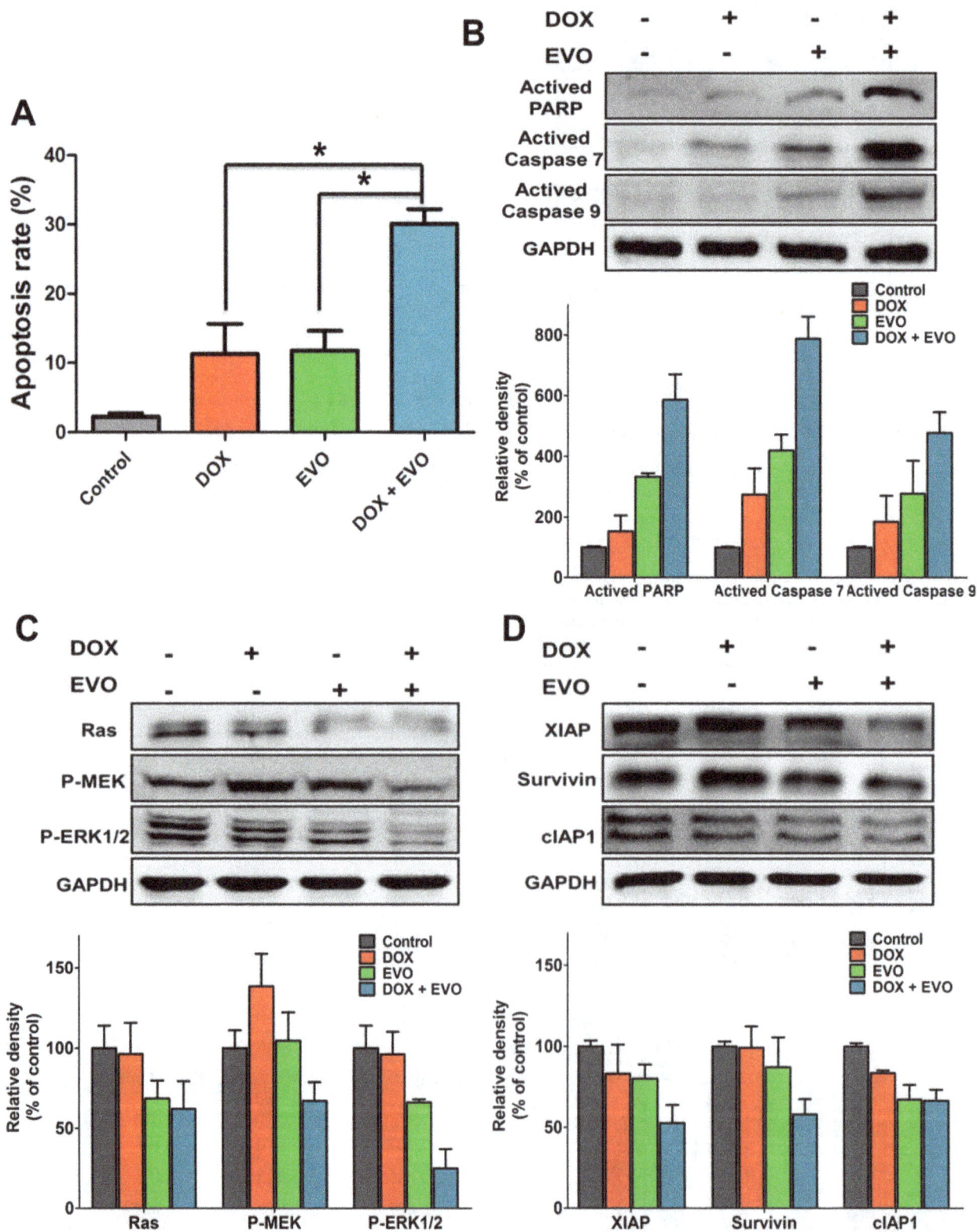

Figure 7. EVO enhanced DOX-induced apoptosis in MCF-7/ADR cancer cells. MCF-7/ADR cells were pretreated with EVO (1 μM) for 12 h, and then incubated with 2 μM of Dox for another 48 h. Apoptotic measurement was Annexin V/PI assay (**A**). Data are expressed as mean ± SE of three independent experiments. * P<0.05. (**B**) The cell lysates were generated for Western blot analysis using antibodies against activated PARP, activated caspase-7, -9 and GAPDH. Examination of the combined effects of DOX and EVO on expression levels of Ras/MEK/ERK cascade (**C**) and IAPs family proteins (**D**). Similar results were obtained in three separate experiments.

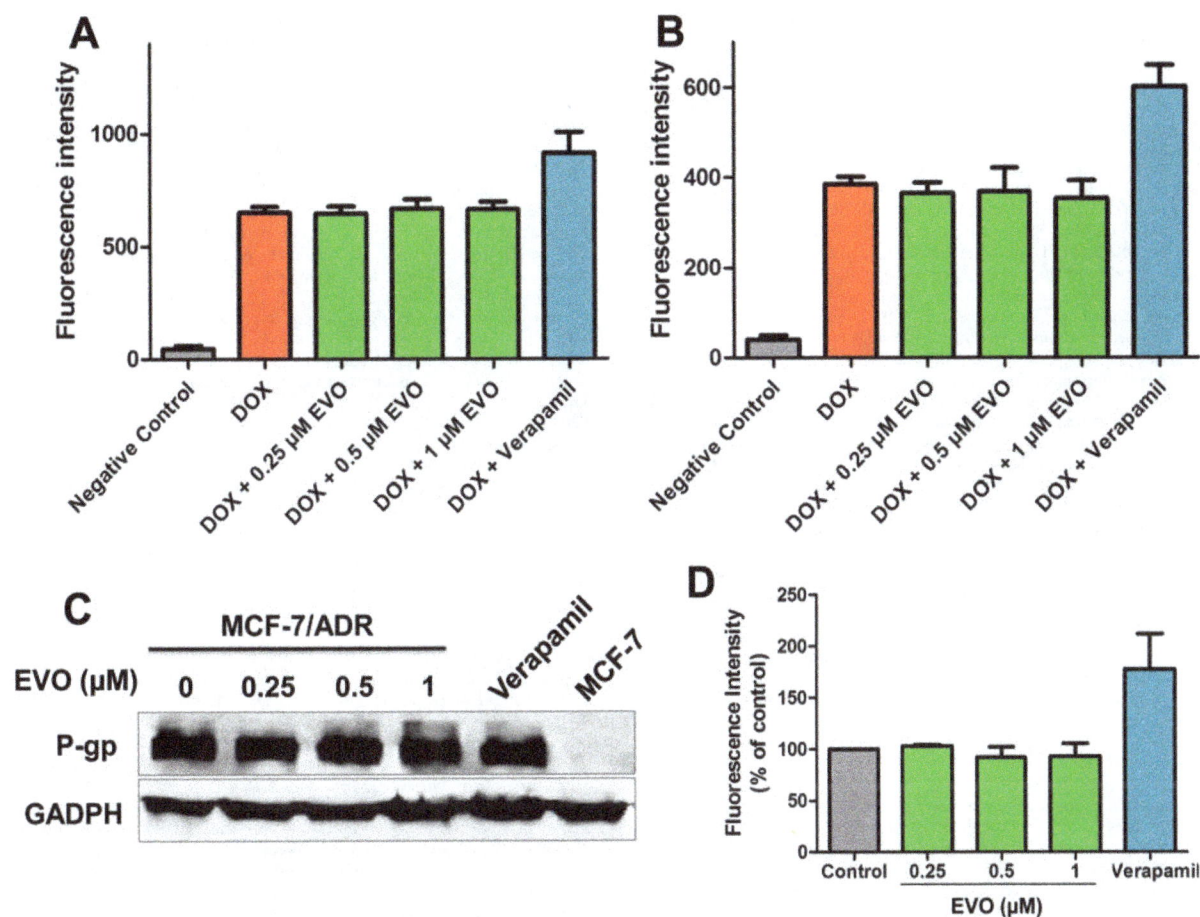

Figure 8. EVO sensitize the effect of DOX without inhibiting P-glycoprotein. MCF-7 (**A**) and MCF-7/ADR (**B**) cells were pretreated with EVO and Verapamil for 12 h, and then incubated Dox (2 μM) for another 4 h, then the intracellular level of Dox was determined using flow cytometry. (**C**) Effects of EVO on the expression levels of P-gp protein in MCF-7/ADR cells. After 24 h treatment of EVO and verapamil, protein levels in cell lysates were analyzed by Western blot. GAPDH was used as an internal control. Similar results were obtained in two or three separate experiments. (**D**) After 12 h treatment, the MDR pump activities were determined using a fluorimetric MDR assay kit (Abcam). Results are expressed as mean ± SE.

nism of EVO to DOX was independent of P-gp inhibition, at least under the experimental conditions presently employed.

Taken together, our data indicate that EVO is proapoptotic, reverses drug resistance and acts synergistically with DOX by inhibiting both IAPs and the Ras/MEK/ERK cascade without inhibiting P-gp. As a natural product, EVO, used alone or in combination with chemotherapeutic agents, may be useful in the treatment of resistant breast cancer.

Author Contributions

Conceived and designed the experiments: SPW MWC YTW. Performed the experiments: SPW LW. Analyzed the data: SPW LW MWC. Contributed reagents/materials/analysis tools: SPW ZFZ LW. Wrote the paper: SPW LW ZS MWC.

References

1. Vaux DL, Silke J (2005) IAPs—the ubiquitin connection. Cell Death Differ 12: 1205–1207.

2. Wang Z, Li Y, Ahmad A, Azmi AS, Kong D, et al. (2010) Targeting miRNAs involved in cancer stem cell and EMT regulation: An emerging concept in overcoming drug resistance. Drug Resist Updat 13: 109–118.

3. Kruh GD (2003) Introduction to resistance to anticancer agents. Oncogene 22: 7262–7264.

4. Krakstad C, Chekenya M (2010) Survival signalling and apoptosis resistance in glioblastomas: opportunities for targeted therapeutics. Mol Cancer 9: 135.

5. Bratton SB, Walker G, Srinivasula SM, Sun XM, Butterworth M, et al. (2001) Recruitment, activation and retention of caspases-9 and -3 by Apaf-1 apoptosome and associated XIAP complexes. EMBO J 20: 998–1009.

6. Plenchette S, Cathelin S, Rebe C, Launay S, Ladoire S, et al. (2004) Translocation of the inhibitor of apoptosis protein c-IAP1 from the nucleus to the Golgi in hematopoietic cells undergoing differentiation: a nuclear export signal-mediated event. Blood 104: 2035–2043.

7. Lu M, Lin SC, Huang Y, Kang YJ, Rich R, et al. (2007) XIAP induces NF-kappaB activation via the BIR1/TAB1 interaction and BIR1 dimerization. Mol Cell 26: 689–702.

8. Rumjanek VM, Vidal RS, Maia RC (2013) Multidrug resistance in chronic myeloid leukaemia: how much can we learn from MDR-CML cell lines? Biosci Rep 33: 875–888.

9. Silva KL, de Souza PS, Nestal de Moraes G, Moellmann-Coelho A, Vasconcelos Fda C, et al. (2013) XIAP and P-glycoprotein co-expression is related to imatinib resistance in chronic myeloid leukemia cells. Leuk Res 37: 1350–1358.

10. Fulda S, Vucic D (2012) Targeting IAP proteins for therapeutic intervention in cancer. Nat Rev Drug Discov 11: 109–124.

11. McCubrey JA, Steelman LS, Kempf CR, Chappell WH, Abrams SL, et al. (2011) Therapeutic resistance resulting from mutations in Raf/MEK/ERK and PI3K/PTEN/Akt/mTOR signaling pathways. J Cell Physiol 226: 2762–2781.

12. Steelman LS, Chappell WH, Abrams SL, Kempf RC, Long J, et al. (2011) Roles of the Raf/MEK/ERK and PI3K/PTEN/Akt/mTOR pathways in controlling

growth and sensitivity to therapy-implications for cancer and aging. Aging (Albany NY) 3: 192–222.

13. McCubrey JA, Steelman LS, Chappell WH, Abrams SL, Franklin RA, et al. (2012) Ras/Raf/MEK/ERK and PI3K/PTEN/Akt/mTOR cascade inhibitors: how mutations can result in therapy resistance and how to overcome resistance. Oncotarget 3: 1068–1111.

14. McCubrey JA, LaHair MM, Franklin RA (2006) Reactive oxygen species-induced activation of the MAP kinase signaling pathways. Antioxidants & Redox Signaling 8: 1775–1789.

15. King CL, Kong YC, Wong NS, Yeung HW, Fong HH, et al. (1980) Uterotonic effect of Evodia rutaecarpa alkaloids. J Nat Prod 43: 577–582.

16. Fei XF, Wang BX, Li TJ, Tashiro S, Minami M, et al. (2003) Evodiamine, a constituent of Evodiae Fructus, induces anti-proliferating effects in tumor cells. Cancer Sci 94: 92–98.

17. Ogasawara M, Matsunaga T, Takahashi S, Saiki I, Suzuki H (2002) Anti-invasive and metastatic activities of evodiamine. Biol Pharm Bull 25: 1491–1493.

18. Shyu KG, Lin S, Lee CC, Chen E, Lin LC, et al. (2006) Evodiamine inhibits in vitro angiogenesis: Implication for antitumorgenicity. Life Sci 78: 2234–2243.

19. Takada Y, Kobayashi Y, Aggarwal BB (2005) Evodiamine abolishes constitutive and inducible NF-kappaB activation by inhibiting IkappaBalpha kinase activation, thereby suppressing NF-kappaB-regulated antiapoptotic and meta-static gene expression, up-regulating apoptosis, and inhibiting invasion. J Biol Chem 280: 17203–17212.

20. Yu H, Jin H, Gong W, Wang Z, Liang H (2013) Pharmacological actions of multi-target-directed evodiamine. Molecules 18: 1826–1843.

21. Yang J, Wu LJ, Tashino S, Onodera S, Ikejima T (2008) Reactive oxygen species and nitric oxide regulate mitochondria-dependent apoptosis and autophagy in evodiamine-treated human cervix carcinoma HeLa cells. Free Radic Res 42: 492–504.

22. Lee TJ, Kim EJ, Kim S, Jung EM, Park JW, et al. (2006) Caspase-dependent and caspase-independent apoptosis induced by evodiamine in human leukemic U937 cells. Mol Cancer Ther 5: 2398–2407.

23. Wang C, Li S, Wang MW (2010) Evodiamine-induced human melanoma A375-S2 cell death was mediated by PI3K/Akt/caspase and Fas-L/NF-kappa B signaling pathways and augmented by ubiquitin-proteasome inhibition. Toxicology in Vitro 24: 898–904.

24. Batist G, Tulpule A, Sinha BK, Katki AG, Myers CE, et al. (1986) Overexpression of a novel anionic glutathione transferase in multidrug-resistant human breast cancer cells. J Biol Chem 261: 15544–15549.

25. Scudiero DA, Shoemaker RH, Paull KD, Monks A, Tierney S, et al. (1988) Evaluation of a soluble tetrazolium/formazan assay for cell growth and drug sensitivity in culture using human and other tumor cell lines. Cancer Res 48: 4827–4833.

26. Chen SY, Hu SS, Dong Q, Cai JX, Zhang WP, et al. (2013) Establishment of Paclitaxel-resistant Breast Cancer Cell Line and Nude Mice Models, and Underlying Multidrug Resistance Mechanisms in Vitro and in Vivo. Asian Pac J Cancer Prev 14: 6135–6140.

27. Lazebnik YA, Kaufmann SH, Desnoyers S, Poirier GG, Earnshaw WC (1994) Cleavage of poly(ADP-ribose) polymerase by a proteinase with properties like ICE. Nature 371: 346–347.

28. Kan SF, Huang WJ, Lin LC, Wang PS (2004) Inhibitory effects of evodiamine on the growth of human prostate cancer cell line LNCaP. Int J Cancer 110: 641–651.

29. Blanc C, Deveraux QL, Krajewski S, Janicke RU, Porter AG, et al. (2000) Caspase-3 is essential for procaspase-9 processing and cisplatin-induced apoptosis of MCF-7 breast cancer cells. Cancer Research 60: 4386–4390.

30. Essmann F, Engels IH, Totzke G, Schulze-Osthoff K, Janicke RU (2004) Apoptosis resistance of MCF-7 breast carcinoma cells to ionizing radiation is independent of p53 and cell cycle control but caused by the lack of caspase-3 and a caffeine-inhibitable event. Cancer Research 64: 7065–7072.

31. Chou TC, Talaly P (1977) A simple generalized equation for the analysis of multiple inhibitions of Michaelis-Menten kinetic systems. J Biol Chem 252: 6438–6442.

32. Rangwala F, Williams KP, Smith GR, Thomas Z, Allensworth JL, et al. (2012) Differential effects of arsenic trioxide on chemosensitization in human hepatic tumor and stellate cell lines. BMC Cancer 12: 402.

33. Saha S, Adhikary A, Bhattacharyya P, Das T, Sa G (2012) Death by design: where curcumin sensitizes drug-resistant tumours. Anticancer Res 32: 2567–2584.

34. Dai Y, Lawrence TS, Xu L (2009) Overcoming cancer therapy resistance by targeting inhibitors of apoptosis proteins and nuclear factor-kappa B. Am J Transl Res 1: 1–15.

35. Yamaguchi Y, Shiraki K, Fuke H, Inoue T, Miyashita K, et al. (2005) Targeting of X-linked inhibitor of apoptosis protein or survivin by short interfering RNAs sensitize hepatoma cells to TNF-related apoptosis-inducing ligand- and chemotherapeutic agent-induced cell death. Oncol Rep 14: 1311–1316.

36. Chawla-Sarkar M, Bae SI, Reu FJ, Jacobs BS, Lindner DJ, et al. (2004) Downregulation of Bcl-2, FLIP or IAPs (XIAP and survivin) by siRNAs sensitizes resistant melanoma cells to Apo2L/TRAIL-induced apoptosis. Cell Death Differ 11: 915–923.

37. Molnar J, Engi H, Hohmann J, Molnar P, Deli J, et al. (2010) Reversal of Multidrug Resistance by Natural Substances from Plants. Current Topics in Medicinal Chemistry 10: 1757–1768.

38. Peng XH, Karna P, O'Regan RM, Liu X, Naithani R, et al. (2007) Down-regulation of inhibitor of apoptosis proteins by deguelin selectively induces apoptosis in breast cancer cells. Mol Pharmacol 71: 101–111.

39. Jia J, Zhu F, Ma X, Cao Z, Li Y, et al. (2009) Mechanisms of drug combinations: interaction and network perspectives. Nat Rev Drug Discov 8: 111–128.

40. Keith CT, Borisy AA, Stockwell BR (2005) Multicomponent therapeutics for networked systems. Nat Rev Drug Discov 4: 71–78.

41. Wang H, Zhao Y, Wu Y, Hu YL, Nan K, et al. (2011) Enhanced anti-tumor efficacy by co-delivery of doxorubicin and paclitaxel with amphiphilic methoxy PEG-PLGA copolymer nanoparticles. Biomaterials 32: 8281–8290.

42. Hu CM, Zhang L (2012) Nanoparticle-based combination therapy toward overcoming drug resistance in cancer. Biochem Pharmacol 83: 1104–1111.

43. L'Ecuyer T, Sanjeev S, Thomas R, Novak R, Das L, et al. (2006) DNA damage is an early event in doxorubicin-induced cardiac myocyte death. American Journal of Physiology-Heart and Circulatory Physiology 291: H1273–H1280.

44. Kim TH, Shin YJ, Won AJ, Lee BM, Choi WS, et al. (2014) Resveratrol enhances chemosensitivity of doxorubicin in multidrug-resistant human breast cancer cells via increased cellular influx of doxorubicin. Biochimica et biophysica acta 1840: 615–625.

45. Khonkarn R, Mankhetkorn S, Talelli M, Hennink WE, Okonogi S (2012) Cytostatic effect of xanthone-loaded mPEG-b-p(HPMAm-Lac2) micelles towards doxorubicin sensitive and resistant cancer cells. Colloids Surf B Biointerfaces 94: 266–273.

2

GSK3A Is Redundant with GSK3B in Modulating Drug Resistance and Chemotherapy-Induced Necroptosis

Emanuela Grassilli[1,2]*, **Leonarda Ianzano**[1], **Sara Bonomo**[1], **Carola Missaglia**[1], **Maria Grazia Cerrito**[1], **Roberto Giovannoni**[1], **Laura Masiero**[1], **Marialuisa Lavitrano**[1]*

1 Department of Surgery and Traslational Medicine, Medical School, University of Milano-Bicocca, via Cadore 48, Monza, Italy, **2** BiOnSil srl, via Cadore 48, Monza, Italy

Abstract

Glycogen Synthase Kinase-3 alpha (GSK3A) and beta (GSK3B) isoforms are encoded by distinct genes, are 98% identical within their kinase domain and perform similar functions in several settings; however, they are not completely redundant and, depending on the cell type and differentiative status, they also play unique roles. We recently identified a role for GSK3B in drug resistance by demonstrating that its inhibition enables necroptosis in response to chemotherapy in p53-null drug-resistant colon carcinoma cells. We report here that, similarly to GSK3B, also GSK3A silencing/inhibition does not affect cell proliferation or cell cycle but only abolishes growth after treatment with DNA-damaging chemotherapy. In particular, blocking GSK3A impairs DNA repair upon exposure to DNA-damaging drugs. As a consequence, p53-null cells overcome their inability to undergo apoptosis and mount a necroptotic response, characterized by absence of caspase activation and RIP1-independent, PARP-dependent AIF nuclear re-localization. We therefore conclude that GSK3A is redundant with GSK3B in regulating drug-resistance and chemotherapy-induced necroptosis and suggest that inhibition of only one isoform, or rather partial inhibition of overall cellular GSK3 activity, is enough to re-sensitize drug-resistant cells to chemotherapy.

Editor: Gerolama Condorelli, Federico II University of Naples, Italy, Italy

Funding: All authors are supported by PON01_02782 from MIUR and F.A.R. grants from the University of Milano-Bicocca to ML. The funders had no role in study design, data collection and analysis, decision to publish, or preparation of the manuscript.

Competing Interests: EG is an employee of the University of Milano-Bicocca spin-off Bionsil srl.

* Email: emanuela.grassilli@unimib.it (EG); marialuisa.lavitrano@unimib.it (ML)

Introduction

Two different GSK3 isoforms, GSK3A and GSK3B, encoded by distinct genes, but 98% identical within their kinase domain, are expressed in mammalian cells [1]. Both isoforms perform similar functions in several settings, but they are not completely redundant as demonstrated by gene knockout studies. In fact, GSK3A is unable to rescue the lethal phenotype of GSK3B null mice: the animals die during embryogenesis as a result of liver degeneration caused by widespread hepatocyte apoptosis, where excessive TNF-alpha-mediated cell death occurs, due to reduced NFkB function [2]. On the other hand, GSK3A null mice are viable and show metabolic defects – such as enhanced glucose and insulin sensitivity and reduced fat mass - which cannot be counteracted by the beta isofom [3]. Moreover, GSK3A KO mice undergo premature death showing acceleration of age-related pathologies, accompanied by marked activation of mTORC1 and associated suppression of autophagy markers, indicating that the alpha isoform is a critical regulator of mTORC1, autophagy, and aging [4].

So far distinct roles for GSK3A and GSK3B have been identified in developmental and differentiation processes [5], as well as in regulation of transcriptional activation [6]. Functional redundancy instead has been demonstrated in the control of several regulatory proteins, in the production of beta-amyloid peptides associated with Alzheimer's disease and in cell cycle and proliferation. In the latter, both isoforms play an anti-proliferative

role by promoting APC-dependent phosphorylation of β-catenin - a transcription factor positively regulating Myc and cyclin D1 expression – therefore targeting it to proteasome-mediated degradation [7]. Either redundant or distinct functions of the two isoforms have been demonstrated in cell survival, depending on the cell type [2,8,9]. In particular, a lot of data are being accumulated about the beta isoform acting as a tumor suppressor in some cancers while potentiating tumoral growth in others: for example, GSK3B activation can be crucial in mediating caspase-dependent apoptosis by contributing to p53 activation in certain epithelial cancers [10], whereas its inhibition arrests pancreatic tumor growth in vivo [11] and is synthetically lethal with MLL oncogene defects in a subset of human leukemia [12]. Moreover, in the experimental systems where GSK3B plays an oncogenic role its targeting has been proved useful, either alone on in combination with chemotherapy, to induce or increase tumor cells death [13,14]. However, very few reports addressed the role of the alpha isoform in cancer cells growth/survival: so far, NFkB-dependent pro-survival effect has been demonstrated to be mediated either by GSK3A or GSK3B in pancreatic cancer cells [9] whereas GSK3A, but not GSK3B, has been identified as a therapeutic target in melanoma [15]. Therefore, very little is known about GSK3A role in cancer cells.

We recently identified a role for GSK3B in drug resistance by finding that its inhibition in p53-null, drug-resistant colon carcinoma cells re-sensitize them to chemotherapy by unleashing RIP1-independent necroptosis in response to DNA damaging agents [16]. Here we report that GSK3A is functionally redundant with GSK3B in modulating drug resistance and chemotherapy-induced necroptosis.

Results

GSK3A silencing in p53-null colon carcinoma cell lines does not affect proliferation but modifies the response to DNA-damaging chemotherapy

To test the role of GSK3A in colon carcinoma cells we first established a stable cell line depleted of the protein by transducing drug-resistant HCT116p53KO cells with retroviruses expressing shRNAs to GSK3A (Fig. 1A). We observed that GSK3A stable silencing in HCT116p53KO did not alter cell proliferation: in fact, when comparing shGSK3A and empty vector-transduced HCT116p53KO we did not find significant differences neither in the growth curve (Fig. 1B) nor in cell cycle distribution (Fig. 1C) and β-catenin activation (Fig. 1D). Next, we assessed the role of GSK3A in the response to chemotherapy and found that its depletion in drug-resistant HCT116p53KO cells abolished colony formation after treatment with 200 μM 5-Fluorouracil (5FU) (Fig. 2A). Accordingly, we observed that, in absence of GSK3A expression, HCT116p53KO cells were resensitized to drug-induced cytotoxicity and showed a cell death response similar to that of parental drug-sensitive HCT116 cells (Fig. 2B); same results were obtained in absence of GSK3B expression. Moreover, stable silencing of GSK3A expression reverted the resistance also to OxPt treatment, another DNA-damaging drug commonly used in colon carcinoma therapy. Notably, GSK3A suppression re-sensitized HCT116p53KO cells to the cytotoxic effect of DNA-damaging drugs to the same extent as GSK3B depletion (Fig. 2C). To fully validate the involvement of GSK3A in drug resistance we inhibited its function by 2 more different means [17] i.e., transient silencing and chemical inhibition. As shown in Fig. 2D transient GSK3A protein depletion by use of siRNA restored cell death in response to 5FU. In order to chemically inhibit GSK3A, but not GSK3B, enzymatic activity we first screened a number of commercially available inhibitors (Fig. S1); in fact, being the ATP-binding pockets of GSK3A and GSK3B very similar, most inhibitors block the activity of both isoforms [18]. GSK3 activity is usually kept off by an inhibitory phosphorylation on Ser (S21 for GSK3A and S9 for GSK3B) that has to be removed to allow phosphorylation on Tyr (T279 for GSK3A and T216 for GSK3B), and therefore enzymatic activation, to occur [5]. Using as a readout the phosphorylation pattern of the two isoforms we found that, in our model system, 20 μM SB216763 was able to strongly reduce T279 (even though not completely) and increase S21 phoshorylation without affecting neither T216 nor S9 phoshorylation indicating that at this concentration it specifically inhibits only the GSK3A isoform. At variance, very low concentrations of other inhibitors - such as BIO and TWS - despite increasing the levels of phospho-S21, but not phospho-S9, abolished both T279 and T216 phosphorylation, indicating that these inhibitors affect the activity of both isoforms, perhaps to a different extent. Interestingly, concentrations of BIO able to completely suppress both T279 and T216 phosphorylation (2 μM), were also cytotoxic (Fig. S2) indicating that blocking completely GSK3 activity is not compatible with survival of cancer cells. To confirm that GSK3A inhibition re-sensitize drug-resistant colon carcinoma cells to chemotherapy, we then treated three cell lines characterized by different genetic background, HCT116p53KO, SW480 and HT-29 drug-resistant cells, with 5FU in the presence of 20 μM SB216763 and 1 μM BIO (Fig. 3). Both inhibitors elicited significant cell death in response to DNA-damaging drugs and,

consistently with an effect also on GSK3B, higher percentage of cell death was observed in BIO- vs SB216763-treated cells (Fig.3 A–D), with the exception of HT-29 cell line. These cells in fact appeared to be intrinsically more resistant to the effect of BIO (Fig.3 E, F) and the concentration had to be increased to 2 μM to obtain percentages of cell death comparable to those observed for HCT116p53KO and SW480 cells.

On the whole, similarly to what observed upon GSK3B protein blockade, also silencing/inhibiting GSK3A does not affect cell proliferation and only modified the response to DNA-damaging chemotherapy.

GSK3A inhibition affects the response to DNA damage and elicits RIP1-independent necroptosis in response to 5FU

Next we investigate whether, similarly to GSK3B, also GSK3A inhibition influences DNA damage response/repair systems. To this end we analysed γH2AX foci formation, as a marker of the DNA damage response [19], and RPA70 foci formation, as a marker of DNA repair [20], in HCT116p53KO cells treated with 5FU. As in the case of GSK3B, also blocking GSK3A, either by silencing (Fig. 4A, B) or by use of a specific inhibitor (Fig. 4C, D) did not affect DNA damage sensing (Fig. 4A, C) as indicated by the formation of γH2AX-positive foci. Similarly to what reported for GSK3B, also GSK3A silencing/inhibition affected the DNA repair response by impairing RPA70 foci formation (Fig. 4B, D).

Finally, we investigated which kind of cell death is induced in response to DNA-damaging drugs when GSK3A function is blocked in p53-null cells: as in the case of GSK3B inhibition, upon 5FU treatment, GSK3A-depleted HCT116p53KO cells underwent caspase-independent (Fig. 5A), PARP1- and tBid-dependent cell death, which was unaffected by RIP1 inhibition (Fig. 5C) and was characterized by PARP-dependent nuclear re-localization of AIF (Fig. 5B, D).

Altogether our data demonstrate that GSK3A isoform, like GSK3B, contributes to cell survival upon treatment with DNA-damaging drugs by suppressing a necroptotic response.

Discussion

Few investigations have addressed the role of GSK3A in cancer cells so far. A redundant role with GSK3B has been described in pancreatic cancer cells where both isoforms are involved in NFkB-dependent pro-survival effect [9]. At variance, GSK3A, but not GSK3B, has been identified as a therapeutic target in melanoma [15] suggesting that, similarly to what has been reported for normal cells, the two isoforms can play both distinct or redundant roles depending on the cancer cell type. Our data demonstrate for the first time that GSK3A is redundant with GSK3B in regulating drug-resistance and chemotherapy-induced necroptosis of p53-null colon cancer cells. In addition, they indicate that inhibition of one isoform is sufficient to bypass drug resistance of p53-null colon cancer cells since both GSK3 isoforms negatively regulate the RIP1-independent necroptotic response elicited by chemotherapy.

From our data GSK3 activity appear to negatively regulate PARP1 in response to 5FU (Fig. 3C and D and ref. 16). Notably, PARP1 is involved in three pathways of DNA repair that are differently affected by p53 absence [21] and directly or indirectly activated by 5FU treatment [22]: base excision repair (BER), non-homologous end joining (NHEJ) and homologous recombination (HR). In fact, in absence of wild type p53, activation of BER, the main repair pathway activated by 5FU, is suppressed whereas NHEJ and HR are active leading to aberrant double strand break repair. Accordingly, it has been reported that after severe

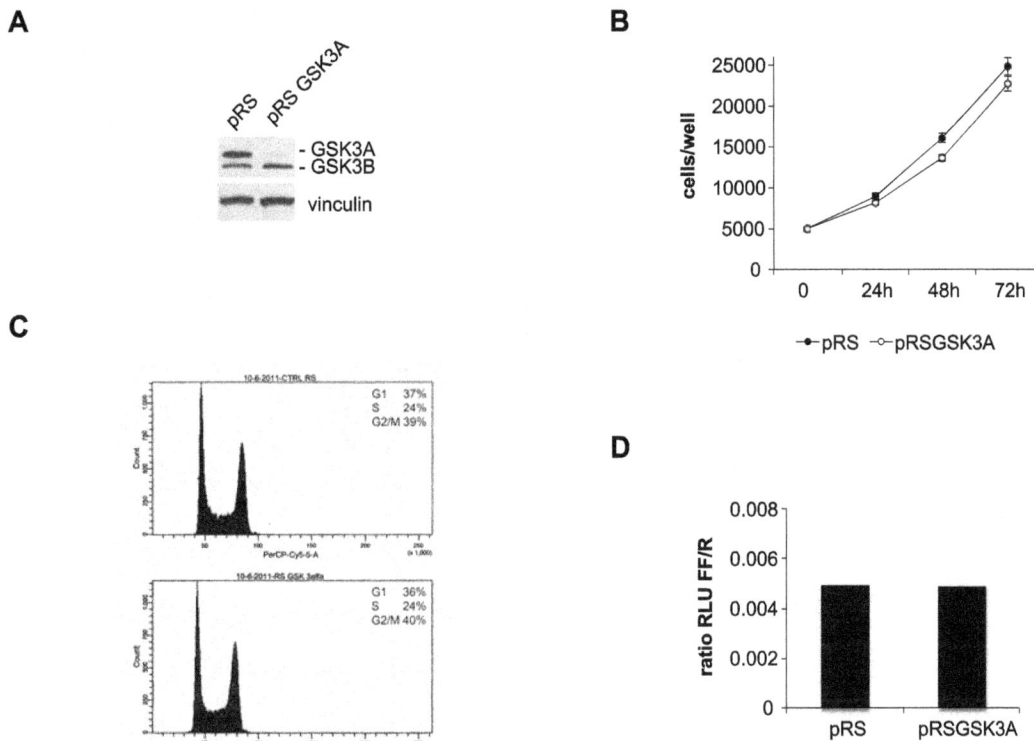

Figure 1. GSK3A silencing in p53-null colon carcinoma cell lines does not affect proliferation or cell cycle. A) Western blot on total lysates (30 µg) from HCT116p53KO cells stably infected with retroviral empty (pRS) and GSK3A shRNA-expressing (pRSGSK3A) vectors. **B)** growth curve of HCT116p53KO-pRS and -pRSGSK3A cells. **C)** DNA content and percentage of cells in G1, S phase and G2/M of HCT116p53KO-pRS and -pRSGSK3Aas evaluated after PI staning and flow cytometric analysis. **D)** β-catenin activity as evaluated by reporter assay 48 hrs after co-transfection with a luciferase-encoding vector driven by a β-catenin-dependent promoter. RLU = Relative Light Units. encoding vector (pRSGSK3B).

genotoxic damage, p53 mutant cells can recover from a G2 arrest and resume proliferation upon DNA re-replication during which aberrant DNA repair occurs [23]. Consistent with the data from the literature, in our model system, RPA70 foci -markers of repair activity - are formed in p53-null drug-resistant cells surviving 5FU treatment but they are strongly impaired in absence of GSK3 activity (Fig. 4), when cells are re-sensitized to the cytotoxic effect of chemotherapy. It is likely that following DNA damage and in absence of GSK3 activity PARP activation (Fig. 5C and D) occurs which is not accompanied by DNA repair (Fig. 4B and D), therefore leading to the triggering of cell death mechanisms.

The finding that both isoforms play redundant roles in the response to chemotherapy is particularly relevant both at clinical and therapeutic level. Due to the high similarity in in the ATP-binding pockets of GSK3A and GSK3B, synthesis of inhibitors able to differentiate between the two isoforms is very difficult [18]. Moreover, when targeting GSK3 it has be kept in mind that a complete inhibition of whole GSK3 activity might be undesirable, based on the observation that GSK3A/B double-knockout cells displayed hyperactivated Wnt/β-catenin signaling [7] which may be oncogenic. On the other hand, it also been demonstrated that only in cells lacking three or all four of the alleles a gene-dosage effect was observed, suggesting that there may be a therapeutic window and dose for GSK3 inhibitors in treating diseases without elevating β-catenin levels and thus a risk of oncogenic events [7]. Due to the redundancy played by GSK3A and GSK3B in the response to DNA-damaging drugs it is reasonable to predict that, when used together with anticancer drugs, GSK3 inhibitors would be particularly effective in abolishing drug resistance even at low

doses since inhibition of only one isoform, or rather partial inhibition of overall cellular GSK3 activity, is enough to re-sensitize drug-resistant cells. Our data using BIO in combination with 5FU (Fig.3 B, D) strongly support this prediction: in fact, when used together with 5FU, concentrations as low as 1 µM BIO (inhibiting GSK3A and partially GSK3B) induce an higher percentage of cell death cells than 20 µM SB216763 (inhibiting only GSK3A). Moreover, in our model system a low concentration of SB216763 is able to specifically inhibit GSK3A, while several reports demonstrate that in different cell lines and/or models higher concentrations of the same inhibitor blocks also GSK3B function [24–27].

In conclusion, we propose that GSK3 inhibition in combination with DNA damaging drugs would be an appealing strategy to induce necroptosis in colon tumors resistant to chemotherapy because of the loss of pivotal apoptosis regulators such as p53.

Materials and Methods

Drugs and reagents

5FU (Teva) and Oxaliplatin (Sanofi-Aventis) were from San Gerardo Hospital, Monza. SB216763, SB415286 and necrostatin-1 were from Sigma-Aldrich. 6-bromoindirubin-3'-oxime, TWS119 and Tideglusib were from Selleck Chemicals

Cell lines and cell culture

Isogenic p53 wild type and p53 knockout HCT116 colon carcinoma cell lines, a kind gift of Dr. Bert Vogelstein (Johns Hopkins University, Baltimore, MD), HT-29 and SW480 were

A

pRS   pRSGSK3A

B

*pRSGSK3A - 5FU vs pRSGSK3A + 5FU p=0.00008
**pRSGSK3B - 5FU vs pRSGSK3B + 5FU p=0.0009

C

*pRSGSK3A - OxPt vs pRSGSK3A + OxPt p=0.003
**pRSGSK3B - OxPt vs pRSGSK3B + OxPt p=0.004

D

* siRNA GSK3A - 5FU vs siRNA GSK3A + 5FU p=0.001

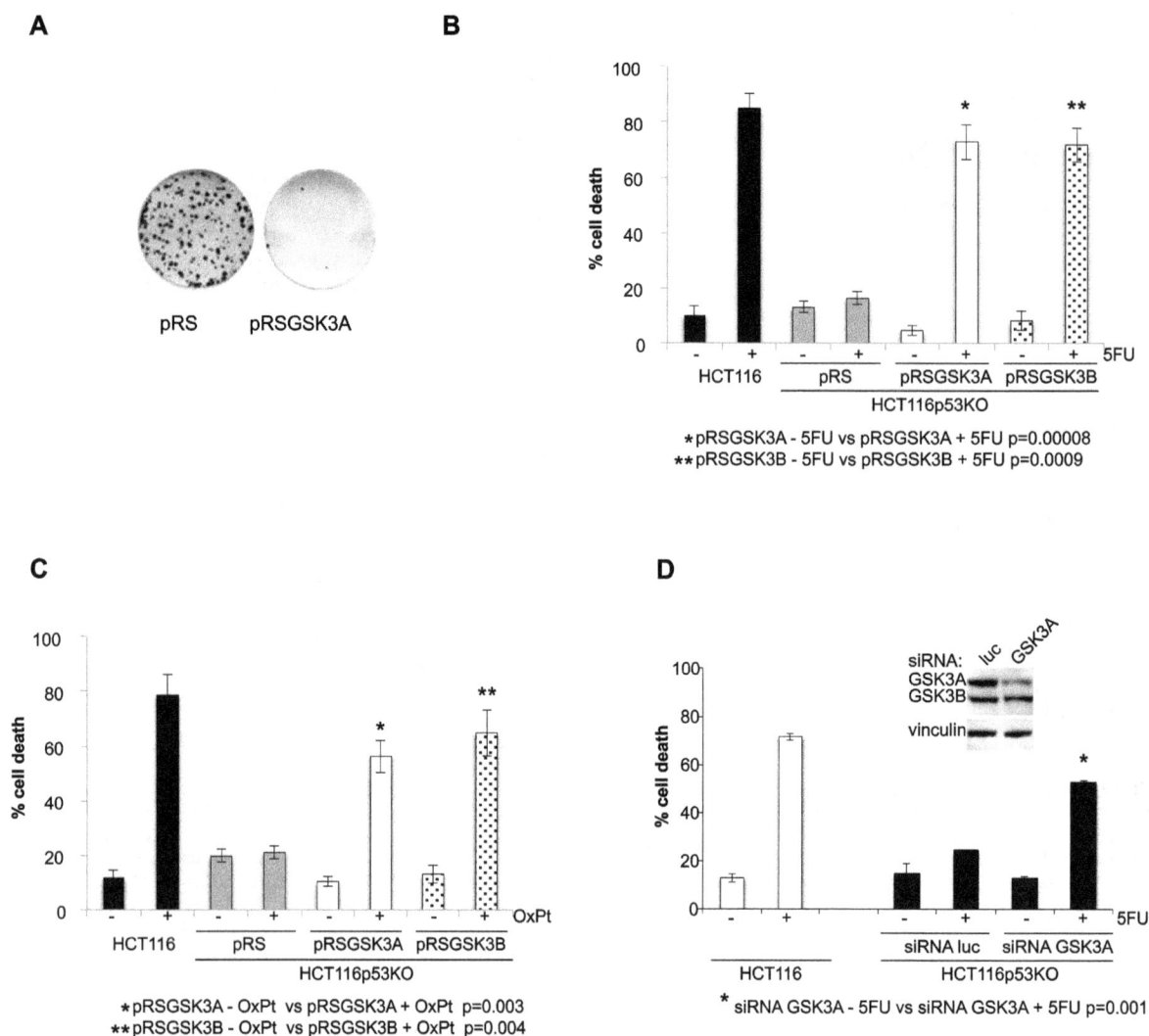

Figure 2. Either stable or transient depletion of GSK3A abolishes drug resistance of p53-null colon carcinoma cell lines. A) colony assay of 5FU-treated HCT116p53KO-pRS and -pRSGSK3A cells. Cells were trypsinized and reseeded at low density 12 hours after 200 μM 5FU treatment. Colony formation was assessed 2 weeks after the reseeding. **B)** percentage of cell death of HCT116p53KO-pRS, -pRSGSK3A and -pRSGSK3B cells treated for 72 hrs with 200 μM 5FU. Drug sensitive HCT116 cells were used as a positive control. **C)** percentage of cell death of HCT116p53KO-pRS, -pRSGSK3A and -pRSGSK3B cells treated for 72 hrs with 50 μM Oxaliplatin (OxPt). Drug sensitive HCT116 cells were used as a positive control. **D)** percentage of cell death of HCT116p53KO upon GSK3A transient silencing and treatment with 200 μM 5FU (72 hrs). In the inset: lysates of HCT116p53KO cells transfected with luciferase (luc)- or GSK3A-specific siRNAs were harvested 24 hs after silencing and GSK3A levels checked by western blot.

from ATCC. All cell lines were maintained in McCoy medium (Invitrogen) supplemented with 10% fetal bovine serum (Invitrogen) and 1% penicillin-streptomycin at 37°C in 5% CO2. Cell lines stably interfered for GSK3A were obtained by retroviral infection and selection with the appropriate antibiotic as previously described [25]. GSK3A siRNA were purchased from Qiagen (#S100288554), Luciferase siRNA from Eurofins MWG Operon, (#GL2).

Cell viability

Cells were seeded overnight at 70% confluency and the next morning treated or not with the indicated drugs and inhibitors. 72 hrs later dead cells were counted - triplicate wells in each experiment - after Trypan blue staining. In experiments using inhibitors, after overnight seeding cells were pre-incubated for 2 hrs before 5FU addition. Graphs shown throughout the paper

represent the average of three to five independent experiments. Average ±SEMs is plotted in the graphs.

Colony assay

3×10^5 cells/well were seeded in 6-well plate, let adhere overnight and treated with 200 μM 5FU for 12 hs. Cells were then trypsinized, counted, and reseeded at a low density (1000 cells/well in 6-well plate) in triplicate; medium was replaced every 3 days, and after 2 weeks colonies were fixed and stained in 1% crystal violet, 35% ethanol.

Caspase assay

4×10^4 cells/well were seeded in triplicate in 96-well plate, let adhere overnight and treated with 200 μM 5FU for 72 hrs before evaluating active caspase-3/7 by the Caspase-Glo3/7 Assay System (Promega) according to the manufacturer's instructions.

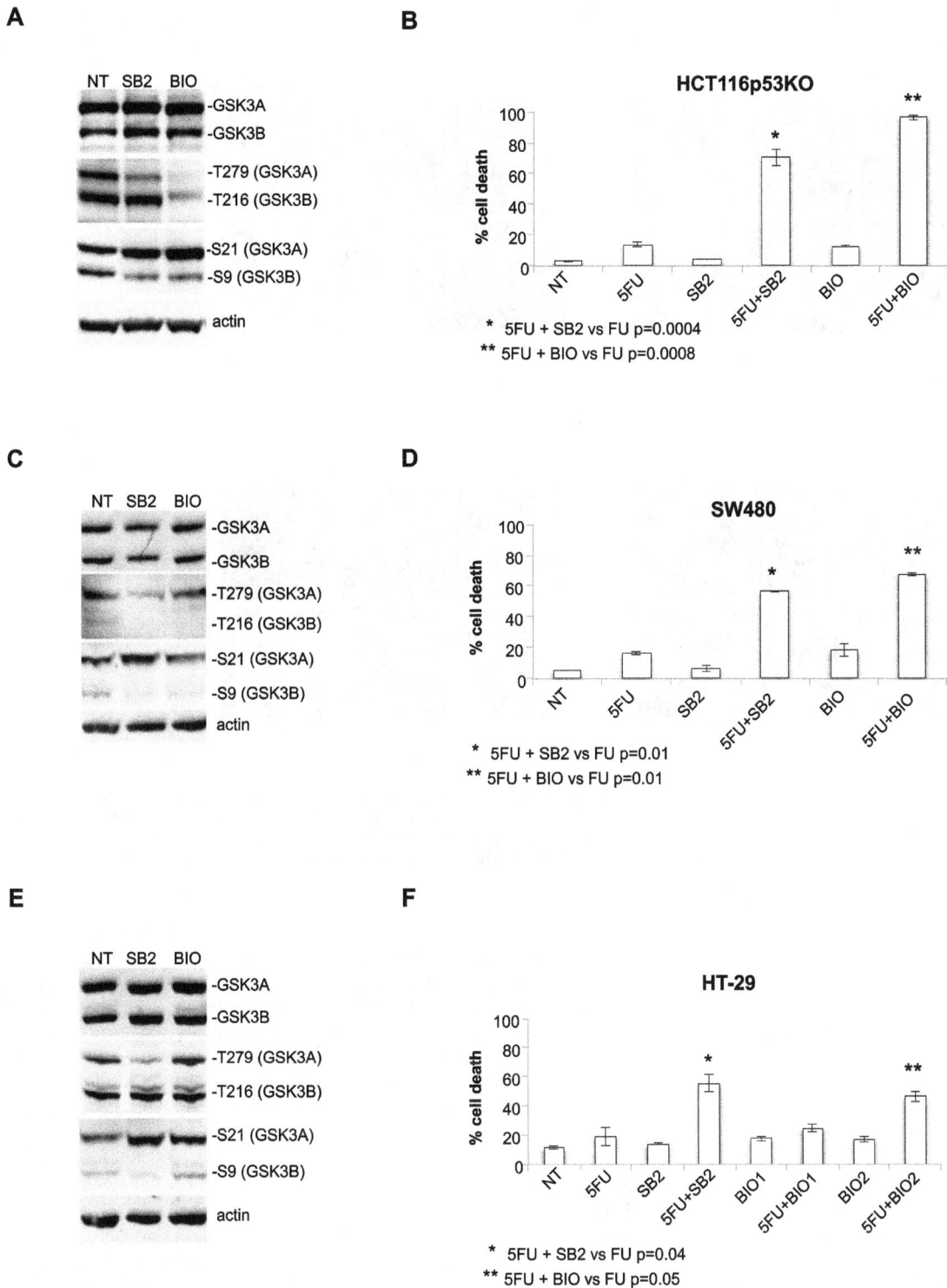

Figure 3. Chemical inhibition abolishes drug resistance of p53-null colon carcinoma cell lines. A, C, E Lysates of HCT116p53KO (**A**) and SW480 (**C**) cells were harvested 24hs after treatment with 1 μM 6-bromoindirubin-3'-oxime (BIO) and 20 μM SB216763 (SB2) GSK3 inhibitors; lysates of HT-29 (**E**) cells were harvested 24 hs after treatment with 2 μM 6-bromoindirubin-3'-oxime (BIO) and 20 μM SB216763 (SB2) GSK3 inhibitors; specificity of the inhibitor for GSK3A was assessed by checking GSK3A activation/inactivation checked by western blot using a mix of pSer21-GSK3A and pSer9-GSK3B antibodies and antibody cross-reacting with both pTyr279-GSK3A and pTyr216-GSK3B. **B, D, F**) percentage of cell death of HCT116p53KO(**B**), SW480 (**D**) and HT-29 (**F**) treated with 200 μM 5FU in presence and in absence of the indicated inhibitors (72 hrs).

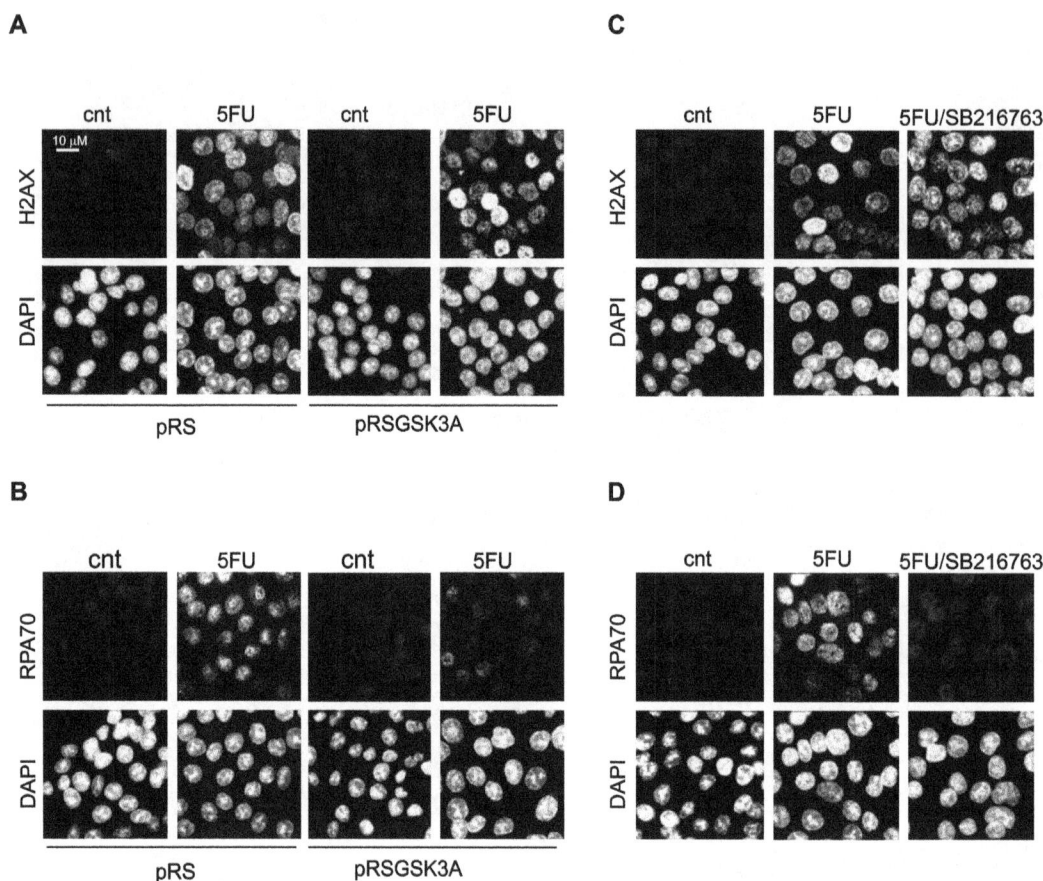

Figure 4. GSK3A inhibition abolishes drug resistance of p53-null colon carcinoma cells by affecting the response to DNA damage. HCT116p53KO cells stably infected with empty (pRS) and GSK3A shRNA-encoding vector (pRSGSK3A) untreated (cnt) or treated for 18 hrs with 200 μM 5FU (5FU) and stained with anti-γH2AX antibody (**A**) or anti-RPA70 antibody (**B**) and counterstained with DAPI. HCT116p53KO untreated (cnt), treated for 18 hrs with 200 μM 5FU (5FU) or with 200 μM 5FU+10 μM SB216763 and stained with anti-γH2AX antibody (**C**) or anti-RPA70 antibody (**D**) and counterstained with DAPI.

Cell proliferation

1×10^4 cells/well were seeded in triplicate in 96-well plate and starting the following day (day 0) proliferation was evaluated each 24 hrs by CellTiter 96 AQueous Non-Radioactive Cell Proliferation Assay (Promega) according to the manufacturer's instructions.

Flow Cytometric Analysis

Exponentially growing cells were trypsinized, washed twice with cold PBS, fixed in ice-cold 96% ethanol, washed twice with cold PBS and incubated overnight at 4°C with propidium iodide (10 μg/mL) and RNase A (12.5 μg/mL) in PBS. Fluorescence intensity of 1×10^4 cells/sample was determined with a FACSCalibur instrument and data analyzed using Modfit Cell Cycle Analysis (Becton Dickinson) as previously described [16].

Reporter assay

0.2 μg TopFlash +0.2 μg pGL4.75 reporters were transfected in 5×10^4 cells/well seeded in triplicate in a 96-well plate and reporter activity was evaluated 48 hrs later by Dual-Glo Luciferase Assay (Promega) according to the manufacturer's instructions.

Western blot analysis

Cells were lysed in high-salt lysis buffer (Hepes 50 mM, pH 7.5, NaCl 500 mM, DTT 1 mM, EDTA 1 mM, 0.1% NP40) supplemented with 1% protease inhibitor cocktail (PIC, Sigma-Aldrich) and Western blots performed as described [25] using the following antibodies: anti-GSK3A/Bsc-7921) and anti-pTyr279/216-GSK3A/Bsc-11758) from Santa Cruz Biotechnology, anti-pSer9-GSK3B (clone D85E12) and anti-pSer21-GSK3A, (clone 36E9) from Cell Signaling, vinculin (SAB4200080) from Sigma-Aldrich.

Immunofluorescence

Cells were fixed with 4% paraformaldehyde in phosphate-buffered saline. Permeabilization and staining with anti-AIF (sc-13116, SantaCruz Biotechnology), anti-γH2AX (Ab 22551, Abcam), anti-RPA70 (clone 2H10, Sigma-Aldrich) was performed as described [28]. Cells were counterstained with DAPI before microscopic examination using 60× magnification and a Nikon Eclipse 80i microscope. Images were acquired using Genikon (Nikon) software and processed with Adobe Photoshop.

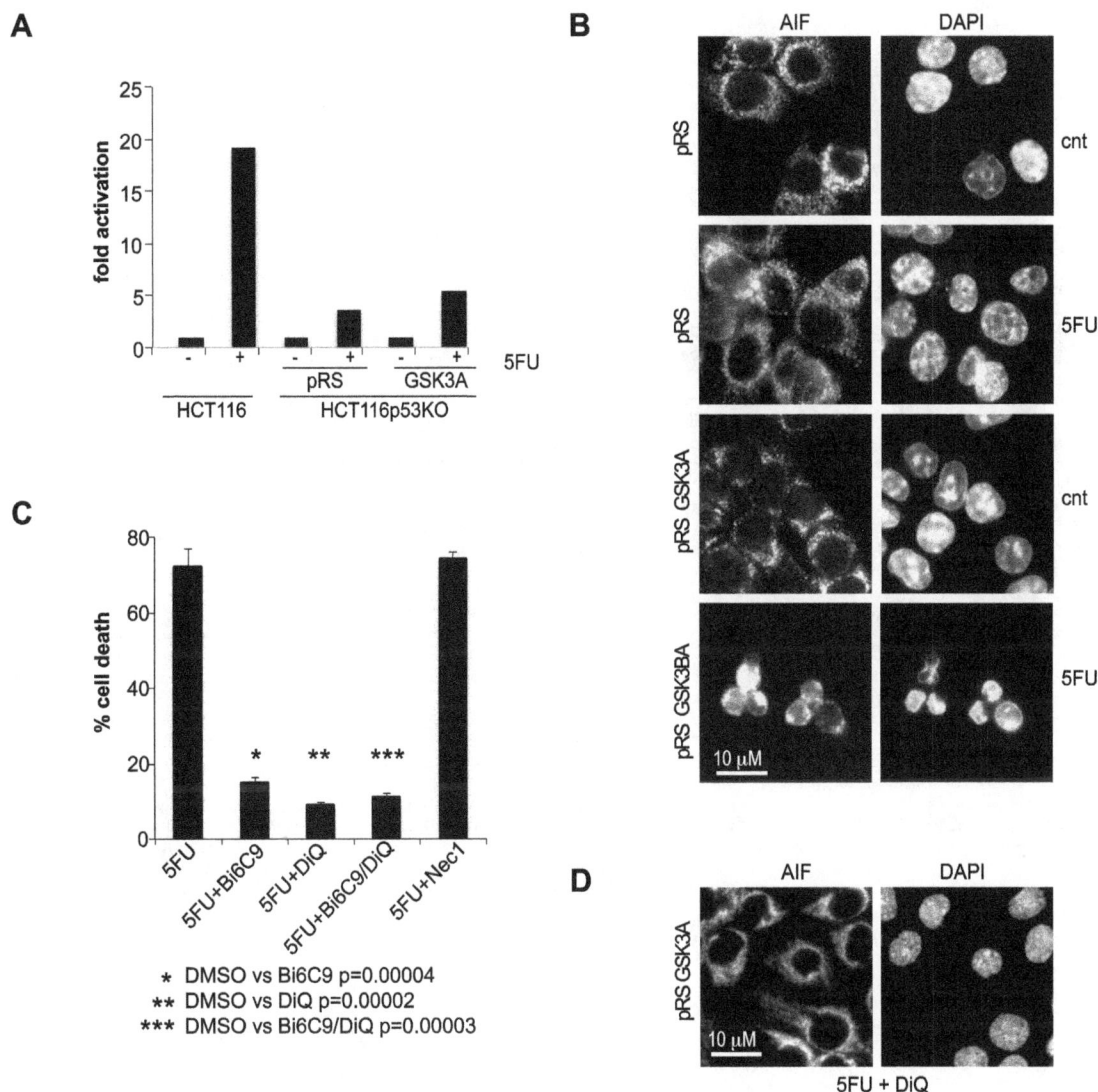

Figure 5. p53-null, GSK3B-silenced colon carcinoma cells treated with 5FU die by RIP1-independent necroptosis. A) caspase-3/7 activation in HCT116p53KO-pRS and -pRSGSK3A cells treated with 200 µM 5FU for 72 hrs. HCT116 were used as control. Values indicate the fold increase of enzymatic activity of treated cells relative to the untreated cells arbitrarily set as 1. A representative experiment is shown. **B)** HCT116p53KO-pRS and -pRSGSK3A treated for 30 hrs with 200 µM 5FU and stained with anti-AIF antibody as well as DAPI. **C)** percentage of cell death of HCT116p53KO-pRSGSK3A after 72 hs treatment with 200 µM 5FU in presence of Bid inhibitor (20 µM Bi6C9), PARP1 inhibitor (100 µM DiQ), Bi6C9+DiQ or Necrostatin-1 (20 µM Nec1). **D)** HCT116p53KO-pRSGSK3A treated for 30 hrs with 200 µM 5FU in presence of 100 µM DiQ and stained with anti-AIF antibody as well as DAPI.

Statistical analysis

T test was applied to evaluate statistically significant differences between series of samples subjected to different experimental treatments, $p \leq 0.05$ was considered significant.

Supporting Information

Figure S1 Isoform specificity of different chemical inhibitors of GSK3. Lysates of HCT116p53KO cells were harvested 24 hs after treatment with different GSK3 inhibitors and GSK3A/B activation/inactivation checked by western blot: a mix of pSer21-GSK3A and pSer9-GSK3B antibodies and antibody cross-reacting with both pTyr279-GSK3A and pTyr216-GSK3B were used to assess the specificity of the inhibitor for GSK3A. BIO: 6-bromoindirubin-3′-oxime, TWS: TWS119, SB2: SB216763, SB4: SB415286.
(EPS)

Figure S2 Inhibition of both GSK3 isoforms is toxic. A) Lysates of HCT116p53KO and SW480 cells were harvested 24 hs after treatment with 2 µM BIO. Inhibition of GSK3A/B was assessed by western blot using a mix of pSer21-GSK3A and pSer9-GSK3B antibodies and an antibody cross-reacting with both pTyr279-GSK3A and pTyr216-GSK3B. **B)** percentage of cell death of HCT116p53KO and SW480 cells treated in presence and in absence of 2 µM BIO (72 hrs).
(EPS)

Author Contributions

Conceived and designed the experiments: EG. Performed the experiments: LI SB CM MGC RG LM. Analyzed the data: EG ML. Wrote the paper: EG ML.

References

1. Rayasam GV, Tulasi VK, Sodhi R, Davis JA, Ray A (2009) Glycogen synthase kinase 3: more than a namesake. Br J Pharmacol 156: 885–898.

2. MacAulay K, Doble BW, Patel S, Hansotia T, Sinclair EM, et al. (2007) Glycogen synthase kinase 3alpha-specific regulation of murine hepatic glycogen metabolism. Cell Metab 6: 329–337.

3. Hoeflich KP, Luo J, Rubie EA, Tsao MS, Jin O, et al. (2000) Requirement for glycogen synthase kinase-3beta in cell survival and NF-kappaB activation. Nature 406: 86–90.

4. Zhou J, Freeman TA, Ahmad F, Shang X, Mangano E, et al. (2013) GSK-3α is a central regulator of age-related pathologies in mice. J Clin Invest 123: 1821–1832.

5. Forde JE, Dale TC (2007) Glycogen synthase kinase 3: A key regulator of cellular fate. Cell Mol Life Sci 64: 1930–1944.

6. Liang MH, Chuang DM (2006) Differential roles of glycogen synthase kinase-3 isoforms in the regulation of transcriptional activation. J Biol Chem 281: 30479–30484.

7. Doble BW, Patel S, Wood GA, Kockeritz LK, Woodgett JR (2007) Functional redundancy of GSK-3alpha and GSK-3beta in Wnt/beta-catenin signaling shown by using an allelic series of embryonic stem cell lines. Dev Cell 12: 957–971.

8. Piazza F, Manni S, Tubi LQ, Montini B, Pavan L, et al. (2010) Glycogen Synthase Kinase-3 regulates multiple myeloma cell growth and bortezomib-induced cell death. BMC Cancer 10: 526–540.

9. Wilson W 3rd, Baldwin AS (2008) Maintenance of constitutive IkappaB kinase activity by glycogen synthase kinase-3alpha/beta in pancreatic cancer. Cancer Res 68: 8156–8163.

10. Beurel E, Jope RS (2006) The paradoxical pro- and anti-apoptotic actions of GSK3 in the intrinsic and extrinsic apoptosis signaling pathways. Prog Neurobiol 79: 173–189.

11. Ougolkov AV, Fernandez-Zapico ME, Bilim VN, Smyrk TC, Chari ST, et al. (2006) Aberrant nuclear accumulation of glycogen synthase kinase-3beta in human pancreatic cancer: association with kinase activity and tumor dedifferentiation. Clin Cancer Res, 12: 5074–81.

12. Wang Z, Smith KS, Murphy M, Piloto O, Somervaille TC, et al. (2008) Glycogen synthase kinase 3 in MLL leukaemia maintenance and targeted therapy. Nature 455: 1205–1209.

13. Mills CN, Nowsheen S, Bonner JA, Yang ES (2011) Emerging roles of glycogen synthase kinase 3 in the treatment of brain tumors. Front Mol Neurosci 4: 47–53.

14. Mishra R (2010) Glycogen synthase kinase 3 beta: can it be a target for oral cancer. Mol Cancer 9: 144–149.

15. Madhunapantula SV, Sharma A, Gowda R, Robertson GP (2013) Identification of glycogen synthase kinase 3α as a therapeutic target in melanoma. Pigment Cell Melanoma Res 26: 886–99.

16. Grassilli E, Narloch R, Federzoni E, Ianzano L, Pisano F, et al. (2013) Inhibition of GSK3B bypass drug resistance of p53-null colon carcinomas by enabling necroptosis in response to chemotherapy. Clin Cancer Res 19: 3820–3831.

17. Sigoillot FD, King RW (2011) Vigilance and validation: keys to success in RNAi screening. ACS Chem Biol 6: 47–60.

18. Meijer L, Flajolet M, Greengard P (2004) Pharmacological inhibitors of glycogen synthase kinase 3. Trends Pharmacol Sci 25: 471–480.

19. Bonner WM, Redon CE, Dickey JS, Nakamura AJ, Sedelnikova OA, et al. (2008) GammaH2AX and cancer. Nat Rev Cancer 8: 957–67.

20. Oakley GG, Patrick SM (2010) Replication protein A: directing traffic at the intersection of replication and repair. Front Biosci 15: 883–900.

21. Gatz SA, Wiesmüller L (2006) p53 in recombination and repair. Cell Death Differ 13: 1003–1016.

22. Thorn CF, Marsh S, Carrillo MW, McLeod HL, Klein TE, et al. (2011) PharmGKB summary: fluoropyrimidine pathways. Pharmacogenet Genomics. 21: 237–42.

23. Ivanov A, Cragg MS, Erenpreisa J, Emzinsh D, Lukman H, et al. (2003) Endopolyploid cells produced after severe genotoxic damage have the potential to repair DNA double strand breaks. J Cell Sci 116: 4095–106.

24. Tanioka T, Tamura Y, Fukaya M, Shinozaki S, Mao J, et al. (2011) Inducible nitric-oxide synthase and nitric oxide donor decrease insulin receptor substrate-2 protein expression by promoting proteasome-dependent degradation in pancreatic beta-cells: involvement of glycogen synthase kinase-3beta. J Biol Chem 286: 29388–29396.

25. Schütz SV, Schrader AJ, Zengerling F, Genze F, Cronauer MV, et al. (2011) Inhibition of glycogen synthase kinase-3β counteracts ligand-independent activity of the androgen receptor in castration resistant prostate cancer. PLoS One, 6: e25341.

26. Deng H, Dokshin GA, Lei J, Goldsmith AM, Bitar KN, et al. (2008) Inhibition of glycogen synthase kinase-3beta is sufficient for airway smooth muscle hypertrophy. J Biol Chem 283: 10198–10207.

27. Giannopoulou M, Dai C, Tan X, Wen X, Michalopoulos GK, et al. (2008) Hepatocyte growth factor exerts its anti-inflammatory action by disrupting nuclear factor-kappaB signaling. Am J Pathol 173: 30–41.

28. Grassilli E, Ballabeni A, Maellaro E, Del Bello B, Helin K (2004) Loss of MYC confers resistance to doxorubicin-induced apoptosis by preventing the activation of multiple serine protease- and caspase-mediated pathways. J Biol Chem 279: 21318–21326.

3

DNA Repair Biomarkers XPF and Phospho-MAPKAP Kinase 2 Correlate with Clinical Outcome in Advanced Head and Neck Cancer

Tanguy Y. Seiwert[1,6]*, XiaoZhe Wang[3], Jana Heitmann[1], Vivian Villegas-Bergazzi[3], Kam Sprott[3], Stephen Finn[3], Esther O'Regan[3], Allan D. Farrow[3], Ralph R. Weichselbaum[4,6], Mark W. Lingen[5,6], Ezra E. W. Cohen[1,6], Kerstin Stenson[2], David T. Weaver[3], Everett E. Vokes[1,6]

1 Department of Medicine, Section of Hematology/Oncology, The University of Chicago, Chicago, Illinois, United States of America, 2 Department of Surgery, Section of Head and Neck Surgery, The University of Chicago, Chicago, Illinois, United States of America, 3 On-Q-ity Inc., Waltham, Massachusetts, United States of America, 4 Department of Radiation Oncology, The University of Chicago, Chicago, Illinois, United States of America, 5 Department of Pathology, The University of Chicago, Chicago, Illinois, United States of America, 6 The University of Chicago Comprehensive Cancer Center, Chicago, Illinois, United States of America

Abstract

Background: Induction chemotherapy is a common therapeutic option for patients with locoregionally-advanced head and neck cancer (HNC), but it remains unclear which patients will benefit. In this study, we searched for biomarkers predicting the response of patients with locoregionally-advanced HNC to induction chemotherapy by evaluating the expression pattern of DNA repair proteins.

Methods: Expression of a panel of DNA-repair proteins in formalin-fixed paraffin embedded specimens from a cohort of 37 HNC patients undergoing platinum-based induction chemotherapy prior to definitive chemoradiation were analyzed using quantitative immunohistochemistry.

Results: We found that XPF (an ERCC1 binding partner) and phospho-MAPKAP Kinase 2 (pMK2) are novel biomarkers for HNSCC patients undergoing platinum-based induction chemotherapy. Low XPF expression in HNSCC patients is associated with better response to induction chemoradiotherapy, while high XPF expression correlates with a worse response (p = 0.02). Furthermore, low pMK2 expression was found to correlate significantly with overall survival after induction plus chemoradiation therapy (p = 0.01), suggesting that pMK2 may relate to chemoradiation therapy.

Conclusions: We identified XPF and pMK2 as novel DNA-repair biomarkers for locoregionally-advanced HNC patients undergoing platinum-based induction chemotherapy prior to definitive chemoradiation. Our study provides insights for the use of DNA repair biomarkers in personalized diagnostics strategies. Further validation in a larger cohort is indicated.

Editor: Apar Kishor Ganti, University of Nebraska Medical Center, United States of America

Funding: This work was supported by an ASCO Translational Professor ship award (EEV), the Grant Achatz and Nick Kokonas/Alinea Head and Neck Cancer Research Fund (EV, TYS), and a Flight Attending Medical Research Institute Young Clinical Scientist Award (FAMRI, YCSA)(TYS). The funders had no role in study design, data collection and analysis, decision to publish, or preparation of the manuscript.

Competing Interests: X Wang, V Villegas-Bergazzi, and DT Weaver were employees of On-Q-ity. K Sprott, S Finn, E O'Regan, DA Farrow were consultants for On-Q-ity.

* Email: tseiwert@medicine.bsd.uchicago.edu

Introduction

Head and neck squamous cell carcinoma (HNSCC) is the 6th most common malignant neoplasm worldwide and accounts for 45.000 new cases in the US every year [1,2]. For practical purposes, head and neck cancer is divided into three clinical stages: early, locoregionally-advanced, and metastatic or recurrent. Treatment approaches can vary depending on the disease stage. The vast majority of patients (~60%) presenting with locoregionally-advanced disease require aggressive multimodality therapy. Reported long-term survival rates ranges between 50–70% [3,4]. Induction or neoadjuvant chemotherapy is increasingly used prior to definitive local therapy (i.e. surgery/chemoradiotherapy/radiation) and FDA approved for this indication. Induction chemotherapy is associated with high response rates, symptomatic relief, and a reduction in distant metastatic failures. Moreover, several groups including ours have reported a clear association between response to induction chemotherapy and improved overall survival [5–7]. Despite a high degree of activity, a recent phase III study failed to show benefit of adding induction chemotherapy to chemoradiotherapy in an unselected patient population [8]. Subgroup analysis suggested potential benefit in certain high-risk populations, but in the absence of a suitable biomarker validation of hypotheses will be difficult and expensive.

A meta-analysis also confirmed a small survival advantage with induction chemotherapy despite heterogeneity of the included therapies [9]. Unfortunately, there is currently no validated method to predict which patients will benefit from this therapy and it remains unclear how to select patients for this potentially beneficial as well as potentially toxic therapy. Biomarkers could help to improve patient selection in the future.

DNA repair proteins play an essential role in maintaining genome stability and have been implicated in tumorigenesis. Patients with chromosomal instability syndromes such as Fanconi anemia (FA), ataxia telangiectasia (AT), Bloom's syndrome or Werner syndrome show defects in DNA repair and an associated increased risk and poor prognosis for cancer including head and neck cancers [10–17]. Cancer cells exhibit genomic instability and are often defective in one of six major DNA repair pathways namely: base excision repair (BER), nucleotide excision repair (NER), mismatch repair (MMR), homologous recombination (HR), nonhomologous endjoining (NHEJ), and translesion DNA synthesis (TLS). Chemotherapy and most chemotherapeutic agents damage DNA and lack of adequate repair induces tumor cell death.

Therefore, it is crucial to identify DNA repair biomarkers that can predict which patients benefit from induction chemotherapy in locoregionally-advanced head and neck cancer.

Previous reports suggest that ERCC1 is a potential biomarker for platinum-based therapy [18–20]. The ERCC1 protein binds to XPF to form a heterodimer, which is a DNA specific endonuclease structure that stabilizes one another *in vivo* and is responsible for the 5′ incision during nucleotide excision repair [21]. Levels of ERCC1 are significantly reduced in XPF deficient cells and vice versa [22]. This biomarker has not been adopted for HNSCC in part due to controversy surrounding the specificity of the employed antibody [23,24]. Other studies found, that resistance towards platinum-based chemotherapy correlates with protein or mRNA levels of ERCC1 and XPF [21,25,26].

In this study, we investigated a panel of DNA repair proteins in five major DNA repair pathways using immunohistochemistry (IHC) and a digital pathology platform to evaluate whether the expression pattern of DNA repair proteins at the biopsy stage can predict tumor response in patients with locoregionally-advanced HNSCC undergoing induction chemotherapy prior to definitive chemoradiation. Our study shows that XPF is highly variable among head and neck cancers with a wide dynamic range: Low levels of expression of XPF correlate with better response to induction chemoradiotherapy, while high levels of XPF expression are associated with a worse response. Furthermore, pMK2, a kinase that has been reported to be critical for post-transcriptional regulation of gene expression as part of DNA damage response [27], is significantly associated with overall survival after induction plus chemoradiation therapy. Our results indicate that the analysis of change in DNA repair pathways may be clinically valuable in HNC.

Materials and Methods

Patient cohorts

Biopsy specimens (formalin-fixed, paraffin embedded tumor samples) from 37 patients with stage IV locoregionally-advanced HNSCC treated at the University of Chicago were evaluated from whole sections. The HNSCC patient biopsies had been obtained from a primary excision or biopsy prior to therapy. Written informed consent was obtained from all donors or the next of kin for the use of these samples in research approved under University of Chicago IRB protocol 8980 and 15410A. All patients had been treated with induction chemotherapy consisting of two cycles of paclitaxel and carboplatin for a total of eight weeks. We subsequently performed an interim assessment, followed by

paclitaxel, 5-fluorouracil, hydroxyurea and radiotherapy-based regimens (FHX) based chemoradiotherapy and finally we evaluated for response [28,29]. We analyzed the patient samples regarding their HPV-status by staining for p16 (Santa Cruz JC-8).

Treatment evaluation

Response evaluation was performed in the interval between induction chemotherapy and consecutive chemoradiotherapy by CT scan and/or clinical examination by an ENT specialist and best response was assessed. Response criteria were defined as complete response (CR) [14], progressive response (PR) and stable disease (SD) based on RECIST criteria [6,30].

Cell lines

The simian virus 40-transformed fibroblasts GM08437 (XPF−/−, Coriell Institute) cells and HeLa cells were grown in Dulbecco's modified Eagle's medium supplemented with 10% heat-inactivated fetal calf serum (FCS) in a humidified 5% CO_2 incubator at 37°C.

Immunohistochemistry (IHC)

The whole sections of the samples were stained by IHC using antibodies against XPF (SPM228)/ERCC1 (8F1) (AbCam), FANCD2 (Santa Cruz), PAR, γH2AX (Millipore), MLH1 (AbSerotec) and phospho-MAPKAP Kinase2 (pMK2) (Cell Signaling Technology). Tissue sections were deparaffinized/rehydrated using standard techniques. Heat-induced epitope retrieval was performed and the tissues were stained with antibodies overnight at 4°C. Primary antibodies were omitted for negative controls. Hematoxylin was used as nuclear counter-stain. Two-fold antibody dilution ranges were established, and antigen retrieval conditions were set such that antibody was in excess and discriminated between control cancer tissues and between low and high expression levels. Renaissance TSATM (Tyramide Signal Amplification) Biotin System (Perkin Elmer) was used for detection of XPF and FANCD2. Super Sensitive TM IHC Detection System (BioGenex) was used for detection of PAR, PARP1, MLH1, pMK2, γH2AX and ERCC1.

IHC Scoring

The IHC stained tissues on the slides were scanned into a digital pathology platform (Aperio). Quality of staining pattern was pathology reviewed. Intensity of nuclear staining, and/or localization of the marker into both nuclear and cytoplasmic compartments was determined. Three tumor regions of interest in a whole section were selected by pathologists in order to minimize the effects of IHC staining variation. Scanned slides were then evaluated by pathologists and machine-based digital image analysis (Aperio). The percentage (0–100%) of tumor cells with positive staining Quantity (Q) and intensity (I) for each marker were independently scored by two trained pathologists (VVB, SF), who were blinded from clinical history. A nuclear score was reported for XPF, ERCC1, FANCD2, MLH1, PARP1, PAR and γH2AX. The nuclear and cytoplasmic compartments were scored separately for pMK2. Staining quantity (Q) was scored 0 to 4: no nuclear staining $= 0$; 1–9% of cells with nuclear stain $= 1$; 10–39% $= 2$; 40–69% $= 3$; and 70–100% $= 4$. Staining intensity (I) was classified from 0 to 3, with $0 =$ negative, $1+ =$ weak, $2+ =$ intermediate, $3+ =$ strong. Final scores were obtained by multiplying the quantity and staining intensity scores (IxQ) [31]. Machine-based image analyses were established based on modified macros of the Aperio IHC nuclear algorithm to score the intensity/quantity of positive tumor nuclei. Marker outputs in 0,

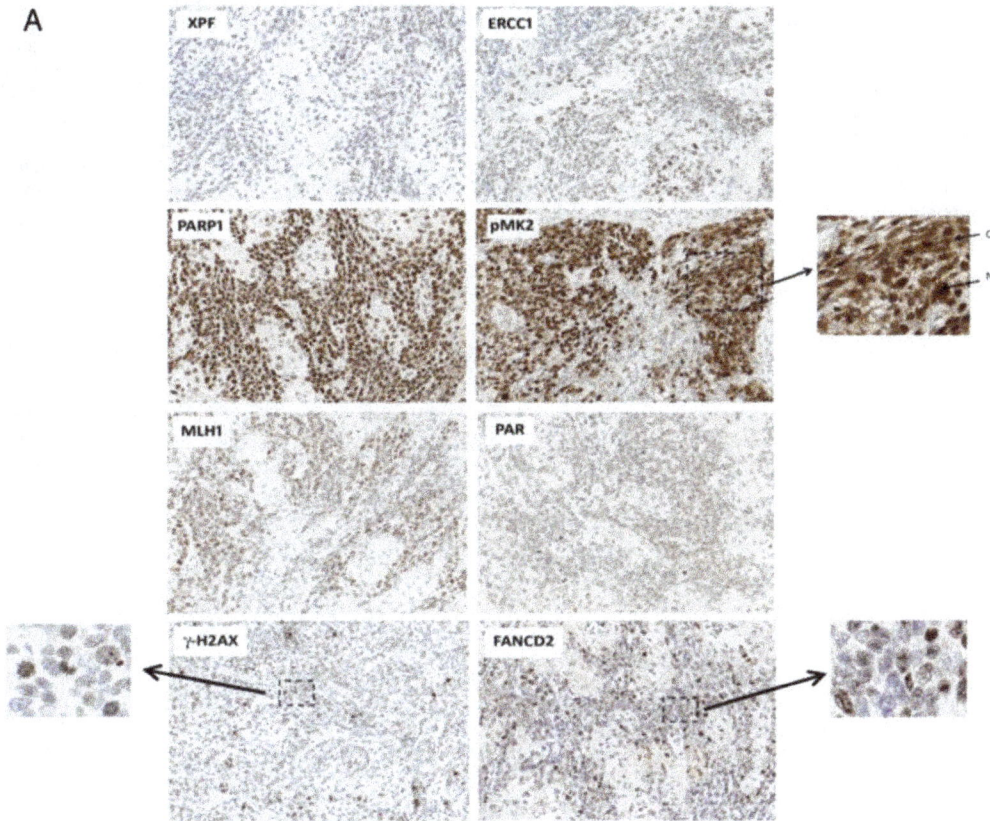

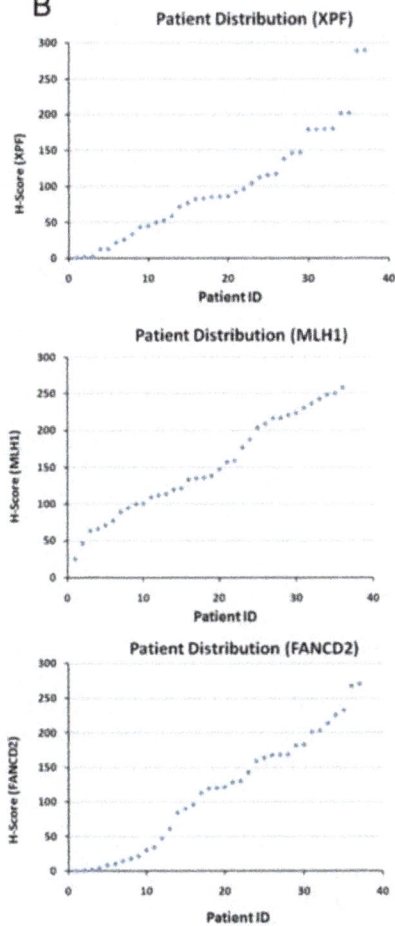

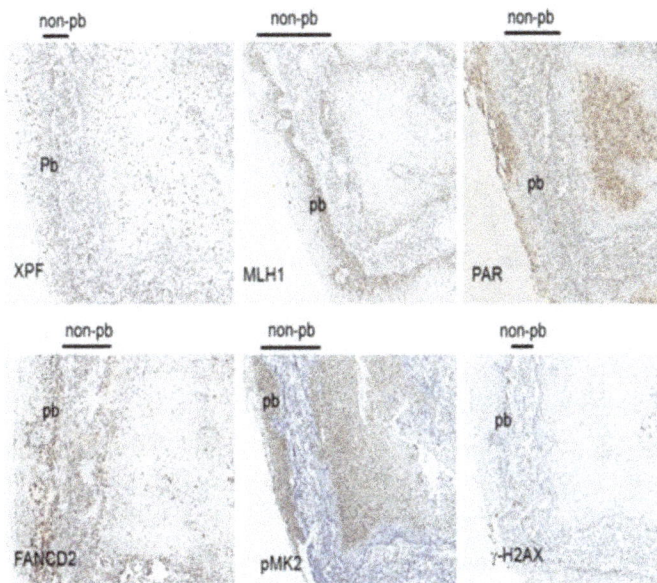

Figure 1. Immunohistochemistry (IHC) staining pattern of the DNA repair biomarkers. A. The FFPE whole sections from 37 HNSCC patient samples were stained by IHC using the antibodies against DNA repair biomarkers (XPF, ERCC1, FANCD2, MLH1, pMK2, PAR, PARP1) according to the protocol described in *Materials and Methods*. The stained tissue on the slide was scanned into a digital pathology platform (Aperio) and images were viewed digitally, magnification 10X. As noted, subcellular localization of pMK2 is in either Nuclear (N), or Nuclear (N) + Cytoplasmic (C), staining patterns of pMK2 in these cancer tissues are shown as indicated, magnification 20X. Nuclear foci in head neck cancer cells were shown for γH2AX and FANCD2 in the lower panel as indicated, magnification 40X. B. Examples of varying biomarker expression in head and neck cancer tissue specimens stained with XPF, FANCD2, MLH1 are shown. Patient distribution of XPF, FANCD2, MLH1 scores are plotted. C. Differences in the staining intensity and distribution of XPF (NER), MLH1 (MMR), PAR (BER), FANCD2 (FA/HR), pMK2 and γH2AX (DDR) in parabasal (pb) and nonparabasal (non-pb) layer cells from specimens of one representative HNSCC patient were shown as indicated.

1+, 2+, and 3+ bins were combined in a weighting algorithm to create a relative intensity score (H-score) from 0–300 [32].

Immunoblotting

Immunoblotting for XPF, ERCC1, and β-Actin was done using standard methodology as previously described [33–37]. Antibodies used for immunoblotting were anti-XPF (SPM228, AbCam), anti-ERCC1 (8F1, AbCam/Santa Cruz), and anti-β-Actin (H-170, Santa Cruz). Nine head and neck cancer cell lines (SCC58, SCC61, SCC35, SCC28, SQ20B, SCC9, HN5, SCC68, SCC25), kindly provided by Dr. Ralph Weichselbaum and Dr. Mark Lingen, were used.

Statistical Analysis

Biomarker scoring was correlated with clinical data to assess for correlation with outcome. A set of optimal threshold marker values was determined by univariate analysis for each marker that yielded

Figure 2. Association of XPF scoring by pathologist scores versus machine assisted image analysis and quantitation. Comparisons are made between alternative scoring strategies for immunohistochemistry with the XPF for each head and neck cancer patient. Machine assisted scoring for XPF was determined based on percentage of nuclei with 1+ (weak), 2+ (medium), 3+ (high) intensity Pathologist scores were Intensity (I). Correlation plots as shown are computed for similarity with an R-value of 0.79.

the highest discrimination to separate Complete response (CR), Partial Response (PR), Stable Disease (SD) groups for induction chemotherapy and overall survival. Multivariate analysis was not feasible due to the small sample number. Univariate Cox proportional hazards models were constructed for each of the markers (single marker models) to examine their potential predictive powers. Discriminant and partition analysis was also conducted to maximally separate the dataset samples into groups.

Statistical outputs for p-value (Positive predictive value), Apparent Error Rate (AER), Receiver Operator Characteristics (ROC) and Area Under Curve (AUC). ROC is a graphical plot of the sensitivity vs. (1-specificity) for a binary classifier system as its discrimination of true positives, in this case, it is 1-specificity (fraction of CR/PR called SD/PD) versus sensitivity (fraction of SD/PD called SD/PD). AUC is a measure of how well two classes of data separate under a testing scheme. Sensitivity, Specificity, Positive Predictive Power, Negative Predictive Power, Relative Risk (RR) and Odds Ratio were computed in the alternative models.

To assess the association of the biomarker scores to overall patient survival, thresholds for each biomarker were determined, which separated patients into two groups. These thresholds were selected by choosing the biomarker value that generated the minimum survival curve p-value when patients with scores above the threshold were compared to patients below the threshold. Thresholds that created a minimum group size of less than 10% of all samples were not considered reliable and excluded from analysis.

Survival curves for the low- and high-risk groups were compared using Kaplan-Meier models and the p-value reported. Additionally, the AER, AUC, ROC curve, sensitivity, specificity, positive predictive value, negative predictive value, and relative risk are reported.

Results

Significant variations of DNA repair proteins expression in multiple DNA repair pathways in head and neck cancer

DNA repair pathways are important for the cellular response to chemotherapy and radiation. Eight selected DNA repair proteins in five major DNA repair pathways were evaluated by IHC in a cohort of 37 patients; an IHC staining example for each biomarker is shown in Figure 1A. Pathologists' scores and machine-based assessment of IHC staining intensities in annotated tumor zones were used to evaluate protein expression differences among patient samples. Expression of DNA repair proteins varies between tumor specimens as shown graphically in the patient distribution for the markers (Figure 1B). Subcellular localization of pMK2 varies between nuclear only, or nuclear + cytoplasmic localization depending on the patient tumor. Several biomarkers such as FANCD2 and γH2AX proteins have a distinct pattern in the nucleus indicative of activation of the FA/Homologous recombination (HR) or DNA Damage Response (DDR) pathway (Figure 1A) in these HNSCC tumors. Biomarkers in different

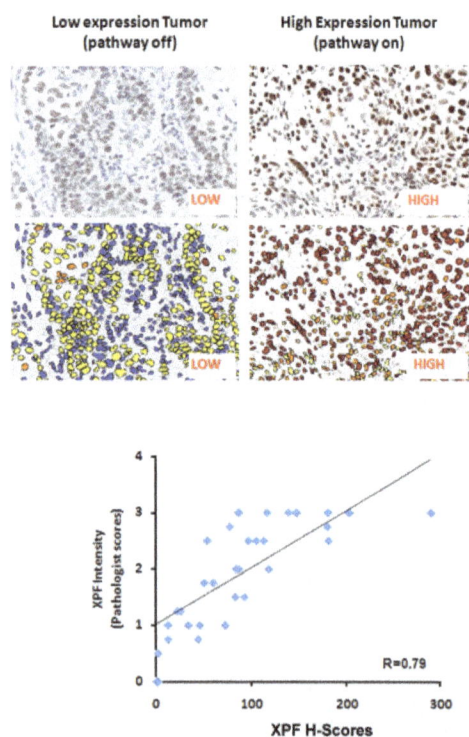

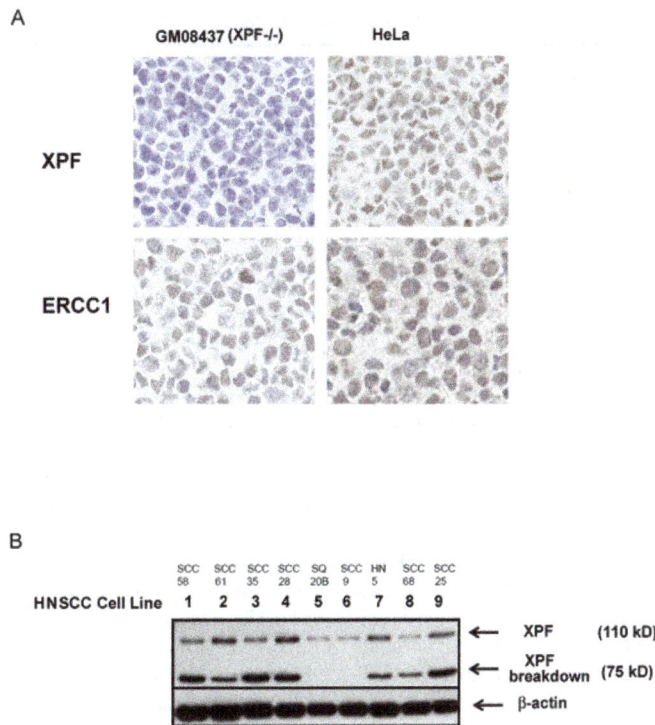

Figure 3. Immunohistochemistry (IHC) staining pattern of XPF and ERCC1 by using anti-XPF (SPM228) and ERCC1 (8F1) antibodies and XPF expression in HNSCC cell lines. A. FFPE blocks of HeLa and GM08437 (XPF deficient cell) pellets were used as negative and positive controls, XPF (SPM228) and ERCC1 (8F1) antibodies were then applied to the sections by immunohistochemistry according to the IHC method for tumor, and nuclear staining patterns of XPF and ERCC1 were shown. B. Nine head and neck cancer cell lines were analyzed by immunoblotting for expression of XPF. XPF and XPF breakdown proteins were detected by an anti-XPF monoclonal antibody (SPM228) with cell lines 5 and 6 showing low expression. β-Actin (Santa Cruz) was used as a protein loading control. The names of the cell lines are listed.

DNA repair pathways such as XPF (NER), MLH1 (MMR), PAR (BER), FANCD2 (FA/HR), pMK2 and γH2AX (DDR) were found to have differences in the nuclear or cytoplasmic staining intensity and distribution between parabasal (pb) and non-parabasal (non-pb) layer cells for certain specimens, suggestive of a variable expression of these DNA repair biomarkers (Figure 1C).

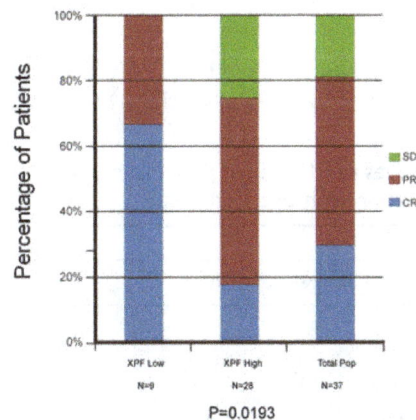

Figure 4. Univariate analysis of XPF biomarker scores shows improved response prediction to induction chemotherapy in head and neck cancer. The chart shows that univariate analysis of the XPF biomarker scores relative to the discrimination between Responder subgroups. The primary outcome measurement was response to induction chemotherapy.

An example shown here is the nuclear staining pattern of NER biomarker XPF in two representative cancers by IHC. Low or negative intensity of XPF nuclear staining indicates that NER pathway is off, and high intensity of XPF staining indicates that NER pathway is on (Figure 2). To test the correlations between pathologist scores, machine-guided and image analysis, we compared IHC stained XPF, which were analyzed by two pathologists, who were blinded to tumor samples, and machine-based algorithm in this study (Figure 2) with R2 value of 0.79.

Highly variable XPF expression in head and neck cancer

In our study, we determined specificity of the XPF (SPM228) and ERCC1 (8F1) antibodies by IHC using formalin fixed, paraffin-embedded blocks of HeLa (positive control) and XPF deficient cell pellets. Other XPF and ERCC1 antibodies were evaluated (data not shown/proprietary). SPM228 was chosen due to high degree of specificity, and 8F1 chosen as it is the most widely used ERCC1 antibody. Our result showed that specific nuclear staining by a monoclonal antibody against XPF (SPM228) was detected in HeLa cells but not in XPF deficient cells, in contrast, nuclear staining by the ERCC1 8F1 antibody was found in both HeLa and XPF deficient cells, indicating that this SPM228 antibody is XPF specific and suitable for detection of XPF by IHC, and ERCC1 8F1 recognizes additional non-specific nuclear proteins and is unable to specifically detect ERCC1 in specimens (Figure 3A).

We evaluated XPF expression in both, p16(+) and p16(−) samples and did not detect a significant difference (178 versus 165, NS).

Table 1. List of DNA repair proteins in univariate analysis of the correlation with response to induction chemotherapy.

Biomarker	ROC plot/AUC value	% Correct Responders at 100% SD/PD Correct	P value (CR/PR vs SD)
XPF	0.783	60	0.0193
ERCC1	0.569	7	0.41
pMK2	0.707	47	0.266
MLH 1	0.545	23	0.616
PARP 1	0.571	20	0.918
PAR	0.509	17	0.872
FANCD2	0.571	13	0.952
γ-H2AX	0.519	N/A	0.629

Higher AUC value means better correlations with response to induction chemotherapy. P values of CR/PR versus SD are shown.

We then measured the level of XPF expression in lysates of nine HNSCC cell lines by immunoblot. Two bands of XPF at 110 kD and 75 kD were found consistently, with the 75 kD band recognizing full length XPF and the other band representing a cleavage product of XPF (XPF breakdown) (Figure 3B). We also found that levels of expression of XPF dramatically vary among nine HNSCC cell lines (Figure 3B). A wide dynamic range of XPF expression in the cohort in our study is also shown in a patient distribution plot (Figure 1B). Taken together, our results demonstrate that levels of XPF expression detected by the SPM228 antibody vary significantly in head and neck cell lines and patient specimens, and that the monoclonal antibody SPM228 can be used to specifically detect XPF expression by Western blot and IHC.

XPF is associated with response to induction chemotherapy for head and neck cancer patients

Eight DNA repair biomarkers stained on 37 patient specimens by IHC were analyzed for their ability to predict response to induction chemotherapy. Of the 37 HNC patients treated with induction chemotherapy in the study, complete response (CR) [14] was observed in 11 patients (29.7%), 19 patients (51.4%) obtained a partial response (PR), and seven patients (18.9%) had a stable disease (SD). We found that low levels of XPF expression in HNC patients were significantly associated with better response to induction chemotherapy (p = 0.02) (Figure 4). Moreover, all of

seven patients who had SD had high levels of XPF expression (Figure 3, Table 1). In contrast, ERCC1 detected by the commonly used antibody (clone 8F1) in our cohort set did not correlate with response, and other markers such as PARP1, PAR, MLH1, pMK2, γH2AX, FANCD2, also failed to correlate (Table 1). Our results suggest that XPF is the preferred NER biomarker to predict response to induction chemotherapy in HNSCC patients.

pMK2 correlates with overall survival to chemoradiation therapy

We then evaluated association of the DNA repair biomarkers to overall survival for this cohort of patients. pMK2 did not correlate with response to induction chemotherapy (Table 1), but it correlated strongly with overall survival: low pMK2 expression was associated with better overall survival (p = 0.01) (Figure 5); pMK2 differentiated a subgroup with improved survival potentially related to chemoradiation therapy, suggesting that pMK2 may relate to chemoradiation therapy. In contrast, XPF was found not to correlate with overall survival (p = 0.08). For several other markers in DNA repair such as PARP1, PAR, MLH1, γH2AX, ERCC1, FANCD2, the same analysis failed to reach statistical significance (Table 2). Further study of pMK2 is needed.

Discussion

Chemotherapy induces DNA-damage in tumor cells. Therefore the ability to repair such damage using specific DNA repair

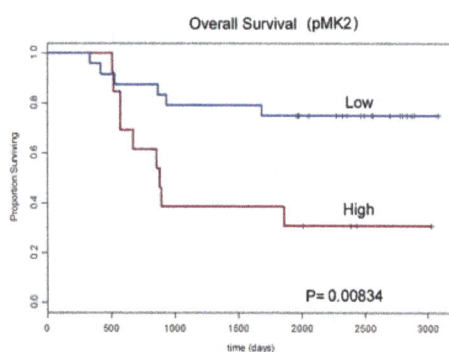

Figure 5. Correlation of expression levels of pMK2 with overall survival. Overall survival estimated by best response to induction chemotherapy using Kaplan-Meier survival curves based on the nuclear staining intensity and quantitation of pMK2 determined by pathologists' scores as NQ (Nuclear Quantity).

Table 2. List of p values of DNA repair proteins in univariate analysis of the correlation with overall survival.

Biomarker	P value (Overall survival)
XPF	0.0791
ERCC1	0.0873
pMK2	0.00834
MLH 1	0.0474
PARP 1	0.200
PAR	0.141
FANCD2	0.0357
γ-H2AX	0.266

pathways is likely predictive of drug sensitivity/resistance, and treatment outcome. Thus, diagnostic DNA repair biomarkers hold potential to significantly change diagnostic strategies and affect therapeutic decision-making and treatment planning for patients with head and neck cancer. In our study, we evaluated eight DNA repair biomarkers in five different DNA repair pathways by immunohistochemistry in locoregionally-advanced head and neck cancer. Significant variations in multiple DNA repair pathways were observed in HNSCC tumors suggesting that clinical decisions may be influenced by a DNA repair biomarker profile (Figures 1, 2). Among all of the DNA repair biomarkers that we analyzed, XPF was the single best marker to predict response to induction chemotherapy by univariate analysis; low levels of expression of XPF in head and neck cancer patients were associated with better response to induction chemotherapy. High levels of XPF expression in head and neck patients correlated with worse response to platinum based chemotherapy consistent with prior reports [38]. By contrast ERCC1 (8F1), detected by the commonly used antibody (clone 8F1), in our cohort set did not correlate with response, which may relate to its poorer specificity (Figures 3 and 4, Table 1). ERCC1 (8F1) performance was not adequate in our study and we hypothesize that the decreased specificity can be compensated by larger sample sizes as seen in other studies [18–20]. Furthermore it is possible that the ERCC1 8F1 measures something different than ERCC1, which correlates with survival.

While patient response to induction chemotherapy is a potential predictor of good overall outcome as reported by several groups [4,5,39–41], overall survival remains clinically most meaningful. pMK2 was found to correlate significantly (p = 0.01) with overall survival. Since pMK2 does not appear to relate to induction response it may be a potential marker of treatment success for concurrent chemoradiation (Figure 5, Table 2) consistent with preclinical data [42].

Given the heterogeneity of head and neck cancer, and the intricately connected network of six major DNA repair pathways, it is unreasonable to anticipate that meaningful diagnostic testing can rely on a single, specific marker. As our study suggests, markers for induction and chemoradiation are likely different. Furthermore, compensation of DNA repair in the absence of one repair pathway by another pathway suggests the possibility that multiple markers may be necessary to optimally assess responsiveness. Such a DNA repair response signature will have to be evaluated by our group, using a larger cohort and may allow improved assessment of HNC heterogeneity and complexities of DNA repair networks.

In conclusion, our study provides an established method to measure DNA repair biomarkers and other biomarkers using quantitative immunohistochemistry to identify and evaluate functional changes to DNA repair and damage signaling pathways as a valuable tool for personalized diagnostics. Our results indicate usefulness of XPF as a biomarker to predict which patients benefit from which treatments with induction chemotherapy. Specifically XPF proved superior to ERCC1 (8F1) testing. XPF may also have value to predict overall treatment success, which potentially relates to its role for prediction of induction response [25]. Furthermore, our results suggest that pMK2 is a potential marker for chemoradiation as it did not correlate with induction response, but did correlate strongly with overall survival. Further validation of these markers in a larger cohort of advanced head and neck cancer patients is imperative and our observations are largely hypothesis-forming at this point, but are consistent with other literature [38]. Ultimately, multiple markers may be necessary to optimally assess tumor specimens, and provide the most information to treating physicians.

Acknowledgments

Flight Attendant Medical Research Institute (FAMRI) YCSA (TYS), Cancer Research Foundation YIA (TYS), ASCO translational professorship award (EEV). We would like to thank Dr. Brian E. Ward for his continued support.

Author Contributions

Conceived and designed the experiments: EEV TS XW RRW DW. Performed the experiments: TS XW VVB K. Sprott SF EO MWL. Analyzed the data: MWL DTW DAF TS JH. Contributed reagents/materials/analysis tools: RRW MWL EEV EEC XW K. Stenson. Wrote the paper: TS JH.

References

1. Ferlay J, Shin H-R, Bray F, Forman D, Mathers C, et al. (2010) Estimates of worldwide burden of cancer in 2008: GLOBOCAN 2008. Int J Cancer 127: 2893–2917. Available: http://www.ncbi.nlm.nih.gov/pubmed/21351269. Accessed 2012 Oct 4.

2. Jemal A, Siegel R, Ward E, Hao Y, Xu J, et al. (n.d.) Cancer statistics, 2009. CA Cancer J Clin 59: 225–249. Available: http://www.ncbi.nlm.nih.gov/pubmed/19474385. Accessed 2012 Oct 25.

3. Seiwert TY, Salama JK, Vokes EE (2007) The chemoradiation paradigm in head and neck cancer. Nat Clin Pract Oncol 4: 156–171. Available: http://www.ncbi.nlm.nih.gov/pubmed/17327856. Accessed 2012 Oct 25.

4. Salama JK, Seiwert TY, Vokes EE (2007) Chemoradiotherapy for locally advanced head and neck cancer. J Clin Oncol 25: 4118–4126. Available: http://www.ncbi.nlm.nih.gov/pubmed/17827462. Accessed 2012 Oct 25.

5. Salama JK, Stenson KM, Kistner EO, Mittal BB, Argiris A, et al. (2008) Induction chemotherapy and concurrent chemoradiotherapy for locoregionally advanced head and neck cancer: a multi-institutional phase II trial investigating three radiotherapy dose levels. Ann Oncol 19: 1787–1794. Available: http://www.ncbi.nlm.nih.gov/pubmed/18539617. Accessed 2012 Oct 25.

6. Vokes EE, Kies MS, Haraf DJ, Stenson K, List M, et al. (2000) Concomitant chemoradiotherapy as primary therapy for locoregionally advanced head and neck cancer. J Clin Oncol 18: 1652–1661. Available: http://www.ncbi.nlm.nih.gov/pubmed/10764425. Accessed 2012 Oct 25.

7. Fakhry C, Westra WH, Li S, Cmelak A, Ridge JA, et al. (2008) Improved survival of patients with human papillomavirus-positive head and neck squamous cell carcinoma in a prospective clinical trial. J Natl Cancer Inst 100: 261–269. Available: http://www.ncbi.nlm.nih.gov/pubmed/18270337. Accessed 2012 Oct 25.

8. Haddad R, O'Neill A, Rabinowits G, Tishler R, Khuri F, et al. (2013) Induction chemotherapy followed by concurrent chemoradiotherapy (sequential chemoradiotherapy) versus concurrent chemoradiotherapy alone in locally advanced head and neck cancer (PARADIGM): a randomised phase 3 trial. Lancet Oncol 14: 257–264. Available: http://www.ncbi.nlm.nih.gov/pubmed/23414589. Accessed 2012 Oct 25.

9. Pignon JP, Bourhis J, Domenge C, Designé L (2000) Chemotherapy added to locoregional treatment for head and neck squamous-cell carcinoma: three meta-analyses of updated individual data. MACH-NC Collaborative Group. Meta-Analysis of Chemotherapy on Head and Neck Cancer. Lancet 355: 949–955. Available: http://www.ncbi.nlm.nih.gov/pubmed/10768432. Accessed 2012 Oct 25.

10. Alter BP, Joenje H, Oostra AB, Pals G (2005) Fanconi anemia: adult head and neck cancer and hematopoietic mosaicism. Arch Otolaryngol Head Neck Surg 131: 635–639. Available: http://www.ncbi.nlm.nih.gov/pubmed/16027289. Accessed 2012 Oct 25.

11. Van Waes C (2005) Head and neck squamous cell carcinoma in patients with Fanconi anemia. Arch Otolaryngol Head Neck Surg 131: 640–641. Available: http://www.ncbi.nlm.nih.gov/pubmed/16027290. Accessed 2012 Oct 25.

12. Rosenberg PS, Socié G, Alter BP, Gluckman E (2005) Risk of head and neck squamous cell cancer and death in patients with Fanconi anemia who did and did not receive transplants. Blood 105: 67–73. Available: http://www.ncbi.nlm.nih.gov/pubmed/15331448. Accessed 2012 Oct 25.

13. He Y, Chen Q, Li B (2008) ATM in oral carcinogenesis: association with clinicopathological features. J Cancer Res Clin Oncol 134: 1013–1020. Available: http://www.ncbi.nlm.nih.gov/pubmed/18288488. Accessed 2012 Oct 25.

14. Van Zeeburg HJT, Snijders PJF, Pals G, Hermsen MAJA, Rooimans MA, et al. (2005) Generation and molecular characterization of head and neck squamous cell lines of fanconi anemia patients. Cancer Res 65: 1271–1276. Available: http://www.ncbi.nlm.nih.gov/pubmed/15735012. Accessed 2012 Oct 25.

15. Berkower AS, Biller HF (1988) Head and neck cancer associated with Bloom's syndrome. Laryngoscope 98: 746–748. Available: http://www.ncbi.nlm.nih.gov/pubmed/3290604. Accessed 2012 Oct 25.

16. Iguchi H, Takayama M, Kusuki M, Sunami K, Nakamura A, et al. (2004) A possible case of Werner syndrome presenting with multiple cancers. Acta Otolaryngol Suppl: 67–70. Available: http://www.ncbi.nlm.nih.gov/pubmed/15513515. Accessed 2012 Oct 25.

17. Friedlander PL (2001) Genomic instability in head and neck cancer patients. Head Neck 23: 683–691. Available: http://www.ncbi.nlm.nih.gov/pubmed/11443752. Accessed 2012 Oct 25.

18. Olaussen KA, Dunant A, Fouret P, Brambilla E, André F, et al. (2006) DNA repair by ERCC1 in non-small-cell lung cancer and cisplatin-based adjuvant chemotherapy. N Engl J Med 355: 983–991. Available: http://www.ncbi.nlm.nih.gov/pubmed/16957145. Accessed 2012 Oct 25.

19. Jun HJ, Ahn MJ, Kim HS, Yi SY, Han J, et al. (2008) ERCC1 expression as a predictive marker of squamous cell carcinoma of the head and neck treated with cisplatin-based concurrent chemoradiation. Br J Cancer 99: 167–172. Available: http://www.pubmedcentral.nih.gov/articlerender.fcgi?artid = 2453006&tool = pmcentrez&rendertype = abstract. Accessed 2012 Oct 25.

20. Kang S, Ju W, Kim JW, Park NH, Song YS, et al. (2006) Association between excision repair cross-complementation group 1 polymorphism and clinical outcome of platinum-based chemotherapy in patients with epithelial ovarian cancer. Exp Mol Med 38: 320–324. Available: http://www.ncbi.nlm.nih.gov/pubmed/16819291. Accessed 2012 Oct 25.

21. McNeil EM, Melton DW (2012) DNA repair endonuclease ERCC1-XPF as a novel therapeutic target to overcome chemoresistance in cancer therapy. Nucleic Acids Res: 1–15. Available: http://www.ncbi.nlm.nih.gov/pubmed/22941649. Accessed 2012 Oct 25.

22. Biggerstaff M, Szymkowski DE, Wood RD (1993) Co-correction of the ERCC1, ERCC4 and xeroderma pigmentosum group F DNA repair defects in vitro. EMBO J 12: 3685–3692. Available: http://www.pubmedcentral.nih.gov/articlerender.fcgi?artid = 413645&tool = pmcentrez&rendertype = abstract. Accessed 2012 Oct 25.

23. Niedernhofer LJ, Bhagwat N, Wood RD (2007) ERCC1 and non-small-cell lung cancer. N Engl J Med 356: 2538–40; author reply 2540–1. Available: http://www.ncbi.nlm.nih.gov/pubmed/17568038. Accessed 2012 Oct 25.

24. Bhagwat NR, Roginskaya VY, Acquafondata MB, Dhir R, Wood RD, et al. (2009) Immunodetection of DNA repair endonuclease ERCC1-XPF in human tissue. Cancer Res 69: 6831–6838. Available: http://www.pubmedcentral.nih.gov/articlerender.fcgi?artid = 2739111&tool = pmcentrez&rendertype = abstract. Accessed 2012 Oct 25.

25. Köberle B, Ditz C, Kausch I, Wollenberg B, Ferris RL, et al. (2010) Metastases of squamous cell carcinoma of the head and neck show increased levels of nucleotide excision repair protein XPF in vivo that correlate with increased chemoresistance ex vivo: 1277–1284. doi:10.3892/ijo

26. Chiu T-J, Chen C-H, Chien C-Y, Li S-H, Tsai H-T, et al. (2011) High ERCC1 expression predicts cisplatin-based chemotherapy resistance and poor outcome in unresectable squamous cell carcinoma of head and neck in a betel-chewing area. J Transl Med 9: 31. Available: http://www.pubmedcentral.nih.gov/articlerender.fcgi?artid = 3072326&tool = pmcentrez&rendertype = abstract. Accessed 2012 Oct 25.

27. Vugt MATM Van, Wang X, Linding R, Ong S, Weaver D, et al. (2011) NIH Public Access. 40: 34–49. doi:10.1016/j.molcel.2010.09.018.DNA

28. Haraf DJ, Rosen FR, Stenson K, Argiris A, Mittal BB, et al. (2003) Induction chemotherapy followed by concomitant TFHX chemoradiotherapy with reduced dose radiation in advanced head and neck cancer. Clin Cancer Res 9: 5936–5943. Available: http://www.ncbi.nlm.nih.gov/pubmed/14676118. Accessed 2012 Oct 25.

29. Vokes EE, Stenson K, Rosen FR, Kies MS, Rademaker AW, et al. (2003) Weekly carboplatin and paclitaxel followed by concomitant paclitaxel, fluorouracil, and hydroxyurea chemoradiotherapy: curative and organ-preserving therapy for advanced head and neck cancer. J Clin Oncol 21: 320–326. Available: http://www.ncbi.nlm.nih.gov/pubmed/12525525. Accessed 2012 Oct 25.

30. Michiels S, Le Maître A, Buyse M, Burzykowski T, Maillard E, et al. (2009) Surrogate endpoints for overall survival in locally advanced head and neck cancer: meta-analyses of individual patient data. Lancet Oncol 10: 341–350. Available: http://www.ncbi.nlm.nih.gov/pubmed/19246242. Accessed 2012 Oct 25.

31. Nanni S, Benvenuti V, Grasselli A, Priolo C, Aiello A, et al. (2009) Endothelial NOS, estrogen receptor beta, and HIFs cooperate in the activation of a prognostic transcriptional pattern in aggressive human prostate cancer. J Clin Invest 119: 1093–1108. Available: http://www.pubmedcentral.nih.gov/articlerender.fcgi?artid = 2673846&tool = pmcentrez&rendertype = abstract. Accessed 2012 Oct 25.

32. Alexander BM, Sprott K, Farrow DA, Wang X, D'Andrea AD, et al. (2010) DNA repair protein biomarkers associated with time to recurrence in triple-negative breast cancer. Clin Cancer Res 16: 5796–5804. Available: http://www.ncbi.nlm.nih.gov/pubmed/21138871. Accessed 2012 Oct 25.

33. Ma PC, Kijima T, Maulik G, Fox EA, Sattler M, et al. (2003) c-MET mutational analysis in small cell lung cancer: novel juxtamembrane domain mutations regulating cytoskeletal functions. Cancer Res 63: 6272–6281. Available: http://www.ncbi.nlm.nih.gov/pubmed/14559814. Accessed 2012 Oct 25.

34. Jagadeeswaran R, Ma PC, Seiwert TY, Jagadeeswaran S, Zumba O, et al. (2006) Functional analysis of c-Met/hepatocyte growth factor pathway in malignant pleural mesothelioma. Cancer Res 66: 352–361. Available: http://www.ncbi.nlm.nih.gov/pubmed/16397249. Accessed 2012 Oct 25.

35. Jagadeeswaran R, Surawska H, Krishnaswamy S, Janamanchi V, Mackinnon AC, et al. (2008) Paxillin is a target for somatic mutations in lung cancer: implications for cell growth and invasion. Cancer Res 68: 132–142. Available: http://www.pubmedcentral.nih.gov/articlerender.fcgi?artid = 2767335&tool = pmcentrez&rendertype = abstract. Accessed 2012 Oct 25.

36. Ma PC, Jagadeeswaran R, Jagadeesh S, Tretiakova MS, Nallasura V, et al. (2005) Functional expression and mutations of c-Met and its therapeutic inhibition with SU11274 and small interfering RNA in non-small cell lung cancer. Cancer Res 65: 1479–1488. Available: http://www.ncbi.nlm.nih.gov/pubmed/15735036. Accessed 2012 Oct 25.

37. Seiwert TY, Jagadeeswaran R, Faoro L, Janamanchi V, Nallasura V, et al. (2009) The MET receptor tyrosine kinase is a potential novel therapeutic target for head and neck squamous cell carcinoma. Cancer Res 69: 3021–3031. Available: http://www.pubmedcentral.nih.gov/articlerender.fcgi?artid = 2871252&tool = pmcentrez&rendertype = abstract. Accessed 2012 Oct 25.

38. Vaezi A, Wang X, Buch S, Gooding W, Wang L, et al. (2011) XPF expression correlates with clinical outcome in squamous cell carcinoma of the head and neck. Clin Cancer Res 17: 5513–5522. Available: http://www.pubmedcentral.nih.gov/articlerender.fcgi?artid = 3156890&tool = pmcentrez&rendertype = abstract. Accessed 2014 March 12.

39. Haddad R, Tishler R, Wirth L, Norris CM, Goguen L, et al. (2006) Rate of pathologic complete responses to docetaxel, cisplatin, and fluorouracil induction chemotherapy in patients with squamous cell carcinoma of the head and neck. Arch Otolaryngol Head Neck Surg 132: 678–681. Available: http://www.ncbi.nlm.nih.gov/pubmed/16785415. Accessed 2012 Oct 25.

40. Dietz A, Rudat V, Dreyhaupt J, Pritsch M, Hoppe F, et al. (2009) Induction chemotherapy with paclitaxel and cisplatin followed by radiotherapy for larynx organ preservation in advanced laryngeal and hypopharyngeal cancer offers moderate late toxicity outcome (DeLOS-I-trial). Eur Arch Otorhinolaryngol 266: 1291–1300. Available: http://www.ncbi.nlm.nih.gov/pubmed/18972123. Accessed 2012 Oct 25.

41. Pointreau Y, Garaud P, Chapet S, Sire C, Tuchais C, et al. (2009) Randomized trial of induction chemotherapy with cisplatin and 5-fluorouracil with or without docetaxel for larynx preservation. J Natl Cancer Inst 101: 498–506. Available: http://www.ncbi.nlm.nih.gov/pubmed/19318632. Accessed 2012 Oct 25.

42. Reinhardt HC, Hasskamp P, Schmedding I, Morandell S, van Vugt MATM, et al. (2010) DNA damage activates a spatially distinct late cytoplasmic cell-cycle checkpoint network controlled by MK2-mediated RNA stabilization. Mol Cell 40: 34–49. Available: http://www.pubmedcentral.nih.gov/articlerender.fcgi?artid = 3030122&tool = pmcentrez&rendertype = abstract. Accessed 2014 Feb 20.

4

Relationship between P53 Status and Response to Chemotherapy in Patients with Gastric Cancer: A Meta-Analysis

Hai-Yuan Xu[1], Wen-Lin Xu[2], Li-Qiang Wang[1], Min-Bin Chen[1], Hui-Ling Shen[3]*

1 Department of Medical Oncology, Kunshan First People's Hospital Affiliated to Jiangsu University, Kunshan, People's Republic of China, 2 Department of Central Laboratory, Zhenjiang Fourth People's Hospital Affiliated to Jiangsu University, Zhenjiang, People's Republic of China, 3 Department of Medical Oncology, Zhenjiang First People's Hospital Affiliated to Jiangsu University, Zhenjiang, People's Republic of China

Abstract

Background: Previous studies have yielded conflicting results regarding the relationship between p53 status and response to chemotherapy in patients with gastric cancer. We therefore performed a meta-analysis to expound the relationship between p53 status and response to chemotherapy.

Methods/Findings: Thirteen previously published eligible studies, including 564 cases, were identified and included in this meta-analysis. p53 positive status (high expression of p53 protein and/or a mutant p53 gene) was associated with improved response in gastric cancer patients who received chemotherapy (good response: risk ratio [RR] = 0.704; 95% confidence intervals [CI] = 0.550–0.903; P = 0.006). In further stratified analyses, association with a good response remained in the East Asian population (RR = 0.657; 95% CI = 0.488–0.884; P = 0.005), while in the European subgroup, patients with p53 positive status tended to have a good response to chemotherapy, although this did not reach statistical significance (RR = 0.828, 95% CI = 0.525–1.305; P = 0.417). As five studies used neoadjuvant chemotherapy (NCT) and one used neoadjuvant chemoradiotherapy (NCRT), we also analyzed these data, and found that p53 positive status was associated with a good response in gastric cancer patients who received chemotherapy-based neoadjuvant treatment (RR = 0.675, 95% CI = 0.463–0.985; P = 0.042).

Conclusion: This meta-analysis indicated that p53 status may be a useful predictive biomarker for response to chemotherapy in gastric cancer. Further prospective studies with larger sample sizes and better study designs are required to confirm our findings.

Editor: Klaus Roemer, University of Saarland Medical School, Germany

Funding: This work was supported by the National Natural Science Foundation (No. 81101677,81070423). The funders had no role in study design, data collection and analysis, decision to publish, or preparation of the manuscript.

Competing Interests: The authors have declared that no competing interests exist.

* E-mail: shenhuiling0826@163.com

Introduction

It is estimated that gastric cancer is the fourth most common cancer in the world [1]. In 2013, an estimated 21,600 new cases will occur and 10,990 cases will eventually die of their disease in the United States [2]. Despite advances in surgical treatment and chemotherapy, prognosis remains poor, particularly as most tumors are diagnosed late and in locally advanced or advanced stages. Currently, due to the ability to shrink cancerous lesions to increase R0 resection rate, neoadjuvant chemotherapy is recommended as the standard treatment for the management of locally advanced gastric cancer [3]. Chemotherapy can also improve the outcome of unresectable gastric cancer. However, some studies suggest that only those patients who respond to neoadjuvant chemotherapy with tolerable toxicity will potentially benefit from this approach, while a proportion of patients fail to respond to neoadjuvant chemotherapy, or even progress during therapy [4–6]. Therefore, predictive markers to identify those patients who would benefit from neoadjuvant chemotherapy are being actively sought.

To date, p53, the most studied gene, may be the primary candidate biomarker for predicting the response of gastric cancer to chemotherapy [7]. The gene encoding p53 is located on chromosome 17p and consists of 11 exons and 10 introns. It has important cellular functions, including in cell cycle regulation, apoptosis, and DNA repair [8,9]. p53 is the gene most frequently mutated in human cancer, with alterations occurring in at least 50% of human malignancies, playing critical roles in their development [10]. Experimental evidence suggests that p53 status is associated with tumor response to genotoxic agents [11–13]. However, data regarding the use of p53 status as a biological marker to predict the response of gastric cancer to chemotherapy are inconclusive [14–19]. Some studies found that patients with p53 mutations or overexpression had higher response rates to chemotherapy than those with normal p53 status; however, other reports drew different conclusions. Therefore, we conducted a meta-analysis to determine the value of p53 status in predicting response to chemotherapy in gastric cancer.

Materials and Methods

Publication Search

Studies were identified by a computerized search of the PubMed, Embase, and Web of Science databases (up to Jun 8, 2013) using the following search terms: 'TP53', 'p53', 'p53 protein', 'p53 mutation', '17p13 gene', 'chemotherapy', 'chemoradiotherapy', and 'gastric cancer'. All potentially eligible studies were retrieved and their references were carefully researched to identify other eligible studies. When multiple studies of the same patient population were identified, the published report with the largest sample size was included.

Inclusion and Exclusion Criteria

Studies selected in this meta-analysis fulfilled all of the following criteria: (a) studies evaluating p53 status for predicting the response to chemotherapy or chemoradiotherapy in gastric cancer; (b) studies involving clinical or pathological therapeutic response; (c) retrospective or prospective cohort study; (d) studies including adequate data to allow the estimation of a risk ratio (RR) with 95% confidence intervals (95% CI); and (e) studies in English or Chinese. Reviews, letters to the editor, and articles published in books were excluded.

Data Extraction and Definitions

Using the inclusion criteria listed above, the following information was extracted from each study: the first author's surname, the publication year, the country of origin, the number of patients analyzed, the treatment, the methods of detection, p53 positive (overexpression or mutation) rate, the type of therapeutic response, the response criteria, and the main outcomes. This information was entered in tables showing the clinical or pathological response to chemotherapy with respect to p53 status. Data was carefully extracted from all eligible publications by two investigators. Any disagreement between the investigators was resolved by discussion until a consensus was reached. If they failed to reach an agreement, a third investigator was consulted to resolve the discrepancies.

As previously reported [20], the definitions and standardizations for 'p53' and 'response to therapy' used in our study followed those of the study by Pakos et al. [21]. For consistency, we used 'p53 status' to refer to both gene and protein markers. p53 positive status indicates patients with high expression of p53 protein and/ or mutations in the p53 gene. Good response was defined as complete response (CR) and partial response (PR), or grade 1b+2+3. Poor response was defined as stable disease (SD) and progress disease (PD), or grade 0+ 1a according to the guidelines for the clinical and pathologic studies on gastric carcinoma by the JRSGC (Japanese Research Society for Gastric Carcinoma), WHO (World Health Organization), or RECIST (Response Evaluation Criteria in Solid Tumors) criteria [22–25]. The response classification is detailed in Table 1.

Statistical Analysis

The software STATA version 12 (StataCorp, College Station, TX) was used to perform the data analysis. We assessed and quantified statistical heterogeneity for each pooled estimate using the I^2 statistic, and p>0.10 was defined as no heterogeneity. The pooled RR was calculated using a fixed-effects model (the Mantel–Haenszel method) or a random-effects model (the DerSimonian and Laird method), according to the heterogeneity results. Pooled analysis was performed using the Mantel-Haenszel model and reported as RR with 95% CIs. The significance of the pooled RR was determined by the z test and P<0.05 was considered statistically significant. χ^2 and z represented the test statistics of the I^2 statistic for heterogeneity and z test for the significance of the pooled RR respectively. The Begg's funnel plot and Egger's test were employed to estimate potential publication bias. We also performed sensitivity analysis by omitting each study or specific studies to find potential outliers.

Results

Eligible Studies

Using different combinations of key terms, a total of 240 articles were retrieved by a literature search of the PubMed, Embase, and Web of Science databases. As indicated in the search flow diagram (Figure 1), 13 studies were finally included in this meta-analysis [15–19,26–33]. The characteristics of the eligible studies are summarized in Table 2. Five used NCT, one used NCRT, and seven used CT (Table 2). The sample sizes in eligible studies ranged from 23–131 patients (median = 36, mean = 43, standard deviation [SD] = 28). Overall, the eligible studies included 564 patients. Five studies were conducted in European populations (167 patients) [15,16,27,28,31], whereas eight were in East Asian populations (397 patients) [17–19,26,29,30,32,33].

Relationship between p53 Status and Response to Chemotherapy in Gastric Cancer

Among the studies of gastric cancer patients who received chemotherapy, 13 (involving 564 patients) contributed data to the calculation of total OR (total OR = clinical OR + pathological OR). p53 positive status was significantly associated with improved total OR among patients treated with chemotherapy (RR = 0.704; 95% CI = 0.550–0.903; P = 0.006, Figure 2). With respect to studies reporting both clinical and pathological responses, the latter data was used, but the clinical response data was also examined with similar results (data not shown). p53 protein expression measured by immunohistochemistry (IHC) does not directly correspond to p53 mutation detected by gene sequencing [15,16]. As all studies included in this meta-analysis employed IHC-based protein detection, and only two employed both IHC and molecular genetic analysis, we adopted the data generated using IHC and also conducted statistical analysis for the molecular genetic data with similar results (RR = 0.720; 95% CI = 0.565–0.916; P = 0.008).

Subgroup Analysis

East Asian and European subgroups were also analyzed separately (Table 3). p53 positive status was associated with improved response in gastric cancer patients who received chemotherapy in the East Asian subgroup (RR = 0.657, 95% CI = 0.488–0.884; P = 0.005; Figure 3). In the European subgroup, however, patients with p53 positive status tended to have high response rates to chemotherapy, but the results did not reach statistical significance (RR = 0.828, 95% CI = 0.525–1.305; P = 0.417).

As five studies used NCT and one used NCRT, we also analyzed these data, and found that p53 positive status was associated with improved response in gastric cancer patients who received chemotherapy-based neoadjuvant treatment (RR = 0.675, 95% CI = 0.463–0.985, P = 0.042; Figure 4).

Table 1. Criteria for response evaluation and standard definitions.

Criteria	Poor response	Standard definition	Complete response
		Good response	
WHO[25]	NC+PD, <50% decrease in tumor load	PR+CR, >50% decrease in tumor load	CR, disappearance of all known disease
RECIST[24]	PD+SD, <30% disease regression	PR+CR, >30% disease regression	CR, 100% disease regression
JRSGC[22,23,34]	PD+SD, Grade 0+1,viable cancer cells account for more than 1/3	PR, Grade 2+3, viable cancer cells account for less than 1/3	CR, Grade 3, no residual viable tumor cells
Sirak et al.[27]	Inoperable tumor after NCRT	Reduction of at least one T-stage level and/or finding of intense tumor regression on histopathologic examination	pCR, absence of tumor cells in the primary site
Cascinu et al.[28]	NR	>50% reduction in the visible tumor or complete disappearance of tumor but positive histology on biopsy of the previously involved area	Complete resolution of the endoscopically visible tumor and a negative biopsy of the original site of the tumor.
Giatromanolaki et al.[31]	25–49% reduction in tumor size	50–95% reduction in tumor size	Disappearance of a measurable lesion

WHO, World Health Organization; RECIST, Response Evaluation Criteria in Solid Tumors; JRSGC, Japanese Research Society for Gastric Carcinoma; CR, complete response; PR, partial response; PD, progressive disease; SD, stable disease; NR, no record; NC, no change.

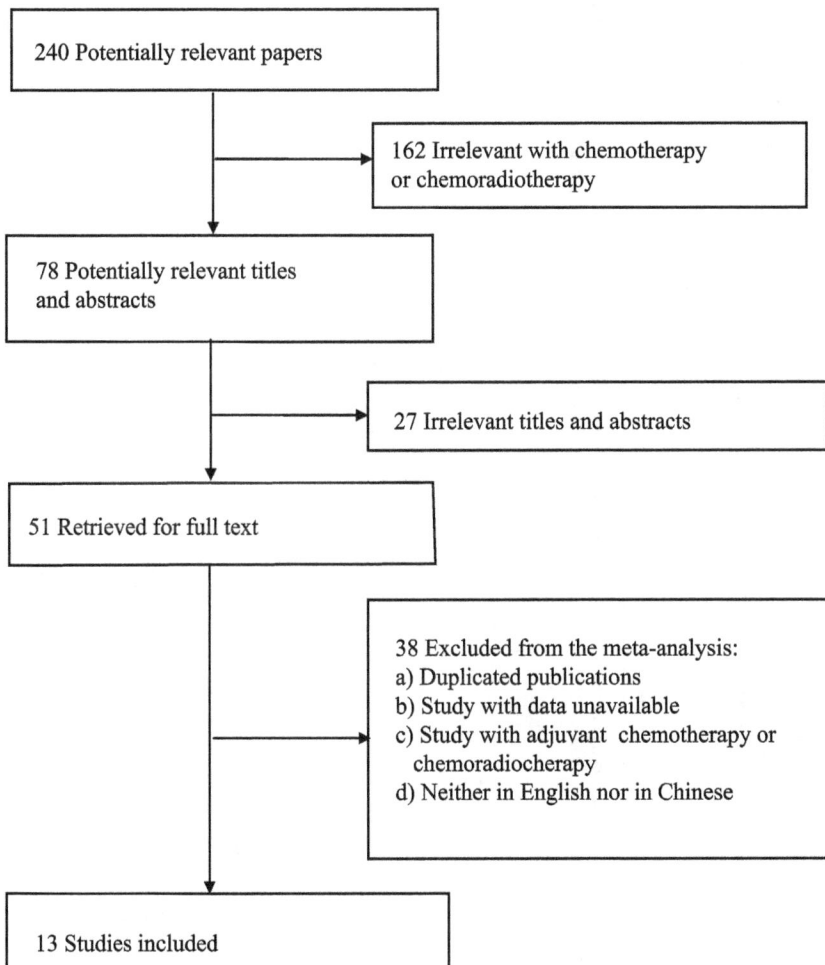

Figure 1. Flow diagram illustrating the screening and selection process.

Table 2. Characteristics of studies included in the meta-analysis.

Author	Year	Country	Cases	Treatment	Detection	p53 (%)	Response	Response criteria	Standard definition response			Response rate (%)	
									Poor response	Good response	Complete response	Good response	Complete response
Qu et al.[32]	2013	China	53	NCT	IHC	53%	clinical	RECIST	PD+SD	PR	CR	53%	0
Sirak et al. [27]	2009	Czech republic	36	NCRT	IHC	63%	pathologic	Sirak et al.	Inoperable	Down-staging	pCR	47%	22%
Kamoshida et al. [26]	2007	Japan	38	NCT	IHC	39%	pathologic	JRSGC	grade 0+1a	grade 1b+2	grade 3	34%	0
Boku et al. [17]	2007	Japan	131	CT	IHC	43%	clinical	WHO/JRSGC	PD+SD	PR+CR	NR	28%	NR
Nagashima et al. [18]	2005	Japan	55	CT	IHC	44%	clinical	WHO	PD+SD	PR+CR	NR	55%	NR
Bataille et al. [16]	2003	Germany	25	NCT	IHC/gene	56%	pathologic	JRSGC	grade 0+1	grade 2	grade 3	44%	28%
Ott et al. [15]	2003	Germany	48	NCT	IHC/gene	35%	clinical	WHO	PD+SD	PR	NR	40%	NR
Giatromanolaki et al. [31]	2001	Greece	28	CT	IHC	25%	clinical	Kamoshida et al.	MR	PR	CR	36%	NR
Kikuyama et al. [30]	2001	Japan	28	CT	IHC	46%	clinical	WHO/JRSGC	PD+SD	PR	CR	36%	4%
Yeh et al. [19]	1999	Taiwan	30	CT	IHC	20%	clinical	WHO	PD+SD	PR+CR	NR	50%	NR
Boku et al. [29]	1998	Japan	39	CT	IHC	38%	clinical	WHO/JRSGC	PD+NC	PR+CR	NR	33%	NR
Cascinu et al. [28]	1998	Italy	30	NCT	IHC	53%	clinical	Cascinu et al.	NR	PR	CR	40%	10%
Nakata et al. [33]	1998	Japan	23	CT	IHC	61%	clinical	JRSGC	PD+NC	PR	CR	43%	9%

CT, chemotherapy; NCT, neoadjuvant chemotherapy; NCRT, neoadjuvant chemoradiotherapy; IHC, immunohistochemistry; WHO, World Health Organization; RECIST, Response Evaluation Criteria in Solid Tumors; JRSGC, Japanese Research Society for Gastric Carcinoma; CR, complete response; PR, partial response; PD, progressive disease; SD, stable disease; NR, no record; NC, no change.

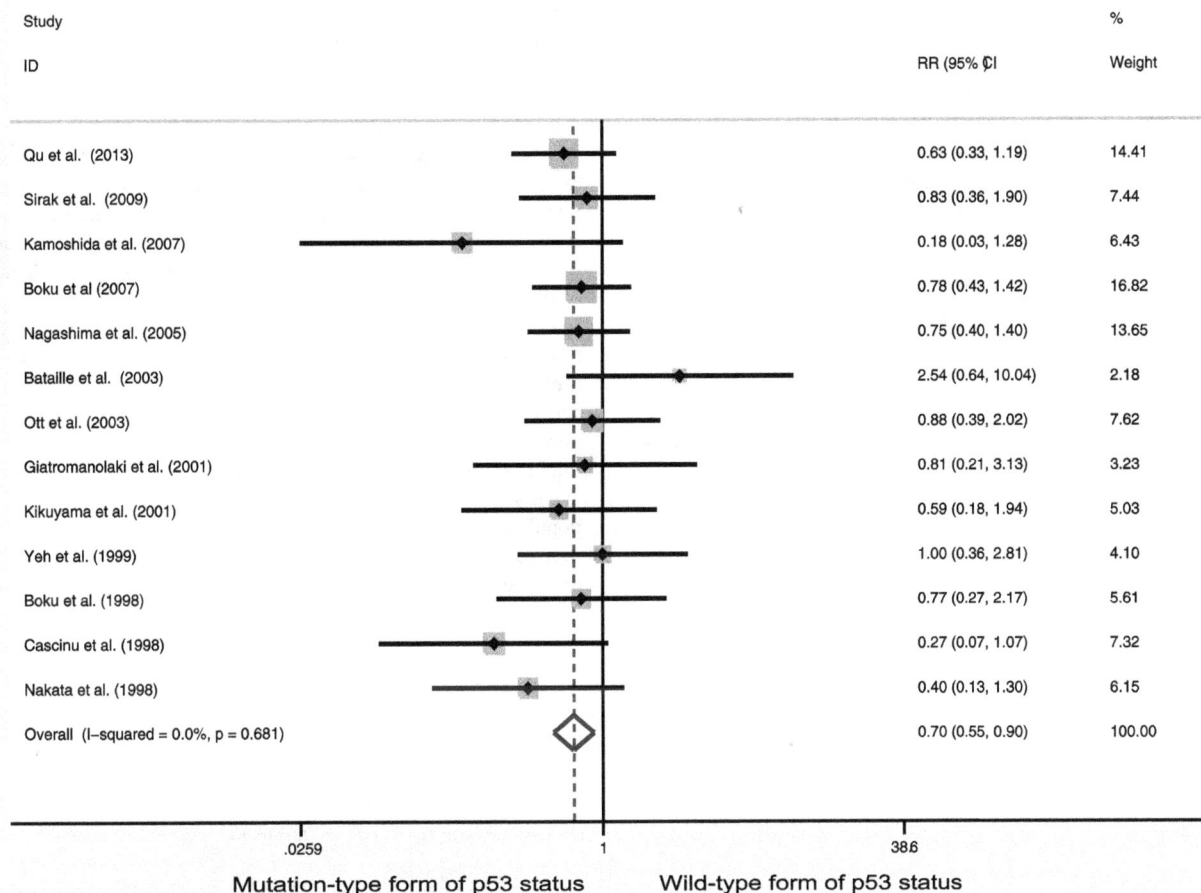

Figure 2. Forest plots of RR estimated for the relationship between p53 status and good response among gastric cancer patients treated with chemotherapy.

Publication Bias and Sensitivity Analysis

The Begg's funnel plot and Egger's test were employed to estimate the publication bias of the literature included in this study. The shape of the funnel plot showed no obvious evidence of asymmetry (Figure 5), and the Egger's test indicated an absence of publication bias (P>0.05). In addition, sensitivity analysis was conducted to assess the influence of individual studies on the summary effect. No individual study dominated this meta-analysis, and the removal of any single study had no significant effect on the overall results (data not shown).

Discussion

p53 status plays a key role in the response to many anticancer drugs. However, no consistent conclusion regarding the effect of p53 mutations on the sensitivity or resistance of gastric cancers to anticancer drugs has been reported. To date, the majority of available clinical reports involve small sample sizes, and were therefore unable to determine the value of p53 status for predicting the response to chemotherapy. Thus, we conducted a meta-analysis of 13 studies to systematically evaluate the association

between p53 status and response to chemotherapy in a large population with gastric cancer.

Our results show that p53 positive status may predict response to chemotherapy in patients with gastric cancer. p53 positive status was associated with improved total OR. Stratification according to ethnicity showed that p53 positive status was significantly associated with increased OR in East Asian populations. In addition, with respect to neoadjuvant chemotherapy, our results showed that p53 positive status was associated with good response.

Although we did our utmost to perform a comprehensive analysis, some limitations remain in this study. Firstly, the meta-analysis may have been influenced by publication bias, as we limited the literature search to studies performed in English or Chinese, and we did not explore conference proceedings or abstract books. Although we attempted to identify all relevant data, some missing data are inevitable. However, using statistical methods, no publication bias was detected, suggesting that the pooled results are likely to be unbiased. Second, in this meta-analysis we used data derived from IHC-based detection of p53, which was performed in all included studies. However, the reported frequencies of positive p53 staining were variable, which may reflect the use of different antibodies, staining standards,

Table 3. Risk ratio for the association between p53 positive status and good response to chemotherapy.

	N	RR (95% CI)	z	P	χ^2	Ph
All studies	13	0.704 (0.550–0.903)	2.77	0.006	9.25	0.681
Treatment						
CT	7	0.729 (0.525–1.013)	1.89	0.059	1.55	0.956
NCT	5	0.644 (0.422–0.985)	2.03	0.042	7.56	0.109
NCT+NCRT	6	0.675 (0.463–0.985)	2.04	0.042	7.73	0.172
Area						
East Asian	8	0.657 (0.488–0.884)	2.78	0.005	3.58	0.827
European	5	0.828 (0.525–1.305)	0.81	0.417	5.14	0.273
Type of measurement						
IHC	13	0.704 (0.550–0,903)	2.77	0.006	9.25	0.681
IHC + gene	11+2	0.720 (0.565–0.916)	2.67	0.008	9.91	0.624

Subgroup analysis was performed when at least five studies were in a subgroup.
N, number of studies; z, the test statistics of z test; P, p value of the z test; χ^2, the test statistics of I^2 statistic for heterogeneity; Ph, p value of the I^2 statistic.

criteria for positivity, and the inclusion of differently selected groups of gastric cancer patient groups. Third, the evaluation criterion of response to treatment among the studies was highly variable. Standardization is therefore of great importance for obtaining an accurate assessment of the clinical significance of p53 status. Despite our considerable efforts to standardize definitions, some variability among studies was inevitable. In addition, many other factors that could affect tumor sensitivity to treatment, such as tumor size, histological subtype, patient age, chemotherapy regimen, dose of chemotherapy or radiation, and courses of treatment, could not be obtained in sufficient detail for inclusion in statistical analyses. Fourth, as our analysis was observational in nature, we cannot exclude confounding as a potential explanation of the observed results.

Despite these limitations, this meta-analysis had several advantages. This is the first meta-analysis to evaluate the usefulness of p53 status for predicting the response of gastric cancer patients to chemotherapy. Also, as mentioned above, no publication bias was detected. The results showed that p53 status might be a useful predictive biomarker for evaluating response to chemotherapy in gastric cancer patients, especially in East Asian populations. However, future prospective studies with larger sample sizes, better study designs, and accurate detection methods are required to confirm our findings.

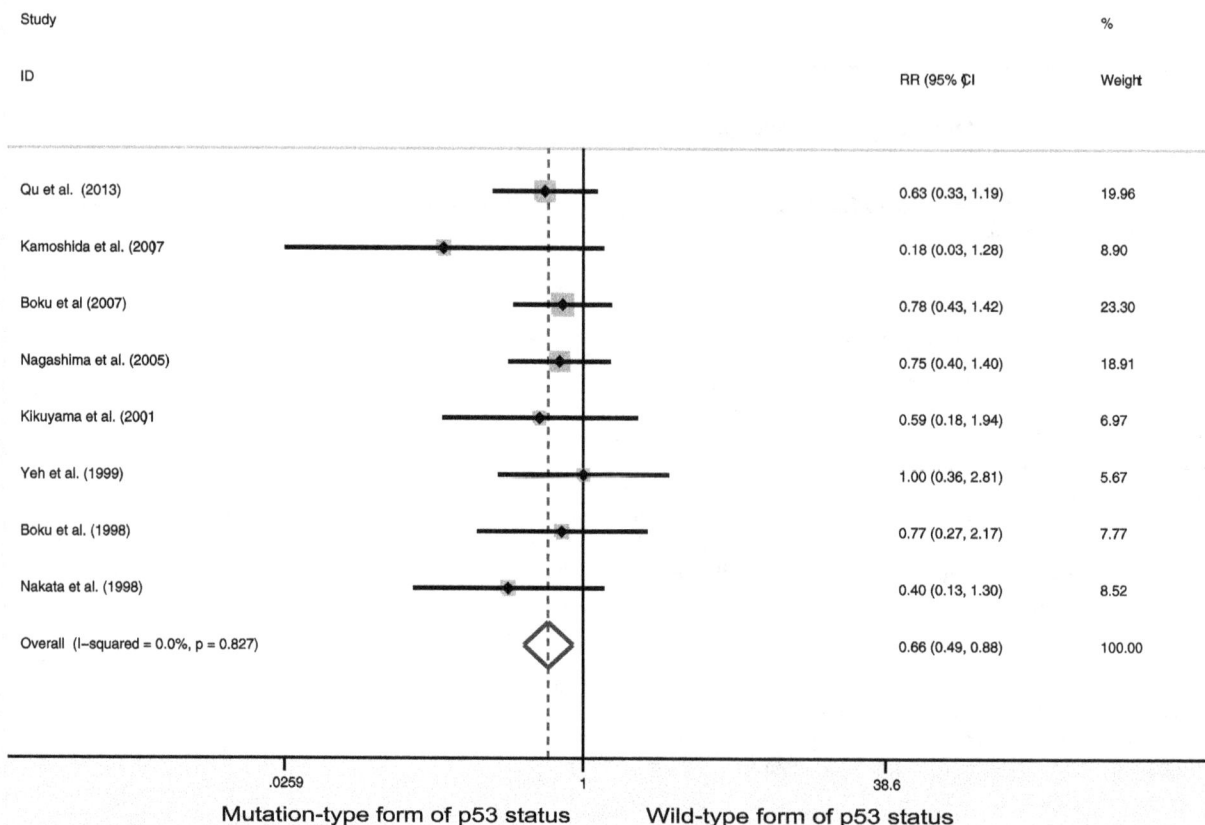

Figure 3. Forest plots of RR estimated for the relationship between p53 status and good response to chemotherapy in East Asian population with gastric cancer.

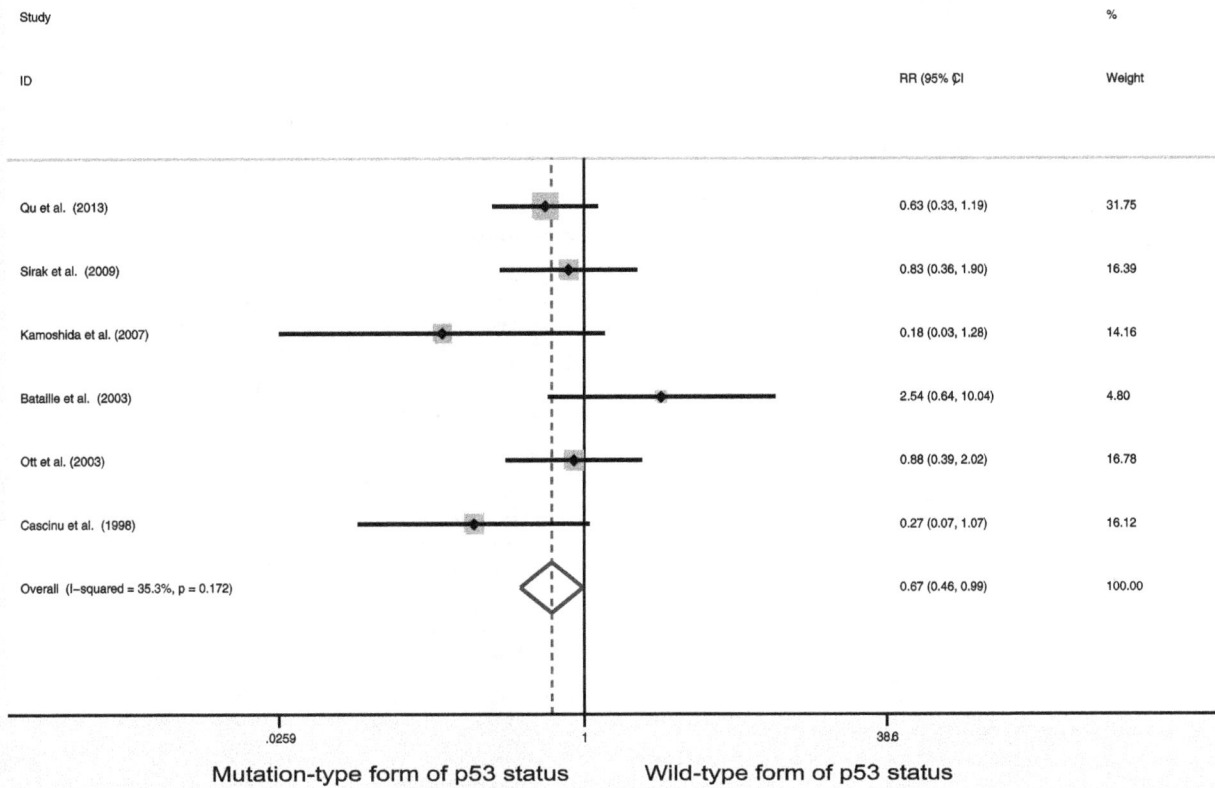

Figure 4. Forest plots of RR estimated for the relationship between p53 status and good response to chemotherapy-based neoadjuvant treatment in patients with gastric cancer.

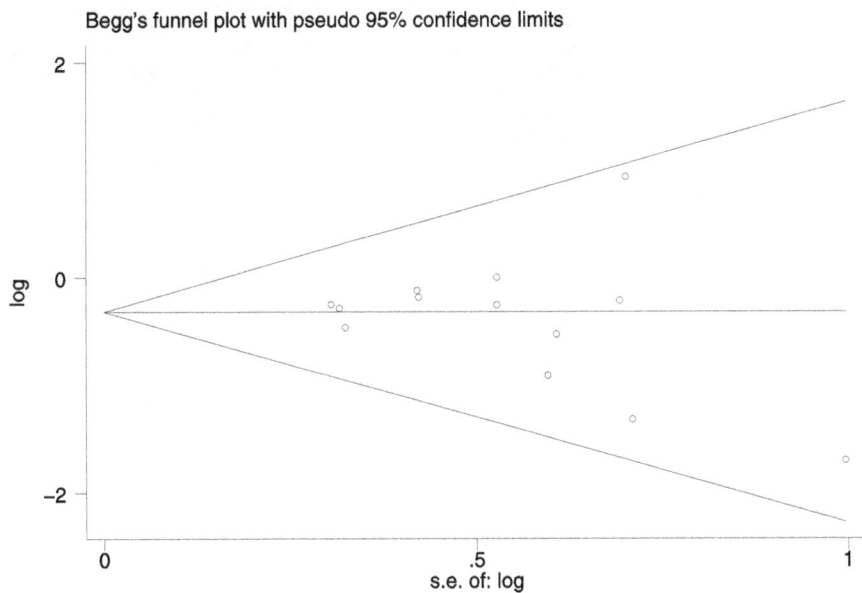

Figure 5. Funnel plot demonstrating that there was no obvious indication of publication bias for the outcome of good response.

Author Contributions

Conceived and designed the experiments: HYX MBC HLS. Performed the experiments: HYX MBC HLS. Analyzed the data: HYX WLX LQW. Contributed reagents/materials/analysis tools: MBC WLX. Wrote the paper: HYX MBC. Helped edit the manuscript: HLS WLX LQW.

References

1. Kamangar F, Dores GM, Anderson WF (2006) Patterns of cancer incidence, mortality, and prevalence across five continents: defining priorities to reduce cancer disparities in different geographic regions of the world. J Clin Oncol 24:2137–2150.

2. Siegel R, Naishadham D, Jemal A (2013) Cancer statistics, 2013. CA Cancer J Clin 63:11–30.

3. Mezhir JJ, Tang LH, Coit DG (2010) Neoadjuvant therapy of locally advanced gastric cancer. J Surg Oncol 101:305–314.

4. Ott K, Sendler A, Becker K, Dittler HJ, Helmberger H, et al. (2003) Neoadjuvant chemotherapy with cisplatin, 5-FU, and leucovorin (PLF) in locally advanced gastric cancer: a prospective phase II study. Gastric Cancer 6:159–167.

5. Cunningham D, Allum WH, Stenning SP, Thompson JN, Van de Velde CJ, et al. (2006) Perioperative chemotherapy versus surgery alone for resectable gastroesophageal cancer. N Engl J Med 355:11–20.

6. Nashimoto A, Yabusaki H, Tanaka O, Sasaki J, Akiyama N (1999) Neoadjuvant chemotherapy in advanced gastric cancer with non-curative factors: a Phase II study with 5-fluorouracil, leucovorin, and cisplatin. Gastric Cancer 2:57–63.

7. Fareed KR, Kaye P, Soomro IN, Ilyas M, Martin S, et al. (2009) Biomarkers of response to therapy in oesophago-gastric cancer. Gut 58:127–143.

8. Lamb P, Crawford L (1986) Characterization of the human p53 gene. Mol Cell Biol 6:1379–1385.

9. Vousden KH, Prives C (2009) Blinded by the Light: The Growing Complexity of p53. Cell 137:413–431.

10. Tewari M, Krishnamurthy A, Shukla HS (2008) Predictive markers of response to neoadjuvant chemotherapy in breast cancer. Surg Oncol 17:301–311.

11. Lowe SW, Bodis S, McClatchey A, Remington L, Ruley HE, et al. (1994) p53 status and the efficacy of cancer therapy in vivo. Science 266:807–810.

12. Lowe SW, Ruley HE, Jacks T, Housman DE (1993) p53-dependent apoptosis modulates the cytotoxicity of anticancer agents. Cell 74:957–967.

13. Weller M (1998) Predicting response to cancer chemotherapy: the role of p53. Cell Tissue Res 292:435–445.

14. Fareed KR, Al-Attar A, Soomro IN, Kaye PV, Patel J, et al. (2010) Tumour regression and ERCC1 nuclear protein expression predict clinical outcome in patients with gastro-oesophageal cancer treated with neoadjuvant chemotherapy. Br J Cancer 102:1600–1607.

15. Ott K, Vogelsang H, Mueller J, Becker K, Muller M, et al. (2003) Chromosomal instability rather than p53 mutation is associated with response to neoadjuvant cisplatin-based chemotherapy in gastric carcinoma. Clin Cancer Res 9:2307–2315.

16. Bataille F, Rummele P, Dietmaier W, Gaag D, Klebl F, et al. (2003) Alterations in p53 predict response to preoperative high dose chemotherapy in patients with gastric cancer. Mol Pathol 56:286–292.

17. Boku N, Ohtsu A, Yoshida S, Shirao K, Shimada Y, et al. (2007) Significance of biological markers for predicting prognosis and selecting chemotherapy regimens of advanced gastric cancer patients between continuous infusion of 5-FU and a combination of 5-FU and cisplatin. Jpn J Clin Oncol 37:275–281.

18. Nagashima F, Boku N, Ohtsu A, Yoshida S, Hasebe T, et al. (2005) Biological markers as a predictor for response and prognosis of unresectable gastric cancer patients treated with irinotecan and cisplatin. Jpn J Clin Oncol 35:714–719.

19. Yeh KH, Shun CT, Chen CL, Lin JT, Lee WJ, et al. (1999) Overexpression of p53 is not associated with drug resistance of gastric cancers to 5-fluorouracil-based systemic chemotherapy. Hepatogastroenterology 46:610–615.

20. Chen MB, Zhu YQ, Xu JY, Wang LQ, Liu CY, et al. (2012) Value of TP53 status for predicting response to neoadjuvant chemotherapy in breast cancer: a meta-analysis. PLoS One 7:e39655.

21. Pakos EE, Kyzas PA, Ioannidis JP (2004) Prognostic significance of TP53 tumor suppressor gene expression and mutations in human osteosarcoma: a meta-analysis. Clin Cancer Res 10:6208–6214.

22. Japanese Research Society for Gastric Cancer. Japanese Classification of Gastric Carcinoma - 1nd English Edition 1st English ed Tokyo: Kanehara 1995,

23. Japanese Research Society of Gastric Cancer. Japanese classificaticion of gastric carcinoma, 1st English ed, p 101–104 Tokyo: Kanehara Shuppan 1999,

24. Therasse P, Arbuck SG, Eisenhauer EA, Wanders J, Kaplan RS, et al. (2000) New guidelines to evaluate the response to treatment in solid tumors. European Organization for Research and Treatment of Cancer, National Cancer Institute of the United States, National Cancer Institute of Canada. J Natl Cancer Inst 92:205–216.

25. WHO: WHO Handbook for Reporting Results of Cancer Treatment, WHO Offset Publication No 48, Geneva:WHO 1979.

26. Kamoshida S, Suzuki M, Shimomura R, Sakurai Y, Komori Y, et al. (2007) Immunostaining of thymidylate synthase and p53 for predicting chemoresistance to S-1/cisplatin in gastric cancer. Br J Cancer 96:277–283.

27. Sirak I, Petera J, Hatlova J, Vosmik M, Melichar B, et al. (2009) Expression of p53, p21 and p16 does not correlate with response to preoperative chemoradiation in gastric carcinoma. Hepatogastroenterology 56:1213–1218.

28. Cascinu S, Graziano F, Del Ferro E, Staccioli MP, Ligi M, et al. (1998) Expression of p53 protein and resistance to preoperative chemotherapy in locally advanced gastric carcinoma. Cancer 83:1917–1922.

29. Boku N, Chin K, Hosokawa K, Ohtsu A, Tajiri H, et al. (1998) Biological markers as a predictor for response and prognosis of unresectable gastric cancer patients treated with 5-fluorouracil and cis-platinum. Clin Cancer Res 4:1469–1474.

30. Kikuyama S, Inada T, Shimizu K, Miyakita M, Ogata Y (2001) p53, bcl-2 and thymidine phosphorylase as predictive markers of chemotherapy in patients with advanced and recurrent gastric cancer. Anticancer Res 21:2149–2153.

31. Giatromanolaki A, Stathopoulos GP, Koukourakis MI, Rigatos S, Vrettou E, et al. (2001) Angiogenesis and apoptosis-related protein (p53, bcl-2, and bax) expression versus response of gastric adenocarcinomas to paclitaxel and carboplatin chemotherapy. Am J Clin Oncol 24:222–226.

32. Qu JJ, Shi YR, Hao FY(2013) Clinical study of the predictors to neoadjuvant chemotherapy in patients with advanced gastric cancer. Zhonghua Wei Chang Wai Ke Za Zhi 16:276–280.

33. Nakata B, Chung KH, Ogawa M, Ogawa Y, Yanagawa K, et al. (1998) p53 protein overexpression as a predictor of the response to chemotherapy in gastric cancer. Surg Today 28:595–598.

34. Japanese Gastric Cancer A (1998) Japanese Classification of Gastric Carcinoma - 2nd English Edition. Gastric Cancer 1:10–24.

5

An 18-Gene Signature for Vascular Invasion Is Associated with Aggressive Features and Reduced Survival in Breast Cancer

Monica Mannelqvist[1], Elisabeth Wik[1,2], Ingunn M. Stefansson[1,2], Lars A. Akslen[1,2]*

1 Centre for Cancer Biomarkers CCBIO, Department of Clinical Medicine, University of Bergen, Norway, 2 Department of Pathology, The Gade Institute, Haukeland University Hospital, Bergen, Norway

Abstract

Aims: Vascular invasion by tumor cells is known to be important for cancer progression. By microarray and qPCR analyses, we earlier identified an 18-gene signature associated with vascular involvement in endometrial cancer. Here, we explored the significance of this vascular invasion signature in multiple series of breast cancer patients.

Methods and Results: The study includes 11 open access gene expression data sets which collectively provide information on 2423 breast cancer patients. The 18-gene signature showed consistent associations with aggressive features of breast cancer, like high tumor grade, hormone receptor negativity, HER2 positivity, a basal-like phenotype, reduced patient survival, and response to neoadjuvant chemotherapy. Also, the vascular invasion signature was associated with several other gene expression profiles related to vascular biology and tumor progression, including the Oncotype DX breast cancer recurrence signature.

Conclusions: The 18-gene vascular invasion signature showed strong and consistent associations with aggressive features of breast cancer and reduced survival.

Editor: Pranela Rameshwar, Rutgers - New Jersey Medical School, United States of America

Funding: The study is funded by the Norwegian Cancer Society, the Research Council of Norway, Helse Vest research and the University of Bergen. The funders had no role in study design, data collection and analysis, decision to publish, or preparation of the manuscript.

Competing Interests: The authors have declared that no competing interests exist.

* E-mail: lars.akslen@gades.uib.no

Introduction

Vascular invasion, *i.e.* tumor cells entering the vascular system, is considered to be an early step in the metastatic process and important for the progress of malignant tumors. When examined on tissue sections as a morphologic marker, the presence of vascular invasion is a strong prognostic factor in breast cancer and other tumor types [1–4]. Recently, we presented a gene expression signature related to vascular invasion in endometrial cancer, being associated with aggressive tumor features and reduced survival [5]. This signature was generated from 57 primary endometrial tumors, and the gene expression pattern was investigated by microarray and qPCR, and subsequently related to the presence of vascular invasion on tissue sections. Finally, 18 significantly and differentially expressed genes were found between tumors with and without such vascular involvement. Here, we explored whether this 18-gene vascular invasion signature was associated with high-grade features and poor survival in breast cancer, and we examined a broad panel of publicly available data sets, collectively representing a total of 2423 patients. The signature genes were investigated in these external data sets and related to clinical data and follow-up information. Briefly, the vascular invasion signature was associated with markers of aggressive breast cancers and reduced survival, and the vascular invasion score was also associated with other published gene signatures related to vascular involvement and tumor progression.

Materials and Methods

Vascular invasion signature

Generation of the 18-gene vascular invasion gene expression signature was originally identified in a prospectively collected patient series of 57 endometrial carcinomas by microarray and qPCR analysis [5]. The vascular invasion signature consists of 7 up-regulated and 11 down-regulated genes (**Table 1**). The vascular invasion signature was based on supervised analyses of gene expression differences related to lymphatic and blood vessel involvement (assessed on HE-sections) [5], and the signature showed significant association with patient survival and aggressive clinico-pathologic features, as well as with vascular and matrix biology.

Gene expression data sets

Publicly available data sets with clinical information on breast cancer patients were found and downloaded from the Gene Expression Omnibus (GEO) website (www.ncbi.nlm.nih.gov/geo). Overall, 11 breast cancer data sets with clinical information were

Table 1. The vascular invasion signature consists of 7 up-regulated and 11 down-regulated genes [5].

Gene symbol	Gene name
Up-regulated genes	
MMP3	Matrix metallopeptidase 3 (stromelysin 1, progelatinase)
TNFAIP6	Tumor necrosis factor, alpha-induced protein 6
FPR2	Formyl peptide receptor 2
IL8	Interleukin 8
ANGPTL4	Angiopoietin-like 4
SERPINE1	Serpin peptidase inhibitor, clade E (nexin, plasminogen activator inhibitor type 1), member 1
COL8A1	Collagen, type VIII, alpha 1
Down-regulated genes	
OGN	Osteoglycin
ATCAY	Ataxia, cerebellar, Cayman type
MAMDC2	MAM domain containing 2
COL4A6	Collagen, type IV, alpha 6
C1orf114	Chromosome 1 open reading frame 114
KLHL13	Kelch-like 13 (Drosophila)
OSR2	Odd-skipped related 2 (Drosophila)
ALDH1A2	Aldehyde dehydrogenase 1 family, member A2
SEMA5A	Sema domain, seven thrombospondin repeats (type 1 and type 1-like), transmembrane domain (TM) and short cytoplasmic domain, (semaphorin) 5A
FGFR2	Fibroblast growth factor receptor 2
ITIH5	Inter-alpha (globulin) inhibitor H5

identified and studied, including a total of 2423 patients. Gene expression data from the following cohorts were analyzed:

GSE1456. A population based breast cancer series from 159 tumors with clinical information on histologic tumor grade, molecular tumor subclasses (as described by Sørlie et al. [6]), recurrence free survival, and breast cancer specific deaths [7].

GSE20271. Gene expression data on 178 breast cancer patients, clinical stage I–III, from 6 different international sites with data on histologic grade, estrogen receptor (ER), progester-

one receptor (PR) and human epidermal growth factor receptor 2 (HER2) status [8].

GSE20194. 230 stage I–III breast cancers from fine-needle aspiration specimens before any therapy, with data on histologic grade, ER, PR, and HER2-status [9].

GSE5460. 129 primary, untreated breast cancers, balanced for nodal status, with information on tumor type and tumor size, histologic grade, lymphatic vascular invasion (LVI), ER-status, HER2-status, and lymph node status [10].

Table 2. Associations between histologic grade and the 18-gene vascular invasion signature score (mean signature score is given).

	Grade				
	1	2	3	p-value[1]	Correlation[6]
GSE25066 (N = 508)	−2.04	−1.31	1.09	<0.001	0.27
GSE22358 (N = 154)	−1.55	−0.82	2.27	0.001	0.31
GSE26639[2] (N = 226)	−1.81	−1.11	1.06	0.001	0.25
GSE1456[3] (N = 159)	−1.23	−1.03	1.32	<0.001	0.25
GSE20271[4] (N = 178)	−2.09	−0.69	0.24	0.006	0.24
GSE 20194[4] (N = 230)	−2.70	−1.21	1.24	<0.001	0.33
GSE5460[5] (N = 129)	−2.57	−0.86	1.39	0.001	0.25

[1]Kruskal-Wallis test, significance level 0.05,
[2]Histologic grade,
[3]Elston & Ellis tumor grade,
[4]Modified Black's nuclear grade,
[5]Modified Bloom–Richardson grade,
[6]Spearman's rho.

Table 3. Associations between ER-status, PR-status, HER2-status and the 18-gene vascular invasion signature score (mean signature score is given).

	ER			PR			HER2		
	Neg	Pos	p-value[1]	Neg	Pos	p-value[1]	Neg	Pos	p-value[1]
GSE22358 (N = 154)	2.53	−1.44	<0.001	1.27	−1.14	0.015	−0.12	2.21	0.041
GSE26639 (N = 226)	1.71	−1.12	<0.001	1.12	−1.52	<0.001	−0.41	0.68	NS
GSE20271 (N = 178)	0.52	−0.52	0.045	0.58	−0.77	0.006	−0.08	0.12	NS
GSE 20194 (N = 230)	1.87	−1.15	<0.001	0.84	−0.98	0.003	−0.19	1.00	0.071
GSE25066 (N = 508)	1.54	−1.08	<0.001	1.11	−1.19	<0.001	-	-	-
GSE7849 (N = 78)	0.75	−0.52	NS	0.89	−0.79	0.038	-	-	-
GSE5460 (N = 129)	2.07	−1.44	<0.001	-	-	-	−0.59	1.87	0.016

[1]Mann-Whitney U test, significance level 0.05.

Table 4. Associations between breast cancer molecular subtypes and the 18-gene vascular invasion signature score (mean signature score is given).

	Molecular subtypes					
	Basal-like	ERBB2	Luminal A	Luminal B	Normal breast-like	p-value[1]
GSE25066 (N = 508)	2.01	1.53	−1.58	−1.58	−1.60	<0.001
GSE22358 (N = 154)	3.38	4.94	−2.28	0.31	−6.68	<0.001
GSE1456 (N = 159)	1.89	3.05	−0.39	1.38	−3.09	<0.001
GSE 20685[2] (N = 327)	5.12[I]	5.81[II]	0.40[III]	1.94[IV]	−0.96[V] −3.91[VI]	<0.001

[1]Kruskal-Wallis test, significance level 0.05,
[2]Molecular subtypes I-VI [12].

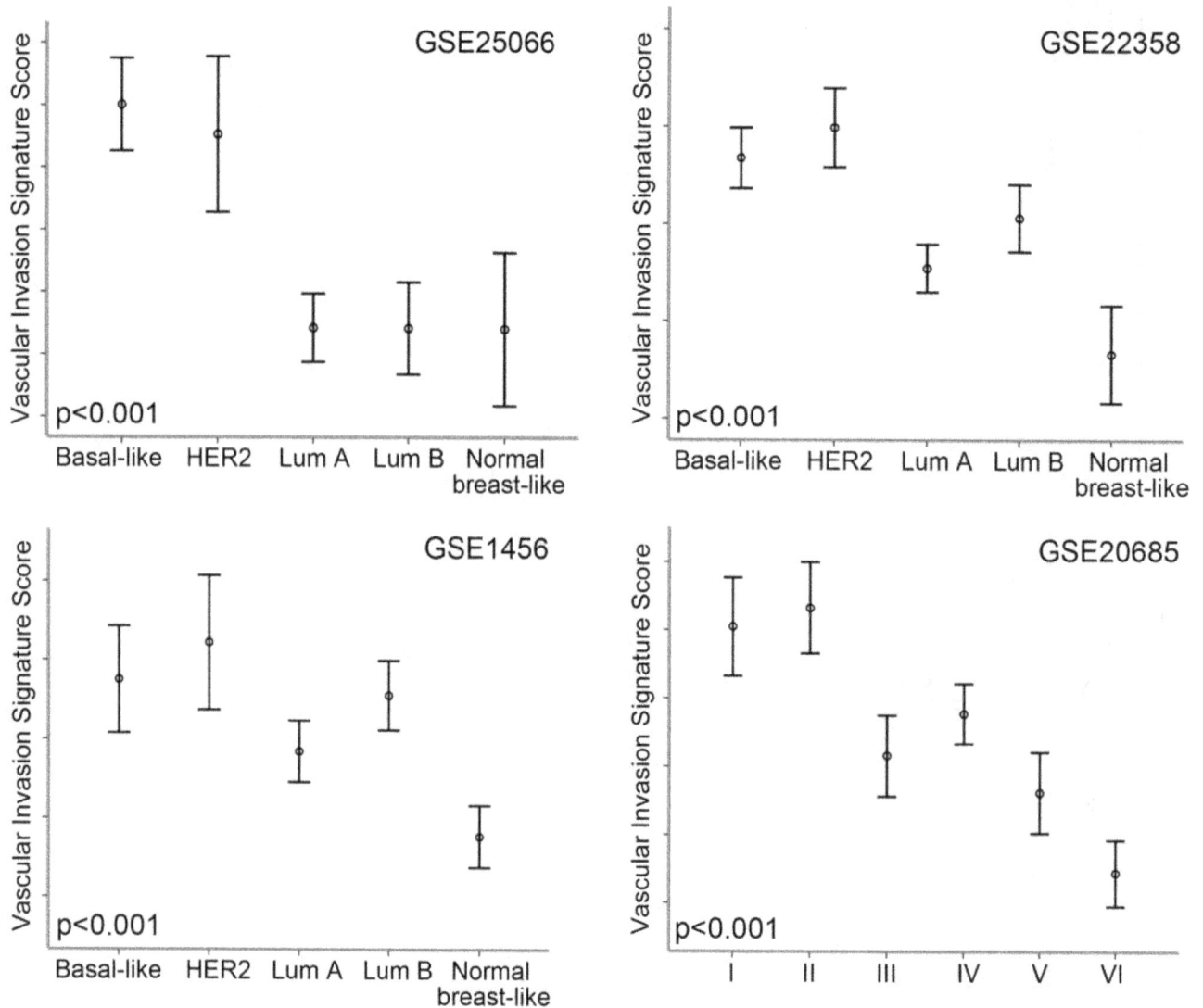

Figure 1. High Vascular Invasion Signature score is associated with Basal-like and HER2 molecular subtypes. High signature score is associated with Basal-like and HER2 molecular subtypes among data sets GSE25066, GSE22358, GSE1456 and GSE20685. Correlations were assessed by Kruskal-Wallis test. Mean expression signature scores indicated by circles, and the bars represent standard error ±2.

GSE7849. 78 tumors from women with early stage breast cancer with information on histological type, nuclear grade, LVI, ER-status, PR-status, lymph node status, and recurrence free survival [11].

GSE20685. 327 primary breast cancers with data on molecular subtypes, recurrence free survival and overall survival. The molecular subtypes were classified in I-VI, where subtypes I and II correspond to the basal-like and HER2 subtypes, subtype III represents a mixture of HER2 and Luminal B, subtype IV is similar to Luminal B, and subtype V and VI correspond to Luminal A tumors [12].

GSE26639. 226 primary breast carcinomas in stage II–III, with data on histologic grade, ER-status, PR-status, and HER2-status [13].

GSE25066. 508 HER2-negative breast cancers with data on tumor subclasses, ER-status, PR-status, and distant relapse free survival [14].

GSE22358. 154 stage II–III breast cancers with data on histologic grade, molecular subtype, ER-status, PR-status, HER2-status, p53 status and response to treatment [15].

GSE17705. 298 ER-positive breast cancers treated with tamoxifen for 5 years with data for distant relapse free survival [16].

GSE12093. 136 ER-positive breast cancer patients treated with tamoxifen with data on disease free survival [17].

Gene expression signatures related to tumor progression

We used the following published gene expression signatures to investigate a possible correlation with the 18-gene vascular invasion score: The *VEGF signature* identifies a compact *in vivo* hypoxia signature highly expressed in metastatic breast tumors. This signature is associated with poor outcome in multiple tumor types [18]. *Wound response signature*; cancer invasion and metastasis have demonstrated similarities with the wound healing process. A published wound response signature predicts increased risk of metastasis and death in several cancers [19]. *NF-κB-regulated genes*

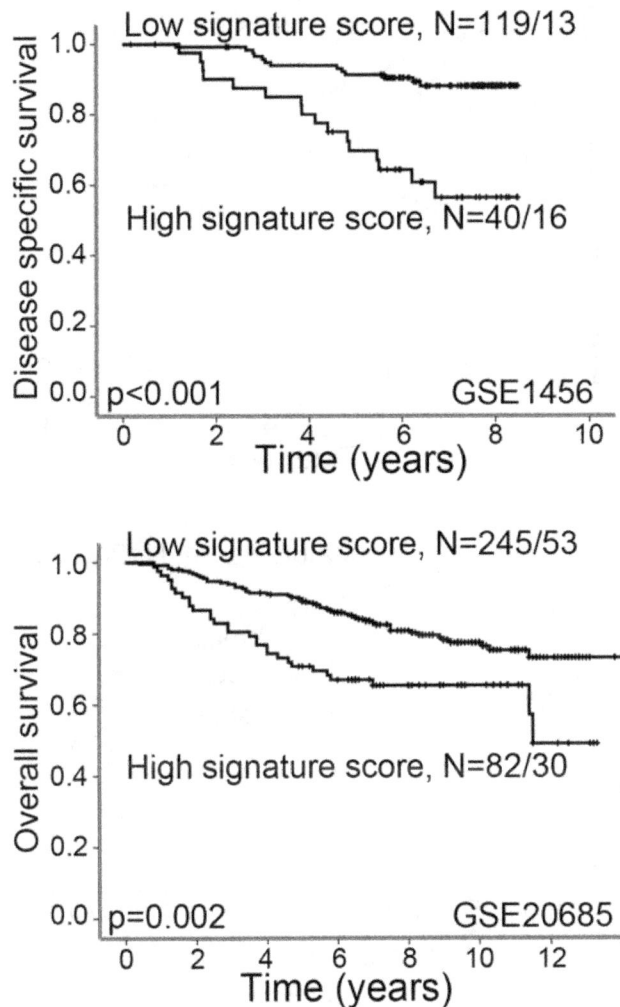

Figure 2. High Vascular Invasion Signature score is associated with reduced survival. High signature score is associated with reduced survival in datasets GSE1456 and GSE20685. Univariate survival analysis was performed by the Kaplan-Meier method (log-rank significance test). For each category, the number of cases is given followed by the number of breast cancer deaths.

are involved in tumor progression like proliferation, invasiveness, angiogenesis, lymphangiogenesis and inflammation. The NF-κB-associated gene signature contains 60 genes and is known to be of importance for tumor progression in inflammatory breast cancer [20]. *Hypoxia gene signature*; tumor hypoxia is an important feature of human cancer progression. This published hypoxia gene signature has demonstrated prognostic importance in breast and ovary cancers [21]. *BMI-1 driven gene signature*; BMI-1 participates in determining the proliferative potential and is required for self-renewal of different stem cells. The BMI-1 driven gene signature shows prognostic impact in many cancers [22]. Tumor stem cells and stemness features are important for tumor progression [23]. *Oncotype DX Recurrence Score* corresponds to the likelihood of breast cancer recurrence. The signature includes 5 reference and 16 cancer related genes [24].

Gene expression signature scores

The genes from the vascular invasion signature and the other signatures, used for correlation studies, were mapped to the breast cancer microarray data sets. A few genes in some of the signatures could not be mapped to some of the data sets. Signature gene expression scores were generated according to the algorithms applied in the papers publishing the specific signatures. For the vascular invasion signature, the hypoxia signature and the BMI-1 driven signature, summarized expression values for the down-regulated genes were subtracted from the sum of expression values for the up-regulated genes. For the wound response signature, a summary expression signature was generated for the activated genes. For the VEGF signature and the NF-κB-regulated genes, a mean expression value from the expression values for the genes in the signature was calculated. For the Oncotype DX recurrence score, the algorithm in the paper was used on the 16 cancer-related genes.

Statistics

Statistical analyses were performed with the PASW statistical software package version 17 (SPSS Inc., Chicago, IL). Correlations between categorical and continuous variables were assessed by non-parametric tests; Mann-Whitney (two categorical groups) or Kruskal-Wallis (>2 categorical groups) with a significance level of 0.05. Spearman's correlation (rho) was also calculated between tumor grade and the vascular invasion score. Linear association between two continuous variables was evaluated by linear regression analysis and Spearman's correlation. Univariate survival analyses were performed using the Kaplan-Meier method (log-rank significance test), and scores were dichotomized based on the upper quartile. Signature scores, together with standard clinico-pathological and molecular variables, were further analyzed by log-log plot to determine how these variables could be incorporated in Cox' proportional hazards regression model, and tested by the backward stepwise likelihood ratio test.

Results

Correlations to histologic grade and lymphatic vascular invasion

Seven of the data sets had information on histologic or nuclear tumor grade [7–10,13–15], and all sets showed significant correlations between high signature score and high tumor grade (**Table 2**).

Two data sets had information on lymphatic vascular invasion (LVI), but there was no significant direct correlation between LVI and the 18-gene signature score (data not shown) [10,11]. As indicated, the original vascular invasion signature was based on vascular invasion as a combination of lymphatic and blood vessel involvement assessed on HE-sections [5].

Increased vascular invasion score is associated with hormone receptor negative tumors

Seven of the data sets had information on ER-status [8–11,13–15], and six of the sets showed significant correlations between high signature score and ER-negative tumors, five of them highly significant ($p<0.001$). The seventh data set did not show a significant correlation (**Table 3**). For PR-status, there was information available in six of the data sets [8,9,11,13–15]. All sets showed a significant association between high signature score and PR-negative tumors (**Table 3**).

Five data sets contained information about HER2-status [8–10,13,15]. Two of them showed a significant correlation between high signature score and HER2-positive tumors, one data set had a borderline significant association, and two data sets did not show any significant association between the signature score and HER2-status (**Table 3**).

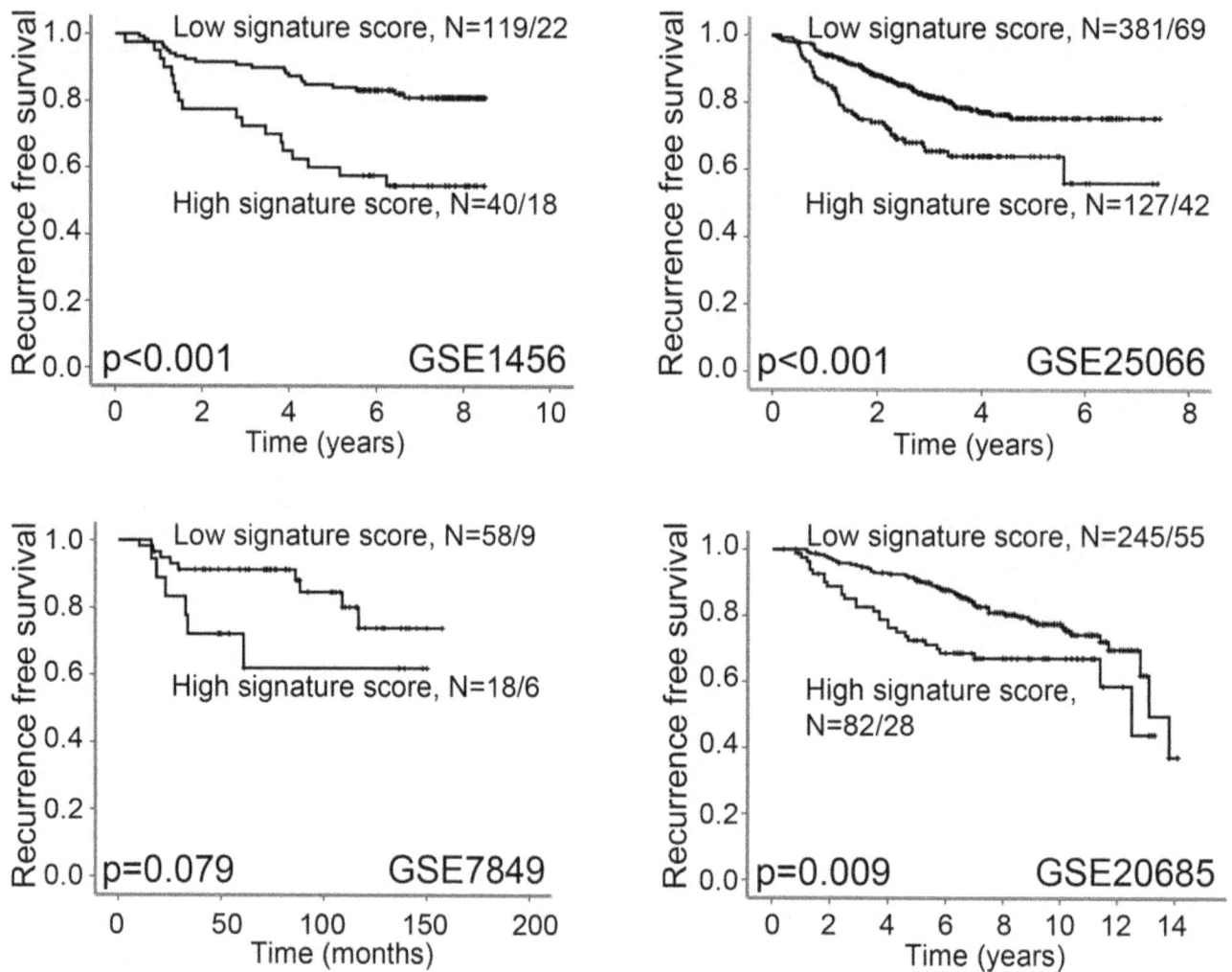

Figure 3. High Vascular Invasion Signature score is associated with reduced recurrence free survival. High signature score is associated with reduced recurrence free survival in data sets GSE1456, GSE2506 and GSE20685. In data set GSE7849, there is a trend between high signature score and reduced recurrence free survival. Survival curves are estimated by the Kaplan-Meier method (log-rank significance test). For each category, the number of cases is given followed by the number of breast cancer deaths.

Table 5. Multivariate survival analysis (Cox' proportional hazards regression model) of the vascular invasion signature score.

Data set	Variables	HR[1]	95% CI[2]	P-value[3]
Disease specific survival				
GSE1456[4]	Vascular invasion score	2.7	1.2–6.1	0.019
	Tumor grade	1.9	1.0–3.9	0.068
Overall survival				
GSE20685[5]	Vascular invasion score	2.0	1.3–3.2	0.002
Recurrence free survival				
GSE1456[4]	Vascular invasion score	1.9	1.0–3.9	0.063
	Tumor grade	1.8	1.1–3.1	0.032
GSE20685[5]	Vascular invasion score	1.8	1.2–2.9	0.010

[1]Adjusted Hazard ratio,
[2]95% confidence interval,
[3]Lratio test, Final model after inclusion of: [4]Vascular invasion score, histologic grade and molecular subtype or [5]Vascular invasion score and molecular subtype.
Data presented for disease specific survival, overall survival and recurrence free survival.

Table 6. Association between the 18-gene signature score and response to treatment (mean signature score is given).

	Response					
GSE22358 (N = 154)	**Neoadjuvant chemotherapy**			**Chemotherapy + trastuzumab**		
	npCR[1]/pCR[2]	NR[3]/PR[4]	p-value[5]	npCR/pCR	NR/PR	p-value[5]
	3.25	−1.15	0.017	3.17	−0.12	0.089
GSE20271 (N = 178)	**FAC treated**			**T/FAC treated**		
	pCR	RD[6]	p-value	pCR	RD	p-value
	0.10	0.21	NS	−0.26	−0.02	NS
GSE 20194 (N = 230)	**Neoadjuvant chemotherapy**					
	pCR	RD	p-value			
	2.18	−0.55	<0.001			

[1]Near-complete pathologic response,
[2]Pathologic complete response,
[3]No response,
[4]Partial respons,
[5]Mann-Whitney U test,
[6]Residual disease.

Increased vascular invasion score is associated with molecular subtypes of breast cancer

Three of the data sets had information on molecular subtypes of breast cancer such as Luminal A, Luminal B, HER2, basal-like, and Normal breast-like [7,14,15]. All data sets showed highly significant correlations between the subtypes and the vascular invasion signature score, p<0.001 (**Table 4**). The most aggressive basal-like and HER2 subtypes showed the highest signature score and Luminal A, Luminal B and normal breast-like the lowest. A fourth data set had molecular subtypes classified from I–VI [12]. When compared with the Sørlie classification [6], the results are similar to the three data sets mentioned above (**Table 4 and Figure 1**).

Increased vascular invasion score is associated with reduced overall and recurrence free survival

Data set GSE1456 had information on breast cancer specific deaths and data set GSE20685 had information on overall survival [7,12]. A high signature score was significantly associated with reduced survival in both these data sets (Kaplan-Meier method, log-rank test, p<0.001 and p = 0.002; **Figure 2**). Also, four data sets had information on recurrence free survival [7,11,12,16]. A high signature score was associated with reduced recurrence free survival in three data sets, whereas the fourth data set showed a trend between reduced recurrence free survival and high signature score (p = 0.079) (**Figure 3**).

Two data sets included ER-positive patients treated with tamoxifen [16,17]. None of these data sets showed a significant association between high signature score and probability of recurrence (data not shown). In data set GSE25066, among patients with ER positive tumors, high vascular invasion score was significantly associated with reduced recurrence free survival, p = 0.03 (data not shown). In data set GSE7849, no such association was found (data not shown).

By multivariate survival analysis, using data sets with patient survival (GSE1456 and GSE20685) or recurrence-free survival (GSE1456, GSE20685, GSE25066 and GSE7849), selected standard clinico-pathologic and molecular variables were included together with the vascular invasion signature score (**Table 5**).

Initially, the vascular invasion score, histologic grade and molecular subtype were included for data set GSE1456, and vascular invasion score and molecular subtype were included for data set GSE20685. Final models showed high vascular invasion signature score to be an independent prognostic marker for decreased survival, with Hazard ratio (HR) of 2.7, p = 0.019, in data set GSE1456. For data set GSE20685, high vascular invasion score showed a HR of 2.0, p = 0.002, for reduced survival (**Table 5**).

For recurrence free survival, data set GSE1456 showed a borderline significance for the signature score, with HR of 1.9, p = 0.063, and in data set GSE20685 vascular invasion signature score is an independent prognostic marker for recurrence free survival with HR = 1.8, p = 0.01. For data sets GSE25066 and GSE7849, the vascular invasion signature was not an independent prognostic factor for recurrence-free survival (data not shown). Since Oncotype DX recurrence score predicts the risk of recurrent disease in breast cancer, this signature was included in multivariate survival analysis in the two data sets where vascular invasion score was a prognostic marker for recurrence free survival. The vascular invasion score still remained an independent prognostic marker for recurrence free survival in data set GSE1456, while in data set GSE20685, Oncotype DX recurrence signature score was an independent prognostic marker, HR = 1.8, p = 0.001 (data not shown).

Correlation to treatment response

GSE20194: In 230 patients with 6 months of preoperative chemotherapy (paclitaxel, 5-fluorouracil, cyclophosphamide and doxorubicin) followed by surgical tumor resection [9], a high vascular invasion signature score showed strong correlation with pathological complete response (pCR) (p<0.001; **Table 6**).

GSE22358. 154 women received either neoadjuvant chemotherapy alone or chemotherapy in combination with trastuzumab [15]. Among patients receiving chemotherapy only, a high signature score showed a significant association with treatment response (p = 0.017). Patients receiving chemotherapy plus trastuzumab showed a borderline significant relation between near complete or complete response and high signature score (p = 0.089) (**Table 6**).

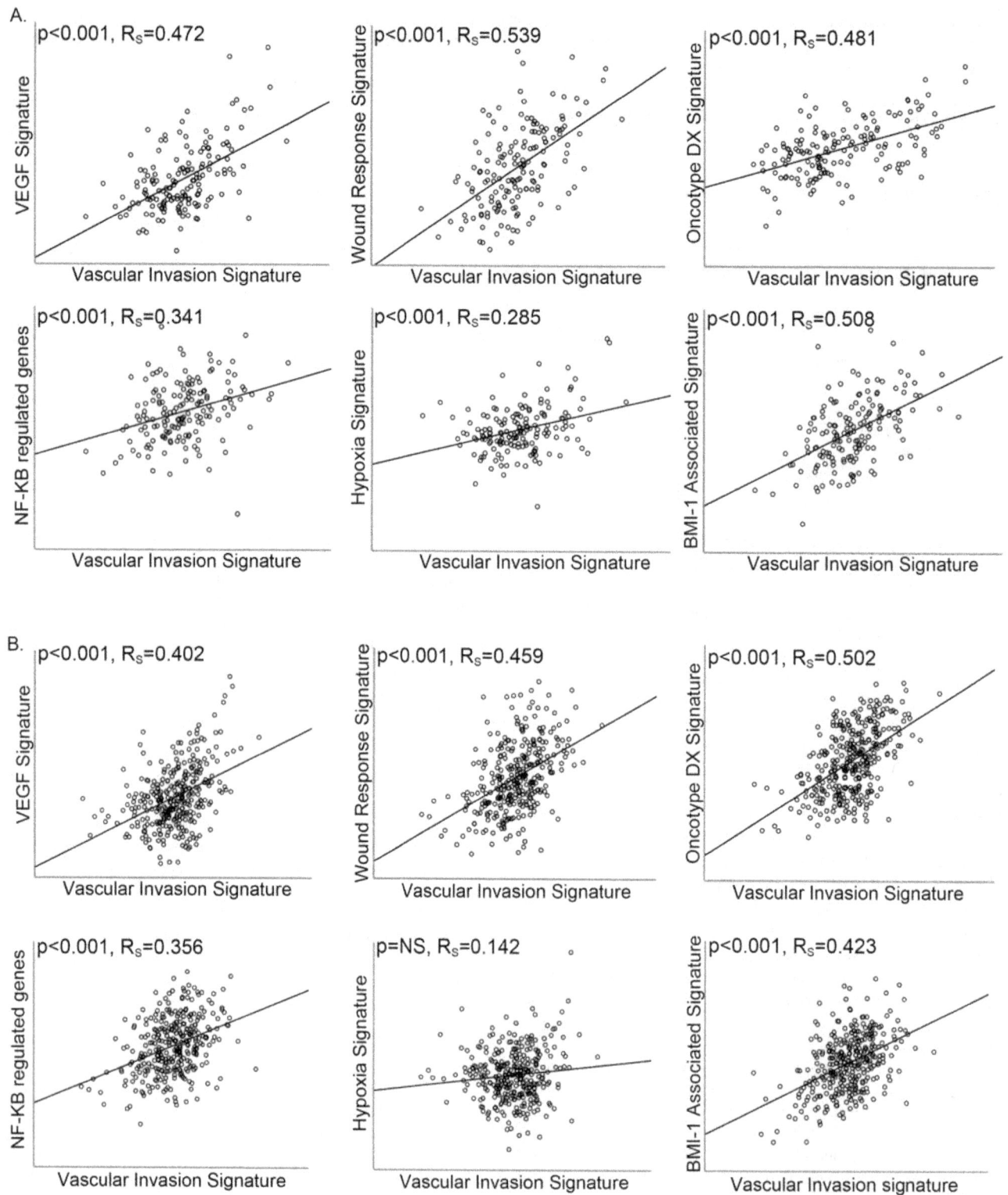

Figure 4. Correlation between the Vascular Invasion Signature and tumor progression signatures. Vascular Invasion Signature score shows a correlation to the VEGF signature, wound response signature, NF-Kβ related genes, hypoxia gene signature, BMI-1 signature and Oncotype DX Recurrence Score in breast cancer data sets; (A) GSE1456 and (B) GSE20685. The Spearman rank correlation test was used for bivariate correlations.

GSE20271. 273 patients were randomly given either weekly paclitaxel ×12 followed by fluorouracil, doxorubicin, and cyclophosphamide × 4 (T/FAC), or alone FAC×6 as neoadjuvant chemotherapy [8]. Of the 273 patients, 178 patients remained for final analysis. Response to the treatment options FAC or T/FAC-treated patients showed no correlation to the 18-gene signature (**Table 6**).

Increased vascular invasion score is associated with other tumor progression signatures

Six gene signatures related to tumor progression were mapped in the two breast cancer data sets with survival information for cancer specific death and overall survival (GSE1456 and GSE20685), and the correlations between the signature scores were explored. In data set GSE1456 (**Figure 4A**), all signatures were significantly correlated to the vascular invasion score, with Rs from 0.29–0.54. In data set GSE20685 (**Figure 4B**), all signatures except the hypoxia score show significant correlation to the vascular invasion score, with Rs from 0.36–0.50.

Discussion

Vascular invasion is a key hallmark of aggressive malignant tumors and is considered an early marker of metastatic spread through the lymphatic or blood vascular networks. In a previous study of endometrial cancer [5], an 18-gene expression signature was established by supervised strategy based on a correlation with microscopic findings of tumor cells entering vascular structures within the tumors. By further characterization of this vascular invasion signature, expression motifs of vascular and matrix biology were found, and the signature was associated with reduced patient survival.

Since the vascular invasion signature appeared to capture important features of aggressive tumors related to tumor-microenvironment interactions, we asked whether the signature could be of value in tumor types separate from those originally studied. Here, in a study including 11 publicly available data sets of breast cancer and information on altogether 2423 patients, we found that the 18-gene vascular invasion signature showed strong associations with features of aggressive breast cancer such as high tumor grade, hormone receptor negativity, HER2 positive tumors, presence of a basal-like phenotype, reduced patient survival and response to neoadjuvant chemotherapy. This association pattern was found in most data sets studied.

However, the small data set GSE7849 did not show significant correlations between the vascular invasion signature score and ER status as well as recurrence free survival. This data set contains a low number of patients with early stage breast cancer. Differences in selection and patient characteristics, in addition to lack of power, might in part explain these negative findings.

Further, a significant association between HER2 and the vascular invasion score was only seen in two of five data sets, whereas ER and PR were associated with the signature in almost all cohorts. Interestingly, HER2 positive breast cancers appear to represent the subgroup with highest frequency of vascular invasion by tumor cells as determined on tissue sections [25]. This could in part explain the lack of significant differences in some series.

We also investigated the vascular invasion signature in three data sets with information on response to treatment. The results were not entirely conclusive, although two of the data sets, including patients treated by neoadjuvant chemotherapy, showed high signature scores in correlation with response.

Our findings support that the 18-gene vascular invasion score reflects tumor-vascular interactions and angiogenesis, by significant associations with gene signatures for VEGF-expression, the wound-response process, NF-κB and tumor hypoxia. In addition, the association with a BMI-1 related signature might indicate a relation with stem cell phenotypes.

The Oncotype DX recurrence score predicts response to chemotherapy and risk of distant recurrence in women with node negative or node positive, ER-positive breast cancer [24,26]. The correlation between our vascular invasion signature score and the Oncotype DX recurrence score further validates that our signature identifies aggressive breast cancers. In multivariate survival analysis, the Oncotype DX recurrence score was included when examining the two data sets where the vascular invasion signature score was an independent prognostic factor for recurrence free survival. In one of these data sets, the vascular signature score maintained an independent association with prognosis, while in the other data set, Oncotype DX was the independent prognostic factor. This might indicate that both signatures capture aggressive tumor subgroups without being completely overlapping. Of note, in this study we investigated Oncotype DX cancer related genes by microarray based data, whereas the approved Oncotype DX test is performed by RT-PCR, hence it is difficult to directly compare the two signature scores.

In an independent experimental study of luminal-like and basal-like breast cancer xenograft models, basal-like tumors consistently showed significantly higher baseline scores of the 18-gene vascular invasion signature, when compared with luminal-like tumors [27]. While no clear associations between the vascular invasion score and treatment response were observed for the basal-like model, significantly higher scores were observed for luminal-like tumors treated with doxorubicin. Interestingly, this result suggests that vascular invasion could be paradoxically increased or selected for in the doxorubicin treated luminal-like tumors [27].

In conclusion, an 18-gene vascular invasion signature showed strong and consistent associations with aggressive features of breast cancer. Our results indicate that this vascular invasion score might reflect important biological characteristics involved in aggressive tumors, probably related to vascular and matrix biology. The practical value of this biomarker, in breast cancer and other tumor types, should be further studied.

Author Contributions

Conceived and designed the experiments: MM EW LAA. Performed the experiments: MM EW. Analyzed the data: MM EW LAA IMS. Contributed reagents/materials/analysis tools: LAA. Wrote the paper: MM LAA IMS EW.

References

1. Mannelqvist M, Stefansson I, Salvesen HB, Akslen LA (2009) Importance of tumour cell invasion in blood and lymphatic vasculature among patients with endometrial carcinoma. Histopathology 54: 174–183.

2. Pinder SE, Ellis IO, Galea M, O'Rouke S, Blamey RW, et al. (1994) Pathological prognostic factors in breast cancer. III. Vascular invasion: relationship with recurrence and survival in a large study with long-term follow-up. Histopathology 24: 41–47.

3. Straume O, Akslen LA (1996) Independent prognostic importance of vascular invasion in nodular melanomas. Cancer 78: 1211–1219.

4. Gardner RE, Tuttle RM, Burman KD, Haddady S, Truman C, et al. (2000) Prognostic importance of vascular invasion in papillary thyroid carcinoma. Arch Otolaryngol Head Neck Surg 126: 309–312.

5. Mannelqvist M, Stefansson IM, Bredholt G, Hellem Bo T, Oyan AM, et al. (2011) Gene expression patterns related to vascular invasion and aggressive features in endometrial cancer. Am J Pathol 178: 861–871.

6. Sorlie T, Perou CM, Tibshirani R, Aas T, Geisler S, et al. (2001) Gene expression patterns of breast carcinomas distinguish tumor subclasses with clinical implications. Proc Natl Acad Sci U S A 98: 10869–10874.

7. Pawitan Y, Bjohle J, Amler L, Borg AL, Egyhazi S, et al. (2005) Gene expression profiling spares early breast cancer patients from adjuvant therapy: derived and validated in two population-based cohorts. Breast Cancer Res 7: R953–964.

8. Tabchy A, Valero V, Vidaurre T, Lluch A, Gomez H, et al. (2010) Evaluation of a 30-gene paclitaxel, fluorouracil, doxorubicin, and cyclophosphamide chemotherapy response predictor in a multicenter randomized trial in breast cancer. Clin Cancer Res 16: 5351–5361.

9. Popovici V, Chen W, Gallas BG, Hatzis C, Shi W, et al. (2010) Effect of training-sample size and classification difficulty on the accuracy of genomic predictors. Breast Cancer Res 12: R5.

10. Lu X, Wang ZC, Iglehart JD, Zhang X, Richardson AL (2008) Predicting features of breast cancer with gene expression patterns. Breast Cancer Res Treat 108: 191–201.

11. Anders CK, Acharya CR, Hsu DS, Broadwater G, Garman K, et al. (2008) Age-specific differences in oncogenic pathway deregulation seen in human breast tumors. PLoS One 3: e1373.

12. Kao KJ, Chang KM, Hsu HC, Huang AT (2011) Correlation of microarray-based breast cancer molecular subtypes and clinical outcomes: implications for treatment optimization. BMC Cancer 11: 143.

13. de Cremoux P, Valet F, Gentien D, Lehmann-Che J, Scott V, et al. (2011) Importance of pre-analytical steps for transcriptome and RT-qPCR analyses in the context of the phase II randomised multicentre trial REMAGUS02 of neoadjuvant chemotherapy in breast cancer patients. BMC Cancer 11: 215.

14. Hatzis C, Pusztai L, Valero V, Booser DJ, Esserman L, et al. (2011) A genomic predictor of response and survival following taxane-anthracycline chemotherapy for invasive breast cancer. JAMA 305: 1873–1881.

15. Gluck S, Ross JS, Royce M, McKenna EF, Jr., Perou CM, et al. (2011) TP53 genomics predict higher clinical and pathologic tumor response in operable early-stage breast cancer treated with docetaxel-capecitabine +/− trastuzumab. Breast Cancer Res Treat.

16. Symmans WF, Hatzis C, Sotiriou C, Andre F, Peintinger F, et al. (2010) Genomic index of sensitivity to endocrine therapy for breast cancer. J Clin Oncol 28: 4111–4119.

17. Zhang Y, Sieuwerts AM, McGreevy M, Casey G, Cufer T, et al. (2009) The 76-gene signature defines high-risk patients that benefit from adjuvant tamoxifen therapy. Breast Cancer Res Treat 116: 303–309.

18. Hu Z, Fan C, Livasy C, He X, Oh DS, et al. (2009) A compact VEGF signature associated with distant metastases and poor outcomes. BMC Med 7: 9.

19. Chang HY, Sneddon JB, Alizadeh AA, Sood R, West RB, et al. (2004) Gene expression signature of fibroblast serum response predicts human cancer progression: similarities between tumors and wounds. PLoS Biol 2: E7.

20. Lerebours F, Vacher S, Andrieu C, Espie M, Marty M, et al. (2008) NF-kappa B genes have a major role in inflammatory breast cancer. BMC Cancer 8: 41.

21. Chi JT, Wang Z, Nuyten DS, Rodriguez EH, Schaner ME, et al. (2006) Gene expression programs in response to hypoxia: cell type specificity and prognostic significance in human cancers. PLoS Med 3: e47.

22. Glinsky GV, Berezovska O, Glinskii AB (2005) Microarray analysis identifies a death-from-cancer signature predicting therapy failure in patients with multiple types of cancer. J Clin Invest 115: 1503–1521.

23. Hanahan D, Weinberg RA (2011) Hallmarks of cancer: the next generation. Cell 144: 646–674.

24. Paik S, Shak S, Tang G, Kim C, Baker J, et al. (2004) A multigene assay to predict recurrence of tamoxifen-treated, node-negative breast cancer. N Engl J Med 351: 2817–2826.

25. Kadivar M, Mafi N, Joulaee A, Shamshiri A, Hosseini N (2012) Breast cancer molecular subtypes and associations with clinicopathological characteristics in Iranian women, 2002- 2011. Asian Pac J Cancer Prev 13: 1881–1886.

26. Albain KS, Barlow WE, Shak S, Hortobagyi GN, Livingston RB, et al. (2010) Prognostic and predictive value of the 21-gene recurrence score assay in postmenopausal women with node-positive, oestrogen-receptor-positive breast cancer on chemotherapy: a retrospective analysis of a randomised trial. Lancet Oncol 11: 55–65.

27. Borgan E, Lindholm EM, Moestue S, Maelandsmo GM, Lingjaerde OC, et al. (2013) Subtype-specific response to bevacizumab is reflected in the metabolome and transcriptome of breast cancer xenografts. Mol Oncol 7: 130–142.

6

Activated cMET and IGF1R-Driven PI3K Signaling Predicts Poor Survival in Colorectal Cancers Independent of KRAS Mutational Status

Jeeyun Lee[1,9], Anjali Jain[3,9], Phillip Kim[3,9], Tani Lee[3], Anne Kuller[3], Fred Princen[3], In-GuDo[4], Suk Hyeong Kim[4], Joon Oh Park[1], Young Suk Park[1], Sharat Singh[3], Hee Cheol Kim[2]*

1 Division of Hematology-Oncology, Department of Medicine, Samsung Medical Center, Sungkyunkwan University School of Medicine, Seoul, Korea, 2 Departments of Surgery, Samsung Medical Center, Sungkyunkwan University School of Medicine, Seoul, Korea, 3 Research and Development, Oncology, Prometheus Laboratories, San Diego, California, United States of America, 4 Pathology, Samsung Medical Center, Sungkyunkwan University School of Medicine, Seoul, Korea

Abstract

Background: Oncogenic mutational analysis provides predictive guidance for therapeutics such as anti-EGFR antibodies, but it is successful only for a subset of colorectal cancer (CRC) patients.

Method: A comprehensive molecular profiling of 120 CRC patients, including 116 primary, 15 liver metastasis, and 1 peritoneal seeding tissue samples was performed to identify the relationship between v-Ki-ras2 Kirsten rat sarcoma viral oncogene homolog (*KRAS*) WT and mutant CRC tumors and clinical outcomes. This included determination of the protein activation patterns of human epidermal receptor 1 (HER1), HER2, HER3, c-MET, insulin-like growth factor 1 receptor (IGF1R), phosphatidylinositide 3-kinase (PI3K), Src homology 2 domain containing (Shc), protein kinase B (AKT), and extracellular signal-regulated kinase (ERK) kinases using multiplexed collaborative enzyme enhanced reactive (CEER) immunoassay.

Results: *KRAS* WT and mutated CRCs were not different with respect to the expression of the various signaling molecules. Poor prognosis in terms of early relapse (<2 years) and shorter disease-free survival (DFS) correlated with enhanced activation of PI3K signaling relative to the HER kinase pathway signaling, but not with the *KRAS* mutational status. *KRAS* WT CRCs were identified as a mixed prognosis population depending on their level of PI3K signaling. *KRAS* WT CRCs with high HER1/c-MET index ratio demonstrated a better DFS post-surgery. c-MET and IGF1R activities relative to HER axis activity were considerably higher in early relapse CRCs, suggesting a role for these alternative receptor tyrosine kinases (RTKs) in driving high PI3K signaling.

Conclusions: The presented data subclassified CRCs based on their activated signaling pathways and identify a role for c-MET and IGF1R-driven PI3K signaling in CRCs, which is superior to KRAS mutational tests alone. The results from this study can be utilized to identify aggressive CRCs, explain failure of currently approved therapeutics in specific CRC subsets, and, most importantly, generate hypotheses for pathway-guided therapeutic strategies that can be tested clinically.

Editor: Hiromu Suzuki, Sapporo Medical University, Japan

Funding: This study was partially supported by Samsung Biomedical Research Institute grant #SS1-B3-011-1. This research was suppoorted by a grant of the Korea Health technology R&D Project through the Korea Health Industry Development Institute(KHIDI), funded by the Ministry of Health & Welfare, Republic of Korea. (Grant Number: HI13C1951). The funders had no role in study design, data collection and analysis, decision to publish, or preparation of the manuscript.

* Email: hckim@skku.edu

⑨ These authors contributed equally to this work.

Introduction

Monoclonal antibodies such as cetuximab and panitumumab that target the epidermal growth factor receptor (EGFR), a human epidermal receptor (HER) family member, have proven to be efficacious in terms of response rate and progression-free survival in combination with standard cytotoxic chemotherapy in metastatic colorectal cancers (CRCs) [1–4]. The EGFR targeting antibodies bind to the extracellular domain of EGFR, leading to

the inhibition of its downstream signaling pathways, including the RAS-RAF-mitogen-activated protein kinase 1 (MAPK1) axis that is mainly involved in cell proliferation, and the v-akt murine thymoma viral oncogene homolog 1 (AKT1) pathway, which is mainly involved in cell survival and tumor invasion [5]. AKT1 is regulated by the upstream phosphatidylinositol 3-kinase (PI3K) signaling pathway.

Mutations in the v-Ki-ras2 Kirsten rat sarcoma viral oncogene homolog (*KRAS*), most frequently detected in codons 12, 13, and

61, occur in approximately 40% of CRC patients [6,7]. *KRAS* mutations have emerged as the key negative predictive factor for treatment response in patients receiving cetuximab [8,9]. These studies have suggested that *KRAS* wild-type (WT) CRC tumors would be responsive to cetuximab; however, up to 65% of patients with *KRAS* WT tumors are still resistant to anti-EGFR monoclonal antibodies [10]. Resistance to anti-EGFR antibodies in a subset of *KRAS* WT CRCs can be explained by the presence of a mutation within the *BRAF* oncogene [8], which is downstream of *KRAS*. The reason for cetuximab non-response in the remaining *KRAS* WT CRCs remains unclear. Furthermore, although *KRAS* mutations are typically associated with non-responsiveness to anti-EGFR antibodies, recent data indicate that *KRAS* G13D mutations may be a positive predictor of cetuximab response [8]. Mutations within the *PIK3CA* gene [10], which is an important regulator of PI3K signaling, are also present in some CRC tumors that can co-occur with *KRAS* or *BRAF* mutations [8,11], thus suggesting their possible influence on responsiveness to targeted therapeutics such as anti-EGFR antibodies but a clear demonstration of such a correlation is lacking [12,13].

From the studies outlined above and given that a large proportion of CRC patients with *KRAS* WT tumors do not respond to cetuximab or panitumumab, it is clear that a simple mutational analysis is insufficient to predict responsiveness to such therapeutics. In addition, since recent studies suggested that the therapeutic responses to PI3K inhibitors were not limited to colorectal cell lines with activating mutations or in patients with mutations [14–16], it is imperative to profile tumors for their predominant as well as potential alternate signaling pathway drivers in addition to the oncogenic mutational analysis. Therefore, we aimed to profile CRC tissues to investigate the correlation between mutational status and various receptor tyrosine kinase (RTK) protein expressions such as HER1, HER2, HER3, c-MET, and insulin-like growth factor 1 receptor (IGF1R). In addition, downstream kinases PI3K, Src homology 2 domain containing (Shc), protein kinase B (AKT), and extracellular signal-regulated kinase (ERK) were determined using the multiplexed immunomicroarray based Collaborative Enzyme Enhanced Reactive (CEER) immunoassay [17–19] in 120 CRC patients from stage I to IV that included 116 primary, 15 liver metastasis, and 1 peritoneal seeding tissue samples. In parallel, somatic mutational analysis scored for mutations within the *KRAS* and *BRAF* oncogenes. CRC tumors with similar oncogenic mutations demonstrated heterogeneity in their signaling pathway profiles.

Patients and Methods

Patient Cohort and Tissue Specimen Procurement

The study was approved by the institutional review board (IRB) at Samsung Medical Center. All clinical investigation was conducted according to the principles expressed in the Declaration of Helsinki. The written informed consent was waived by the IRB due to retrospective analysis and anonymous data. Fresh frozen tissues (n = 120) collected from surgically resected tumors (73 colon, 47 rectum), 15 from metastatic liver tumors and one from peritoneal seeding nodule, were available for final analysis. All fresh frozen tissues were collected within 30 min at the surgical field by a surgeon, were immediately snap-frozen in liquid nitrogen, and stored at −80°C until use. Tumor specimens were confirmed for the presence of tumor >70% area by a pathologist. For the analysis, small pieces of frozen tissues (10-μm sections ×3) were prepared using prechilled razor blades and were then lysed in 100 μL of lysis buffer. The resulting lysates were stored at −80°C until subsequent analysis.

Collaborative Enzyme Enhanced Reactive-Immunoassay (CEER)

CEER uses an antibody microarray-based platform that can measure the expression and activation levels of signal transduction proteins in tumor tissues and surrogate tissues. The selected target is first captured by a target-specific capture antibody followed by co-localization of two additional detector antibodies against the same target, eventually resulting in specific target detection and quantitation. Detailed methods for this technology have been described previously [17–19] and can be found in the File S2. Representative experiments are shown in Fig.S1 in File S1.

Mutation analysis

Genomic DNA was extracted from CRC tissues using the Qiagen Tissue Kit. Samples were screened for mutations in *KRAS*, *BRAF*, and *PIK3CA* genes: G12A/C/D/S/V, G13C/D, and Q61H in *KRAS* and V600E in *BRAF*. The mutational assay was based on the TaqMan real time polymerase chain reaction (PCR) technology in combination with allele specific primers (ASP), blocker, and probe using a modification of the real-time Allele Specific PCR detection method [20]. Briefly, ASPs were used to specifically detect the mutant allele. A blocking oligonucleotide (blocker) complementary to the wild-type sequence was used to suppress any non-specific amplification of the wild-type allele. The PCR mix used for all the assays was GTXpress Master Mix from Life Technologies. All the assays were run on 384-well plates ABI 7900HT Real Time PCR Instrument (Life Technologies).

The percentage of the allelic variant present in unknown samples was calculated using a standard curve. The standard curve was generated for each mutation from the DNA extracted from a cell line positive for that mutation using a series of DNA dilutions (100, 10, 1, 0.1, and 0.01 ng). A list of the positive cell lines used for generating the standard curves is shown in the table below. The DNA from the respective cell lines was extracted using the Qiagen DNeasy Blood & Tissue Kit.

Using the standard curve, the amount of the respective mutation in the unknown DNA sample was calculated from the Ct value that could then be used to calculate the percent allelic variant based on the assumption that the standard cell line is 100% positive for that specific mutation. The allelic variance of the cell lines was determined using primers specific to the wild-type allele. Following are the cell lines used for gene mutations: SW1116 (KRASG12A), NCI-H23(KRASG12C), LS174T (KRASG12D), PSN1(KRASG12R), A549(KRASG12S), SW403(G12V), H1734 (KRASG13C), T84(KRASG13D), H460(KRASQ61H), and HT29 (BRAFV600E).

Statistical analysis

Mann-Whitney *t*-tests, Kaplan-Meier survival analysis, and Pearson correlation analysis were performed using GraphPad Prism version 5 for Mac OS X (GraphPad Software, La Jolla California USA, www.graphpad.com). DFS was determined using the Kaplan–Meier method, and survival curves were compared using the Log-ratio method. Survival was measured from the date of surgery. All tests were two-sided, and P values less than 0.05 were considered significant. Statistical analysis was performed using SPSS 20 software for Windows (SPSS Inc., Chicago, IL).

Results

Patient Characteristics

The characteristics of the 120 CRC patients are provided in Table 1. Seventy-three patients presented with a colon primary,

Activated cMET and IGF1R-Driven PI3K Signaling Predicts Poor Survival in Colorectal Cancers Independent...

47

Table 1. Patient characteristics.

Characteristics	(Total N = 120) (%)
Age	
Median age (range)	61 (31–85)
≤65	68 (56.7)
>65	52 (43.3)
Sex	
Male	73 (60.8)
Female	47 (39.2)
Stage	
I	11 (9.2)
II	38 (31.7)
III	38 (31.7)
IV	33 (27.4)
Histology	
WD	8 (6.7)
MD	99 (82.5)
PD	5 (4.1)
Adenocarcinoma, not specified	8 (6.7)
Primary tumor	
Colon	73 (60.8)
Rectum	47 (39.2)
Curative resection	
Yes	108 (90.0)
No	12 (10.0)
Adjuvant chemotherapy (Colon)	
5-FU based chemotherapy	20 (27.4)
Capecitabine	18 (24.7)
XELOX or XELIRI	13 (17.8)
No adjuvant chemotherapy	22 (30.1)
Adjuvant chemotherapy (Rectum)	
5-FU+RT	28 (59.6)
capecitabine/oxaliplatin+RT	1 (2.1)
5-FU based chemotherapy	2 (4.3)
capecitabine	1 (2.1)
No adjuvant chemotherapy	15 (31.9)
Tissue specimens (from 120 patients)	
Primary (colon or rectum)	116
Liver metastasis	14 (10 paired with primary)
Peritoneal seeding	1 (paired with primary)
KRAS mutational status	
At least one mutation	49 (42%)
KRAS G12S	3
KRAS G12D	19
KRAS G12A	1
KRAS G12V	6
KRAS G12C	7
KRAS G13D	17

The characteristics of the 120 patients used in this study are summarized.
WD: Well differentiated; MD: Moderately differentiated; PD: Poorly differentiated.

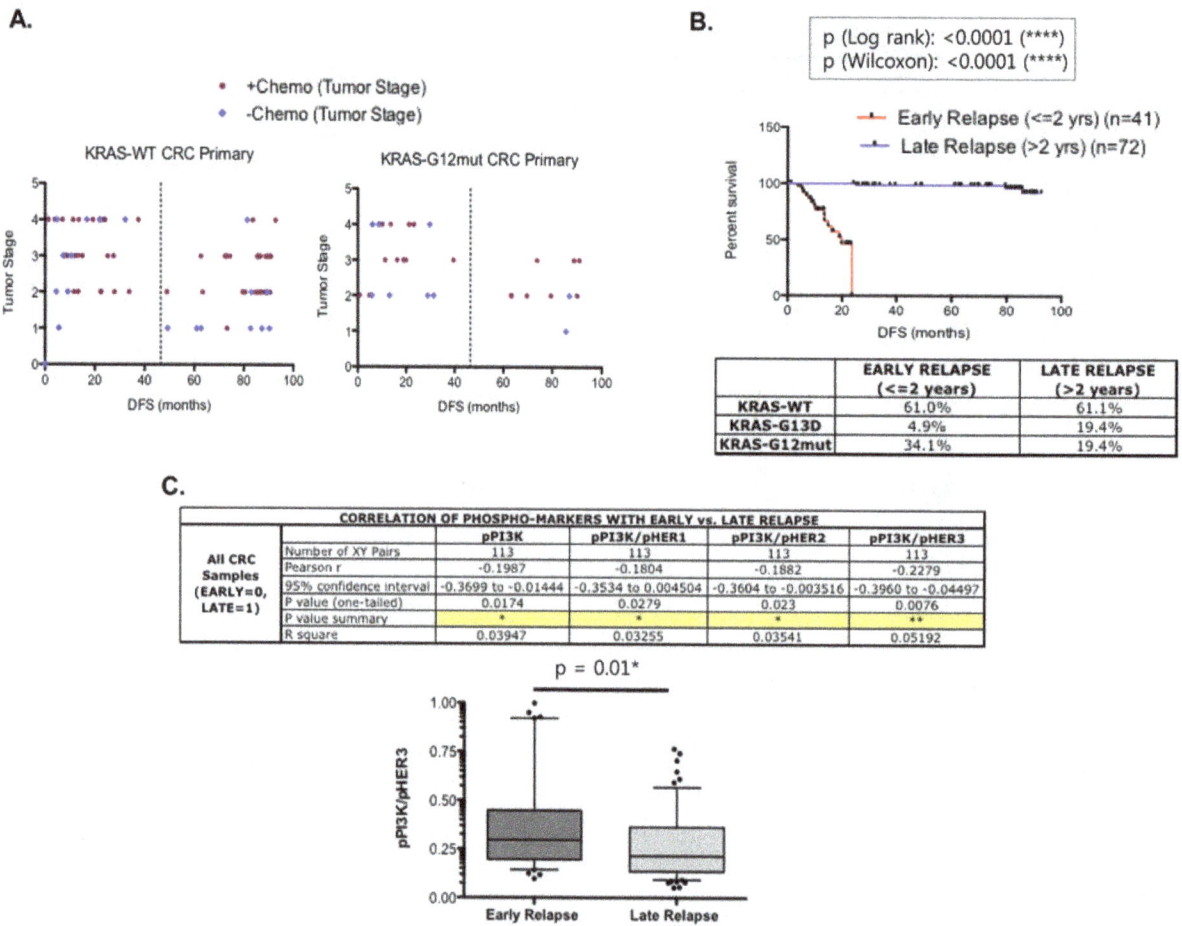

Figure 1. Heterogeneity in colorectal cancers (CRCs). (A) Plot of disease-free survival (DFS) versus tumor stage in *KRAS* WT and G12mut primary CRCs. Each dot represents an individual patient and the brown and blue dots indicate patients that did or did not receive adjuvant chemotherapy, respectively. (B) Comparative DFS curves of CRC samples segregated by their recurrence times post-surgery. DFS for early relapse patients (recurrence ≤2 years) is shown in red and DFS for late relapse patients (recurrence >2 years) is shown in blue. p-Values are indicated. The table below the graph lists the percentage of patients with a specific *KRAS* genotype in each group. (C) Pearson correlation analysis of early vs. late relapse CRCs to the expression of pPI3K, pPI3K/pHER1, pPI3K/pHER2, and pPI3K/pHER3 in the entire CRC cohort. Significant correlations are highlighted in yellow. The plot in the box shows the difference in the pPI3K/pHER3 ratios in early relapse vs. late relapse CRCs.

whereas 47 patients had rectum primary. Approximately 70% of the patients underwent adjuvant chemo- or radiotherapy depending on the primary tumor location. Ten colon-liver metastasis pairs and one colon-peritoneal seeding pair were included in the analysis. All tissues, including paired specimens, were procured at the time of surgery and immediately snap-frozen at the surgical field for future molecular analysis.

Differential signaling pathway activations predicted poor survival better than KRAS mutations

KRAS mutations, with *KRAS* G12D and G13D mutations being the most frequent, were observed in 39% (45/115) of the samples in our CRC patient cohort. In particular, 28/115 patients carried the *KRAS* G12 mutations and 17/115 patients carried the *KRAS* G13D mutations. Mutations in *BRAF*, which is downstream of *KRAS*, were found in 4% (5/115) of the patients. Although *KRAS* G12-mutated CRCs are generally associated with poor prognosis, a considerable percentage of *KRAS* WT CRCs showed low DFS and some *KRAS* G12 mutated CRCs showed high DFS regardless of their tumor stage (Fig. 1A). Tumors in each *KRAS* mutational subtype demonstrated a similar median expression of phosphorylated ERK (pERK), which is downstream

of *KRAS* (Fig. S1). An equivalent percentage of CRC tumors expressed pERK above the median (51.8% in *KRAS* WT, 48.5% in G12 mutated, and 44.4% in G13D mutated tumors).

As expected, the survival curves for the two cohorts were significantly different (Fig. 1B), with the respective median survival times of 19.8 months for early relapse (2 years from surgery) and undefined for late relapse (hazard ratio = 117.5). As shown in Fig. 1C, higher expression of activated PI3K correlated with early relapse and specifically, higher expression of pPI3K/pHER ratios was significantly associated with an early relapse. PI3K is an important downstream signaling effector of the HER kinase axis with direct binding sites on HER3. The cut off value for pPIK3/HER3 ratio was determined as shown in Fig.S2 in File S1. Furthermore, pPI3K/pHER3 expression was significantly higher in CRC tumors that relapsed within 2 years (Fig. 1C). Therefore, enhanced PI3K signaling was observed in CRCs with a shorter DFS or poorer prognosis.

High PI3K signaling is associated with early recurrence in CRC

To gain further insight into the high vs. low pPI3K signaling CRC cohorts, we focused on the CRC sub-cohorts segregated by

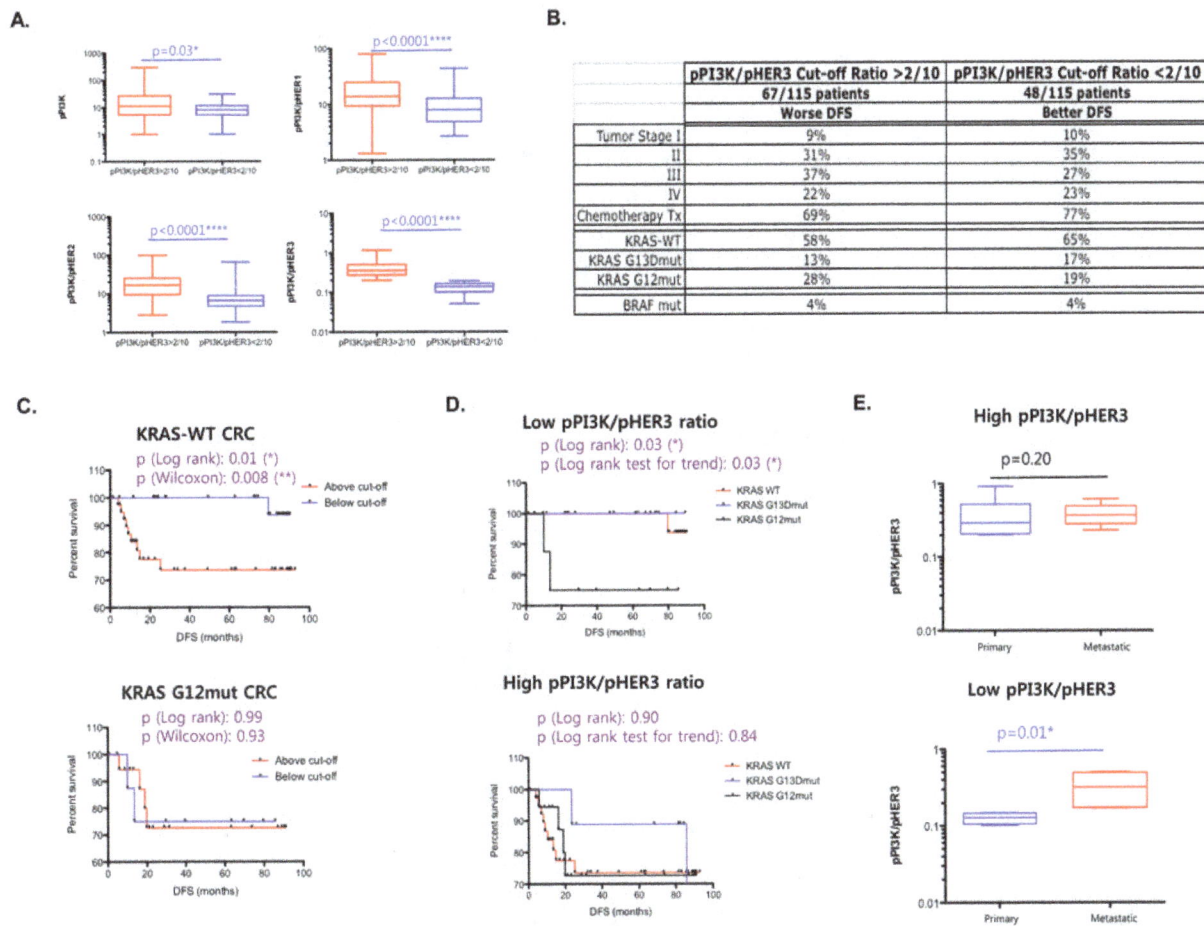

Figure 2. PI3K signaling in colorectal cancers (CRCs). The respective p-values are indicated. (A) Box plots of the Mann–Whitney *t*-test showing the difference in the expression of pPI3K, pPI3K/pHER1, pPI3K/pHER2, and pPI3K/pHER3 between the high pPI3K/pHER3 group and low pPI3K/pHER3 groups. The respective p-values are indicated. (B) Table listing the characteristics of primary CRCs in high PI3K (high pPI3K/pHER3) versus low PI3K (low pPI3K/pHER3) signaling cohorts. Characteristics include segregations based on tumor stage, status of chemotherapy treatment, and mutational status of *KRAS* and *BRAF*. Altogether, 67/115 samples are included in the high PI3K cohort and 48/115 samples are included in the low PI3K cohort. The numbers indicate the percentage of samples within each cohort based on each indicated characteristic. (C) DFS according to pPI3K/pHER3 ratios in *KRAS* WT and *KRAS* G12mut CRCs. (D) Kaplan–Meier survival curves of high PI3K (pPI3K/pHER3) and low PI3K cohorts comparing the DFS of *KRAS* WT, G13Dmut, and G12mut samples. (E) high PI3K (high pPI3K/pHER3) and low PI3K (low pPI3K/pHER3) groups in paired primary and metastatic CRC samples.

the pPI3K/pHER3 ratio (Fig. 2A). Patient characteristics in the high vs. low pPI3K signaling CRC cohorts were well balanced in terms of their tumor stage, chemotherapy treatments, and mutational status of the oncogenes *KRAS* and *BRAF* (Fig. 2B). DFS of *KRAS* WT CRCs with higher pPI3K/pHER3 expression was significantly worse than that of *KRAS* WT CRCs with lower pPI3K/pHER3 expression (Fig. 2C); however, *KRAS* G12mut tumors demonstrated poor DFS regardless of their level of pPI3K expression. Interestingly, DFS comparisons of *KRAS* WT, G13Dmut, and G12mut CRCs within the low pPI3K group showed considerable differences, with *KRAS* WT and *KRAS* G13D tumors having a better survival than the *KRAS* G12mut tumors (Fig. 2D). Despite the dramatic differences in survival observed in the high and low pPI3K/pHER3 groups depending on their *KRAS* WT or G12 mutated genotype, the two groups were very similar in terms of their expression differences of the relevant markers. In other words, pPI3K/pHER1, pPI3K/pHER2, and pPI3K/pHER3 were expressed to considerably higher levels in the high pPI3K/pHER3 group in both *KRAS* WT and G12 mutated CRCs (Fig. S3 in File S1). Note that the pPI3K

expression was not considerably higher, but it was the pPI3K expression relative to the activated HER axis that was higher in the groups showing poor survival.

These data provided evidence that a high pPI3K signaling, which may possibly be driven by upstream signals other than or in addition to the HER axis, is associated with aggressive CRCs with early recurrence. Furthermore, these data clearly demonstrated the heterogeneity within the *KRAS* WT population based on the level of pPI3K expression in these tumors. On the other hand, *KRAS* G12-mutated CRCs typically demonstrated poor survival regardless of the level of pPI3K signaling.

PI3K-driven aggressive CRCs, including metastatic CRCs, show higher c-MET and IGF1R signaling than the HER axis signaling

Since higher pPI3K/pHER ratios correlated with early relapse CRCs, we hypothesized that there should also be a significant difference in pHER/pMET and pHER/pIGF1R ratios if pMET and pIGF1R are responsible for high pPI3K signaling. Next, we

A.

B.

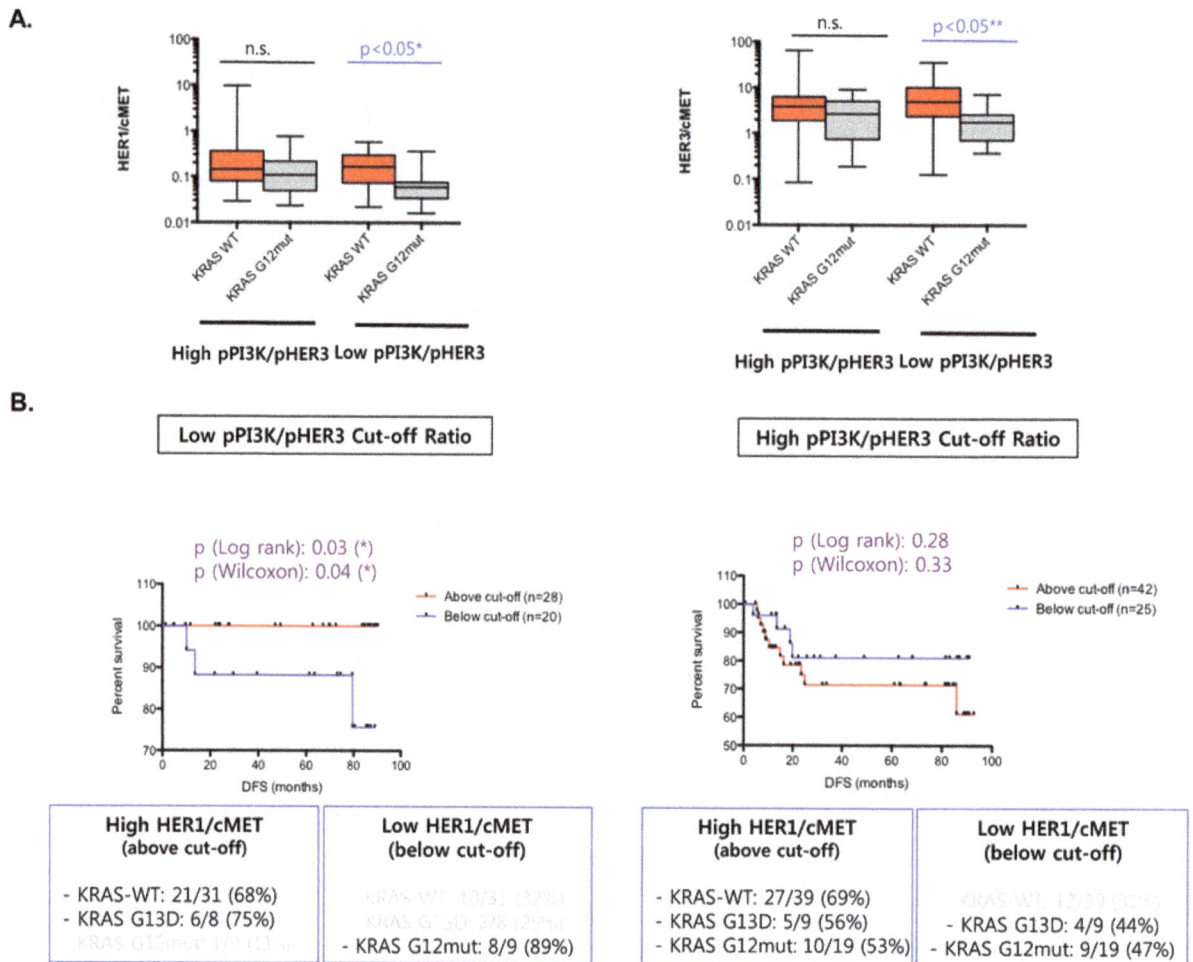

Figure 3. Relative c-MET and IGF1R expression in high and low PI3K signaling colorectal cancer (CRC) cohorts. (A) pMET/T-c-MET ratio was compared between high PI3K (high pPI3K/pHER3) and low PI3K (high pPI3K/pHER3) groups using the Mann–Whitney t-test. The comparison is shown in all CRCs, *KRAS* WT, G13D mutated, and G12 mutated CRCs. Significant differences with p-values are indicated in blue. (B) Comparative expression between high and low PI3K groups for the following markers: pHER1/pMET, pHER2/pMET, pHER3/pMET, pHER1/pIGF1R, pHER2/pIGF1R, and pHER3/pIGF1R. Significant differences with p-values are indicated in blue.

examined these signaling networks in 10 pairs of matched primary-metastatic synchronous samples available in our study cohort. The primary-metastatic CRC pairs were segregated into two groups based on the pPI3K/pHER3 expression ratio of the primary CRC sample in each pair. There was a significant increase in the pPI3K/pHER3 ratio for the matched metastatic samples in the low pPI3K/pHER3 ratio group (Fig. 2E), whereas it remained unchanged between primary and metastatic samples in the high pPI3K/pHER3 ratio group.

Aggressiveness of KRAS G12mut CRCs is correlated with high c-MET expression relative to HER axis members

We then attempted to identify markers that may be differentially expressed between *KRAS* WT and G12mut CRCs in the low pPI3K group. Based on our preliminary observation of high expression of total c-MET and IGF1R in *KRAS* G12mut tumors compared to the *KRAS* WT tumors (Fig. 3A, Fig. S4 in File S1), we examined whether a differential c-MET- or IGF1R-dependent expression may segregate the *KRAS* WT and G12mut subgroups within the low pPI3K/pHER3 ratio group. Relative HER1/c-MET and HER3/c-MET ratios were considerably higher in the *KRAS* WT CRCs than in *KRAS* G12mut tumors (Fig. 3B) in the

low pPI3K/pHER3 group, but not in the high pPI3K/pHER3 group, which was consistent with the DFS differences (Fig. 3A). We investigated whether appropriate ratios of HER1/c-MET (Fig. S5 in File S1) or HER3/c-MET may also segregate the DFS differences observed between the *KRAS* WT and G12mut CRCs within the low pPI3K/pHER3 ratio group. Analysis of the *KRAS* genotypes of the samples in the two sub-cohorts revealed that the majority of the *KRAS* WT and G13D samples were present in the high HER1/c-MET sub-cohort (i.e., HER1 > c-MET), whereas the majority of the *KRAS* G12mut samples were present in the low HER1/c-MET sub-cohort (i.e., HER1 < c-MET) (Fig. 3C). A similar HER1/c-MET cut-off ratio did not segregate the high pPI3K/pHER3 group based on the *KRAS* genotypes (Fig. 3D). Parallel analysis with a HER3/c-MET index resulted in similar but less robust data that did not segregate the KRAS WT and G12mut CRCs as distinctly as the HER1/c-MET index (*data not shown*). These data indicated that the aggressive *KRAS* G12mut tumors are molecularly distinct because they are mostly marked by a high c-MET expression, which is equivalent to or higher than HER1 and HER3 expression.

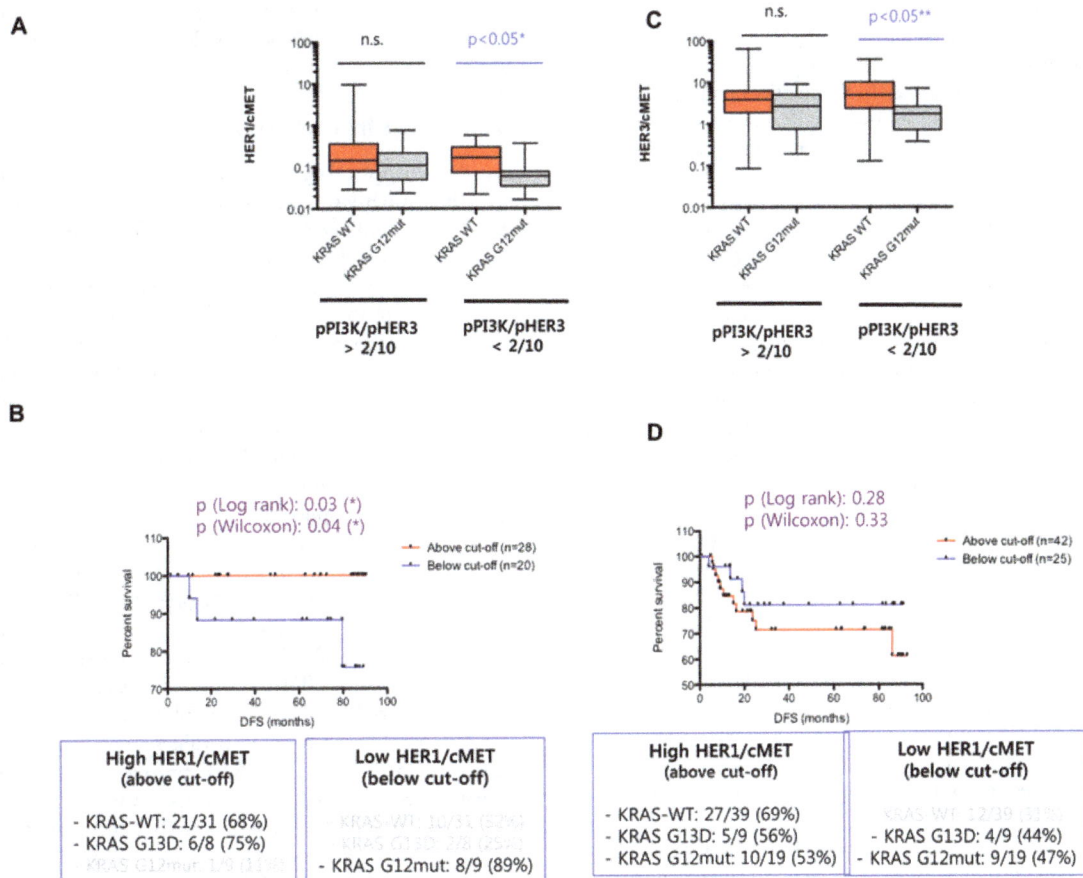

Figure 4. Summary of colorectal cancer (CRC) sub-classifications based on their signaling pathway profiles. Schematic summarizing the sub-classification of CRCs based on their signaling pathway profiles and *KRAS* mutational status. The possible therapeutic options for each sub-class based on their pathway profiles are indicated.

Discussion

This study was based on the hypothesis that the status of activated signaling pathways in *KRAS* WT and mutant CRCs can provide additional information that may be useful for understanding the therapeutic outcomes in these tumors [17–19]. The analysis presented in this study gives evidence that CRC can be sub-classified based on its signaling pathway molecular profiles regardless of the *KRAS* mutational status, as summarized in Fig. 4. Besides providing molecular insights into CRC prognosis, such a pathway-based profiling can have important implications on stratifying the CRC patient population for appropriate therapeutic strategies.

Prognosis of CRC primary tumors post-surgery has been correlated with their *KRAS* mutational status [21]. Although this general trend was also observed in our CRC sample cohort, with *KRAS* WT tumors demonstrating better DFS post-surgery than *KRAS* G12 mutant tumors, it was not significant due to the heterogeneity in the signaling pathways within each *KRAS* mutational subtype, especially in stage II and III CRC tumors regardless of whether or not the patients received chemotherapy. This suggests that *KRAS* mutations confer only part of the advantage needed for tumor cell survival with additional survival signals presumably deriving from multiple signaling pathways. CRCs with high PI3K activity relapsed within 2 years independent of their *KRAS* mutational status and had poor prognosis. Even *KRAS* WT CRCs with high PI3K signaling were as aggressive as

the *KRAS* G12mut CRCs with indistinguishable DFS post-surgery. In contrast, *KRAS* WT CRCs with low PI3K signaling activity demonstrated a better prognosis and could be segregated from the aggressive *KRAS* G12mut CRCs with an appropriate HER1/c-MET index cut-off ratio, because c-MET expression levels were higher in *KRAS* G12mut CRCs. In our study cohort, these *KRAS* WT CRCs constituted ~44% of the total *KRAS* WT population and revealed heterogeneity. Heterogeneity in *KRAS* WT CRC populations has been previously noticed in numerous other studies, because not all *KRAS* WT CRCs are responsive to anti-EGFR antibodies. One possible reason has been described as the presence of *BRAF* mutations. The number of *BRAF*-mutated samples in our cohort was too small to draw any reasonable conclusions; however, 3/5 of *BRAF*-mutated CRCs in the presence of WT *KRAS* demonstrated a high PI3K signaling. Our study provides a possible mechanism for the heterogeneity in *KRAS* WT CRCs and we speculate that 44% of the *KRAS* WT CRCs with low PI3K signaling and high HER1 expression may be those responsive to anti-HER therapies such as anti-EGFR antibodies. Approximately 47% of the CRC samples with *KRAS* G13D mutations were recently suggested to have distinct therapy-based outcome characteristics [8] and were tracked with our *KRAS* WT samples in terms of having low PI3K signaling and a high HER1 expression. The relevance of PI3K signaling and PI3K/mTOR inhibitors has been previously suggested in *KRAS* mutant [22] and *BRAF* mutant [23] CRCs. The results from our study are consistent with these reports and further expand the importance of PI3K signaling in CRCs regardless of their mutational status.

Relatively high c-MET and IGF1R activities compared to HER kinase members activities in aggressive CRCs suggested that these alternative RTKs may be the drivers of the high PI3K signaling. KRAS G12-mutated CRCs were noted to express higher c-MET receptor levels than the HER members that correlated with their poor prognosis. Most compelling evidence in support of c-MET- and IGF1R-driven PI3K activity in aggressive CRCs came from the primary-metastatic sample pairs, in which these markers showed a clear increase in the metastatic counterpart when compared to the matched primary sample, even though the mutational status of the pair remained unchanged. It is important to note that expression differences for single markers did not present meaningful differences but it was the relative expression of pHER signaling to pMET and pIGF1R that revealed considerably differential patterns between CRCs that were more aggressive and relapsed earlier versus the ones that were associated with better prognosis. Currently, there are no tangible options to identify aggressive CRCs and defining therapeutic options to treat them. Mutational tests are the only available strategy, which does not identify the aggressive KRAS WT CRCs. Our study provides evidence for activated signaling pathway profiles that are superior to oncogenic mutational tests alone, because these results can be utilized to identify aggressive CRCs and possibly guide therapeutic strategies. The clinical implication of combinatorial protein profiling and mutational tests in terms of drug sensitivity is currently being tested both in preclinical and prospective clinical studies.

Our study also uncovered a substantial variation in phosphorylated proteomic profiling between matched primary and metastatic CRCs. This was in contrast with genotyping, according to which there was complete concordance between primary and metastatic tumor tissues. This is in line with the results from one of the largest comparison studies between primary and matched liver metastases in 305 CRC patients (concordance rate, 96.4%; 95% confidence interval, 93.6–98.2%) [24]. Furthermore, a recent genomic analysis on 84 patients with primary CRC and liver metastases demonstrated a high concordance rate of >90% between primary and liver metastases for five genes (i.e., KRAS, NRAS, BRAF, PIK3CA, TP53) [25]. One of the most plausible hypotheses for such high concordance rate in the mutational status is that KRAS mutations are the early driving events in CRC progression from adenoma [26]. If these differences in pathway profiling correlate with the treatment responses to specific RTK inhibitors, we may need to biopsy metastatic sites in addition to primary tumors to obtain a more precise prediction of the treatment response. However, our sample size was very small with only ten pairs of primary and metastasis. Hence, more extensive paired analysis is needed to rigorously address this discrepancy in proteomic profiling.

In conclusion, our study demonstrates that there is significant heterogeneity in activated protein signaling pathways despite a similar mutational status in CRC. Therefore, dichotomizing CRC simply as KRAS mutant versus KRAS WT may be an underestimation of the molecular heterogeneity within each subgroup of CRC. Moreover, a more comprehensive signaling pathway profiling, in addition to oncogenic mutational tests, should be performed to obtain a clearer molecular identity of the tumors.

Supporting Information

File S1 Supporting Figures. Figure S1. Profiling of signaling pathway markers in colorectal cancers using CEER. (A) Ranking of pERK expression from high to low in KRAS wild-type, G12 mutated and G13D mutated CRCs is shown in a waterfall plot. pERK expression above the median is represented on the positive y-axis. pAKT expression in each sample is also shown. The table below shows the median pERK CU values in each mutational subgroup of CRC tumors as well as the percentage of tumors that express pERK above the median. (B) CEER immuno-array images for indicated signal transduction proteins in 8 colorectal samples. As represented with a color bar below the immuno-array, a white or a red represents a high level expression or phosphorylation whereas a green or a blue represents a low level expression or phosphorylation of the respective markers. Tumor stage and the KRAS mutational status of each sample are indicated. **Figure S2. Effect of pPI3K/ pHER3 index on disease-free survival in CRCs.** Comparative DFS curves of CRC samples segregated by decreasing pPI3K/pHER3 ratios. DFS for samples above each respective cut-off is shown in red and DFS for samples below each respective cut-off is shown in blue. Respective p-values are indicated. **Figure S3. Characteristics of matched primary-metastatic CRC sample pairs.** Table listing primary tumor characteristics of the 10 matched primary-metastatic CRC pairs segregated by their pPI3K/pHER3 expression ratios. 6 pairs of matched samples are included in the worse DFS group where pPI3K/pHER3 expression was >2/10. Characteristics include number of samples in each tumor stage, whether the patient received chemotherapy and number of samples based on the mutational status of KRAS, BRAF and PIK3CA. **Figure S4. Comparative signaling marker expression between KRAS WT and G12 mutated CRCs.** Box plots showing Mann Whitney t-test based expression differences in total and phosphorylated HER1, HER2, HER3, cMET, IGF1R, pPI3K, pSHC, pAKT and pERK in KRAS WT and G12 mutated CRCs. Significant differences with respective p values are indicated. **Figure S5. DFS segregation based on HER1/cMET index.** Comparative DFS curves of CRC samples within the pPI3K/pHER3<2/10 group segregated by decreasing HER1/cMET ratios. DFS for samples above each respective cut-off is shown in red and DFS for samples below each respective cut-off is shown in blue. Respective p-values are indicated.

File S2 Supplementary Methods.

Author Contributions

Conceived and designed the experiments: JL PK HCK SS. Performed the experiments: PK TL AK FP IGD SHK. Analyzed the data: JL AJ PK SS HCK. Contributed reagents/materials/analysis tools: IGD SHK JOP YSP HCK. Contributed to the writing of the manuscript: JL AJ PK HCK.

References

1. Douillard JY, Siena S, Cassidy J, Tabernero J, Burkes R, et al. (2010) Randomized, phase III trial of panitumumab with infusional fluorouracil, leucovorin, and oxaliplatin (FOLFOX4) versus FOLFOX4 alone as first-line treatment in patients with previously untreated metastatic colorectal cancer: the PRIME study. J Clin Oncol 28: 4697–4705.

2. Starling N, Cunningham D (2005) Cetuximab in previously treated colorectal cancer. Clin Colorectal Cancer 5 Suppl 1: S28–33.

3. Tabernero J, Van Cutsem E, Diaz-Rubio E, Cervantes A, Humblet Y, et al. (2007) Phase II trial of cetuximab in combination with fluorouracil, leucovorin, and oxaliplatin in the first-line treatment of metastatic colorectal cancer. J Clin Oncol 25: 5225–5232.

4. Van Cutsem E, Kohne CH, Hitre E, Zaluski J, Chang Chien CR, et al. (2009) Cetuximab and chemotherapy as initial treatment for metastatic colorectal cancer. N Engl J Med 360: 1408–1417.

5. Bardelli A, Siena S (2010) Molecular mechanisms of resistance to cetuximab and panitumumab in colorectal cancer. J Clin Oncol 28: 1254–1261.

6. Poehlmann A, Kuester D, Meyer F, Lippert H, Roessner A, et al. (2007) K-ras mutation detection in colorectal cancer using the Pyrosequencing technique. Pathol Res Pract 203: 489–497.

7. Raponi M, Winkler H, Dracopoli NC (2008) KRAS mutations predict response to EGFR inhibitors. Curr Opin Pharmacol 8: 413–418.

8. De Roock W, Jonker DJ, Di Nicolantonio F, Sartore-Bianchi A, Tu D, et al. (2010) Association of KRAS p.G13D mutation with outcome in patients with chemotherapy-refractory metastatic colorectal cancer treated with cetuximab. JAMA 304: 1812–1820.

9. Karapetis CS, Khambata-Ford S, Jonker DJ, O'Callaghan CJ, Tu D, et al. (2008) K-ras mutations and benefit from cetuximab in advanced colorectal cancer. N Engl J Med 359: 1757–1765.

10. Allegra CJ, Jessup JM, Somerfield MR, Hamilton SR, Hammond EH, et al. (2009) American Society of Clinical Oncology provisional clinical opinion: testing for KRAS gene mutations in patients with metastatic colorectal carcinoma to predict response to anti-epidermal growth factor receptor monoclonal antibody therapy. J Clin Oncol 27: 2091–2096.

11. De Roock W, Claes B, Bernasconi D, De Schutter J, Biesmans B, et al. (2010) Effects of KRAS, BRAF, NRAS, and PIK3CA mutations on the efficacy of cetuximab plus chemotherapy in chemotherapy-refractory metastatic colorectal cancer: a retrospective consortium analysis. Lancet Oncol 11: 753–762.

12. Gupta S, Ramjaun AR, Haiko P, Wang Y, Warne PH, et al. (2007) Binding of ras to phosphoinositide 3-kinase p110alpha is required for ras-driven tumorigenesis in mice. Cell 129: 957–968.

13. Cantley LC, Neel BG (1999) New insights into tumor suppression: PTEN suppresses tumor formation by restraining the phosphoinositide 3-kinase/AKT pathway. Proc Natl Acad Sci U S A 96: 4240–4245.

14. Juric D, Baselga J (2012) Tumor genetic testing for patient selection in phase I clinical trials: the case of PI3K inhibitors. J Clin Oncol 30: 765–766.

15. Martin-Fernandez C, Bales J, Hodgkinson C, Welman A, Welham MJ, et al. (2009) Blocking phosphoinositide 3-kinase activity in colorectal cancer cells reduces proliferation but does not increase apoptosis alone or in combination with cytotoxic drugs. Mol Cancer Res 7: 955–965.

16. Roper J, Richardson MP, Wang WV, Richard LG, Chen W, et al. (2011) The dual PI3K/mTOR inhibitor NVP-BEZ235 induces tumor regression in a genetically engineered mouse model of PIK3CA wild-type colorectal cancer. PLoS One 6: e25132.

17. Elkabets M, Vora S, Juric D, Morse N, Mino-Kenudson M, et al. (2013) mTORC1 Inhibition Is Required for Sensitivity to PI3K p110alpha Inhibitors in PIK3CA-Mutant Breast Cancer. Sci Transl Med 5: 196ra199.

18. Kim P, Liu X, Lee T, Liu L, Barham R, et al. (2011) Highly sensitive proximity mediated immunoassay reveals HER2 status conversion in the circulating tumor cells of metastatic breast cancer patients. Proteome Sci 9: 75.

19. Ward TM, Iorns E, Liu X, Hoe N, Kim P, et al. (2013) Truncated p110 ERBB2 induces mammary epithelial cell migration, invasion and orthotopic xenograft formation, and is associated with loss of phosphorylated STAT5. Oncogene 32: 2463–2474.

20. Morlan J, Baker J, Sinicropi D (2009) Mutation detection by real-time PCR: a simple, robust and highly selective method. PLoS One 4: e4584.

21. Phipps AI, Buchanan DD, Makar KW, Win AK, Baron JA, et al. (2013) KRAS-mutation status in relation to colorectal cancer survival: the joint impact of correlated tumour markers. Br J Cancer 108: 1757–1764.

22. Ebi H, Corcoran RB, Singh A, Chen Z, Song Y, et al. (2011) Receptor tyrosine kinases exert dominant control over PI3K signaling in human KRAS mutant colorectal cancers. J Clin Invest 121: 4311–4321.

23. Coffee EM, Faber AC, Roper J, Sinnamon MJ, Goel G, et al. (2013) Concomitant BRAF and PI3K/mTOR blockade is required for effective treatment of BRAF(V600E) colorectal cancer. Clin Cancer Res 19: 2688–2698.

24. Knijn N, Mekenkamp LJ, Klomp M, Vink-Borger ME, Tol J, et al. (2011) KRAS mutation analysis: a comparison between primary tumours and matched liver metastases in 305 colorectal cancer patients. Br J Cancer 104: 1020–1026.

25. Vakiani E, Janakiraman M, Shen R, Sinha R, Zeng Z, et al. (2012) Comparative genomic analysis of primary versus metastatic colorectal carcinomas. J Clin Oncol 30: 2956–2962.

26. Vogelstein B, Fearon ER, Hamilton SR, Kern SE, Preisinger AC, et al. (1988) Genetic alterations during colorectal-tumor development. N Engl J Med 319: 525–532.

7

Chemotherapy-Induced Monoamine Oxidase Expression in Prostate Carcinoma Functions as a Cytoprotective Resistance Enzyme and Associates with Clinical Outcomes

Ryan R. Gordon[1,◈], Mengchu Wu[1,◈], Chung-Ying Huang[1], William P. Harris[1], Hong Gee Sim[1], Jared M. Lucas[1], Ilsa Coleman[1], Celestia S. Higano[3,5], Roman Gulati[1], Lawrence D. True[4,5], Robert Vessella[5], Paul H. Lange[5], Mark Garzotto[6,7], Tomasz M. Beer[2], Peter S. Nelson[1,3,4,5]*

1 Divisions of Human Biology and Clinical Research, Fred Hutchinson Cancer Research Center, Seattle, Washington, United States of America, 2 Department of Medicine, Oregon Health and Sciences University, Portland, Oregon, United States of America, 3 Department of Medicine, University of Washington, Seattle, Washington, United States of America, 4 Department of Pathology, University of Washington, Seattle, Washington, United States of America, 5 Department of Urology, University of Washington, Seattle, Washington, United States of America, 6 Department of Urology and Cancer Institute, Oregon Health and Sciences University, Portland, Oregon, United States of America, 7 Section of Urology, Portland VA Medical Center, Portland, Oregon, United States of America

Abstract

To identify molecular alterations in prostate cancers associating with relapse following neoadjuvant chemotherapy and radical prostatectomy patients with high-risk localized prostate cancer were enrolled into a phase I-II clinical trial of neoadjuvant chemotherapy with docetaxel and mitoxantrone followed by prostatectomy. Pre-treatment prostate tissue was acquired by needle biopsy and post-treatment tissue was acquired by prostatectomy. Prostate cancer gene expression measurements were determined in 31 patients who completed 4 cycles of neoadjuvant chemotherapy. We identified 141 genes with significant transcript level alterations following chemotherapy that associated with subsequent biochemical relapse. This group included the transcript encoding monoamine oxidase A (MAOA). *In vitro*, cytotoxic chemotherapy induced the expression of MAOA and elevated MAOA levels enhanced cell survival following docetaxel exposure. MAOA activity increased the levels of reactive oxygen species and increased the expression and nuclear translocation of HIF1α. The suppression of MAOA activity using the irreversible inhibitor clorgyline augmented the apoptotic responses induced by docetaxel. In summary, we determined that the expression of MAOA is induced by exposure to cytotoxic chemotherapy, increases HIF1α, and contributes to docetaxel resistance. As MAOA inhibitors have been approved for human use, regimens combining MAOA inhibitors with docetaxel may improve clinical outcomes.

Editor: Philip C. Trackman, Boston University Goldman School of Dental Medicine, United States of America

Funding: MW was supported by a fellowship from the AUA Foundation. CYH was supported by a fellowship from the DOD CDMRP in Prostate Cancer (PC050489). RG was supported by a fellowship from the DOD CDMRP in Prostate Cancer (PC110257). This work was supported by grants R01CA119125, PC093509, P01CA085859, and the PNW Prostate Cancer SPORE (CA097186). The funders had no role in study design, data collection and analysis, decision to publish, or preparation of the manuscript.

Competing Interests: The authors have declared that no competing interests exist.

* Email: pnelson@fhcrc.org

◈ These authors contributed equally to this work.

Introduction

Despite numerous clinical trials conducted over a span of more than four decades, few interventions have extended survival in patients with advanced castration resistant prostate cancer (CRPC). Among these are the chemotherapeutic agent docetaxel which results in a median life-span extension of about 2 months, though few patients sustain durable complete remissions [1,2]. For several types of solid tumors, notably neoplasms of the breast [3] and colon [4], cytotoxic drugs administered in conjunction with surgery or radiation have demonstrated survival benefits for those clinically-localized tumors with features indicating a predilection

for early micrometastasis, or those with only documented local or regional spread. However, to date no studies have demonstrated a benefit for the addition of chemotherapy to primary surgical or radiotherapy approaches for prostate cancer as determined by outcomes of disease relapse or survival rates. Further, of five clinical studies evaluating neoadjuvant docetaxel alone or combined with other agents prior to prostatectomy, pathological complete responses are extremely rare [5–9]. These results indicate that prostate cancers either exhibit a high degree of intrinsic resistance to taxanes and other cytostatic and cytotoxic drugs, and/or rapidly acquire refractory phenotypes. Defining mechanisms underlying chemotherapy resistance is critical for selecting patients who may optimally benefit from specific regimens, and for designing new therapeutic strategies that either avoid – or specifically target resistance pathways.

To identify molecular changes associated with tumor cell exposure to chemotherapy agents commonly used in the treatment of prostate cancer, we conducted a prospective phase I-II clinical trial of neoadjuvant docetaxel and mitoxantrone in patients with high-risk localized prostate adenocarcinoma [10]. There were no complete pathological responses identified at the time of prosta-tectomy, and thus tumors analyzed after docetaxel and mitoxan-trone exposure are presumably enriched for cells with molecular features contributing to therapy resistance. Although residual viable tumor cells were identified in each case, chemotherapy effects were evident [11]. We previously reported the results of profiling gene expression changes in microdissected tumors acquired in the context of this study and found that post-therapy gene expression varied substantially between individuals [12]. However, the short follow-up interval post-therapy precluded analyses to determine if gene expression changes were associated with tumor recurrence, a situation expected to occur through the survival and subsequent proliferation of subclinical micrometasta-sis present at the time of initial treatment.

In the present study we sought to test the hypothesis that gene expression changes in prostate cancer cells following exposure to cytotoxic chemotherapy would associate with clinical outcomes. The median follow-up of the cohort of prostate cancer patients treated with neoadjuvant docetaxel and mitoxantrone was 40 months at the time of this analysis. Molecular changes associating with relapse included increases in transcripts encoding monoamine oxidase A (MAOA). MAOA is a key enzyme involved in the degradation of the biogenic and dietary monoamine neurotrans-mitters such as 5-hydroxytryptamine (5-HT, or serotonin) and norepinephrine. Amine metabolism is linked to essential cellular processes such as cell growth and differentiation, and the catalytic byproducts of MAOA, such as hydrogen peroxide, are known to cause oxidative damage with implications for cancer, aging and neurodegenerative processes. We previously found that MAOA expression was upregulated in prostate cancers in association with higher Gleason grades [13], but mechanisms modulating cytotoxic drug effects have not been established. Two features of MAOA provided additional rationale for studies of this enzyme in the context of therapy resistance: approved inhibitors of MAOA are currently in routine clinical use for psychiatric illness and the safety and toxicity profiles are established. Second, MAOA enzymatic properties have been exploited to develop positron-emission tomography (PET)-based imaging reagents for localizing MAOA activity in humans. These features provide a clear path for the rapid clinical evaluation of MAOA as a therapeutic target in the context of advanced prostate cancer once sufficient preclinical evidence of roles in therapy resistance are established.

Materials and Methods

Ethics Statement

The clinical trial protocol (NCT00017563) was approved by the Institutional Review Boards of the Oregon Health & Science University, Portland VA Medical Center, Kaiser Permanente Northwest Region, Legacy Health System, and the University of Washington. All patients signed informed consent. All mouse studies were approved by the Fred Hutchinson Cancer Research Center (FHCRC) Institutional Animal Care and Use Committee (IACUC) and performed in accordance with the approved protocols.

Patients and Study Description

Fifty-seven patients with high-risk localized prostate cancer (defined as TNM>cT2b or T3a or PSA≥15 ng/ml or Gleason grade ≥4+3) were recruited between 2001 and 2004 for a phase I-II clinical trial of neoadjuvant chemotherapy. The design of this clinical trial has been previously described [8,10]. The trial identifier is NCT00017563.

Prostate Tissue Collection, Processing and Microarray Profiling of Gene Expression

Details of the tissue collection and gene expression profiling have been previously described in detail [8]. Briefly, transrectal ultrasound-guided needle biopsies were obtained from each patient at study entry and snap-frozen in liquid nitrogen prior to chemotherapy. At radical prostatectomy, cancer-containing tissue samples were snap frozen immediately after prostate removal. Benign and neoplastic epithelial cells were separately acquired by laser-capture microdissection (LCM) using an Arcturus PixCell IIe microscope (Arcturus, Mountain View, CA). Total RNA was extracted from captured epithelium using a Picopure RNA isolation kit according to the manufacturer's instructions (Arcturus Inc., Mountain View, CA), and amplified using the messageAMP aRNA kit (Ambion, Austin, TX). Labeled cDNA probes were hybridized in a head-to-head fashion, pre-chemotherapy versus post-chemotherapy simultaneously to cDNA microarrays as we have previously described [14].

Quantitative reverse transcription PCR

cDNA was synthesized from 1 μg amplified RNA (aRNA) from paired pre- vs. post-treated patient samples, or 1 μg RNA extracted from cultured cells, using 2 μg random hexamers for priming reverse transcription by SuperScript II (200 U per reaction; Invitrogen). Quantitative reverse transcription real-time PCR (qRT-PCR) reactions were done in duplicate, using approximately 5 ng of cDNA, 0.2 μM of each primer, and SYBR Green PCR master mix (Applied Biosystems, Foster City, CA) in a 20 μl reaction volume and analyzed using an Applied Biosystems 7700 sequence detector. Samples were normalized to the cycle threshold value obtained during the exponential amplification of GAPDH. Control reactions with RNA or water as template did not produce significant amplification products. The sequences of primers used in this study were: GAPDH forward, 5′-CCTCAAC-GACCACTTTGTCA-3′; GAPDH reverse, 5′-TTACTCCTTG-GAGGCCATGT-3′; MAOA forward, 5′-AAAGTG-GAGCGGCTACATGG-3′; MAOA reverse, 5′-CAGAAAC-AGAGGGCAGGTTCC-3′; pleiotrophin (PTN) forward: 5′-GGGCAGCAATTTAAATGTTATGACTA-3′; PTN reverse: 5′-ACCCCCATTTTGCTGACTACATT-3′.

Cell Cultures and Treatments

The androgen responsive prostate cancer cell line, LNCaP and androgen insensitive prostate cancer cell line PC3 (both from the American Type Culture Collection, Manassas, VA) were grown in RPMI 1640 supplemented with 10% heat-inactivated fetal bovine serum and 100 IU/ml penicillin (Invitrogen Corp, Carlsbad, CA). The MAOA specific inhibitor, N-Methyl-N-propargyl-3-(2,4-dichlorophenoxy) propylamine hydrochloride (clorgyline), was purchased from Sigma-Aldrich (St Louis, MO). Docetaxel (provided by Sanofi-Aventis, Bridgewater, NJ) was diluted in 70% ethanol and used at 1 nM, 10 nM, and 100 nM concentra-tions for LNCaP cells and 50 nM and 200 nM for PC3 cells. For HIF1a expression studies, VCaP cells were grown in DMEM-F12 with 10% FBS. The MAOA specific inhibitor clorgyline (Sigma-

Aldrich, St Louis, MO) was diluted in 70% ethanol and used at 1 μM concentration. Total RNA was isolated using the RNeasy kit (Qiagen, Valencia, CA). cDNA was synthesized using the SuperScript II Reverse Transcriptase kit (Invitrogen Corp, Carlsbad, CA). qRT-PCR reactions were done in triplicate, using SYBR Green master mix (Applied Biosystems, Foster City, CA) and analyzed using an Applied Biosystems 7700 sequence detector. Samples were normalized to the expression level of GAPDH.

MAOA Expression

The full-length human MAOA cDNA was amplified from human placenta cDNA using the pair of primers, huMAOA_B-stUI_170: GTCCGCGAAAGCATGGAG and huMAOA_E-coRI_1788: GCAGAGAGCATAAGAATTCAACTTCA. The amplification products were first cloned into pCR2.1 and then subcloned into the retro-viral vector pBABE-puro using BstU I and EcoR I sites. pBABE-puro-MAOA as well as the empty vector pBABE-puro were transfected into phoenix retro-viral packaging cells using Lipofectamine 2000 (Invitrogen Corp, Carlsbad, CA). The medium containing retrovirus expressing the vectors was collected and used to infect PC-3 cells followed by puromycin selection and confirmation of MAOA overexpression by both RT-PCR and western blot.

Cell proliferation and apoptosis assays

Cell proliferation was assessed using the MTS dye reduction assay (Promega Corp, Madison, WI). Briefly, 10 μl of MTS reagent was added to each well of the 96-well plate and incubated at 37°C for 60 min. The color change was assessed by measuring the absorbance value of each well at 450 nm with an ELx808 BioTek absorbance microplate reader (BioTek Instruments, Winooski, VT). The Apo-One Caspase-3/7 assay (Promega Corp, Madison, WI) was used to assess apoptosis as per the manufacturer's instructions.

MAO activity assay

MAO enzyme activity was assessed using the MAO-Glo assay (Promega Corp, Madison, WI). Cells were lysed using a passive lysis buffer (Promega Corp, Madison, WI) and a luminogenic MAOA substrate was added to the lysate to yield methyl ester luciferin. After incubating at room temperature for one hour, a detection reagent reconstituted from esterase and luciferase enzymes was added to each well and the luminescence was measured using a Berthold L9505 BioLumat microplate lumi-nometer (Berthold Technologies, Oak Ridge, TN).

Assay for Reactive Oxygen Species (ROS)

ROS was detected by CM-H2DCFDA (Invitrogen Corp, Carlsbad, CA). Cells were trypsinized and washed with PBS, incubated either with 10 μM of DCFDA in PBS or with PBS as a negative control at 37C for 30 min, washed with PBS and returned to media for a 30 min recovery period at 37C. Fluorescent cells in 10^5 cells were counted by flow cytometry. Mean fluorescence intensity was used as a measurement of ROS. The assay was done in a triplicate.

Western blot analysis

Whole cell lysates were prepared using RIPA buffer (25 mM Tris pH 7.6, 150 mM NaCl, 1% NP-40, 1% sodium deoxycho-late, 0.1% SDS) with added protease inhibitors (Roche, India-napolis, IN). Nuclear protein extracts were prepared using the Nuclear/Cytosol Fractionation Kit protocol (Biovision, Mountain

View, CA). Thirty micrograms of protein were subjected to electrophoresis for 45 min at 200 V on a SDS polyacrylamide gel and transferred to a PVDF filter. The filters were blocked with 3% BSA for 1 h and then incubated overnight with anti-MAOA polyclonal antibody, anti- NFkB (Santa Cruz Biotechnology, Santa Cruz, CA), anti-HIF-1α (BD Biosciences, Franklin Lakes, NJ), or with anti-β-actin goat antibody (Promega Corp, Madison, WI). The filters were then incubated with species appropriate horse-radish peroxidase labeled secondary antibodies (Thermo Scientif-ic, Rockford, IL). Immuno blots were visualized using SuperSignal West Pico Chemiluminescent Substrate (Thermo Scientific, Rock-ford, IL).

Xenograft experiments

Mouse xenograft models were generated via subcutaneous injections into the right flank of 8–10 week old male CB17 SCID mice (Taconic, Hudson, NY). Specifically, subcutaneous xeno-grafts were derived utilizing either PC3 cells engineered to stably overexpress MAOA or empty vector controls. Prior to injection cells were grown to 90% confluence, washed once with PBS and resuspended in ice-cold PBS. Animals were anesthetized and 10^6 cells were implanted subcutaneously in 200 microliters of 1:1 PBS:Matrigel solution. Once tumors were established, mice were dosed with 5 mg/kg docetaxel weekly by IP injection. For both treatment arms (MAOA and Control) 12 xenografts were generated and tumor growth was monitored for a period of 4 weeks post injection at which point tumors were excised and snap frozen. Tumor measurements and animal weights were assessed three times weekly and weekly, respectively. Total tumor volumes were calculated with the following formula: $(.5236) \times (L_1) \times (L_2)^2$, where L_1 represents the long axis and L_2 the short axis of the tumor [15]. Total RNA was extracted from frozen tumor sections using the RNeasy Mini RNA isolation kit (Qiagen, Valencia, CA) according to the manufactures protocol and further amplified to incorporate amino-allyl UTP using the MessageAmp II aRNA Kit (Ambion, Austin, TX). Samples were labeled and subsequently hybridized to Agilent 44K whole human genome expression arrays following the manufacturer's protocol (Agilent Technolo-gies Inc., Santa Clara, CA). Data were processed using the Agilent Feature Extraction software, normalized, and filtered to remove probes with average intensity levels of <300. Resulting data were analyzed using the Statistical Analysis of Microarray (SAM) program [16], setting the significance threshold at a q-value of < 0.5.

Statistical analysis

In order to identify genes whose expression was significantly related to biochemical (PSA) relapse free survival, gene expression profiles were analyzed for associations with biochemical relapse (http://linus.nci.nih.gov/BRB-ArrayTools.html). Briefly, we com-puted a statistical significance level for each gene related to biochemical relapse-free survival based on univariate proportional hazards models. Significant gene lists were determined by a threshold of $p<0.01$. The association of expression change of MAOA and time to PSA relapse was analyzed using a Cox proportional hazards model (Stata 8.0, Texus). Multivariate models included age, clinical stage, pathology Gleason grade, baseline PSA level, and post-chemotherapy MAOA expression change. The final model only included factors meeting a significance threshold of $p<0.1$. The statistical significance of assays of MAOA activity, cell proliferation, and apoptosis was evaluated using a Student's t test for 2-group comparisons. A value of $p<0.05$ was considered to be significant. The Statistical Analysis of Microarray (SAM) program was used to analyze expression

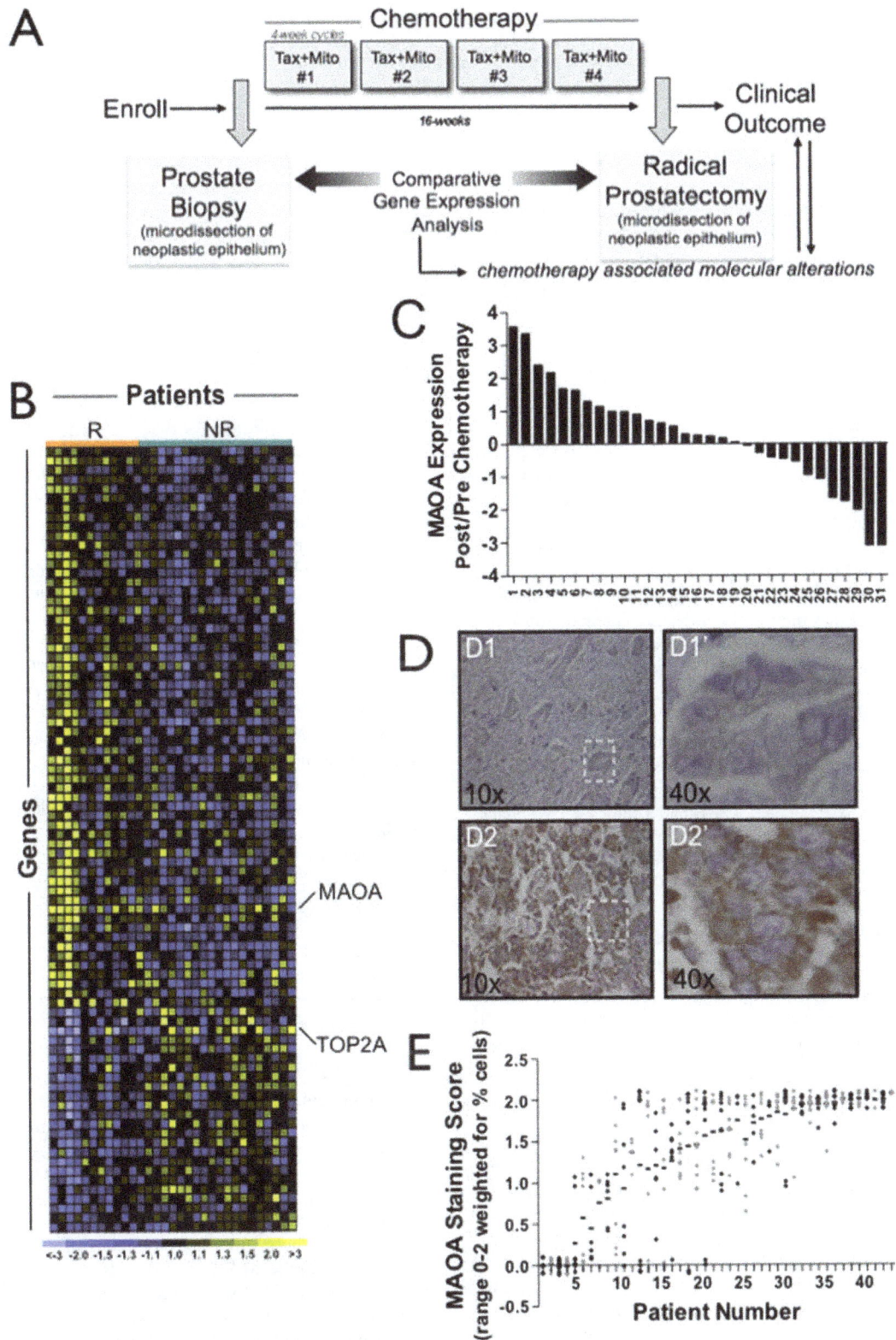

Figure 1. MAOA expression is induced *in vivo* following exposure to docetaxel and mitoxantrone. (A) Schema of the neoadjuvant chemotherapy and prostatectomy trial. (B) Heat-map of gene expression changes in prostate carcinoma cells that associate with biochemical relapse following radical prostatectomy. Columns are 31 patients and rows are 141 genes. Yellow indicates increased expression following chemotherapy. Blue indicates decreased expression and black indicates no change. Grey indicates absent or poor quality data. R is relapse and NR is no relapse. (C) MAOA transcript alterations shown for 31 study participants. Ratios are intra-individual post-treatment versus pre-treatment MAOA transcript abundance measurements determined by qRT-PCR from microdissected neoplastic epithelium. (D) MAOA protein expression determined by immunohistochemistry. Representative images of neoplastic prostate epithelium acquired before (D1) and after (D2) chemotherapy exposure. D1' and D2' indicate higher magnification images. Brown pigment indicates presence of MAOA protein. (E) MAOA protein expression by

immunohistochemistry in prostate cancer metastasis from 44 patients. Each metastasis is indicated by a datapoint with multiple metastasis from the same individual located on the y-axis corresponding to each patient number. Grey and black datapoints alternate for ease of visualization. The horizontal line indicates the mean expression of MAOA across all metastasis for a given individual.

differences between control and MAOA transcript profiles using unpaired, two-sample t tests and controlled for multiple testing by estimation of q-values using the false discovery rate (FDR) method. To determine the association between MAOA and HIF1 changes following chemotherapy Pearson correlations were utilized. Finally, the statistical significance of data generated in the xenograft experiments were evaluated with the Proc GLM (General Linear Model) procedure in SAS (Cary, NC) utilizing a significance threshold of $p<0.05$.

Results

Clinical Trial Design and Patient Characteristics

Patients with high-risk localized prostate cancer (N = 57) were enrolled in a neoadjuvant treatment protocol designed to administer four 28-day cycles of docetaxel 35 mg/m^2 and escalating mitoxantrone doses (Phase I) to a maximum of 4 mg/m^2 administered as 3 weekly doses followed by a 1-week off-treatment period (**Figure 1A**) [8]. Trans-rectal ultrasound-guided prostate biopsies were obtained prior to the first course of treatment. Within one month of completing chemotherapy each patient underwent a radical prostatectomy. We quantitated gene expression changes in benign and neoplastic prostate epithelium from 31 patients who completed the full courses of chemotherapy and for which sufficient tumor in the available pre- and post-therapy tissue samples permitted cell acquisition by microdissection. The attributes of the study participants have been described previously [8]. The median Gleason score was 7 and approximately half of the participants (16/31) had a clinical stage equal to or exceeding T3. No patient had a complete pathological response following chemotherapy. The median follow-up of the cohort was 40 months at the time of this analysis.

Alterations in MAOA Expression Associate with Biochemical Relapse Following Neoadjuvant Chemotherapy and Prostatectomy

We measured gene expression changes in prostate cancer cells exposed to chemotherapy *in vivo* with the hypothesis that these molecular alterations would comprise resistance mechanisms and pathways that could be exploited as therapeutic targets to improve treatment responses. We used laser capture microdissection to acquire enriched populations of neoplastic epithelium from pre-treatment and post-treatment prostate tissue samples and quantitated gene expression changes following chemotherapy by microarray analysis [12]. At a median follow-up time of 40 months, using an intermediate end-point of serum PSA≥0.4 ng/ml and rising as a surrogate indicator of ultimate progression to metastasis [17], 11 out of 31 patients were determined to have biochemical progression. Of the chemotherapy-associated gene expression changes, 141 were significantly associated with PSA relapse-free survival (**Figure 1B** and **Table S1**). Several of these differentially-altered genes have previously been shown to influence chemotherapy resistance in other malignancies. For example, we found that down regulation of topoisomerase II alpha (TOP2A) associated with a higher rate of biochemical recurrence following chemotherapy. Low TOP2A levels have been associated with *in vitro* and *in vivo* resistance to chemotherapeutics including the TOP2A poison doxorubicin [18,19] (**Figure 1B**).

Of those transcripts upregulated in neoplastic epithelial cells following chemotherapy (**Figure 1B**), we focused further on monoamine oxidase A (MAOA), as we previously found MAOA to be upregulated in localized prostate cancers, with higher expression in poorly-differentiated relative to well-differentiated tumors [13]. To confirm the microarray findings, we used qRT-PCR to assess MAOA transcripts in microdissected prostate cancers from the same patient before and after chemotherapy. In 18 of the 31 cases (58%) MAOA expression increased following treatment, and corresponding increases in MAOA protein levels were observed in three of three cases with elevated MAOA transcripts and sufficient tumor material in both pre- and post-treatment samples (**Figure 1C,D**).

We incorporated the magnitude of MAOA mRNA alterations in a univariate Cox Proportional Hazard Model to estimate hazard ratios of several risk factors including age, baseline serum PSA before chemotherapy, pathologic stage, and histological Gleason grade, using time to PSA relapse as the clinical outcome. Of these variables, only greater MAOA transcript change and higher Gleason grade were significantly associated with biochemical failure after chemotherapy and prostatectomy (**Table 1**). In order to measure the net effect of MAOA expression change associated with time to PSA relapse, we further fit MAOA expression change and prostatectomy Gleason grade into a multivariate Cox Proportional Hazard Model (**Table 2**). After adjusting for Gleason grade, the expression change of MAOA was marginally associated with time to PSA relapse (hazard ratio = 1.55, $p = 0.068$): the reduction in hazard ratio suggests that MAOA expression and status of tumor differentiation are associated.

To assess whether MAOA may contribute to therapy resistance in disseminated tumor cells, we evaluated MAOA protein expression in prostate cancer metastasis acquired from 44 men with advanced castration resistant prostate cancer (**Figure 1E**). The majority of patients (90%) had at least one tumor with high MAOA expression (staining score ≥1), and concordant MAOA expression across multiple tumors (range 2–7 tumors per patient) from the same individual was evident.

MAOA Activity is Altered by Chemotherapy and Influences Cell Proliferation *In Vitro*

To determine if chemotherapy directly influenced MAOA expression and to evaluate the influence of MAOA on cellular phenotypes, we measured steady-state MAOA expression in several androgen-sensitive and androgen-insensitive prostate epithelial cell lines. We found that androgen-responsive LNCaP cells expressed the greatest concentrations of MAOA transcripts and protein (**Figure S1A,B**). VCaP cells also expressed relatively high amounts of MAOA compared BPH-1 and 22RV1 prostate epithelial cells while androgen-insensitive DU145 and PC-3 showed limited, but detectable MAOA protein expression. None of the prostate cancer cell lines expressed appreciable levels of MAOB (**Figure S1A**). We treated the LNCaP prostate cancer cell line with increasing concentrations of docetaxel ranging from 1 to 100 nM. After 24 hours, MAOA activity increased significantly at each of the docetaxel concentrations, with higher levels affecting a greater magnitude of MAOA response (**Figure 2A**).

To determine if MAOA expression influences cell phenotypes, we expressed MAOA in PC3 cells, a line which exhibits very

Table 1. Univariate Model of MAOA Expression and Post-Therapy Biochemical Relapse.

Risk Factors	Hazard Ratio	P-value	95% CI
Gleason Grade*	2.02	0.014	1.15–3.56
Age	1.65	0.464	0.43–6.27
Baseline PSA	1.01	0.671	0.97–1.05
MAOA Expression Change *†	1.66	0.027	1.06–2.59

*$p < 0.05$
†MAOA expression in pre-treatment and post-treatment samples was measured by a quantitative real-time PCR. Expression changes were measured by cycle threshold difference ($\triangle$CT) of MAOA between post-treatment and pre-treatment samples.

limited MAOA at baseline. Relative to vector controls, PC3 cells expressing MAOA increased growth by 30% after 5 days in culture (**Figure 2B**). Inhibitors of MAOA enzymatic activity have been developed, including several with approved clinical uses as anti-depressant agents. We determined that the MAOA inhibitor clorgyline could substantially reduce MAOA enzymatic activity in LNCaP cells at concentrations between 0.1–10 µM (**Figure 2C**). The MAOA-induced elevated growth rate in PC3 cells was eliminated by treatment with the MAOA inhibitor clorgyline at doses that effectively suppressed MAOA enzyme activity (**Figure 2D**). In control PC3 cells with absent MAOA expression at baseline, clorgyline had no effect on proliferation (**Figure 2D**). In contrast, clorgyline treatment of LNCaP (**Figure 2E**) and VCaP cells that normally express high steady-state levels of MAOA also resulted in significant growth suppression ($p < 0.05$).

Inhibition of MAOA Activity Modulates Docetaxel Effects on Prostate Cancer Cell Viability

In the neoadjuvant clinical trial of docetaxel and mitoxantrone (**Figure 1A**), increased MAOA expression following chemotherapy associated with biochemical relapse, suggesting MAOA may confer resistance to chemotherapy-induced cell death. In order to determine if inhibition of MAOA modifies chemoresistance, we compared the effects of docetaxel toward wild-type PC3 cells that express very low levels of MAOA, and PC3 cells engineered to express high levels of active MAOA enzyme. In short-term *in vitro* assays of cell viability, the expression of MAOA slightly increased the number of metabolically-active cells after 48 and 72 hours of treatment with 200 nM docetaxel; 8% and 5%, respectively ($p < 0.05$) (**Figure 3A**). The expression of MAOA significantly reduced the cellular apoptotic response to docetaxel as determined by measurements of activated caspase 3 and 7 in the cells ($p < 0.05$) (**Figure 3B**). We next treated LNCAP and VCaP cells expressing high endogenous levels of MAOA with the MAOA inhibitor clorgyline followed one hour later by different concentrations of docetaxel. In both cell lines, clorgyline substantially further reduced the number of viable cells resulting from docetaxel administration, with the most pronounced additive effects seen at

lower concentrations of docetaxel (e.g. ~30% further loss of cell viability at 10^{-9} M docetaxel; $p < 0.05$) (**Figure 3C,D**).

MAOA Expression Increases Reactive Oxygen Species and Activates Components of the HIF1A Program

We next sought to determine mechanisms by which MAOA could influence cellular resistance to chemotherapeutic agents. Monoamine oxidase enzymatic activity regulates oxidative deamination reactions of neurotransmitters such as serotonin, norepinephrine, and dopamine. Byproducts of this reaction include reactive oxygen species (ROS) such as H_2O_2 and hydroxyl radicals (**Figure 4A**). Using a fluorescence-based assay we determined that PC3 cells engineered to express MAOA had significantly higher levels of ROS than control PC3 cells propagated in identical growth medium and assayed at the same cell density (**Figure 4B**). ROS have been shown to activate several signaling programs including NFκB, MAP-kinase, and HIF1A. We determined that relative to control PC3 cells, PC3-MAOA cells expressed elevated levels of nuclear HIF1A (**Figure 4C**). Further, transcripts encoding the known HIF1A target gene, vascular endothelial growth factor (VEGF), and the EMT-associated proteins vimentin (VIM), and pleiotropin (PTN) [20-23] were increased in PC3 cells expressing high MAOA levels (**Figure 4D**). To further evaluate the clinical relevance of MAOA and HIF1A, we assessed whether elevated MAOA levels in prostate cancers treated with neoadjuvant chemotherapy associated with increased HIF1A *in vivo*. We found that MAOA expression following chemotherapy was significantly associated with HIF1A, r = 0.42 ($p = 0.02$) (**Figure 4E**). To further confirm that endogenous HIF1α expression was associated with MAOA activity, we treated high MAOA-expressing VCaP cells with clorgyline, and determined that after 48 hours of clorgyline exposure, HIF1A transcripts decreased more than 4-fold relative to cells treated only with vehicle control (**Figure 4F**).

Table 2. Multivariate Model of MAOA Expression and Post-Therapy Biochemical Relapse.

Risk Factors	Hazard Ratio	P-value	95% CI
Gleason Grade	1.85	0.038	1.03–3.32
MAOA Expression Change ‡	1.55	0.068	0.97–2.47

‡$0.05 < p < 0.1$.

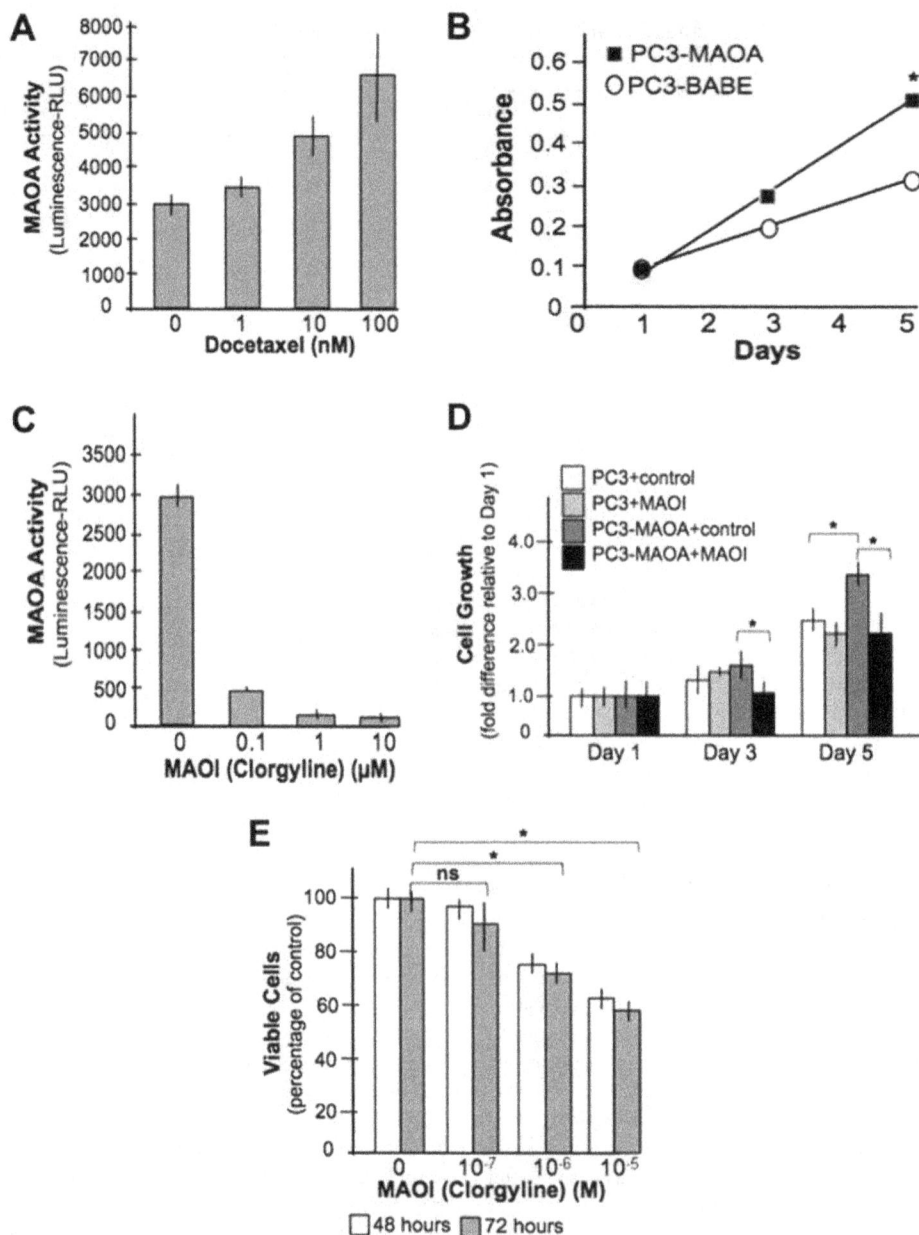

Figure 2. MAOA expression is induced by chemotherapy *in vitro* and promotes cell proliferation. (A) Treatment of LNCaP prostate cancer cells with docetaxel increases MAOA enzyme activity. (B) Over-expression of MAOA increases cell proliferation in PC3 prostate cancer cells. *$p < 0.05$. (C) The irreversible MAOA inhibitor clorgyline reduces MAOA activity in LNCaP cells (*$p < 0.05$). (D) Expression of MAOA in the PC3 prostate cancer cell line (PC3-MAOA) increases cell growth which is inhibited by clorgyline (MAOI). (E) LNCaP cell growth is inhibited by the MAOI clorgyline (*$p < 0.05$).

Elevated MAOA Expression Enhances Tumor Growth *In-vivo* and Alters Transcriptional Profiles

To assess the influence of MAOA activity *in vivo*, we compared the growth of PC3 cells expressing either MAOA or empty vector controls. After implanting tumor cells into CB-17 SCID mice as xenografts, growth rates were monitored for a duration of four weeks. MAOA expression markedly influenced tumor growth with grafts of PC3 cells overexpressing MAOA averaging tumor volumes 5-fold greater than grafts comprised of control PC3 cells ($p < 0.01$) (**Figure 5A**). Furthermore, similar to the *in vitro* cell culture studies, the xenograft tumors overexpressing MAOA had elevated levels of ROS compared to the control PC3 tumors ($p < 0.05$) (**Figure 5B**).

Tumors collected for transcriptional analysis revealed a wide spectrum of gene expression differences between the MAOA and control xenografts, with over 1000 differentially expressed genes at a significance threshold of $Q < 0.1\%$ including upregulation of HIF1α(2-fold) in the MAOA overexpressing tumors (**Figure 5C**). In addition, transcripts encoding several proteins known to be involved in oxygen sensing (TRPA1 [24]), ROS production (S100A8 [25]) and cellular proliferation (TACSTD2/TROP2 [26]; VSNL1 [27]) were substantially upregulated in tumors expressing MAOA (**Figure 5C and 5D**).

Discussion

For reasons that remain unclear, adenocarcinomas arising in the prostate appear to be particularly resistant to the cytotoxic effects of commonly used anti-neoplastic drugs [1,12,28]. To identify resistance mechanisms, we designed a clinical trial to assess molecular features of tumor cells that associate with effects of chemotherapy exposure *in situ*. Among the gene expression changes we found to be altered by treatment, transcript levels of the gene encoding MAOA correlated with clinical relapse as defined by a rising PSA following radical prostatectomy. *In vitro* studies confirmed that docetaxel exposure increased the expression of MAOA in multiple prostate cancer cell lines, and inhibition of MAOA enzymatic activity using MAOA inhibitors enhanced the cytotoxicity of docetaxel.

Monoamine oxidase enzymes function to catalyze oxidative deamination reactions of neurotransmitters. Inhibition of MAO activity results in elevated levels of these amines in the central nervous system, a property responsible for antidepressant effects. Monoamine oxidase is encoded by two isozymes, MAOA and MAOB arranged in opposite orientation on the X chromosome, and expressed in the outer mitochondrial membrane in many diverse tissues throughout the body. MAOB preferentially metabolizes phenylethylamine and dopamine. MAOA metabolizes dopamine, serotonin and norepinephrine, though the dietary sympathomimetic tyramine is also a clinically-relevant substrate. Studies of MAO expression or activity in the context of cell growth, stress responses, apoptosis and neoplasia have primarily focused on cells derived from the central nervous system. Most of the available data indicate that biogenic amines serve as antiapoptotic factors and protect mitochondria against pro-apoptotic events by permitting closure of the mitochondrial permeability transition pore and preventing the initiation or propagation of the pro-apoptotic cascade [29]. In studies of neuronal cells, MAO inhibitors, leading to higher intracellular concentrations of monoamines and reduced production of reaction products such as H_2O_2, function to protect cells from pro-apoptotic stimuli [30-32]. A similar protective effect of MAO inhibitors toward melanoma cells has also been observed [29]. Further, studies of prostate cancer cells have demonstrated that serotonin, an MAO substrate, and serotonin receptor activity, associate with enhanced prostate cancer cell proliferation [33,34].

In contrast to reports indicating that inhibiting MAO activity exerts effects that restrain tumor growth, several lines of evidence support a role for MAO in cancer promotion or progression. We previously found that MAOA expression correlated with prostate tumor cell differentiation status, with higher MAOA levels associated with higher Gleason patterns [13]. Subsequent studies demonstrated that MAOA inhibits prostate cell differentiation [35], and the MAOA inhibitor clorgyline is capable of suppressing pro-oncogenic programs in prostate cancer cells [36]. The expression of several other amine oxidases are increased in various cancer types such as those arising in the lung, breast, liver, and cervix [29]. Of interest, the administration of L-deprenyl, an inhibitor of MAOB, resulted in significant reductions in tumor incidence in a rodent model of carcinogen-induced breast cancer [37]. While a component of the anti-tumor effects were hypothesized to result from indirect activity toward prolactin production as well as neural-immune responses, direct effects of L-deprenyl on tumor cells were not ruled out.

An important area of inquiry centers on defining the mechanism(s) by which monoamine oxidases modulate tumor

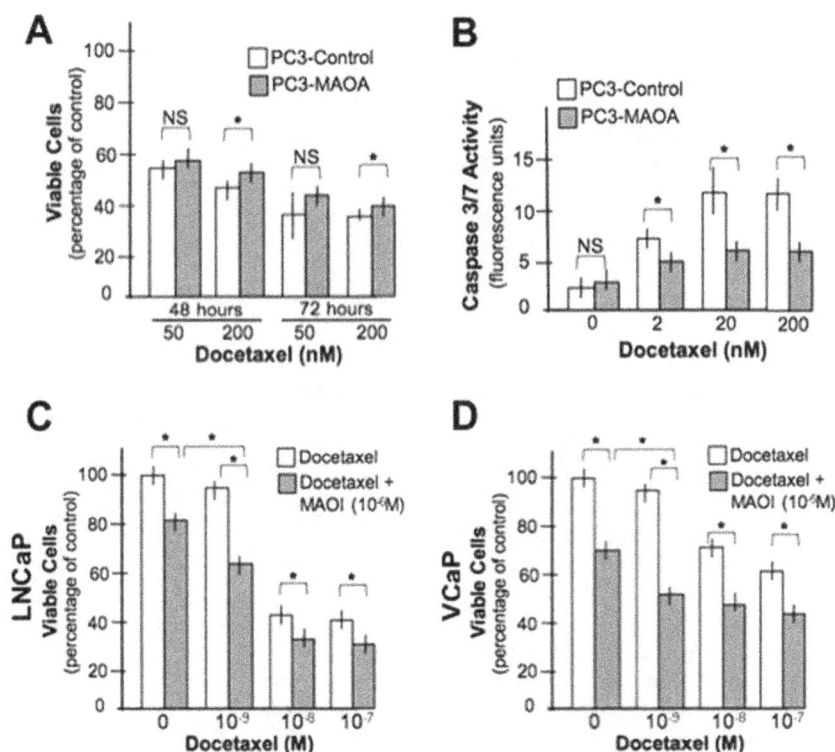

Figure 3. MAOA expression inhibits docetaxel cytotoxicity. (A) PC3 cells expressing MAOA exhibit enhanced cell survival following 48 and 72 hours of exposure to docetaxel (*p<0.05) (B) Elevated MAOA expression reduces cellular apoptosis following exposure to docetaxel. The addition of clorgyline enhances the cytotoxicity of docetaxel toward LNCaP (C) and VCaP (D) prostate cancer cells (*p<0.05).

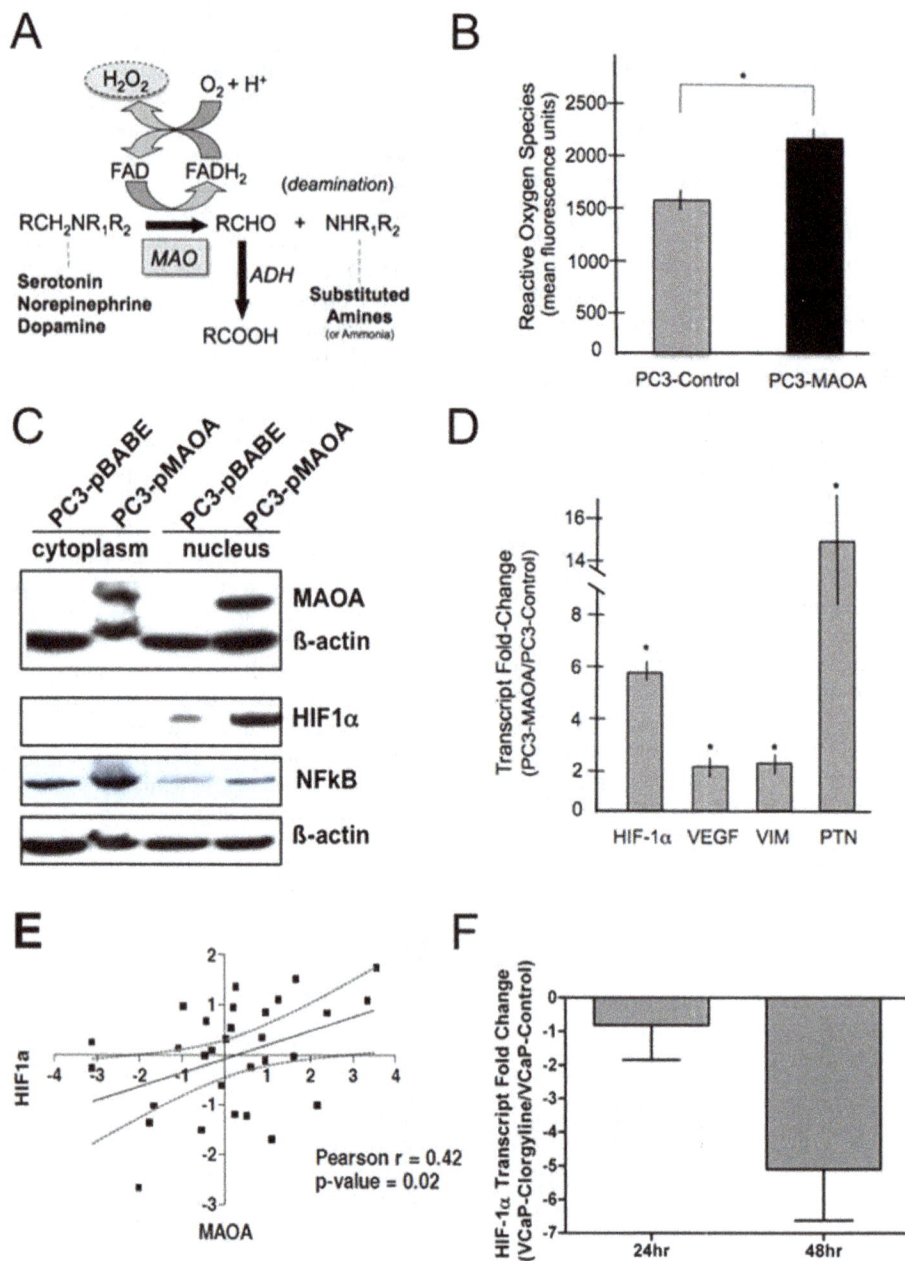

Figure 4. MAOA expression increases ROS and the expression of HIF1α and HIF1α pathway genes. (A) Deamination reaction catalyzed by monoamine oxidase (MAO) enzymes produces H_2O_2 as a reactive oxygen species (ROS) byproduct. (B) ROS levels are increased in PC3 cells expressing MAOA (*$p<0.05$). (C) Expression of MAOA in PC3 cells results in elevated nuclear HIF1α and NFκB protein. (D) Expression of MAOA in PC3 cells results in increased levels of transcripts encoding known HIF1A target genes. (E) Association of MAOA and HIF1 transcript level changes following chemotherapy. Plotted are the Log2 post-chemotherapy versus pre-chemotherapy transcript abundance ratios for each of 31 patients. The Pearson correlation value is 0.42 ($p=0.02$). (F) Treatment of VCaP cells with the MAOA inhibitor clorgyline suppresses HIF1A expression. A four-fold reduction of HIF1A mRNA was quantitated by qRT-PCR at 48 hours relative to vehicle control ($p<0.01$).

growth and chemotherapy resistance, and the corollary studies to determine how inhibitors of MAOA enhance chemotherapy sensitivity. The physiological functions of amine oxidases remain to be completely established, but known byproducts of amine metabolism include H_2O_2 and hydroxyl radicals that have the ability to promote MAP-kinase signaling through redox-sensitive pathways [29]. Our data indicate that one mechanism of therapy resistance links MAOA with the generation of ROS and activation of HIF1α. HIF1α expression – both protein stabilization and transcription, is promoted by elevated cellular ROS [38]. Several

studies have demonstrated that elevated HIF1α enhances cell survival in the context of cytotoxic chemotherapy and radiation [39-41]. Thus, further investigations into MAOA-mediated therapy resistance mechanisms should seek to determine if the primary effects of MAOA inhibition on prostate cancer treatment responses operate through HIF1α versus other ROS-dependent or ROS-independent pathways.

Two additional attributes of MAOA provide further impetus for studies involving therapy for prostate carcinoma. First, tracers for positron emission tomography (PET) imaging of MAOA activity

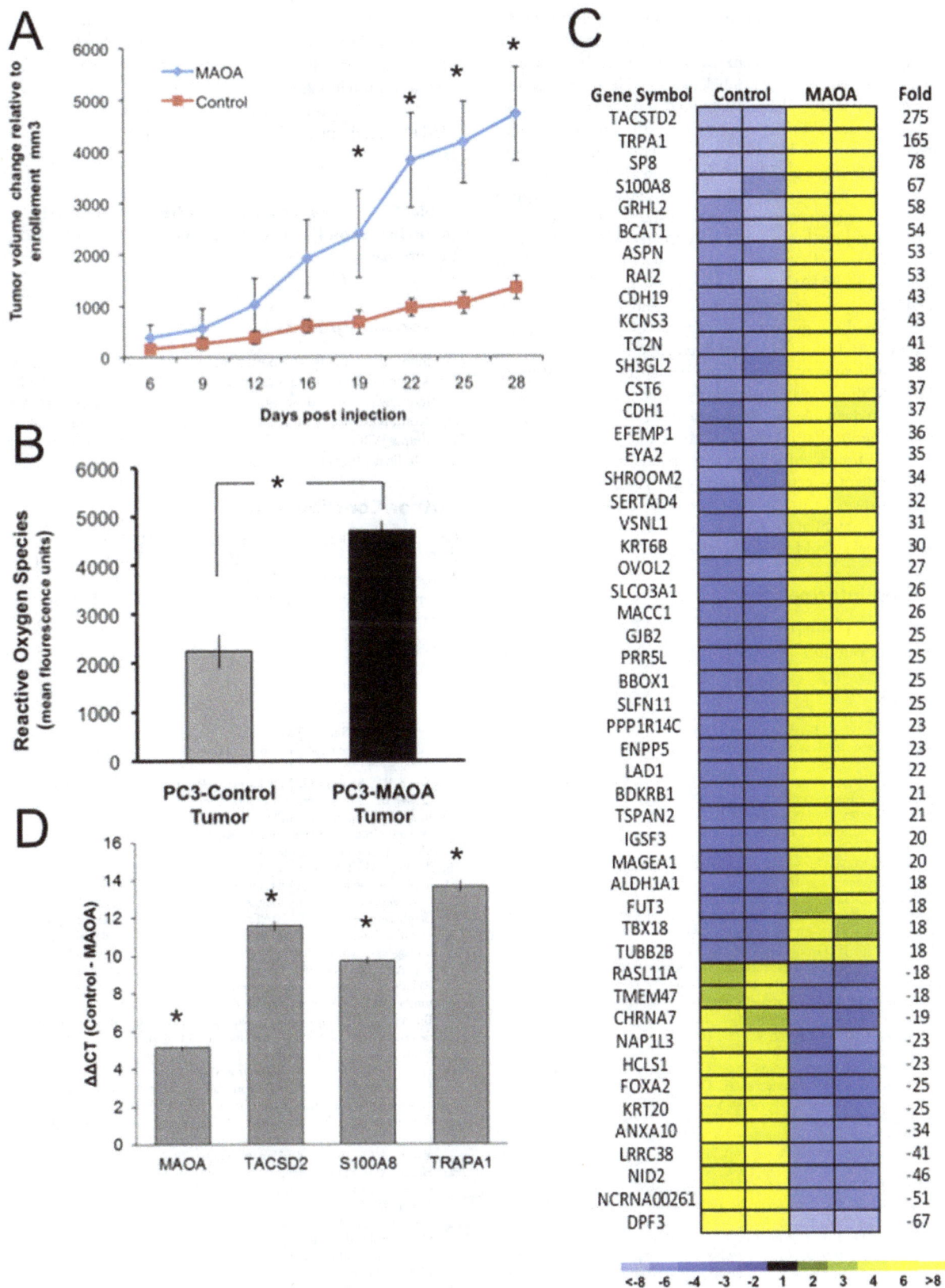

Figure 5. MAOA expression enhances *in-vivo* tumor growth and ROS production. (A) Animals harboring xenograft tumors overexpressing MAOA developed significantly larger tumor burdens over the four week observation period as compared to animals carrying the vector control tumors (*$p<0.01$ at the 28 week timepoint). (B) ROS levels are increased in xenograft tumor cells expressing MAOA (*$p<0.05$). (C) Heatmap of transcripts differentially expressed between PC3 vector control xenografts and PC3-MAOA expressing xenografts. Shown are transcripts increased (yellow) or decreased (blue) between the PC3-control versus PC3-MAOA tumors. (D) Quantitation of transcripts encoding MAOA, TACSD2, S100A8 and TRPA1 by qRT-PCR in PC3-MAOA versus PC3-control xenografts (*$p<0.05$).

have been developed. For example, [11C] clorgyline and L-[11C] deprenyl have been used to image MAOA and MAOB, respectively, in studies of CNS enzyme activity [42]. The MAOA ligand Harmine has also been labeled with [11C] and used to image a subset of neuroendocrine carcinoid and pancreatic tumors [43]. These tracers offer the opportunity to quantitate the on-target effectiveness of inhibitors, as well as overall tumor responses. A second notable feature of MAO involves a recent finding that MAO blockade appears to exhibit differential cytoprotective effects toward benign versus malignant tissues [44]. Nontumorigenic and tumorigenic human cells were treated with MAOA and MAOB inhibitors, and exposed to gamma irradiation or cisplatin chemotherapy. The MAO inhibitors reduced radiation effects in the benign, but not the malignant cells, and MAO inhibition further suppressed the growth of malignant cells relative to those exposed only to radiation. MAO inhibitors also reduced cell death due to chemotherapy exposure in the benign but not malignant cells. Though the selective and irreversible MAOA inhibitor clorgyline is not available for clinical use due to adverse side-effect profiles, compounds that inhibit both MAOA and MAOB such as phenelzine and tranylcypromine, or reversible competitive inhibitors with excellent selectivity toward MAOA such as moclobemide, are approved for use as antidepressants in several countries. Exploiting their potential to enhance the effectiveness of therapies for prostate cancer could be evaluated rapidly.

Supporting Information

Figure S1 A. Transcript levels of MAOA and MAOB in prostate cancer cell lines as determined by microarray hybridization. MAOB levels were at the lowest limit of detection across all cell lines. B. Western blot analysis of MAOA protein expression in prostate cancer cell lines. The detection of b-actin protein was used as a protein loading control. MAOA protein levels generally corresponded to the transcript levels across these lines through MAOA protein in PC-3 was detectable only with very prolonged exposures.

Table S1 **Genes associated with biochemical relapse following neoadjuvant chemotherapy and radical prostatectomy.**

Acknowledgments

We thank the patients who participated in this study for their altruism. We thank Alex Moreno for administrative assistance, David Gifford for assistance with tissue dissections, Gang Wang for MAOA mRNA studies, and Roman Gulati, Ruth Etzioni and Sarah Hawley for statistical analyses. We thank William Ellis and support staff in the Departments of Urology and Medical Oncology for contributions to patient care.

Author Contributions

Conceived and designed the experiments: RRG MW CYH WPH PSN. Performed the experiments: RRG MW CYH WH HGS JL IC LT. Analyzed the data: RRG MW CYH WPH JL IC RG PSN. Contributed reagents/materials/analysis tools: RV PL MG TB CH. Wrote the paper: RRG MW PSN.

References

1. Tannock IF, de Wit R, Berry WR, Horti J, Pluzanska A, et al. (2004) Docetaxel plus prednisone or mitoxantrone plus prednisone for advanced prostate cancer. N Engl J Med 351: 1502–1512.
2. Petrylak DP, Tangen CM, Hussain MH, Lara PN Jr, Jones JA, et al. (2004) Docetaxel and estramustine compared with mitoxantrone and prednisone for advanced refractory prostate cancer. N Engl J Med 351: 1513–1520.
3. Shannon C, Smith I (2003) Is there still a role for neoadjuvant therapy in breast cancer? Crit Rev Oncol Hematol 45: 77–90.
4. O'Connell MJ (2004) Current status of adjuvant therapy for colorectal cancer. Oncology (Williston Park) 18: 751–755; discussion 755–758.
5. Dreicer R, Magi-Galluzzi C, Zhou M, Rothaermel J, Reuther A, et al. (2004) Phase II trial of neoadjuvant docetaxel before radical prostatectomy for locally advanced prostate cancer. Urology 63: 1138–1142.
6. Febbo PG, Richie JP, George DJ, Loda M, Manola J, et al. (2005) Neoadjuvant docetaxel before radical prostatectomy in patients with high-risk localized prostate cancer. Clin Cancer Res 11: 5233–5240.
7. Hussain M, Smith DC, El-Rayes BF, Du W, Vaishampayan U, et al. (2003) Neoadjuvant docetaxel and estramustine chemotherapy in high-risk/locallyad-vanced prostate cancer. Urology 61: 774–780.
8. Beer TM, Garzotto M, Lowe BA, Ellis WJ, Montalto MA, et al. (2004) Phase I study of weekly mitoxantrone and docetaxel before prostatectomy in patients with high-risk localized prostate cancer. Clinical cancer research: an official journal of the American Association for Cancer Research 10: 1306–1311.
9. Chi KN, Chin JL, Winquist E, Klotz L, Saad F, et al. (2008) Multicenter phase II study of combined neoadjuvant docetaxel and hormone therapy before radical prostatectomy for patients with high risk localized prostate cancer. J Urol 180: 565–570; discussion 570.
10. Garzotto M, Myrthue A, Higano CS, Beer TM (2006) Neoadjuvant mitoxantrone and docetaxel for high-risk localized prostate cancer. Urologic oncology 24: 254–259.
11. O'Brien C, True LD, Higano CS, Rademacher BL, Garzotto M, et al. (2011) Histologic changes associated with neoadjuvant chemotherapy are predictive of nodal metastases in patients with high-risk prostate cancer. Am J Clin Pathol 133: 654–661.
12. Huang CY, Beer TM, Higano CS, True LD, Vessella R, et al. (2007) Molecular alterations in prostate carcinomas that associate with in vivo exposure to chemotherapy: identification of a cytoprotective mechanism involving growth differentiation factor 15. Clin Cancer Res 13: 5825–5833.
13. True L, Coleman I, Hawley S, Huang CY, Gifford D, et al. (2006) A molecular correlate to the Gleason grading system for prostate adenocarcinoma. Proceedings of the National Academy of Sciences of the United States of America 103: 10991–10996.

14. Wright GW, Simon RM (2003) A random variance model for detection of differential gene expression in small microarray experiments. Bioinformatics 19: 2448–2455.
15. Singh RP, Sharma G, Mallikarjuna GU, Dhanalakshmi S, Agarwal C, et al. (2004) In vivo suppression of hormone-refractory prostate cancer growth by inositol hexaphosphate: induction of insulin-like growth factor binding protein-3 and inhibition of vascular endothelial growth factor. Clinical cancer research: an official journal of the American Association for Cancer Research 10: 244–250.
16. Tusher VG, Tibshirani R, Chu G (2001) Significance analysis of microarrays applied to the ionizing radiation response. Proceedings of the National Academy of Sciences of the United States of America 98: 5116–5121.
17. Stephenson AJ, Kattan MW, Eastham JA, Dotan ZA, Bianco FJ Jr, et al. (2006) Defining biochemical recurrence of prostate cancer after radical prostatectomy: a proposal for a standardized definition. J Clin Oncol 24: 3973–3978.
18. Fry AM, Chresta CM, Davies SM, Walker MC, Harris AL, et al. (1991) Relationship between topoisomerase II level and chemosensitivity in human tumor cell lines. Cancer Res 51: 6592–6595.
19. Burgess DJ, Doles J, Zender L, Xue W, Ma B, et al. (2008) Topoisomerase levels determine chemotherapy response in vitro and in vivo. Proc Natl Acad Sci U S A 105: 9053–9058.
20. Higgins DF, Kimura K, Bernhardt WM, Shrimanker N, Akai Y, et al. (2007) Hypoxia promotes fibrogenesis in vivo via HIF-1 stimulation of epithelial-to-mesenchymal transition. J Clin Invest 117: 3810–3820.
21. Cannito S, Novo E, Compagnone A, Valfre di Bonzo L, Busletta C, et al. (2008) Redox mechanisms switch on hypoxia-dependent epithelial-mesenchymal transition in cancer cells. Carcinogenesis 29: 2267–2278.
22. Haase VH (2009) Oxygen regulates epithelial-to-mesenchymal transition: insights into molecular mechanisms and relevance to disease. Kidney Int 76: 492–499.
23. Perez-Pinera P, Alcantara S, Dimitrov T, Vega JA, Deuel TF (2006) Pleiotrophin disrupts calcium-dependent homophilic cell-cell adhesion and initiates an epithelial-mesenchymal transition. Proc Natl Acad Sci U S A 103: 17795–17800.
24. Takahashi N, Kuwaki T, Kiyonaka S, Numata T, Kozai D, et al. (2011) TRPA1 underlies a sensing mechanism for O2. Nature chemical biology 7: 701–711.
25. Ghavami S, Eshragi M, Ande SR, Chazin WJ, Klonisch T, et al. (2010) S100A8/A9 induces autophagy and apoptosis via ROS-mediated cross-talk between mitochondria and lysosomes that involves BNIP3. Cell research 20: 314–331.
26. Cubas R, Zhang S, Li M, Chen C, Yao Q (2010) Trop2 expression contributes to tumor pathogenesis by activating the ERK MAPK pathway. Molecular cancer 9: 253.

27. Xie Y, Chan H, Fan J, Chen Y, Young J, et al. (2007) Involvement of visinin-like protein-1 (VSNL-1) in regulating proliferative and invasive properties of neuroblastoma. Carcinogenesis 28: 2122–2130.

28. Magi-Galluzzi C, Zhou M, Reuther AM, Dreicer R, Klein EA (2007) Neoadjuvant docetaxel treatment for locally advanced prostate cancer: a clinicopathologic study. Cancer 110: 1248–1254.

29. Toninello A, Pietrangeli P, De Marchi U, Salvi M, Mondovi B (2006) Amine oxidases in apoptosis and cancer. Biochimica et biophysica acta 1765: 1–13.

30. Yi H, Akao Y, Maruyama W, Chen K, Shih J, et al. (2006) Type A monoamine oxidase is the target of an endogenous dopaminergic neurotoxin, N-methyl(R)salsolinol, leading to apoptosis in SH-SY5Y cells. J Neurochem 96: 541–549.

31. Maragos WF, Tillman PA, Chesnut MD, Jakel RJ (1999) Clorgyline and deprenyl attenuate striatal malonate and 3-nitropropionic acid lesions. Brain Res 834: 168–172.

32. Maragos WF, Young KL, Altman CS, Pocernich CB, Drake J, et al. (2004) Striatal damage and oxidative stress induced by the mitochondrial toxin malonate are reduced in clorgyline-treated rats and MAO-A deficient mice. Neurochem Res 29: 741–746.

33. Dizeyi N, Bjartell A, Nilsson E, Hansson J, Gadaleanu V, et al. (2004) Expression of serotonin receptors and role of serotonin in human prostate cancer tissue and cell lines. Prostate 59: 328–336.

34. Siddiqui EJ, Shabbir M, Mikhailidis DP, Thompson CS, Mumtaz FH (2006) The role of serotonin (5-hydroxytryptamine1A and 1B) receptors in prostate cancer cell proliferation. J Urol 176: 1648–1653.

35. Zhao H, Nolley R, Chen Z, Reese SW, Peehl DM (2008) Inhibition of monoamine oxidase A promotes secretory differentiation in basal prostatic epithelial cells. Differentiation.

36. Zhao H, Flamand V, Peehl DM (2009) Anti-oncogenic and pro-differentiation effects of clorgyline, a monoamine oxidase A inhibitor, on high grade prostate cancer cells. BMC Med Genomics 2: 55.

37. ThyagaRajan S, Felten SY, Felten DL (1998) Antitumor effect of L-deprenyl in rats with carcinogen-induced mammary tumors. Cancer Lett 123: 177–183.

38. Jung SN, Yang WK, Kim J, Kim HS, Kim EJ, et al. (2008) Reactive oxygen species stabilize hypoxia-inducible factor-1 alpha protein and stimulate transcriptional activity via AMP-activated protein kinase in DU145 human prostate cancer cells. Carcinogenesis 29: 713–721.

39. Patiar S, Harris AL (2006) Role of hypoxia-inducible factor-1alpha as a cancer therapy target. Endocr Relat Cancer 13 Suppl 1: S61–75.

40. Harada H, Kizaka-Kondoh S, Li G, Itasaka S, Shibuya K, et al. (2007) Significance of HIF-1-active cells in angiogenesis and radioresistance. Oncogene 26: 7508–7516.

41. Dewhirst MW, Cao Y, Moeller B (2008) Cycling hypoxia and free radicals regulate angiogenesis and radiotherapy response. Nat Rev Cancer 8: 425–437.

42. Fowler JS, Logan J, Volkow ND, Wang GJ, MacGregor RR, et al. (2002) Monoamine oxidase: radiotracer development and human studies. Methods 27: 263–277.

43. Orlefors H, Sundin A, Fasth KJ, Oberg K, Langstrom B, et al. (2003) Demonstration of high monoaminoxidase-A levels in neuroendocrine gastro-enteropancreatic tumors in vitro and in vivo-tumor visualization using positron emission tomography with 11C-harmine. Nucl Med Biol 30: 669–679.

44. Seymour CB, Mothersill C, Mooney R, Moriarty M, Tipton KF (2003) Monoamine oxidase inhibitors l-deprenyl and clorgyline protect nonmalignant human cells from ionising radiation and chemotherapy toxicity. Br J Cancer 89: 1979–1986.

8

An Individual Patient Data Meta-Analysis on Characteristics and Outcome of Patients with Papillary Glioneuronal Tumor, Rosette Glioneuronal Tumor with Neuropil-Like Islands and Rosette Forming Glioneuronal Tumor of the Fourth Ventricle

Annika Schlamann[1,9]**, André O. von Bueren**[2,9]**, Christian Hagel**[3]**, Isabella Zwiener**[4]**, Clemens Seidel**[1]**, Rolf-Dieter Kortmann**[1]**, Klaus Müller**[1]*

1 Department for Radiation Oncology, University of Leipzig Medical Center, Leipzig, Saxony, Germany, 2 Department of Pediatrics and Adolescent Medicine, Division of Pediatric Hematology and Oncology, University of Göttingen Medical Center, Göttingen, Lower Saxony, Germany, 3 Department of Neuropathology, University of Hamburg Eppendorf Medical Center, Hamburg, Germany, 4 Institute for Medical Biostatistics, Epidemiology and Informatics, University of Mainz Medical Center, Mainz, Rhineland-Palatinate, Germany

Abstract

Background and Purpose: In 2007, the WHO classification of brain tumors was extended by three new entities of glioneuronal tumors: papillary glioneuronal tumor (PGNT), rosette-forming glioneuronal tumor of the fourth ventricle (RGNT) and glioneuronal tumor with neuropil-like islands (GNTNI). Focusing on clinical characteristics and outcome, the authors performed a comprehensive individual patient data (IPD) meta-analysis of the cases reported in literature until December 2012.

Methods: PubMed, Embase and Web of Science were searched for peer-reviewed articles reporting on PGNT, RGNT, and GNTNI using predefined keywords.

Results: 95 publications reported on 182 patients (PGNT, 71; GNTNI, 26; RGNT, 85). Median age at diagnosis was 23 years (range 4–75) for PGNT, 27 years (range 6–79) for RGNT, and 40 years (range 2–65) for GNTNI. Ninety-seven percent of PGNT and 69% of GNTNI were located in the supratentorial region, 23% of GNTNI were in the spinal cord, and 80% of RGNT were localized in the posterior fossa. Complete resection was reported in 52 PGNT (73%), 36 RGNT (42%), and 7 GNTNI (27%) patients. Eight PGNT, 3 RGNT, and 12 GNTNI patients were treated with chemo- and/or radiotherapy as the primary postoperative treatment. Follow-up data were available for 132 cases. After a median follow-up time of 1.5 years (range 0.2–25) across all patients, 1.5-year progression-free survival rates were 52±12% for GNTNI, 86±5% for PGNT, and 100% for RGNT. The 1.5-year overall-survival were 95±5%, 98±2%, and 100%, respectively.

Conclusions: The clinical understanding of the three new entities of glioneuronal tumors, PGNT, RGNT and GNTNI, is currently emerging. The present meta-analysis will hopefully contribute to a delineation of their diagnostic, therapeutic, and prognostic profiles. However, the available data do not provide a solid basis to define the optimum treatment approach. Hence, a central register should be established.

Editor: Robert K. Hills, Cardiff University, United Kingdom

Competing Interests: The authors have declared that no competing interests exist.

* Email: klaus.müller@medizin.uni-leipzig.de

9 These authors contributed equally to this work.

Background

In the most recent update of the World Health Organization (WHO) classification of central nervous system (CNS) tumors [29,30], three new entities have been added to the repertoire of glioneuronal tumors: papillary glioneuronal tumor (PGNT) (WHO grade I), rosette-forming glioneuronal tumor of the fourth ventricle (RGNT) (WHO grade I), and rosetted glioneuronal tumor with neuropil-like islands (GNTNI) (WHO grade II/III) [29,40]. PGNT, a mixed tumor consisting of glial und neuronal histological differentiation, shows a typical structure of GFAP-positive psedopapillae surrounded by an interpapillary (neuronal) zone [2]. Necroses and elevated mitotic activities are rarely seen [3].

The biphasic histopathology, consisting of neurocytic and glial architecture, is also typical for RGNT [29,30]. Neurocytes of the neuronal component shape rosettes with eosinophilic, synaptophysin-positive cores and perivascular pseudorosettes. The glial part of the tumor, showing similar features like pilocytic astrocytoma, represents the larger portion [39]. In contrast, GNTNI shows features of a high-grade glioma, mostly interpreted as astrocytic [43], but ependymal or oligodendroglial differentiation is possible [12]. Dispersed in this glial component, the most prominent feature of these tumors, rosetted neuropil-like islands, can be found [37].

Although morphological, immunohistochemical, and molecular features have been intensively investigated over recent years [29,30], clinical features, current treatment approaches, and prognosis are still elusive. The pertinent literature on the topic is primarily limited to single- case reports or small case series and do not provide a comprehensive overview. In 2009, Allende et al. aimed to summarize the pathological and clinical findings of PGNT, RGNT, and GNTNI [3]. However, a major methodological shortcoming of their review is based on the fact that a systematic literature search was not performed. Accordingly, their findings may be biased by the authors' personal opinions or the selection of publications included in their analysis. In particular, the variety of articles published during the past four years may contribute valuable new information toward the understanding of the three previously mentioned entities. The purpose of this individual patient data meta-analysis was to increase the current knowledge about clinical features, treatment, and outcome of PGNT, RGNT and GNTNI.

Materials and Methods

Scientific question

The purpose of the present IPD meta-analysis was to assess the clinical characteristics and outcome of the patients with PGNT, RGNT and GNTNI reported in the literature.

Search strategy and selection criteria

The authors searched PubMed, Embase and Web of Science from January 1998 to December 2012 (the last update to all databases was on December, 17, 2012) for published articles with predefined search terms without language restrictions. The search was assisted by an experienced librarian (Mrs. Christiane Hofmann; library of the University of Leipzig). The keywords were (1) (papillary) AND (glioneuronal OR glioneural) AND (tumor OR tumour OR neoplasm), (2) (rosette forming OR rosetted) AND (glioneuronal OR glioneural) AND (tumor OR tumour OR neoplasm), (3) neuronal AND (glioneuronal OR glioneural) AND (tumor OR tumour OR neoplasm); (1) OR (2) OR (3). The process of publication retrieval and in- and exclusion of cases is displayed in a PRISMA (preferred reporting itmens for systematic review and meta-analysis) flow chart [34] (Fig. 1).

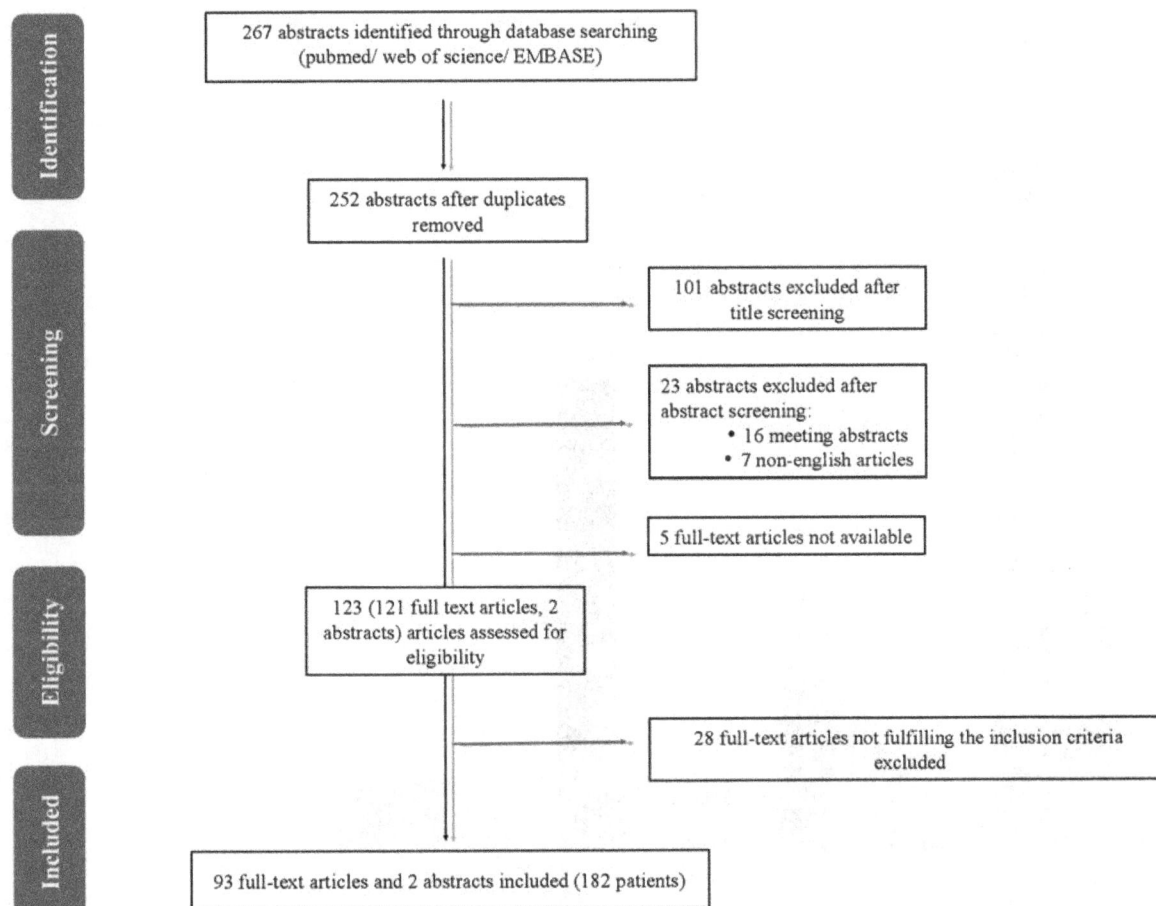

Figure 1. Systematic literature search. Procedure of publication retrieval and in- and exclusion of cases is displayed in a PRISMA (preferred reporting items for systematic reviews and meta-analyses) flow chart.

Table 1. Limitation of this study - non-English articles.

	Language	Case report (y/n)	Number of cases[a]	Abstract y/n	Language of abstract	Information delivered
1	Polish	n/s	n/s	**no**	n/s	–
2	Chinese	yes	1	**no**	n/s	–
3	Russian	yes	1	**yes**	English	histology, age+gender of patient, tumor location, **no symptoms/treatment/PFS/OS**
4	Chinese	yes	1	**no**	n/s	–
5	Chinese	yes	1	**yes**	English	age+gender of patient, symptoms, MRI-character (solid/cystic), tumor location, histology, treatment, follow-up
6	Chinese	yes	2	**no**	n/s	–
7	Chinese	yes	2	**no**	n/s	–
8	Japanese	no	0	**yes**	English	WHO classification 2007
9	Slovakian	no	0	**yes**	English	WHO classification 2007

Note: n/s – not specified; y/n – yes/no.
[a]Provided by title of the article or abstract if available.

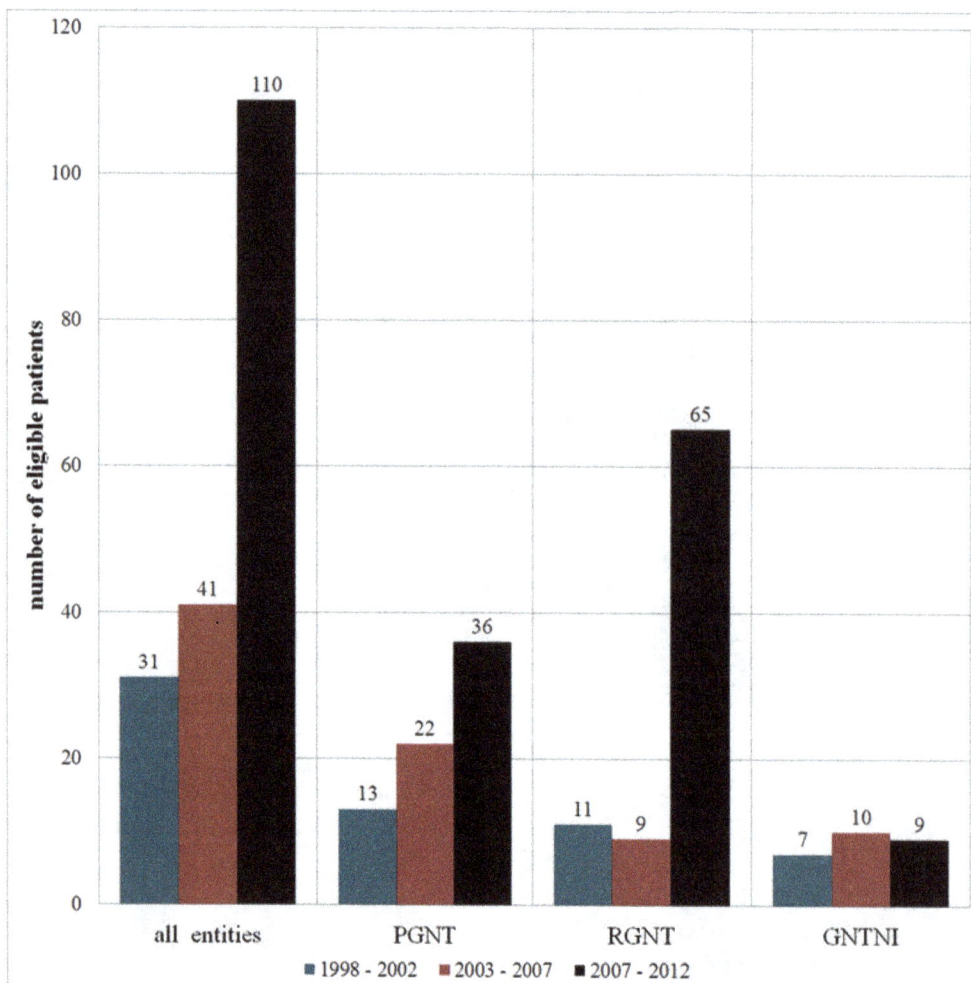

Figure 2. Number of published case reports. There is an increasing number of case reports over the last years.

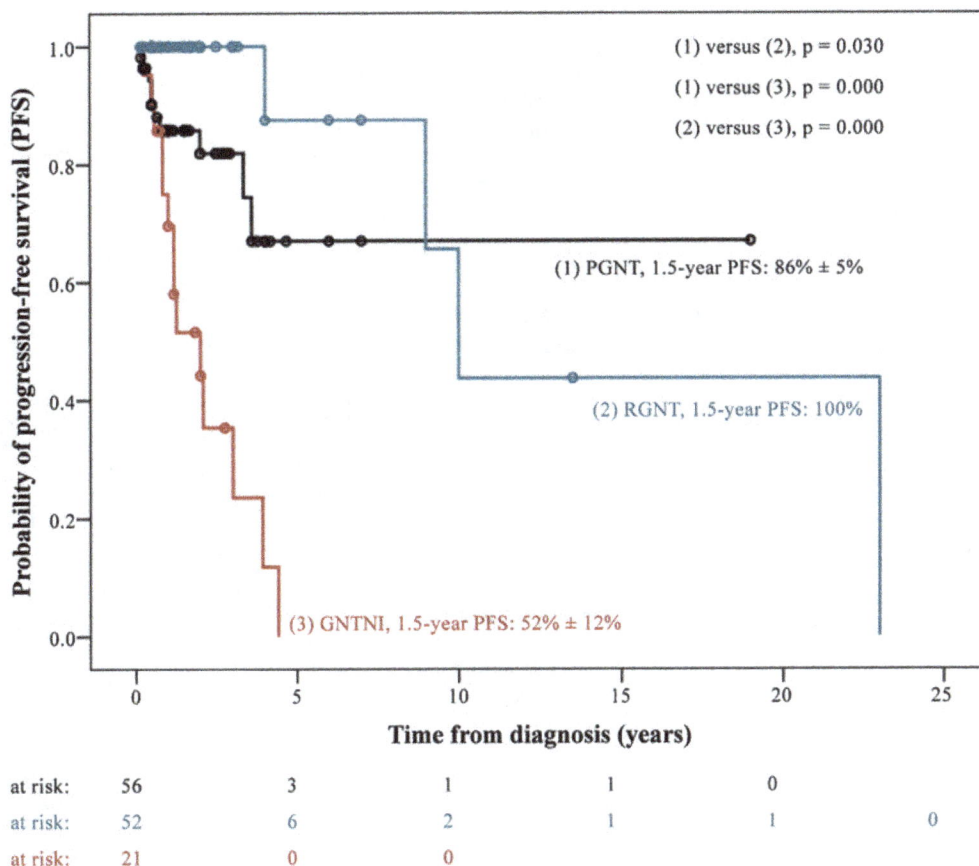

Figure 3. Kaplan-Meier Plot PFS.

The authors identified 267 hits from a search of PubMed, Embase, and Web of Science databases. These were imported in reference management software (endnote.com X6.0.1). Titles and abstracts were reviewed by one researcher (AS). Duplications were excluded (n = 15). In addition to the obvious duplicates (e.g. same articles twice), we identified identical cases by reviewing investigators in the study and patient characteristics. Results obtained on the same cohort of cases in multiple publications were collected only once, similar as described in a previos study [32], by including the largest series of patients.

Furthermore the authors excluded 101 abstracts because the subjects were not related to the aforementioned search terms. Case- series or cohort studies reporting on papillary glioneuronal tumor (PGNT) (WHO grade I), rosette-forming glioneuronal tumor of the fourth ventricle (RGNT) (WHO grade I), and rosetted glioneuronal tumor with neuropil-like islands (GNTNI) (WHO grade II/III) were included.

Another 16 meeting abstracts were excluded as well as five abstracts with insufficient data for which no full-text was available despite interlibrary loan. One exception was made, including one abstract providing sufficient information about one case without the available full-text.

Nine non-English articles in Polish, Chinese, Russian, Japanese and Slovakian were found. For eight of these nine articles, no full-texts were available; however there was one article with an English abstract and available Chinese full-text. For inclusion, the authors translated this article and contacted the authors of the study to receive sufficient data for the meta-analysis. For three articles the English abstracts were disposable, of which two were reviews and

did not include original data. Those two reviews were therefore excluded. The remaining abstract (case report) was included, despite limited data. To complete the limited data we contacted the authors of the study, but no responses were received in time. The remaining five articles were excluded because neither the full-texts nor the abstract were available (Table 1).

Overall, the authors assessed 123 eligible articles, 121 full-texts, and 2 abstracts. Possible additional studies were traced by checking the reference lists of selected publications, but they did not provide any further articles. Papers were reviewed by two authors (AS and AOvB). Disagreements were resolved through discussion and consensus with a third author (CH and/or KM). In case of uncertainty with regard to histopathological diagnosis, CH assessed whether diagnoses were based on mandatory analysis for the 2007 WHO classification of tumors of the central nervous system: Data from five patients whose tumor could not be histologically categorized according to the 2007 WHO grading system were excluded (part of the 28 excluded full-texts). The following criteria were used: (1) published immunohistochemistry, (2) growth pattern as described by WHO 2007 classification, and (3) case report considered as typical example by authors.

Data collection, quality control, and data synthesis

Information on the symptoms at diagnosis, histopathological diagnoses, patient characteristics, MRI findings, treatments, and outcomes were recorded on a standard data extraction form.

To ensure correct histopathological diagnosis according to the criteria defined by the 2007 WHO classification of tumors of the central nervous system, articles published before 2007 were

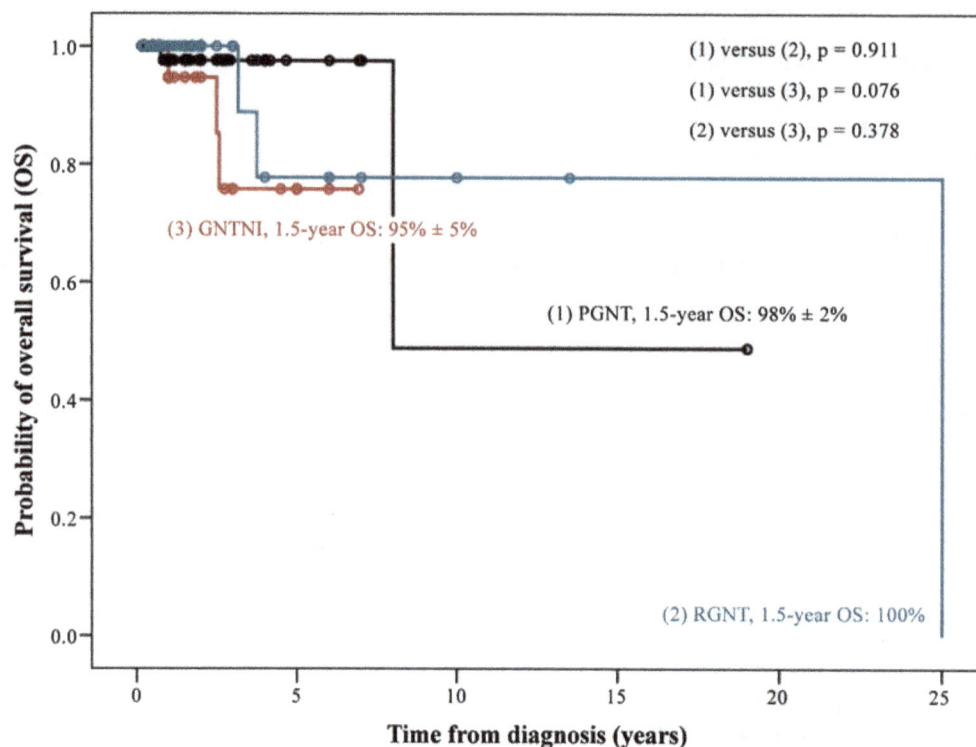

Figure 4. Kaplan-Meier Plot OS.

included only if they were cited in the 2007 WHO classification of tumors of the central nervous system ("blue book") or after a detailed assessment of the description of the analysis was performed to diagnose a case by an experienced neuropathologist (CH) in order to check whether criteria to diagnose a case according to the 2007 WHO classification of tumors of the central nervous system are fulfilled.

Any obvious errors (plausibility tests), inconsistencies with publication, inconsistencies between variables, or extreme values were discussed with the authors (CH and KM) and corrected where necessary.

Statistics

Study- level data were collected (95 studies; 182 patients). Because of the small number of patients per study, the study-level characteristics are not presented for each individual case report or case series. A one-stage approach according to Simmonds et al. was used to pool all data into a single master database [44].

PFS was defined, as described elsewhere [18], as the time from date of diagnosis to first progression or relapse or tumor-related death. Last contact (without an observed event) or death unrelated to progression or relapse required censoring.

For overall survival (OS) death by any cause was taken into account. Survival times were calculated from the date of diagnosis onwards. The Kaplan–Meier method was used to estimate PFS and OS rates. PFS estimates were compared by means of the log rank test. In some cases the date of diagnosis differed from the date of surgery. Therefore, the influence of the extent of resection on the PFS was not assessed. In addition to the assessment by means

of the Kaplan-Meier method and the log rank test, each variable was tested individually in a Cox proportional hazards model using the change in log likelihood from the null model. All analyses are exploratory; therefore, no significance level was fixed. All analyses were performed using SPSS, version 20 (SPSS Inc., Chicago, IL, USA).

Ethical standards

This manuscript is in accordance with the ethical standards established in the 1964 Declaration of Helsinki and its subsequent amendments.

Results

The authors evaluated the full text articles of 95 publications reporting on 182 patients with PGNT (n = 71), RGNT (n = 85), and GNTNI (n = 26) (Fig. 2). A detailed description of references containing patient data is provided in File S1.

Clinical characteristics and first-line treatment

PGNT. In total, we assessed 71 patients with PGNT. Thirty-three (46.5%) were male. Median age at diagnosis was 23 years (range, 4–75 years). The majority of PGNT (97.2%) were located in the supratentorial region. Primary metastatic dissemination was evident in one case (Table 2). In 64 out of 71 patients (90.1%) diagnosis was preceded by neurological symptoms, most frequently headache, seizures, and nausea/vomiting (Table 3). Complete resection was reported in 52 cases. Two patients received adjuvant radiation therapy after complete tumor resection (1x focal RT with

Table 2. Clinical Characteristics of ....

Characteristics	PGNT (n = 71)		RGNT (n = 85)		GNTNI (n = 26)	
	n	%	n	%	n	%
Gender						
Male	33/71	46.5	39/85	45.9	17/26	65.4
Female	38/71	53.5	46/85	54.1	9/26	34.6
Age at diagnosis						
Median (range)	23.0 years (4.0–75.0 years)		27.0 years (6.0–79.0 years)		40.0 years (2.0–65.0 years)	
Children (<18 years)	25/71	35.2	18/85	21.2	6/26	23.1
Adults (≥18 years)	46/71	64.8	67/85	78.8	20/26	76.9
Patients <26 years	42/71	59.2	40/85	47.1	8/26	30.8
Patients ≥26 years	29/71	40.8	45/85	52.9	18/26	69.2
Tumor location						
supratentorial	69/71	97.2	13/85	15.3	18/26	69.2
Posterior fossa	1/71	1.4	68/85	80.0	–	–
Spinal	–	–	1/85	1.2	6/26	23.1
More than one area	1/71	1.4	3/85	3.5	2/26	7.7
Primary metastasis	1/71	1.4	6/85	7.1	4/26	15.4
Proliferation index (Ki-67)						
Ki-67 reported	55/71	77.5	64/85	75.3	24/26	92.3
Median (range) (%)	1.8 (0.5–50.0)		1.0 (0.4–4.9)		4.0 (1.0–20.0)	
>1.6%	27/55	49.1	18/64	28.1	21/24	87.5
≤1.6%	28/55	50.9	46/64	71.9	3/24	12.5
Tumor size (cm), reported	51/71	71.8	36/85	42.4	5/26	19.2
median (range)	4.0 (1.0–9.0)		3.0 (0.5–9.6)		4.5 (3.5–6.0)	
>3.5 cm	30/51	58.8	8/36	22.2	3/5	60.0
≤3.5 cm	21/51	41.2	28/36	77.8	2/5	40.0
Character in imaging, reported	61/71	85.9	51/85	60.0	26/26	100.0
solid	5/61	8.2	19/51	37.3	19/26	73.1
cystic parts	56/59	91.8	32/51	62.7	7/26	26.9
Extent of tumor resection						
Complete resection	52/65	80.0	36/63	57.1	7/25	28.0
Incomplete resection	13/65	20.0	27/63	42.9	18/25	72.0
Not reported	6/71	8.5	22/85	25.9	1/26	3.8
Follow-up time of survivors						
Median (range)	1.5 years (0.2–19.0 years)		1.2 years (0.2–13.5 years)		1.7 years (0.6–7.0 years)	
Outcome						
Assessable for PFS	57/71	80.3	52/85	61.2	21/26	80.8
Disease progressions	10/57	17.5	4/52	7.7	14/21	66.7
Assessable for OS	57/71	80.3	52/85	61.2	23/26	88.5
Deaths	2/57	3.5	3/52	5.8	3/23	13.0

55 Gy, 1x no RT details available). Six patients with incomplete tumor resection underwent adjuvant radiotherapy (n = 2), chemotherapy (n = 1), or both (n = 3). RT details were not reported except in one case (focal RT with 45 Gy). The outcome was reported in 57 out of 71 patients. Ten patients progressed and two patients died. The median follow-up time of surviving patients was 1.5 years (0.2–19.0 years) (Table 2). The 1.5-year PFS and OS rates were 86% ±5% and 98% ±2% (2-year PFS were 82% ±6% and OS 98% ±2%, respectively) (Figs. 3 and 4).

RGNT. The authors evaluated 85 patients [men, 39 (45.9%)] with RGNT. The median age at diagnosis was 27 years (range, 6–79 years). Eighty percent of the tumors were located in the infratentorial region. Six patients presented with primary metastatic spread (Table 2). In 58 out of 85 cases (68.2%) the diagnosis was preceded by neurological symptoms, most frequently headache, abnormalities of gait and coordination, and nausea and vomiting (Table 3). Complete resection was achieved in at least 36 cases. Three patients with incomplete tumor resection received focal RT (total doses 46, 55, and 57 Gy, respectively). The

Table 3. Initial symptoms and radiology features.

Characteristics	PGNT (n =71)		RGNT (n =85)		GNTNI (n =26)	
	n	%	n	%	n	%
Information about initial symptoms provided	66/71	93.0	66/85	77.6	26/26	100.0
symptomatic	64/66	97.0	58/66	87.9	26/26	100.0
headache	39/64	60.9	43/58	74.1	3/26	11.5
nausea/vomiting	15/64	23.4	15/58	25.9	2/26	7.7
abnormality of gait and coordination	3/64	4.7	18/58	31.0	2/26	7.7
papilloedema or optic atrophy	8/64	12.5	6/58	10.3	0/26	0.0
seizures	21/64	32.8	2/58	3.4	17/26	65.4
visual disturbance	12/64	18.8	9/58	15.5	0/26	0.0
Radiology						
Character in imaging, reported	61/71	85.9	51/85	60.0	26/26	100.0
solid	5/71	7.0	19/51	37.3	19/26	73.1
cystic	8/61	13.1	11/51	21.6	0/26	0.0
cystic with mural nodule	23/61	37.7	0/51	0.0	5/26	19.2
cystic and solid	25/61	41.0	21/51	41.2	2/26	7.7
enhancement, reported	63/71	88.7	61/85	71.8	26/26	100.0
enhancement	60/63	95.2	44/61	72.1	14/26	53.8
density in MR-imaging T1	44/71	62.0	52/85	61.2	12/26	46.2
hypointens	41/44	93.2	48/52	92.3	11/12	91.7
hyperintens	3/44	6.8	–	–	1/12	8.3
isointens	–	–	4/52	7.7	–	–
density in MR-imaging T2	39/71	54.9	47/85	55.3	12/26	46.2
hypointens	0/39	0.0	–	–	1/12	8.3
hyperintens	39/39	100.0	40/47	85.1	11/12	91.7
isointens	–	–	7/47	14.9	–	–

outcome was reported in 52 out of 85 patients (61.2%). Four patients progressed and three patients died. The median follow-up time of surviving patients was 1.2 years (0.2–13.5 years) (Table 2). The PFS and OS rates at 1.5 and 2 years after diagnosis were 100%, respectively (Figs. 3 and 4).

GNTNI. Twenty-six patients with GNTNI were investigated. Seventeen (65.4%) were male. The median age at diagnosis was 40 years (range, 2–65 years).

Tumors were in the supratentorial (69.2%) and spinal (23.1%) regions. Four patients showed initial metastases (Table 2). All patients were symptomatic when diagnosed with seizures and headache being the most frequent clinical signs (Table 3). Gross total resection was not achievable in 18 out of 26 patients. Ten with incomplete (n = 9) or unknown extent of tumor resection (n = 1) underwent adjuvant focal radiotherapy (n = 4), irradiation of the craniospinal axis (n = 1, disseminated disease), or focal radiotherapy and chemotherapy (n = 5). The maximum RT doses were reported in five cases (2 × 60 Gy, 50 Gy, 59.4 Gy, and 50.4 Gy). Two patients underwent adjuvant treatment (chemotherapy, n = 1; RT and chemotherapy, n = 1) despite complete tumor resection. The outcome was reported in 21 patients. Fourteen patients progressed and three patients died. The median follow-up time of surviving patients was 1.7 years (0.6–7.0 years) (Table 2). Progression-free and overall survival rates at 1.5 years after diagnosis were 52% ±12% and 95% ±5%, respectively (Figs. 3 and 4). Two-year PFS was 44% ±12% and OS 95% ±5%.

Evaluation of potential prognostic factors for PFS across all three entities

Univariable analyses, Kaplan-Meier method and log rank test. Neither gender (p = 0.315) nor age (cut-off of 18 years; p = 0.846; cut-off of 26 years as median age for all patients: p = 0.575) had an on PFS. In contrast, univariable survival analyses identified histology (p<0.001), WHO grading (p<0.001), the Ki-67 proliferation index (cut-offs of 1.6 and 5.0%, respectively) (1.6%, p = 0.002; 5.0%, p<0.001), the maximum tumor diameter as measured on imaging [cut-off 3.5 cm (median size of tumor) (p = 0.028)], and the occurrence of cystic tumor parts (p = 0.015) as critical factors for PFS. Patients with primary metastatic disease tended to progress earlier (p = 0.054) (Fig. 3, Table 4).

Cox proportional hazards regression analysis (continuous variables). In the univariable cox regression analysis age (p = 0.128, hazard ratio = 1.02 per year, 95% CI: 0.99–1.04) and the maximum tumor diameter (p = 0.057, hazard ratio = 1.338 per cm, 95% CI: 0.992–1.805) did not influence PFS, whereas the proliferation index of Ki-67 (p = 0.003, hazard ratio = 1.10 per %, 95% CI: 1.03–1.18) did.. As an example, a 1% increase in Ki-67 positive tumor cells extended the risk of progression by 10% and a 10% increase in Ki-67 positive tumor cells by 259% (1.1^{10}). For the categorical variables (WHO grading, gender, primary metastasis and the occurrence of cystic tumor parts), the results delivered by the Kaplan-Meier method and the log rank test were confirmed (Table 5).

Table 4. Impact of potential prognostic factors on progression.

Factor	n =	2-year PFS (%)	1.5-year PFS (%)	p =
Histology				
Assessable for PFS	130/180 (71.4%)			
PGNT	57/130 (43.8%)	82±6	86±5	**0.000**
RGNT	52/130 (40.0%)	100	100	
GNTNI	21/129 (16.2%)	44±12	52±12	
WHO Grade				
Assessable for PFS	130/182 (71.4%)			
WHO °I	109/130 (83.8%)	90±4	93±3	**0.000**
WHO ° II/III	21/130 (16.2%)	44±12	52±12	
Gender				
Assessable for PFS	130/182 (71.4%)			
Male	62/130 (47.7%)	79±7	86±5	0.315
Female	68/130 (52.3%)	82±5	82±5	
Age				
Accessible for PFS	130/182 (71.4%)			
Children (<18 years)	39/130 (30.0%)	77±8	83±7	0.846
Adults (≥18 years)	91/130 (70,0%)	82±5	85±4	
Patients <26 years	68/130 (52.3%)	83±6	86±5	0.575
Patients ≥26 years	62/130 (47.7%)	78±7	82±6	
Primary metastasis				
Accessible for PFS	130/182 (71.4%)			
yes	9/130 (6.9%)	51±20	51±20	**0.054**
no	121/130 (93.1%)	83±4	87±4	
Proliferation index (Ki-67) (%)				
Accessible for PFS	111/182 (61.0%)			
>1.6	50/111 (45.0%)	92±5	92±5	**0.002**
≤1.6	61/111 (55.0%)	66±8	73±7	
≥5	93/111 (83.8%)	44±13	53±12	**0.000**
<5	18/111 (16.2%)	88±5	90±4	
Maximum tumor diameter (cm)				
Accessible for PFS	73/182 (40.1%)			
>3.5	36/73 (49.3%)	81±7	81±7	**0.028**
≤3.5	37/73 (50.7%)	97±3	97±3	
Appearance on imaging	137/182 (75.3%)			
Accessible for PFS	113/182 (62.1%)			
Exclusively solid	31/113 (27.4%)	68±11	76±9	**0.015**
cystic parts	82/113 (72.6%)	85±5	87±4	

Discussion

General aspects

PGNT, RGNT, and GNTNI have been raising more and more awareness in (clinical) neuro-oncology over recent years. This was particularly underscored by the special recognition given to them in the latest update of the WHO classification of CNS tumors [29,30,40]. Meanwhile, a considerable number of case reports and small case series have been published (Fig. 2). Now, studies extracting and subsequently interpreting the available data are highly needed. Recently, Zhang et al. assessed a total of 41 RGNT patients reported in the literature between 2002 and 2012 [52]. However, comparable studies for PGNT and GNTNI do not exist

so far to the best of our knowledge. The aim of the present study is to provide a comprehensive meta-analysis for all three entities. Through a systematic literature search, we were able to generate a data set containing 71 cases of PGNT, 85 cases of RGNT, and 26 cases of GNTNI.

PGNT

PGNT is a rare tumor of the central nervous system, first described by Komori et al. in 1998 [24]. Histopathological features, including biphasic components of glial and neuronal pattern as well as radiological characteristics such as frequent occurrence of a cystic lesion with mural nodule (39%, Table 3) or

Table 5. Cox Regression.

Factor	p =	hazard ratio (HR)	95% confidence interval (HR)
WHO Grade			
°I			
°II/III	**0.000**	0.137	0.062–0.305
Gender			
Male	0.320	0.675	0.312–1.463
Female			
Age	0.128	1.017	0.995–1.039
Primary metastasis			
yes			
no	0.069	0.316	0.091–1.095
Proliferation index (Ki-67) (%)	**0.003**	1.102	1.033–1.175
Maximum tumor diameter (cm)	0.057	1.338	0.992–1.805
Appearance on imaging			
Exclusively solid	**0.020**	2.659	1.168–6.052
Cystic parts			

mixed solid-cystic lesions (39%, Table 3) with ring-like enhancement in MRI, are able to facilitate the diagnosis [9,50]. However, the differentiation among ganglioglioma, pleomorphic xanthoastrocytoma, pilocytic astrocytoma and dysembryoplastic neuroepithelial tumor can sometimes be challenging [7,39,49].

When defined as a WHO grade I tumor, a benign course and an excellent prognosis can be assumed, especially when presenting with a low proliferation index or after gross total tumor resection (GTR). This study's PGNT showed a 1.5-year PFS of 86% ±5% and a 1.5-year OS of 98% ±2%, respectively (Figs. 3 and 4). Even cases with an elevated proliferation index showed a favorable course [6,10,20,22,23,35]. As a single exception to the rule one case of PGNT recurred despite GTR and low proliferation [23]. Therefore, no certain correlation between outcome and the extent of the tumor resection or the proliferation index can be made, which might give the impression that genetic alterations of PGNT may be a key issue for our understanding [28].

PGNT mostly occurs in young adults, but with a wide range in age (median age 23.0 years, Table 2). Initial symptoms can be seen in almost every case (64/71 patients, 90%, Table 3), resulting in physical examination and diagnostic services such as CT or MRI. At the time of diagnosis, a median tumor size of 4.0 cm (range 1.0–9.0) was shown in radiological imaging. In most cases enhancement of the tumor was reported (60/71 patients, 85%, Table 3), in addition to hyperintensity in T2-MR imaging (Table 3).

Most patients (80%, Table 2) received GTR and had an excellent prognosis, indicating that this is the first-choice treatment for PGNT [10,11,13,27,38]. Any additional therapy such as radiotherapy or chemotherapy appears to be necessary only in a minority of patients. Whether adjuvant treatment was administered for PGNT patients was reported in 31 (chemotherapy) and 35 (radiotherapy) out of 71 cases (45 and 49%, respectively). Four patients received chemotherapy (6% of all cases), all after STR, and seven patients got radiotherapy (10% of all cases; five after STR, two after GTR). However, there might be the possibility that more patients received adjuvant therapy than the authors are aware because of the low rate of reported data. Possible reasons for adjuvant treatment include high proliferation index, inoperability

and progressive disease [16,47]. Regular radiological monitoring is necessary to detect any recurrence of tumor. In this case, surgical intervention should be considered first [8].

RGNT

First described as dysembryoplastic neuroepithelial tumor (DNT) of the cerebellum by Kuchelmeister et al. in 1995 [26], Komori et al. defined RGNT as a specific disease in 2002 [25]. RGNT is a rare tumor of the central nervous system, typically arising in the III and IV ventricles. An increasing number of patients are now known with RGNT outside the characteristic location, such as in the pineal region, optic chiasm, spinal cord and septum pellucidum [5,19,42,45,51]. Radiologically, a solid or mixed solid/cystic tumor can be found in 37 and 41%, respectively, usually enhancing (72% of 61 reported cases), with hyper-intense signals in T2-MRI (85%) and iso- or hypo- intense signals in T1-MRI (92%, Table 3) [52]. Similar to PGNT, RGNT histologically consists of both glial and neuronal components [43]. Pseudorosettes are the most characteristic feature. Against the background of a histological similarity to DNT, some publications discussed that RGNT might be the infratentorial version of cerebral DNT [25,26]. Differential diagnoses include pilocytic astrocytoma, ependymoma, oligodendroglioma, central neurocytoma and DNT, of course [43,51]. Thus, a distinct diagnosis might be demanding.

Occurring primarily in young adulthood (median age 27.0 years), one case of a 79-year-old patient provides some evidence that this tumor may also occur in older persons [31].

Classified as a WHO grade I tumor, RGNT is characterized by a favorable prognosis upon surgical resection: a 1.5-year PFS and OS of 100% was achieved in RGNT patients in this study's data set (Figs. 3 and 4). However, local recurrences have been reported as well as disseminated disease in 7% (Table 2) [15,48], leading to the hypothesis that GTR is the treatment of first choice. As far as the authors are aware, only about half of the patients received GTR, leaving many cases with subtotal resection (STR) (Table 2). Some authors even recommended performing a biopsy only [25,48]. Zhang et al. (2013) could not show any difference in survival when comparing patients with GTR versus STR [52], which might be the result of the small number of cases.

Even though it is challenging because of the delicate tumor location, surgery seems to remain the most important first-line therapy, whereas radiotherapy should be considered as adjuvant treatment for progressive or disseminated diseases as well as definitive treatment in case of inoperability [25,48,52]. Data about given adjuvant treatment for RGNT was reported in 76% of this study's cases: Three patients received radiotherapy, which is 4% of all cases (all after STR), but no chemotherapy was given (data not shown). The robustness of this information might be slightly limited because of the possibility that more patients may have received chemotherapy and/or radiotherapy.

GNTNI

In 1999, Teo et al. described GNTNI as a scarce tumor that differs from PGNT and RGNT [46]. Characterized as a WHO grade II or III tumor, it is the only one of these three entities that is not part of the glioneuronal tumor category [3]; instead, it is categorized as astrocytoma [29,30]. GNTNI appears with a biphasic histology consisting of neurocytic cells that surround distinctive oval neuropil-rich islands and fibrillary, protoplasmic, or gemistocytic astrocytes as part of the glial component [1,2,41]. This glial part exposes anaplastic features such as increased cellularity, frequent mitosis and necrosis, nuclear pleomorphism, high proliferation index, and/or microvascular proliferation. In this study's analysis, GNTNI showed a median proliferation index of 4.0% (range 1.0–20.0%), compared with a median proliferation index of 1.6% for PGNT and 1.0% for RGNT (Table 2). This might help to differentiate this tumor from both PGNT and RGNT. Differential diagnoses include ependymomas (with neuropil-like islands), oligodendrogliomas (with neurocytic differentiation), or RGNT.

Most of these tumors are located in the supratentorial region (69%); however, spinal (23%) and even disseminated disease at primary diagnosis (8%) have been described by authors frequently (Table 2) [17,21,37,41]. Showing variable contrast enhancement (Table 3), GNTNIs appear mostly as solid tumor in 73%, or, a smaller amount of 19%, cystic with a mural nodule with T2-hyperintensity (92%) and T1-hypointensity (92%) (Table 3) [4].

GNTNI shows an unfavorable prognosis when compared with RGNT and PGNT (1.5-year PFS 52% ±12%, 1.5-year OS 95% ±5%; Figs. 3 and 4), which is reflected in the histomorphology and the grading. Most of all published cases have been treated with incomplete resection (72%, Table 2). Again, this increases the risk of local recurrence. The best therapy for patients with GNTNI remains a serious challenge. Radiotherapy and chemotherapy as adjuvant treatments after resection are important and constitute a cornerstone of the treatment that should be discussed for every patient. A total of 21 out of 26 (81%) cases reported about adjuvant treatment: seven patients received chemotherapy (27% of all cases) and 11 patients radiotherapy (42% of all cases) (data not shown). Most patients received adjuvant treatment after an incomplete resection of the tumor (10/11 radiotherapy and 5/7 chemotherapy). For disseminated disease, a definitive radiotherapy or radiochemotherapy is conceivable but must be considered as an experimental approach. Even though much remains uncertain, treatment of GNTNI may include the cornerstones of the treatment of diffuse astrocytoma, because of the histopathological similarity.

Limitations of this study

To the author's knowledge, we generate the first analysis containing progression-free and overall-survival for these three entities. It turns out that PGNT, RGNT and GNTNI demonstrate good survival rates. However, the authors cannot fully eliminate several limitations of the study.

First, the follow-up period is too short to draw definitive conclusions. Therefore, a registry study is needed for these rare tumors to collect follow-up data over a longer period.

Second, without a doubt, the patients in this study underwent very heterogeneous treatments. This may bias outcome and prognosis.

Third, unfortunately the authors failed to find every single full-texts for every abstract or hit, especially for the non-English case studies. Thus, two of the 95 case-series or cohort studies were assessed by abstracts only, and seven non-English hits were excluded entirely, resulting in another limitation of this study.

Statistical limitations

On univariate analyses the authors identified a variety of potential risk factors for PFS (Fig. 3, Table 3). However, it is highly improbable that all these factors are independent of each other. The simultaneous s of several variables on survival times are usually investigated by means of the Cox proportional hazard regression model. However, for the results to be reliable, the number of events (e.g. disease progressions or relapses) must be high enough. For each variable investigated, at least 10 events are required [36]. If the number of events is small, only a few exploratory variables can be investigated simultaneously [53]. In the present study there were only 28 cases of disease progressions or relapses (Table 2). This indicates that a maximum of two variables could be included in a multivariate Cox regression model.

In this study, the benefit of complete tumor resection and other treatment-related factors for progression-free survival was not investigated, because these variables were mostly unknown at the beginning of survival time (i.e., at diagnosis). To investigate a variable that is still elusive at the beginning of survival time or that changes over time, a time-dependent Cox regression must be used. For example, if the authors wish to know whether cancer patients' cumulative dose of chemotherapy affects the length of time until the tumor progresses, they cannot stipulate the cumulative dose as a known quantity at the outset. Patients who survive longer will generally receive a higher total dose. However, this high cumulative dose is not the cause of longer disease control. To allow for this, the cumulative dose must be included in a Cox regression as a time-dependent variable. Time-dependent Cox regression is a procedure that requires particularly detailed information about the starting date of therapy, which is generally not provided by case series/reports extracted from literature. [14,53].

Limitations inherent to the concept of IPD meta-analyses

In addition, several limitations of this study are inherently in the concept of individual patient data (ITP) meta-analyses. First, there certainly was a selection bias, because the cases reported might have been published because of their rare or uncommon presentation and outcomes. Second, the data were gathered from different institutions during a relatively long period of time, and significant advances may have simultaneously occurred in diagnostic and therapeutic approaches. Last but not least, not all data assessed were available for every patient, which further restricts the number of variables assessable in a multivariate model [33].

Conclusions

The clinical understanding of the three new members of the family of glioneuronal tumors - PGNT, RGNT and GNTNI - is currently in evolution. The present meta-analysis will hopefully contribute to a narrower diagnostic, therapeutic, and prognostic profile. However, the available data do not provide a solid basis to define the optimum treatment approach. It is proposed to establish a central register.

Acknowledgments

The authors wish to thank their librarian, Mrs. Christiane Hofmann, for her meticulous literature search. Mrs. Hofmann, an experienced librarian, operated the search with PubMed, Embase, and Web Of Science.

We thank Britt Scott for proofreading the manuscript.

Author Contributions

Conceived and designed the experiments: KM AOB RDK. Performed the experiments: AS KM AOB CH. Analyzed the data: AS KM IZ. Contributed reagents/materials/analysis tools: AS KM AOB CH. Wrote the paper: AS KM. Manuscript editing: AOB CH IZ CS RDK.

References

1. Adachi J, Nishikawa R, Hirose T, Matsutani M (2005) Mixed neuronal-glial tumor of the fourth ventricle and successful treatment of postoperative mutism with bromocriptine: case report. Surg Neurol 63: 375–379.
2. Agarwal S, Sharma MC, Singh G, Suri V, Sarkar C, et al. (2012) Papillary glioneuronal tumor - a rare entity: report of four cases and brief review of literature. Childs Nerv Syst 28: 1897–1904.
3. Allende DS, Prayson RA (2009) The expanding family of glioneuronal tumors. Adv Anat Pathol 16: 33–39.
4. Amemiya S, Shibahara J, Aoki S, Takao H, Ohtomo K (2008) Recently established entities of central nervous system tumors: review of radiological findings. J Comput Assist Tomogr 32: 279–285.
5. Anan M, Inoue R, Ishii K, Abe T, Fujiki M, et al. (2009) A rosette-forming glioneuronal tumor of the spinal cord: the first case of a rosette-forming glioneuronal tumor originating from the spinal cord. Hum Pathol 40: 898–901.
6. Atri S, Sharma MC, Sarkar C, Garg A, Suri A (2007) Papillary glioneuronal tumour: a report of a rare case and review of literature. Childs Nerv Syst 23: 349–353.
7. Barnes NP, Pollock JR, Harding B, Hayward RD (2002) Papillary glioneuronal tumour in a 4-year-old. Pediatr Neurosurg 36: 266–270.
8. Benesch M, Eder HG, Sovinz P, Raith J, Lackner H, et al. (2006) Residual or recurrent cerebellar low-grade glioma in children after tumor resection: is re-treatment needed? A single center experience from 1983 to 2003. Pediatr Neurosurg 42: 159–164.
9. Bisson EF, Pendlebury WW, Horgan MA (2005)Glioneuronal tumor with unique imaging and histologic features. J Neurooncol 72: 89–90.
10. Bouvier-Labit C, Daniel L, Dufour H, Grisoli F, Figarella-Branger D (2000) Papillary glioneuronal tumour: clinicopathological and biochemical study of one case with 7-year follow up. Acta Neuropathol 99: 321–326.
11. Broholm H, Madsen FF, Wagner AA, Laursen H (2002) Papillary glioneuronal tumor - a new tumor entity. Clin Neuropathol 21: 1–4.
12. Buccoliero AM, Castiglione F, Degl'innocenti DR, Moncini D, Paglierani M, et al. (2012) Glioneuronal tumor with neuropil-like islands: clinical, morphologic, immunohistochemical, and molecular features of three pediatric cases. Ped Dev Pathol 15: 352–360.
13. Celli P, Caroli E, Giangaspero F, Ferrante L (2006) Papillary glioneuronal tumor. Case report and literature review. J Neurooncol 80: 185–189.
14. Collett D (2003) Modelling survival data in medical research. 2nd edition ed. London: Chapman and Hall.
15. Ellezam B, Theeler BJ, Luthra R, Adesina AM, Aldape KD, et al. (2012) Recurrent PIK3CA mutations in rosette-forming glioneuronal tumor. Acta neuropathol 123: 285–287.
16. Epelbaum S, Kujas M, Van Effenterre R, Poirier J (2006) Two cases of papillary glioneuronal tumours. Br J Neurosurg 20: 90–93.
17. Fraum TJ, Barak S, Pack S, Lonser RR, Fine HA, et al. (2012) Spinal cord glioneuronal tumor with neuropil-like islands with 1p/19q deletion in an adult with low-grade cerebral oligodendroglioma. J Neurooncol 107: 421–426.
18. Friedrich C, Müller K, von Hoff K, Kwiecien R, Rutkowski S, et al. (2014) Adults with CNS primitive neuroectodermal tumors/pineoblastomas: results of multimodal treatment according to the pediatric HIT 2000 protocol. J Neurooncol 116: 567–575.
19. Frydenberg E, Laherty R, Rodriguez M, Ow-Yang M, Steel T (2010) A rosette-forming glioneuronal tumour of the pineal gland. J Clin Neurosci 17: 1326–1328.
20. Gelpi E, Preusser M, Czech T, Slavc I, Prayer D, et al. (2007) Papillary glioneuronal tumor. Neuropathology 27: 468–473.
21. Harris BT, Horoupian DS (2000) Spinal cord glioneuronal tumor with "rosette" neuropil islands and meningeal dissemination: a case report. Acta neuropathol 100: 575–579.
22. Ishizawa T, Komori T, Shibahara J, Ishizawa K, Adachi J, et al. (2006) Papillary glioneuronal tumor with minigemistocytic components and increased prolifer-ative activity. Hum Pathol 37: 627–630.
23. Javahery RJ, Davidson L, Fangusaro J, Finlay JL, Gonzalez-Gomez I, et al. (2009) Aggressive variant of a papillary glioneuronal tumor. Report of 2 cases. J Neurosurg Pediatr 3: 46–52.
24. Komori T, Scheithauer BW, Anthony DC, Rosenblum MK, McLendon RE, et al. (1998) Papillary glioneuronal tumor: a new variant of mixed neuronal-glial neoplasm. Am J Surg Pathol 22: 1171–1183.
25. Komori T, Scheithauer BW, Hirose T (2002) A rosette-forming glioneuronal tumor of the fourth ventricle: infratentorial form of dysembryoplastic neuroepithelial tumor? Am J Surg Pathol 26: 582–591.
26. Kuchelmeister K, Demirel T, Schlorer E, Bergmann M, Gullotta F (1995) Dysembryoplastic neuroepithelial tumour of the cerebellum. Acta neuropathol 89: 385–390.
27. Lamszus K, Makrigeorgi-Butera M, Laas R, Westphal M, Stavrou D (2003) September 2002: 24-year-old female with a 6-month history of seizures. Brain Pathol 13: 115–117.
28. Lavrnic S, Macvanski M, Ristic-Balos D, Gavrilov M, Damjanovic D, et al. (2012) Papillary glioneuronal tumor: unexplored entity. J Neurol Surg A Cent Eur Neurosurg 73: 224–229.
29. Louis DN, Ohgaki H, Wiestler OD, Cavenee WK, Burger PC, et al. (2007) The 2007 WHO classification of tumours of the central nervous system. Acta neuropathol 114: 97–109.
30. Louis DN, Ohgaki H, Wiestler OD, Cavenee WK, Burger PC, et al (2007) WHO Classification of tumours of the central nervous system. Lyon, IARC Press.
31. Lu JQ, Scheithauer BW, Sharma P, Scott JN, Parney IF, et al. (2009) Multifocal complex glioneuronal tumor in an elderly man: an autopsy study: case report. Neurosurgery 64: E1193–1195.
32. Malats N, Bustos A, Nascimento CM, Fernandez F, Rivas M, et al. (2005) P53 as a prognostic marker for bladder cancer: a meta-analysis and review. Lancet Oncol 6: 678–686.
33. Mazloom A, Hodges JC, Teh BS, Chintagumpala M, Paulino AC (2012) Outcome of patients with pilocytic astrocytoma and leptomeningeal dissemina-tion. Int J Radiat Oncol Biol Phys 84: 350–354.
34. Moher D, Liberati A, Tetzlaff J, Altman DG, Group P (2009) Preferred reporting items for systematic reviews and meta-analyses: the PRISMA statement. J Clin Epidemiol 62: 1006–1012.
35. Newton HB, Dalton J, Ray-Chaudhury A, Gahbauer R, McGregor J (2008) Aggressive papillary glioneuronal tumor: case report and literature review. Clin Neuropathol 27: 317–324.
36. Peduzzi P, Concato J, Feinstein AR, Holford TR (1995) Importance of events per independent variable in proportional hazards regression analysis. II. Accuracy and precision of regression estimates. J Clin Epidemiol 48: 1503–1510.
37. Poliani PL, Sperli D, Valentini S, Armentano A, Bercich L, et al. (2009) Spinal glioneuronal tumor with neuropil-like islands and meningeal dissemination: histopathological and radiological study of a pediatric case. Neuropathology 29: 574–578.
38. Prayson RA (2000) Papillary glioneuronal tumor. Arch Path Lab Med 124: 1820–1823.
39. Rainov NG, Wagner T, Heidecke V (2010) Rosette-forming glioneuronal tumor of the fourth ventricle. Cent Eur Neurosurg 71: 219–221.
40. Rosenblum MK (2007) The 2007 WHO Classification of Nervous System Tumors: newly recognized members of the mixed glioneuronal group. Brain Pathol 17: 308–313.
41. Ruppert B, Welsh CT, Hannah J, Giglio P, Rumboldt Z, et al. (2011) Glioneuronal tumor with neuropil-like islands of the spinal cord with diffuse leptomeningeal neuraxis dissemination. J Neurooncol 104: 529–533.
42. Scheithauer BW, Silva AI, Ketterling RP, Pula JH, Lininger JF et al. (2009) Rosette-forming glioneuronal tumor: report of a chiasmal-optic nerve example in neurofibromatosis type 1: special pathology report. Neurosurgery 64: E771–772.
43. Shah MN, Leonard JR, Perry A (2010) Rosette-forming glioneuronal tumors of the posterior fossa. J Neurosurg Pediatr 5: 98–103.

44. Simmonds MC, Higgins JP, Stewart LA, Tierney JF, Clarke MJ, et al. (2005) Meta-analysis of individual patient data from randomized trials: a review of methods used in practice. Clin Trials 2: 209–217.

45. Solis OE, Mehta RI, Lai A, Mehta RI, Farchoukh LO, et al. (2011) Rosette-forming glioneuronal tumor: a pineal region case with IDH1 and IDH2 mutation analyses and literature review of 43 cases. J Neurooncol 102: 477–484.

46. Teo JG, Gultekin SH, Bilsky M, Gutin P, Rosenblum MK (1999) A distinctive glioneuronal tumor of the adult cerebrum with neuropil-like (including "rosette") islands: report of 4 cases. Am J Surg Pathol 23: 502–510.

47. Vaquero J, Coca S (2007) Atypical papillary glioneuronal tumor. J Neurooncol 83: 319–323.

48. Wang Y, Xiong J, Chu SG, Liu Y, Cheng HX, et al (2009) Rosette-forming glioneuronal tumor: report of an unusual case with intraventricular dissemination. Acta neuropathol 118: 813–819.

49. Williams SR, Joos BW, Parker JC, Parker JR (2008) Papillary glioneuronal tumor: a case report and review of the literature. Ann Clin Lab Sci 38: 287–292.

50. Xiao H, Ma L, Lou X, Gui Q (2011) Papillary glioneuronal tumor: radiological evidence of a newly established tumor entity. J Neuroimaging 21: 297–302.

51. Xiong J, Liu Y, Chu SG, Chen H, Chen HX, et al. (2012) Rosette-forming glioneuronal tumor of the septum pellucidum with extension to the supratentorial ventricles: rare case with genetic analysis. Neuropathology 32: 301–305.

52. Zhang J, Babu R, McLendon RE, Friedman AH, Adamson C (2013) A comprehensive analysis of 41 patients with rosette-forming glioneuronal tumors of the fourth ventricle. J Clin Neurosci 20: 335–341.

53. Zwiener I, Blettner M, Hommel G (2011) Survival analysis: part 15 of a series on evaluation of scientific publications. Dtsch Arztebl Int 108: 163–169.

9

Model of Tumor Dormancy/Recurrence after Short-Term Chemotherapy

Shenduo Li[1], Margaret Kennedy[1], Sturgis Payne[1], Kelly Kennedy[1], Victoria L. Seewaldt[2], Salvatore V. Pizzo[1], Robin E. Bachelder[1]*

1 Department of Pathology, Duke University Medical Center, Durham, North Carolina, United States of America, 2 Department of Medicine, Duke University Medical Center, Durham, North Carolina, United States of America

Abstract

Although many tumors regress in response to neoadjuvant chemotherapy, residual tumor cells are detected in most cancer patients post-treatment. These residual tumor cells are thought to remain dormant for years before resuming growth, resulting in tumor recurrence. Considering that recurrent tumors are most often responsible for patient mortality, there exists an urgent need to study signaling pathways that drive tumor dormancy/recurrence. We have developed an *in vitro* model of tumor dormancy/recurrence. Short-term exposure of tumor cells (breast or prostate) to chemotherapy at clinically relevant doses enriches for a dormant tumor cell population. Several days after removing chemotherapy, dormant tumor cells regain proliferative ability and establish colonies, resembling tumor recurrence. Tumor cells from "recurrent" colonies exhibit increased chemotherapy resistance, similar to the therapy resistance of recurrent tumors in cancer patients. Previous studies using long-term chemotherapy selection models identified acquired mutations that drive tumor resistance. In contrast, our short term chemotherapy exposure model enriches for a slow-cycling, dormant, chemo-resistant tumor cell sub-population that can resume growth after drug removal. Studying unique signaling pathways in dormant tumor cells enriched by short-term chemotherapy treatment is expected to identify novel therapeutic targets for preventing tumor recurrence.

Editor: Irina U. Agoulnik, Florida International University, United States of America

Funding: National Cancer Institute R21 CA141223, www.cancer.gov; National Cancer Institute R01 CA155664, www.cancer.gov; Department of Defense Congressionally Directed Medical Research W81XWH-12-1-0478, cdmrp.army.mil/; Department of Defense Congressionally Directed Medical Research W81XWH-13-1-0404, cdmrp.army.mil/. The funders had no role in study design, data collection and analysis, decision to publish, or preparation of the manuscript.

Competing Interests: The authors have delcared that no competing interests exist.

* E-mail: robin. bachelder@duke.edu

Introduction

Despite the apparent efficacy of chemotherapy in "shrinking" primary tumors, chemotherapy-resistant tumor cells are thought to contribute to future tumor recurrence, the leading cause of patient mortality [1]. The identification of proteins that confer chemotherapy resistance has historically relied on studies of signaling pathways supported by tumor cells subjected to long-term, high dose drug selection [2,3]. These long-term selection models select for mutations/epigenetic modifications that result in acquired expression/activity of proteins involved in therapy resistance. The clinical relevance of these long term selection models remains controversial [4].

Other models propose that tumors are heterogeneous, consisting of therapy-sensitive and therapy-resistant tumor cell subpopulations [5,6,7,8,9,10]. According to these models, following chemotherapy treatment, chemo-resistant tumor cells exist in a dormant (sleeping) state for many years before resuming growth, resulting in tumor recurrence. Methods are needed to enrich for dormant tumor cells, allowing for studies of their unique signaling properties. Such studies will be critical to defining logical therapeutic targets for preventing tumor recurrence.

Using short term chemotherapy treatment to enrich for drug-resistant tumor cells, we have developed an *in vitro* model of tumor recurrence. In this model, short-term exposure of breast and prostate tumor cells to clinically-relevant chemotherapy classes/doses enriches for a population of slow-cycling (dormant) tumor cells. Chemotherapy-enriched dormant tumor cells resume proliferation approximately ten days after chemotherapy withdrawal, forming colonies resembling a tumor recurrence. Colonies emanating from chemotherapy-enriched dormant cells exhibit increased resistance to the original chemotherapy insult, similar to recurrent tumors in cancer patients. Contrasting with evolution models of therapy resistance, the existence of drug-resistant tumor cell subpopulations in the original tumor suggests that we can effectively eliminate tumor recurrence by implementing combination therapies [chemotherapy (targeting proliferative cells)+therapy targeting drug-resistant tumor cells].

Materials and Methods

Cell Culture/Reagents

SUM159 cells were obtained from Duke Cell Culture Facility and maintained in Ham's F-12 medium containing 5% heat-inactivated FBS, 5 µg/ml insulin, and 1 µg/ml hydrocortisone. DU145 prostate cancer cells were obtained from the Duke Cell Culture Facility and maintained in RPMI 1640 containing 10% heat-inactivated FBS.

A.

B.

C.

D.

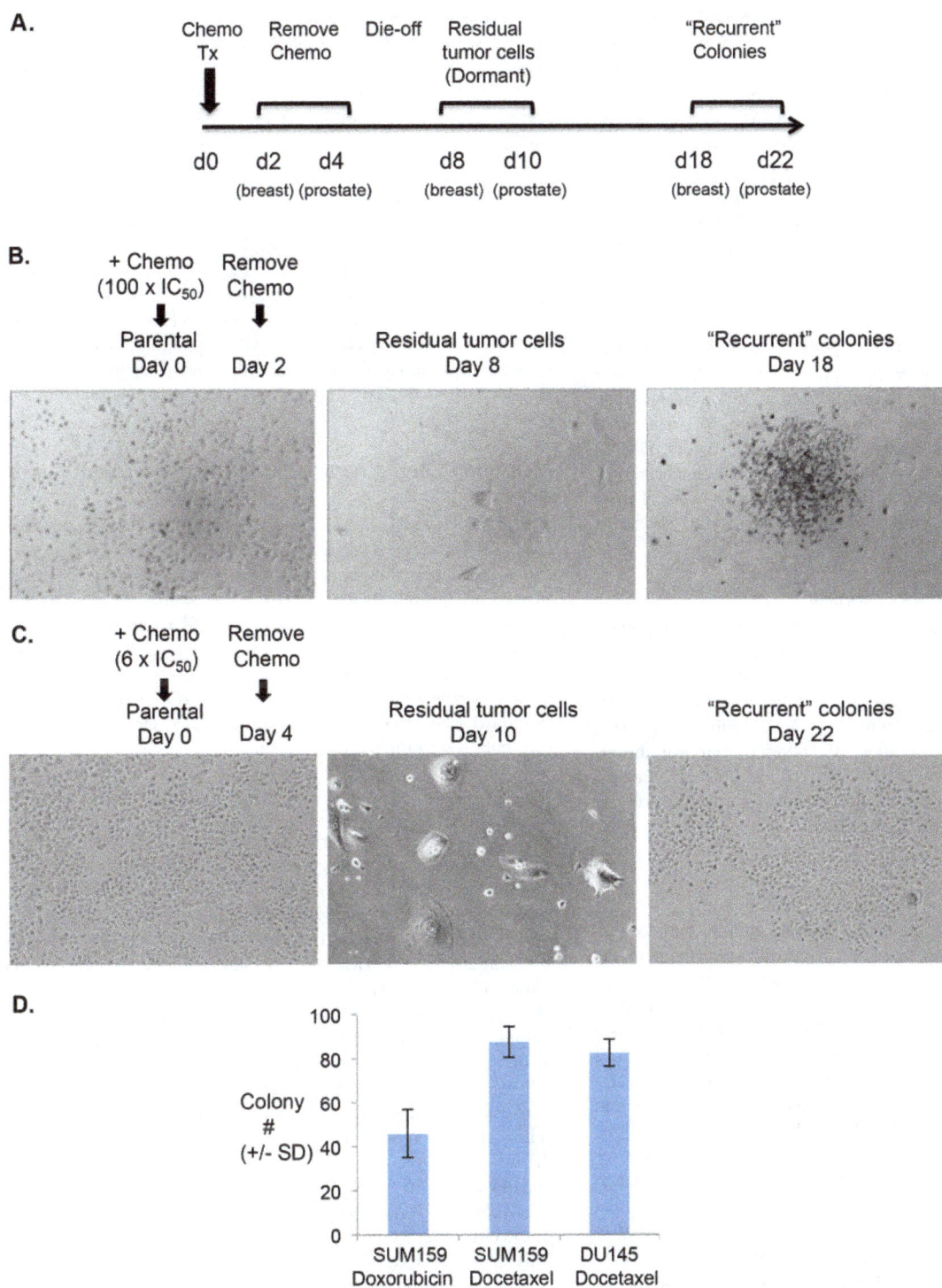

Figure 1. *In vitro* **model of tumor dormancy/recurrence after short-term chemotherapy treatment. A.** Schematic of experimental tumor dormancy/recurrence model. Breast (SUM159) or prostate (DU145) tumor cells were treated short term (breast 2 d; prostate 4 d) with chemotherapy *in vitro*. After 8 d (breast) or 10 d (prostate), dormant tumor cells (breast d8; prostate d10) were observed. Over time (breast d18; prostate d22), these dormant tumor cells resumed growth, establishing "recurrent" colonies. **B.** SUM159 breast tumor cells (Parental, left panel; 4X) were incubated with Docetaxel (100 nM; 100 fold IC_{50}) for 2 d, after which chemotherapy was removed and fresh culture medium added. Residual tumor cells were imaged on d8 after treatment (Residual tumor cells, middle panel; 4X). Colonies evolving from residual tumor cells were imaged on d18 ("Recurrent" colonies, right panel; 4X). Similar results were obtained using SUM159 cells incubated with Doxorubicin (Dox) for 2 d (1 µg/ml; 100 fold IC_{50}; data not shown). **C.** DU145 prostate cancer cells (Parental, left panel; 4X) were incubated with Docetaxel (10 nM) for 4 d, after which chemotherapy was removed and fresh culture medium added. Residual tumor cells were imaged on d10 after treatment (Residual tumor cells, middle panel; 10X). Colonies were imaged on d22 ("Recurrent" colonies, right panel; 4X). **D.** SUM159 were incubated with Doxorubicin or Docetaxel as in "B". Recurrent colonies were counted using crystal violet on d18. Likewise, DU145 cells were incubated with Docetaxel as in C. Recurrent colonies were counted using crystal violet on d22. Results are representative of at least three independent trials.

Time Course- Cell Death Following Acute Chemotherapy Treatment

SUM159 were incubated with doxorubicin (1 μM) for 2 d, after which chemotherapy was removed, and new media added. Photographs were taken using an Olympus inverted microscope with a Canon EOS Rebel T4I. Final magnifications were 4X and 10X. Viable cell number was determined by performing trypan blue stains on cells harvested at 6 h, d1, d2, d3, and d7 post-chemotherapy treatment. Alternatively, DU145 tumor cells were incubated with docetaxel (10 nM). Chemotherapy was removed after 4 d. Viable cell number was determined as above for chemotherapy-treated SUM159 cells.

Time Course- Regrowth of Chemo-residual Tumor Cells

Six days after chemotherapy removal, SUM159 cells were harvested with trypsin-EDTA, and replated in 96 well plates (1000 cells/well). Tumor cell proliferation was assessed on a daily basis by measuring thymidine uptake. For the DU145 model, DU145 cells were harvested with accutase six days after chemotherapy removal, and replated in 96 well plates (1000 cells/well). Tumor cell proliferation was assessed on a daily basis by measuring thymidine uptake.

Evolution of "Recurrent" Colonies

SUM159 dormant cells were harvested 5–6 d after chemotherapy removal with trypsin-EDTA, and re-plated in 6-well plates (10^5 cells/well). Media was changed every 3–4 d. Recurrent colonies (d18–d22) were stained with crystal violet and colonies containing >50 cells were counted. DU145 dormant cells were harvested with accutase 6 d after chemotherapy removal and re-plated in 6-well plates (2.5×10^3 cells/well). Media was changed every 5–6 d. Recurrent colonies were stained with crystal violet on d22 and counted using the GelCount.

Western Blots

Cells were harvested using trypsin-EDTA, washed with PBS, incubated in RIPA buffer on ice for 20 min, and then subjected to high speed centrifugation to obtain total cellular protein in the soluble fraction. For nuclear protein extraction, harvested cells were first incubated in cytosolic lysis buffer (10 mM HEPES, 10 mM KCl, 1.5 mM $MgCl_2$, 0.5% NP40, and proteinase inhibitors) on ice for 20 min, centrifuged, and the supernatants were collected as cytosolic protein lysates. The residual pellets were washed with cytosolic lysis buffer once, and then incubated in nuclear lysis buffer (50 mM TRIS, 1% SDS, and proteinase inhibitors) plus Benzonase (Sigma, St. Louis, MO) on ice for 20 min. The supernatants after centrifugation were collected as nuclear protein extracts. Protein concentrations were determined by BCA assay. Equivalent amounts of protein were subjected to SDS-polyacrylamide gel electrophoresis (PAGE) and immuno-blotted with the following primary antibodies, followed by the approprimate species IRDye-conjugated secondary antibody (Invitrogen): p21 (Cell Signaling), GAPDH (GenScript), Actin (Sigma). Proteins were detected using Odyssey infrared imaging system (LI-COR, Lincoln, NE).

Thymidine Uptake

Cells were plated in 96-well plates (2×10^3 cells/well). After overnight incubation, cells were incubated with 0.5 μCi/well [Methyl-^{3}H]-Thymidine (Perkin Elmer) for 4–6 hs before harvesting onto glass-fiber filters. [^{3}H]-Thymidine incorporation was measured as counts per minute (CPM) using a Tri-Carb 2100TR time-resolved liquid scintillation counter (Perkin Elmer).

Alamar Blue

Cells were plated in 96-well black, clear bottom plates (2×10^3 cells/well) in 100 μl complete medium. After 6 h, 10 μl/well alamarBlue (Life Technologies) reagent was added and, after 3 hs, fluorescence was measured using a Cytation3 plate reader (BioTek).

PKH Labeling Study

SUM159 and DU145 cells were labeled using the PKH26 Red Fluorescent Cell Linker Kit (Sigma) according to the manufacturer's instructions. The labeled SUM159 cells were treated with doxorubicin (1 μg/ml) to generate chemotherapy enriched dormant cells, as described above. Likewise, PKH26-labelled DU145 were treated with docetaxel (10 nM) to generate chemotherapy-enriched dormant cells, as described above. Labelled cells were detected using the Guava EasyCyte Plus flow cytometer (Millipore).

Measuring Chemotherapy Sensitivity of Recurrent Tumor Cells

SUM159 and DU145 "recurrent" colonies (as described above) were re-plated in T75 tissue culture flasks and grown as a monolayer. Parental tumor cells and recurrent tumor cells were plated in 96-well plates (2×10^3 cells/well). After overnight incubation, cells were incubated with media only, doxorubicin, or docetaxel at the indicated concentrations for 2 d. [Methyl-^{3}H]-Thymidine was added (0.5 μCi/well) 6 h before harvesting onto glass-fiber filters. [^{3}H]-Thymidine incorporation was measured as described above. Data were reported as fold change relative to cells cultured in media alone.

Results

Several studies indicate that drug-resistant, slow-cycling tumor cells are represented at low frequency in human tumors, and are therapy resistant [5,6]. The contribution of these cells to tumor recurrence following chemotherapy treatment is not known. We investigated the hypothesis that short-term exposure of tumor cells to chemotherapy enriches for a slow-cycling, chemo-resistant tumor cell sub-population that can, over time, resume growth, thus resembling tumor recurrence. To test this hypothesis, we exposed human breast (SUM159) and prostate (DU145) tumor cells to acute chemotherapy treatment (Fig. 1A). SUM159 breast tumor cells were exposed to Docetaxel (100 nM; 100-fold IC_{50}) or Doxorubicin (1 μg/mL; 100-fold IC_{50}). DU145 prostate tumor cells were exposed to Docetaxel (10 nM; 6-fold IC_{50}). Chemotherapy was removed on d2 for SUM159 cells and on d4 for DU145 cells, and fresh culture medium was added. After 8 days (SUM159) or 10 days (DU145), the majority of tumor cells were dead. However, we noted that a small number of residual tumor cells remained (Fig. 1B and 1C). These residual tumor cells appeared to be non-proliferative, as indicated by the fact that their numbers did not increase for several days (data not shown). Approximately 10 d after chemotherapy removal, these residual tumor cells resumed proliferation (Fig. 3C) and eventually formed colonies, resembling a tumor recurrence (Fig. 1B–1D).

Tumor dormancy has been defined as a condition in which residual cancer cells stop dividing [11]. It is thought that these cells remain dormant for a prolonged period before receiving signals (intrinsic or extrinsic) that cause them to resume growth and establish recurrent tumors. Fitting this definition of dormancy, both breast tumor cells and prostate tumor cells surviving short term chemotherapy in our model represented a sub-population of cells that did not take up appreciable thymidine (Fig. 2A), but were

A.

B.

C.

D.

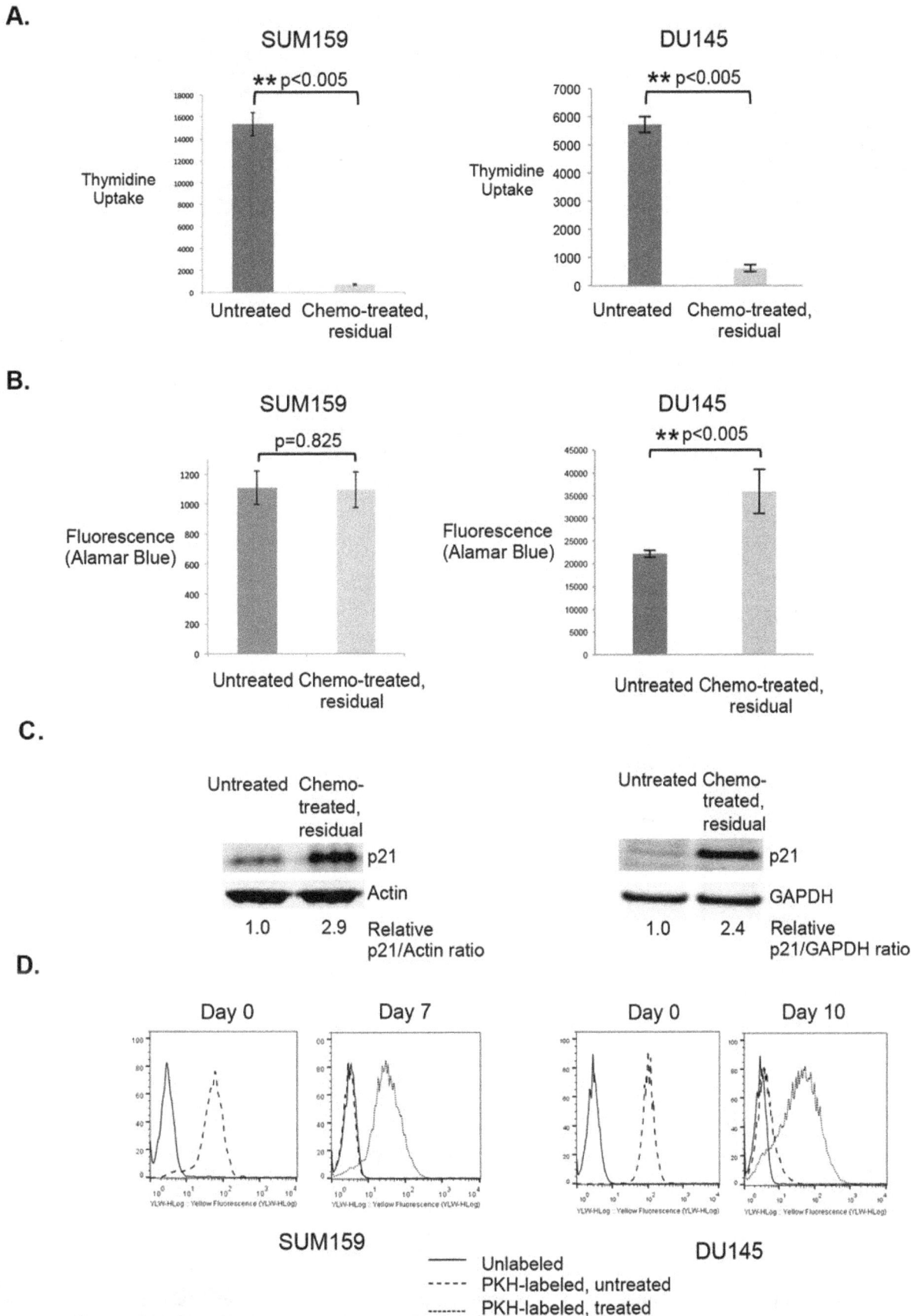

Figure 2. Chemotherapy enriches for dormant tumor cells. A and B. SUM159 breast and DU145 prostate cancer cells were exposed to acute Doxorubicin or Docetaxel treatment, respectively (as described in Fig. 1). Residual tumor cells surviving short-term chemotherapy treatment were

harvested on d8 (breast) or d10 (prostate), and seeded at 2000 cells/well in triplicate wells of a 96 well plate. Proliferation was determined by thymidine incorporation (+/−SD). Cell viability was assessed by alamar blue (fluorescence +/− SD) (**B**). Statistical significance for (A) and (B) was determined using a two-tailed student's t-test, with p<0.05 being considered significant. p≤0.05 (*); p≤0.005 (**). **C.** Total cellular protein was extracted from parental and residual, chemo-resistant tumor cells, and equivalent amounts were immunoblotted with p21 antibody, followed by IrDye-conjugated secondary antibody. Protein loading was assessed using Actin or GAPDH antibodies. Protein bands were detected by infrared imaging. Protein bands were quantified using Image J software (NIH), and the relative ratio of p21 to loading control is shown for each lane. Similar results were obtained in 3 independent trials. **D.** SUM159 or DU145 tumor cells were stained with the label-retaining dye PKH26, and labeling efficiency was assessed by flow cytometry on Day 0. PKH26-labelled SUM159 cells were either left untreated (- - - -) or incubated for 2 d with Doxorubicin (1 µg/ml; −−). PKH26-labelled DU145 cells were either left untreated (- - - -) or incubated for 4 d with Docetaxel (10 nM; −−). The % label-retaining cells was determined on d7 (SUM159) or d10 (DU145) after treatment. Note that at the time of harvest, the majority of untreated cells (proliferative) had lost the dye, whereas slow-cycling dormant cells enriched by chemotherapy had retained the dye.

A.

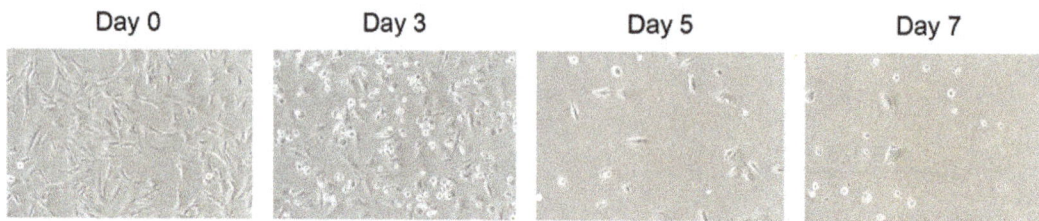

B.

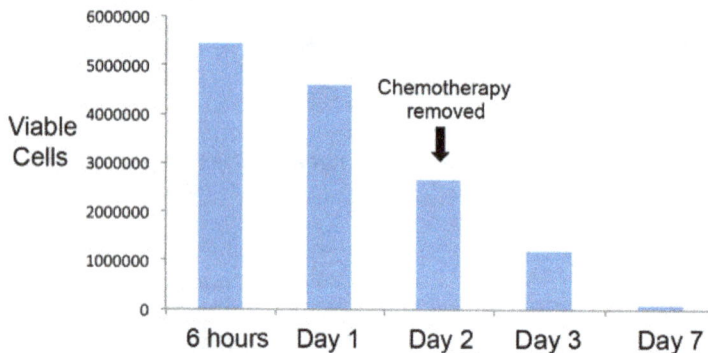

C.

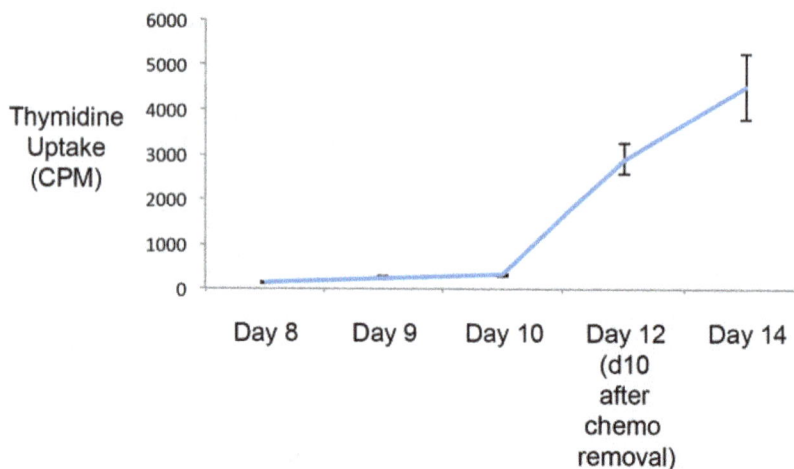

Figure 3. Kinetics of "recurrent" colony growth. SUM159 tumor cells were incubated with Doxorubicin (2d) as indicated in Fig. 1. **A and B.** Kinetics of cell die-off were assessed by imaging representative fields (**A**) as well as by counting viable cells using trypan blue (**B**) at the indicated times post-chemotherapy treatment. **C.** Proliferative status of residual tumor cells was measured over time by performing thymidine incorporation assays on cells (2000 cells/well) harvested at the indicated times post-chemotherapy treatment.

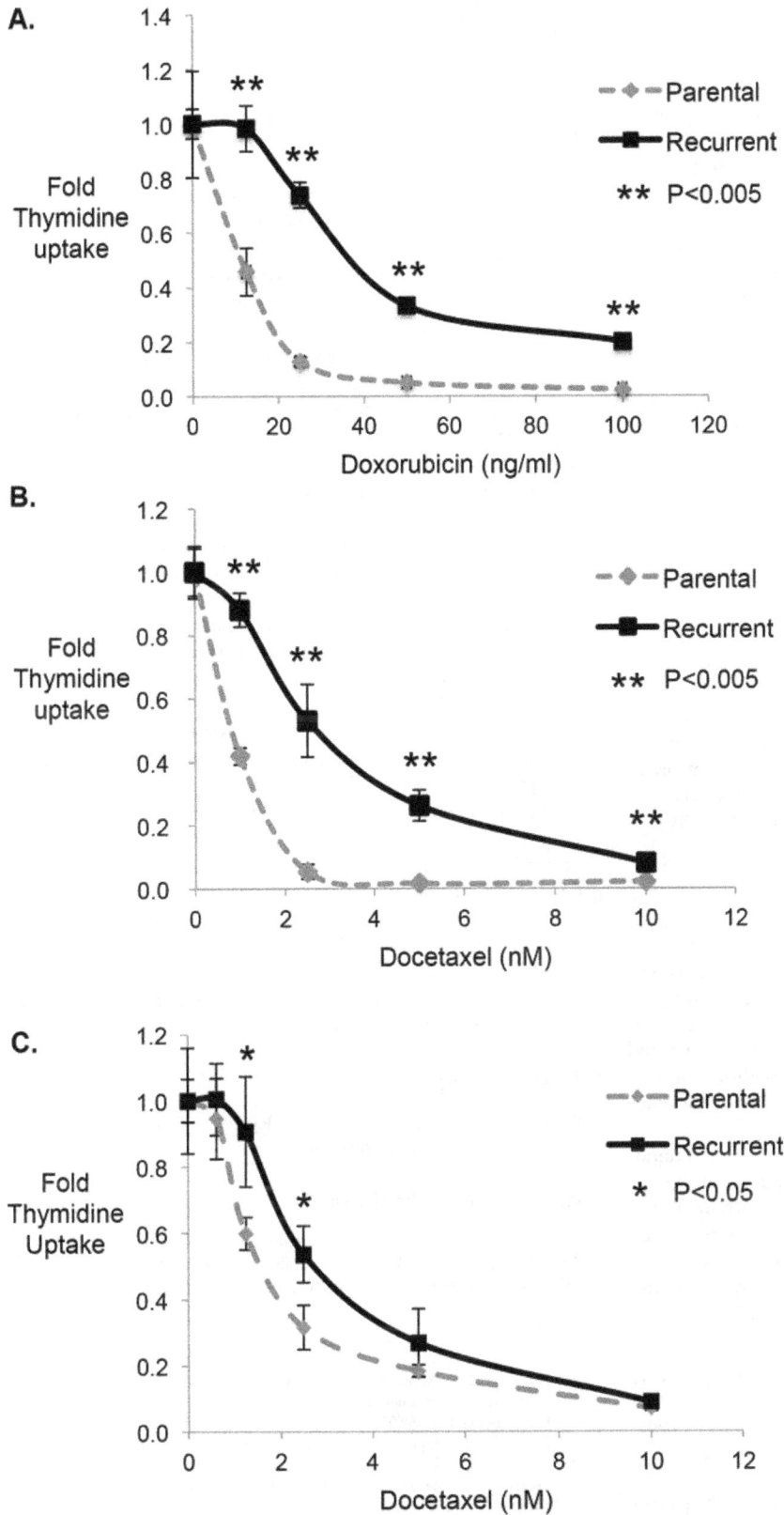

Figure 4. Tumor cells from recurrent colonies are more resistant to chemotherapy than parental tumor cells. A and B. SUM159 breast tumor cells were incubated with Doxorubicin (**A**) or Docetaxel (**B**) as in Fig. 1. Residual tumor cells were allowed to grow in the absence of chemotherapy, resulting in the evolution of "recurrent" colonies. Tumor cells from recurrent colonies, as well as parental tumor cells, were re-challenged with the indicated concentrations of Doxorubicin (**A**) or Docetaxel (**B**). Chemo-sensitivity was assessed by thymidine incorporation. Data for each point are expressed as fold change relative to cells cultured in media only. n = 4, error bars represent S.D., *p<0.05, **p<0.005. **C.** DU145 prostate tumor cells were incubated with Docetaxel as in Fig. 1. Residual tumor cells were allowed to grow in the absence of chemotherapy, resulting

in the evolution of "recurrent" colonies. Tumor cells from recurrent colonies and parental tumor cells were re-challenged with the indicated concentrations of Docetaxel. Chemo-sensitivity was assessed by thymidine incorporation, as in A and B.

metabolically active, as indicated using an alamar blue assay (Fig. 2B). Notably, chemo-residual DU145 prostate cancer cells exhibited increased alamar blue positivity compared to parental DU145 cells, suggesting that these enriched cells may have elevated metabolism. Chemo-residual tumor cells also expressed increased levels of p21 (Fig. 2C), a cell cycle arrest protein. Contrasting with parental tumor cells, chemotherapy-enriched tumor cells were slow-cycling, as indicated by their retention of the lipophilic dye PKH26 (Fig. 2D).

We next sought to determine the time after chemotherapy removal that dormant tumor cells resumed growth after chemotherapy removal. The number of viable breast tumor cells decreased for five days after chemotherapy removal, as demonstrated in Fig. 3A and B. However, residual tumor cells did not resume proliferation until approximately 10 days after chemotherapy removal, as assessed by thymidine uptake (Fig. 3C). Similar kinetics of growth were observed using the DU145/docetaxel prostate cancer model (data not shown).

Recurrent tumors are frequently detected in cancer patients many years after initial chemotherapy treatment, and these tumors are chemo-refractory. Similar to recurrent tumors in patients, recurrent tumor cells evolving in our model from chemotherapy-enriched dormant cells exhibited increased chemotherapy resistance (Fig. 4). Increased therapy resistance was observed in both recurrent breast tumor cells (Fig. 4A and B) and in recurrent prostate tumor cells (Fig. 4C). Notably, resistant recurrent breast tumor colonies were observed independent of the class of chemotherapy treatment (taxane vs anthracycilne) (Fig. 4A and 4B).

Discussion

Our results demonstrate that dormant, chemo-resistant tumor cells can be enriched from human breast and prostate tumor cell lines by short-term chemotherapy treatment. DNA-damaging (Doxorubicin) and microtubule-modifying (Docetaxel) chemotherapies, representing standard treatment regimens for breast and prostate cancer patients respectively, enriched for these dormant cells at clinically relevant doses [12,13], indicating broad relevance to patient treatment (Fig. 1).

The current study focused on the ability of these dormant tumor cells to resume growth upon chemotherapy withdrawal, resembling the process of tumor recurrence. Notably, "recurrent" tumor cells evolving after chemotherapy withdrawal were more resistant to subsequent chemotherapy challenge than parental tumor cells. The therapy resistance of recurrent tumor cells in our model

resembles therapy resistance of recurrent tumors in cancer patients [4].

The resistant phenotype of "recurrent" tumor cells evolving from our chemotherapy-enriched dormant cells contrasts with the reversibly-resistant phenotype of tumor cells subjected to long-term drug selection [6,14]. To date, we have observed continued resistance of our "recurrent" breast tumor lines for 50 days after chemotherapy withdrawal (representing approximately 40 doubling times for these cells; data not shown). The irreversible resistance of these drug resistant tumor cells has important implications for patient treatment. Specifically, the existence of irreversible drug resistant phenotypes in the original tumor argues against models suggesting that recurrent tumors arising in patients after a gap in treatment ("drug holiday") may benefit from retreatment with the same therapy [4]. Studies are ongoing to determine if "recurrent" tumor cells from our in vitro model remain chemo-refractory for months after therapy withdrawal.

We are currently defining resistance mechanisms (DNA repair, drug efflux) of recurrent tumor cells evolving from our short term chemotherapy enrichment model. Notably, recurrent colonies exhibiting increased chemotherapy resistance relative to parental tumor cells were obtained regardless of the chemotherapy class studied [DNA-damaging (Doxorubicin) or microtubule-modifying (Taxane)]. This finding raises the important possibility that chemo-resistant tumor cells may be cross-resistant to multiple chemotherapy classes, a topic of current investigation.

Our in vitro model of tumor dormancy/recurrence is important because it enriches for a dormant tumor cell population that is normally under-represented in the parental tumor cell line. Current studies in the lab are focused on identifying novel signaling pathways that drive tumor dormancy/recurrence using this short-term chemotherapy enrichment strategy. These studies have the potential to identify: 1) logical therapeutic targets in chemo-resistant, dormant tumor cell populations, and 2) biomarkers that predict recurrence-free survival.

Acknowledgments

We thank Drs. Rupa Ray, Gustaaf de Ridder, and George Cianciolo for their useful comments on these studies.

Author Contributions

Conceived and designed the experiments: SL MK SP KK REB. Performed the experiments: SL MK SP KK. Analyzed the data: SL MK SP KK VLS SVP REB. Wrote the paper: SL KK REB.

References

1. Weiss RB, Woolf SH, Demakos E, Holland JF, Berry DA, et al. (2003) Natural history of more than 20 years of node-positive primary breast carcinoma treated with cyclophosphamide, methotrexate, and fluorouracil-based adjuvant chemotherapy: a study by the Cancer and Leukemia Group B. Journal of clinical oncology: official journal of the American Society of Clinical Oncology 21: 1825–1835.

2. Calcagno AM, Salcido CD, Gillet JP, Wu CP, Fostel JM, et al. (2010) Prolonged drug selection of breast cancer cells and enrichment of cancer stem cell characteristics. Journal of the National Cancer Institute 102: 1637–1652.

3. Puhr M, Hoefer J, Schafer G, Erb HH, Oh SJ, et al. (2012) Epithelial-to-mesenchymal transition leads to docetaxel resistance in prostate cancer and is mediated by reduced expression of miR-200c and miR-205. The American journal of pathology 181: 2188–2201.

4. Kuczynski EA, Sargent DJ, Grothey A, Kerbel RS (2013) Drug rechallenge and treatment beyond progression–implications for drug resistance. Nature reviews Clinical oncology 10: 571–587.

5. Moore N, Houghton J, Lyle S (2012) Slow-cycling therapy-resistant cancer cells. Stem cells and development 21: 1822–1830.

6. Sharma SV, Lee DY, Li B, Quinlan MP, Takahashi F, et al. (2010) A chromatin-mediated reversible drug-tolerant state in cancer cell subpopulations. Cell 141: 69–80.

7. Fillmore CM, Kuperwasser C (2008) Human breast cancer cell lines contain stem-like cells that self-renew, give rise to phenotypically diverse progeny and survive chemotherapy. Breast cancer research: BCR 10: R25.

8. Iliopoulos D, Hirsch HA, Wang G, Struhl K (2011) Inducible formation of breast cancer stem cells and their dynamic equilibrium with non-stem cancer cells via IL6 secretion. Proceedings of the National Academy of Sciences of the United States of America 108: 1397–1402.

9. Li X, Lewis MT, Huang J, Gutierrez C, Osborne CK, et al. (2008) Intrinsic resistance of tumorigenic breast cancer cells to chemotherapy. Journal of the National Cancer Institute 100: 672–679.

10. Shipitsin M, Campbell LL, Argani P, Weremowicz S, Bloushtain-Qimron N, et al. (2007) Molecular definition of breast tumor heterogeneity. Cancer cell 11: 259–273.

11. Lin WC, Rajbhandari N, Wagner KU (2014) Cancer Cell Dormancy in Novel Mouse Models for Reversible Pancreatic Cancer: A Lingering Challenge in the Development of Targeted Therapies. Cancer research 74: 2138–2143.

12. Brunsvig PF, Andersen A, Aamdal S, Kristensen V, Olsen H (2007) Pharmacokinetic analysis of two different docetaxel dose levels in patients with non-small cell lung cancer treated with docetaxel as monotherapy or with concurrent radiotherapy. BMC cancer 7: 197.

13. Liu J, Zheng H, Tang M, Ryu YC, Wang X (2008) A therapeutic dose of doxorubicin activates ubiquitin-proteasome system-mediated proteolysis by acting on both the ubiquitination apparatus and proteasome. American journal of physiology Heart and circulatory physiology 295: H2541–2550.

14. Williams KP, Allensworth JL, Ingram SM, Smith GR, Aldrich AJ, et al. (2013) Quantitative high-throughput efficacy profiling of approved oncology drugs in inflammatory breast cancer models of acquired drug resistance and re-sensitization. Cancer letters 337: 77–89.

10

Evolution of Treatment Regimens in Multiple Myeloma: A Social Network Analysis

Helen Mahony[1], Athanasios Tsalatsanis[1], Ambuj Kumar[1], Benjamin Djulbegovic[1,2]*

1 Department of Internal Medicine, Division of Evidence-Based Medicine & Health Outcomes Research, University of South Florida, Tampa, Florida, United States of America, **2** H. Lee Moffitt Cancer Center & Research Institute, Department of Hematology and Health Outcomes and Behavior, Tampa, Florida, United States of America

Abstract

Background: Randomized controlled trials (RCTs) are considered the gold standard for assessing the efficacy of new treatments compared to standard treatments. However, the reasoning behind treatment selection in RCTs is often unclear. Here, we focus on a cohort of RCTs in multiple myeloma (MM) to understand the patterns of competing treatment selections.

Methods: We used social network analysis (SNA) to study relationships between treatment regimens in MM RCTs and to examine the topology of RCT treatment networks. All trials considering induction or autologous stem cell transplant among patients with MM were eligible for our analysis. Medline and abstracts from the annual proceedings of the American Society of Hematology and American Society for Clinical Oncology, as well as all references from relevant publications were searched. We extracted data on treatment regimens, year of publication, funding type, and number of patients enrolled. The SNA metrics used are related to node and network level centrality and to node positioning characterization.

Results: 135 RCTs enrolling a total of 36,869 patients were included. The density of the RCT network was low indicating little cohesion among treatments. Network Betweenness was also low signifying that the network does not facilitate exchange of information. The maximum geodesic distance was equal to 4, indicating that all connected treatments could reach each other in four "steps" within the same pathway of development. The distance between many important treatment regimens was greater than 1, indicating that no RCTs have compared these regimens.

Conclusion: Our findings show that research programs in myeloma, which is a relatively small field, are surprisingly decentralized with a lack of connectivity among various research pathways. As a result there is much crucial research left unexplored. Using SNA to visually and analytically examine treatment networks prior to designing a clinical trial can lead to better designed studies.

Editor: Yu-Kang Tu, National Taiwan University, Taiwan

Funding: The authors have no support or funding to report.

Competing Interests: The authors have declared that no competing interests exist.

* Email: bdjulbeg@health.usf.edu

Introduction

Multiple myeloma (MM) is a hematological malignancy, which accounts for 1% of cancer deaths and 10% of all hematological malignancies in the US. [1] Several advances in the treatment of MM have been possible due to testing of newer agents in randomized controlled trials (RCTs). As a result of these advancements, MM has transformed into a chronic disease.

The first randomized controlled trial (RCT) in MM was published in 1966. [2] Since then over 300 RCTs have been published and nearly half have been conducted in an induction and transplant setting. [3] While there is a vast body of research involving RCTs in MM as well as systematic reviews and meta-analyses [4–7], there has been no formal assessment of patterns of treatment discoveries in the context of RCTs. That is, it is not known how a new treatment regimen makes its way through the translational cycle to be tested in an RCT. Understanding the

process of this translational cycle, specifically in relation to the choice of new regimens for the treatment of MM in RCTs, is important and has several benefits. At the highest level, it can provide investigators interested in assessing the efficacy of similar treatment regimens with collaborative opportunities, thereby avoiding duplication of research efforts. Avoiding duplication can result in not only consolidation of research efforts and allocation of limited resources, but can also lead to averting patients from participating in trials where the answers to the treatment efficacy may already be known.

Using methodologies that provide analytical as well as visual representations of existing research in MM, prior to conducting new RCTs, could lead to better designed studies and enable researchers to address more relevant clinical and research questions. In this paper, we propose using social network analysis (SNA) to study the patterns of interactions between treatment regimens in RCTs, to identify potential limitations, and draw future research directions. SNA provides a "bird's-eye view" of the overall RCT universe, which enables us to examine relationships, directions, and importance of different treatment regimens in the network. Such an approach could allow industry and government to save valuable healthcare dollars by focusing resources on relevant research.

We have previously reported on a preliminary SNA on RCTs of autologous stem cell transplant (ASCT) and novel agents for MM [8]. Our analyses showed that research programs in myeloma, which is a relatively small field, were surprisingly decentralized and various research pathways suffered by lack of connectivity. We hypothesize that this finding is attributed to lack of interaction among researchers performing RCTs and the absence of policies that enforce consolidation of the totality of existing evidence prior to designing new RCTs. In this paper, we expand our initial analyses to include all RCTs of induction or ASCT among patients with MM and we illustrate a novel application of SNA to study the topology of RCT treatment networks.

Methods

Dataset

We searched MEDLINE for any relevant RCTs published until April 2012 using the searching strategies described by Haynes et al. [9] No limits of any kind were imposed. Abstracts from the American Society of Hematology and the American Society of Clinical Oncology were also searched. All references from relevant publications were scanned manually to identify additional candidate studies. Any MM RCT studying the treatment regimens of induction or ASCT was eligible for our analysis. We extracted data on treatments used for experimental arm and control arm, year of publication, funding type, and number of patients enrolled. For funding type, we categorized the funding source into the broad categories of public, private for profit, or private not for profit. If the funding source were a mix of these categories, funding type was recorded as mixed. For publications that did not report a funding source, we labeled their funding type as unclear.

Social networks

A social network is represented as a set of nodes denoting different entities such as individuals or organizations and their interactions denoted as ties [10,11]. SNA is the theoretical framework developed to understand social networks and to reveal hidden and potentially useful information regarding entities and their interactions. SNA has been used extensively to explain phenomena such as (among others) scientific interaction [12], information exchange [13], and treatment success [14]. In this paper, we use SNA to study the RCTs of MM universe focusing on the treatment regimen interactions as they appear in each RCT. Such modeling can provide an in-depth understanding of how treatments and comparisons are distributed and identify the factors associated with development of research questions. [10] We define a treatment network as the set of nodes denoting each treatment tested in an RCT connected with ties denoting a direct comparison between treatments in RCTs (Figure S1 in File S1). The direction of a tie in the treatment network is used to distinguish treatments as experimental and as control. That is, the ties are directed away from the experimental node and toward the control node. Using SNA we can measure the properties of the entire treatment network as well as the properties of each node individually. [15] These measures help us understand how nodes interact and identify opportunities and constraints for future research.

Node-level properties

Not all nodes in a network are of the same importance. Nodes with a certain position in the network can interact easier/harder with particular nodes and faster/slower with others. To measure the ability of the node to interact with other nodes in the network or to facilitate interactions between nodes we use the *centrality* measures of *degree*, *closeness*, and *betweenness*. In general, centrality measures describe key attributes of the position of a node representing a treatment regimen in the treatment network. [10] Degree measures the number of different comparisons a treatment regimen has participated in; closeness measures the ease at which a treatment regimen can reach other treatment regimens in a network [16], and it is directly associated with the ability to extract information about regimen superiority outside an RCT environment (i.e. indirect meta-analyses); betweenness [17] represents the ability of a treatment regimen to link other treatment regimens, a property that is particularly desirable in indirect meta-analyses. Degree and closeness are further classified into *in-* and *out-degree* and *in-* and *out-closeness* respectively. In the RCT network, in- and out-degree show the number of times a particular regimen has been participating in an RCT as control or experimental respectively. In-closeness shows the easiness at which a node can be reached and out-closeness the easiness at which a node can reach others in the network. When measuring degree and closeness we need to differentiate between control and experimental treatments. Therefore, degree and closeness calculations are performed on the directed treatment networks. On the other hand, when measuring betweenness, we are interested only in the position of the node. Therefore, betweenness calculations were performed on the undirected networks. Note that directed and undirected networks have the same structure (i.e. same number of nodes and number of ties); however, directed networks are represented with directional ties, while undirected networks are represented with bidirectional ties.

Network level properties

Network level properties are associated with the topology of the entire treatment network. We compute measures such as the network's *density*, *maximum geodesic distance*, *clustering coefficient*, *centrality measures*, *KeyPlayer function*, and the *Girvan-Newman Algorithm* as indicators of the network structure. [10] Density reports the actual treatment interactions in the network as a fraction of all possible interactions (e.g. each regimen is compared to all other regimens). A density value of 15% to 25% indicates that a very small portion of all available comparisons have been achieved and that any changes to the interactions between treatments would have a profound effect on the cohesion of the network. [10] Conversely, values greater than 50% demonstrate that a significant number of comparisons have been made and that changes to interactions will have no or little effect on the cohesion of the network. The maximum geodesic distance corresponds to the network's diameter and it measures the maximum distance between any two treatments in the network. The clustering coefficient is the degree at which treatments in the network form clusters. [10] The clustering coefficient takes values between 0 and 1 where 1 indicates a fully connected network (e.g. each treatment is connected to all the rest). Smaller values of clustering coefficient reveal a rather random pattern of connectivity. [10] The network level centralization measures such as closeness, betweenness, and degree provide an overall impression of network centrality. Interpretation of the network level centralization values is similar to their node level centrality counterparts. For example, a network with low betweenness does not facilitate sharing of information. The Girvan-Newman

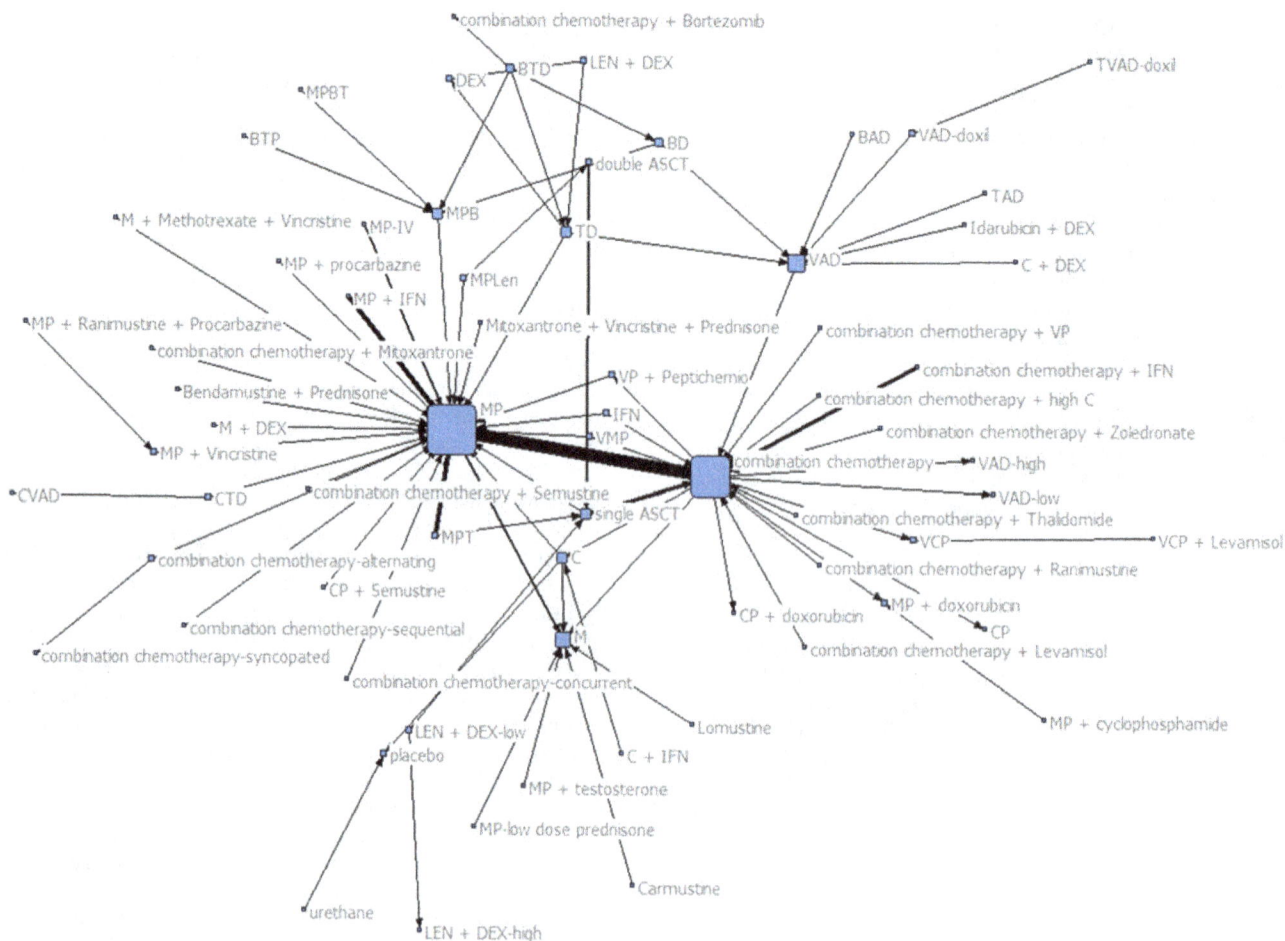

Figure 1. Connected component of RCT treatment network. Each node is associated with a treatment tested in an RCT and each tie denotes a comparison between two treatments. The width of the ties among treatments denotes the number of times two treatments have been tested in RCTs. The network represents the connected component of the network depicted in Figure S1 in File S1 and it is comprised of 155 treatment comparisons. The most frequently tested comparison is between *combination therapy* and *MP*.

Algorithm identifies *communities* of treatment regimens. Communities are loosely connected groups of tightly interconnected nodes. [18] The existence of multiple communities may be an indicator of research in isolation. The KeyPlayer function determines the optimal set of treatments in the sense that if an optimal set of nodes were to be removed from the network, this would have a crippling effect. Additionally, the KeyPlayer function determines the most well-connected treatment regimens. Changes to these regimens can influence other treatment regimens. [19]

2-mode networks

In addition to the treatment network described in the previous subsections we formed and studied a different category of networks. 2-Mode networks are used to report and analyze the relationships between two different classes of entities. While the treatment network presented previously is used to analyze the relationships between all treatment regimens, the 2-mode network is built to analyze the relationships between treatment regimens and an additional entity such as the funding source or the publication year. We have generated two 2-mode networks. The first 2-mode network (treatment – year) provides a visual association of treatment regimens and the decade they have been used. Similarly, the second 2-mode network (treatment –funding)

provides a representation of the funding mechanisms used for each regimen. In the 2-mode networks, the direction of the ties is formed from the experimental and control nodes towards either year of publication or funding type.

Data analysis

The main analysis included calculation of the following measures: *betweenness, density, clustering coefficient, closeness, degree, Girvan-Newman Algorithm, KeyPlayer, maximum geodesic distance* and *distance* among treatments. For the analysis of the node-level and network level properties, we included only treatment regimens from the connected component of the treatment network (e.g. disregarded isolated sets of nodes). The first well-designed RCT of ASCT versus chemotherapy was published in 1996. [20] In order to examine the effect of the first important breakthrough (ASCT) on the evolution of treatment regimens, we also conducted a subgroup analysis of trials published in 1996 or later. Additionally, a time series analysis of the networks with trials from 1996 to 2012 was conducted to compare network properties through time. All networks ware analyzed with UCINET 6 [21] and KeyPlayer 1.44 [19]. Visual representations of the networks were created with NetDraw 2.119. [21]

89

Table 1. Abbreviations of Treatment Regimens.

Abbreviation	Name of Treatment Regimens
M	melphalan
P	prednisone
C	cyclophosphamide
V	vincristine
MP	melphalan, prednisone
ASCT	autologous stem cell transplant
LEN	lenalidomide
DEX	dexamethasone
TD	thalidomide, dexamethasone
MPT	melphalan, prednisone, thalidomide
MPB	melphalan, prednisone, bortezomib
MPLen	melphalan, prednisone, lenalidomide
BTP	bortezomib, thalidomide, prednisone
BD	bortezomib, dexamethasone
VAD	vincristine, doxorubicin, dexamethasone
MPBT	melphalan, prednisone, bortezomib, thalidomide
TAD	thalidomide, doxorubicin, dexamethasone
TVAD	thalidomide, vincristine, doxorubicin, dexamethasone
BTD	bortezomib, thalidomide, dexamethasone
CTD	cyclophosphamide, thalidomide, dexamethasone
VP	vincristine, prednisone
Q	quinine
IFN	interferon
Combination chemotherapy	vincristine, doxorubicin, melphalan, cyclophosphamide, prednisone
	vincristine, BCNU, doxorubicin, melphalan, prednisone
	vincristine, BCNU, melphalan, cyclophosphamide, prednisone
	vincristine, BCNU, doxorubicin, dexamethasone
	BCNU, doxorubicin, melphalan, cyclophosphamide
	BCNU, melphalan, cyclophosphamide, prednisone
	vincristine, BCNU, doxorubicin, prednisone
	vincristine, doxorubicin, cyclophosphamide, prednisone

Table 2. Node-level properties of RCT treatment network (connected component).

Treatment	Betweenness	In-Closeness	Out-Closeness	In-Degree	Out-Degree
MP	1399.8	4.572	1.471	72	4
Combination chemotherapy	1129.5	2.209	1.753	23	39
VAD	451.3	1.694	1.779	7	1
TD	264.3	1.493	1.838	3	4
MPB	207.167	1.538	1.492	4	1
C	197	2.293	1.515	2	4
Single ASCT	188.5	1.538	1.779	7	9
M	262.0	5.732	1.449	11	0
VAD-doxil	67	1.471	1.805	1	1

Table 3. Distances between selected treatment regimens.

Measure	Value
Distance from:	
MPT to combination chemotherapy	2
MPB to combination chemotherapy	2
MPLen to combination chemotherapy	2
MPT to MPB	2
MPT to MPLen	2
MPB to MPLen	2
MPT to single ASCT	1
MPB to single ASCT	2
MPLen to single ASCT	2

Results

Study selection

We found 135 trials which examined induction or ASCT therapies among patients with MM. Because of multi-arm RCTs, these 135 trials represented 165 comparisons and enrolled 36,869 patients. The entire treatment network is shown in Figure S1 in File S1. Figure 1 depicts the connected portion (connected component) of the entire treatment network that includes 155 comparisons and disregards the unconnected regimens. The treatment regimen abbreviations are listed in Table 1.

Node-level properties

Table 2 shows selected node-level properties for treatment regimens in the network depicted in Figure 1. The tie thickness, in Figure 1, denotes the frequency that two trials have been compared in an RCT. For example, the treatment regimen of *combination chemotherapy* was frequently compared to the treatment regimen of *MP*. The size of a node represents the number of different comparisons a regimen has been included in (node degree). The larger the size of the node, the greater the number of trials the associated treatment was compared to. The treatment participated in most trials was *MP* followed by *combination chemotherapy*. Also, based on the measures for in- and out-degree we see that MP (in-degree of 72) and combination

chemotherapy (in-degree of 23) are the regimens used most often as controls in RCTs. Combination chemotherapy has also been frequently used as experimental therapy in RCTs (out-degree of 39).

Regarding closeness (measured using directed network), all nodes had small, relatively similar closeness measures demonstrating a large distance between each node in the network and all other nodes in the network (Table 2). The node-level betweenness (measured using undirected network) was largest for the treatment regimens of *combination chemotherapy, MP,* and *VAD,* indicating that these regimens and those directly connected to them are excellent candidates for indirect meta-analysis.

Distances between selected treatment regimens (undirected network) are reported in Table 3. The majority of the distance between many important treatment regimens (e.g. *MP* to *combination chemotherapy; MPT* to *MPB; MPT* to *MPLen; MPB* to *MPLen;* and *MPB* to *single ASCT*) is equal to 2. This demonstrates that these treatment regimens can reach each other in two "steps", a property of significance in indirect meta-analyses. This also indicates that these treatment regimens have never been tested in a head-to-head comparison in an RCT.

Network level properties

The network level properties of *density, geodesic distance, clustering coefficient,* and the *centrality* measures are reported in Table 4. The density of the network was low, indicating there is

Table 4. Results of network level analysis for myeloma treatment network.

Measure	RCT network	Erdos-Renyi (random network) value
Density (%)	2.5	2.5
Average Geodesic Distance	3	4.33
Maximum Geodesic Distance	6	10
Clustering Coefficient	3.4	0.025
Network Centralization Metrics		
Betweenness	55.3	78
in-Closeness	1.69	24.1
out-Closeness	1.59	24.1
in-Degree	2.36	4.2
out-Degree	2.13	4.2

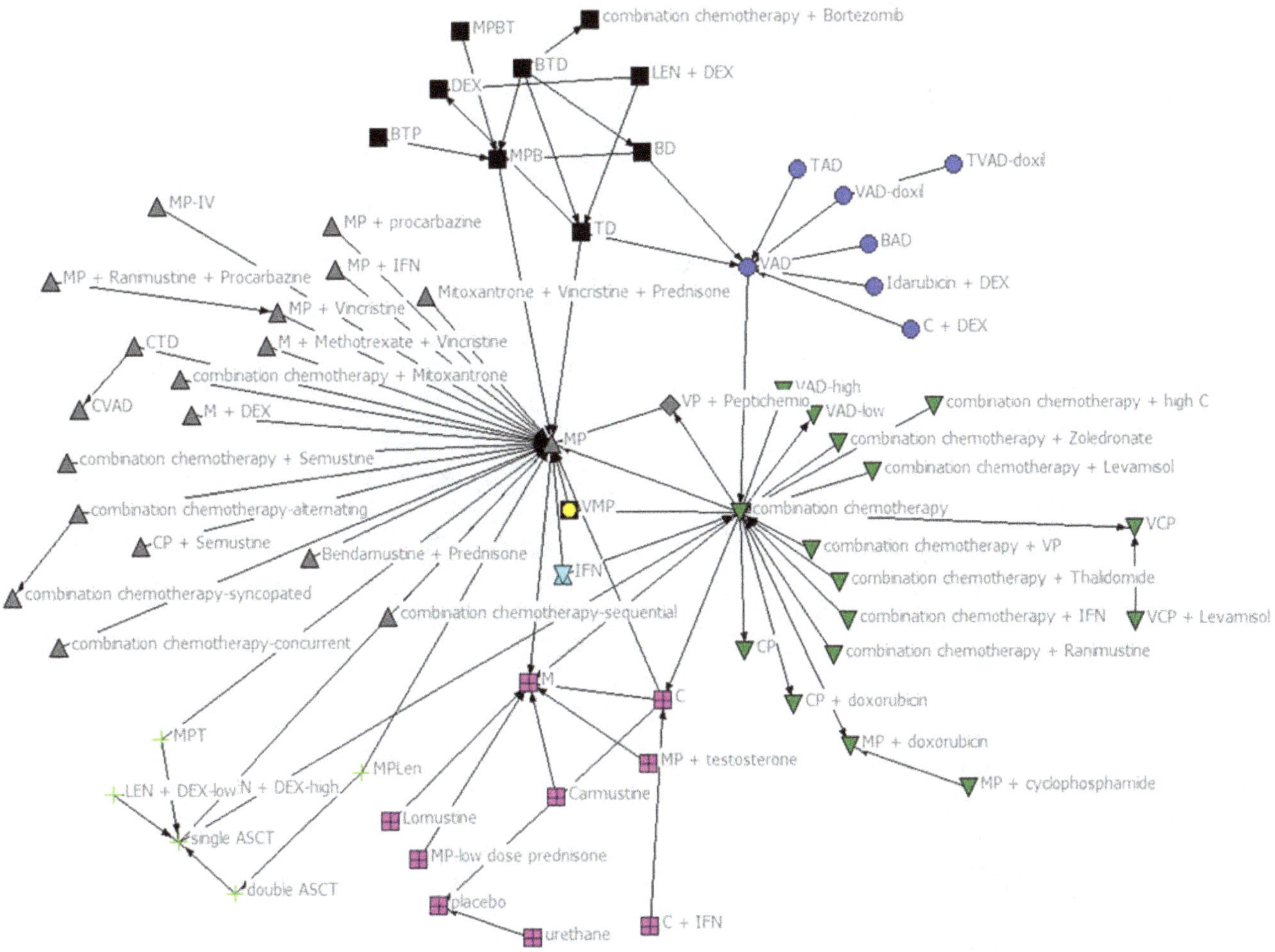

Figure 2. Girvan-Newman Algorithm. The algorithm identified 9 research communities that are loosely connected with each other.

little cohesion among the treatments studied. The maximum geodesic distance was equal to 6, indicating that all connected treatments could reach each other in six "steps" within the same pathway of development. All centrality measures are much lower than a similar random network (e.g. Erdos-Renyi with same number of nodes and same density). This shows that the RCT network is decentralized.

The KeyPlayer function identified that the treatment regimens of *MP*, *combination chemotherapy*, and *VAD* are vital to the network. The Girvan-Newman Algorithm (Figure 2) identified 9 research communities that are loosely connected with each other. These communities would be completely disconnected if the nodes: *MP*, *combination chemotherapy*, and *VAD* were to be removed.

For our subgroup analysis, we focused on trials published in 1996 or later to determine the effect of the publication by Attal et al., [20] on evolution of treatment regimens. The associated network is shown in Figure S2 in File S1. The KeyPlayer function identified again the *combination chemotherapy*, *MP*, and *VAD* as vital to the network. As in the complete treatment network, the Girvan-Newman Algorithm (Figure 3) shows that there are six research communities that are loosely connected to each other. A visual inspection of Figure 3 shows that these communities would be completely disconnected if the MP, combinational chemotherapy, TD and VAD therapies were to be removed.

2-mode network

Figure 4 demonstrates trends in treatment regimens over time and Figure S4 in File S1 displays the treatment comparisons by funding source. In these figures, degree is represented by the size of the node i.e. the larger the node the more comparisons are directed toward that node. All treatment comparisons were used in these networks, which included 165 comparisons.

In Figure 4, the largest number of treatment regimens was studied in the decades of the 1990s and 2000s, which corresponds to these nodes being the largest out of the six decades in which RCTs of MM patients have existed. As shown in Figure S4 in File S1, the highest number of comparisons came from trials which were publicly funded while the fewest trials were funded by private for profit funding organizations. Out of the 47 trials which did not report funding source, the majority (77%) were trials reported in either abstracts only (full publication not available) at the time this search was conducted or in trials published prior to 1996 when the CONSORT statement [22] was published.

The funding trends have changed for RCTs conducted after 1996. Figure 5 demonstrates the results of our subgroup analysis, where it is clear that the majority of RCTs are funded by both public and private entities (mixed). However, there are many trials that did not clearly report their funding mechanisms. The number of these trials is larger than the trials with mixed funding

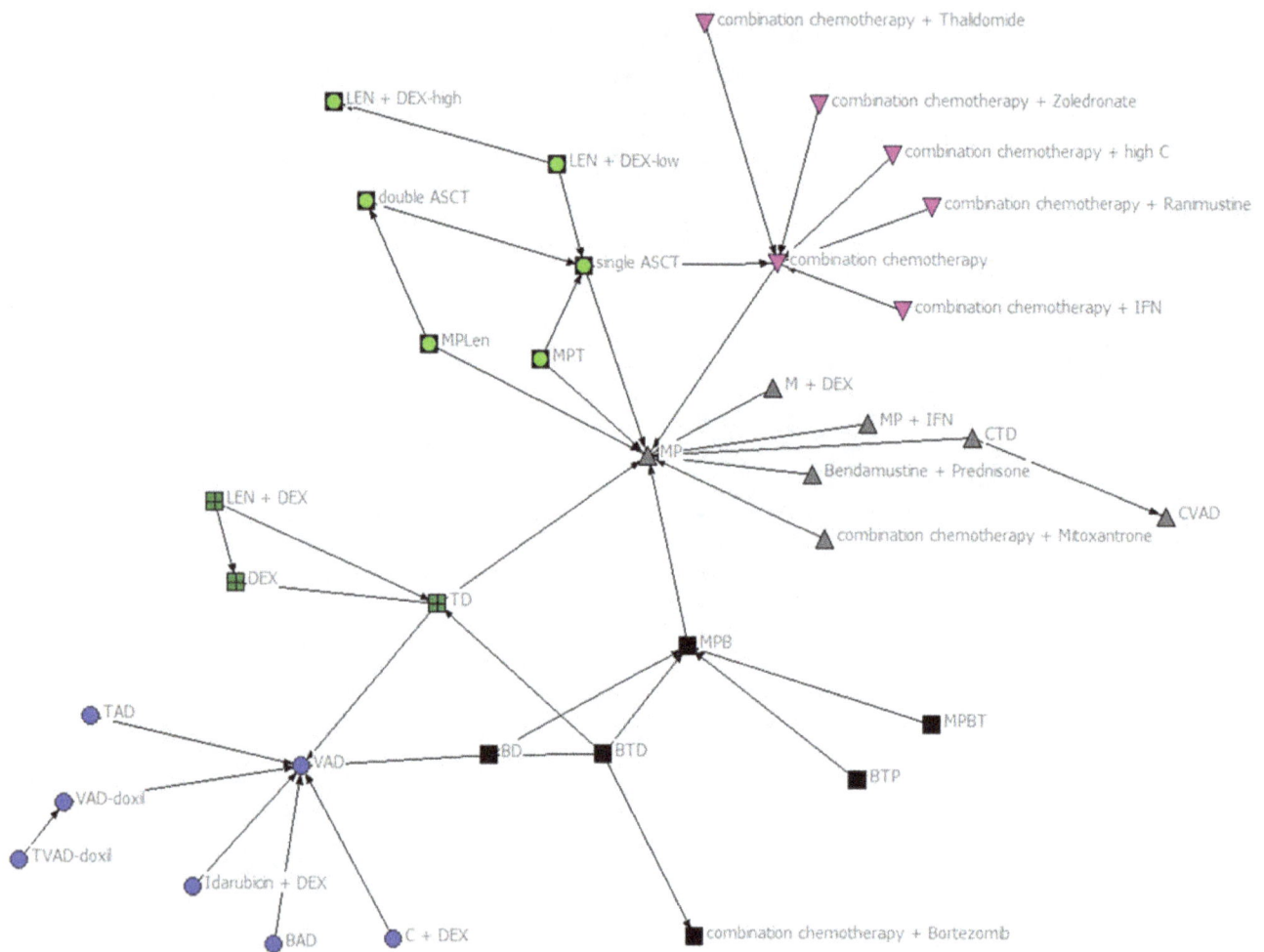

Figure 3. Girvan-Newman Algorithm of RCTs published 1996–2012. The algorithm 6 research communities that are loosely connected with each other.

(Figure 6). Even though the evidence is missing, we believe that these trials have been funded by private entities.

Finally, Figure 6 presents the evolution of different centrality measures as the treatment network is constructed over time (Figure S3 in File S1). It is interesting to note that even with the addition of multiple treatment regimens over time, there is very little change in the network's centrality, which stresses the fact that there is no coordinated research effort in MM.

Discussion

We have analyzed a diverse network of induction and transplant treatment regimens compared in RCTs. Our main finding is that new therapies are compared against established treatments over and over again and not proceeding within a logical framework of testing the most relevant hypotheses. This is demonstrated by the low closeness at both the node and network level and the high betweenness for *MP*, *combination chemotherapy*, *VAD*, and *single ASCT* that do not fully extend to novel agents such as bortezomib, lenalidomide, and thalidomide. This is further exemplified by the fact that there are no direct comparisons between many new regimens, which draws future research directions for RCTs in indirect meta-analysis.

One surprising finding was that through the KeyPlayer function and Girvan-Newman Algorithm we identified two newer treatment regimens, *TD* and *MPB*, which in addition to *combination chemotherapy* and *VAD*, are crucial in maintaining the network structure. However, lenalidomide was not identified as being important in the network even though it is widely used in contemporary practice as first line treatment. These findings point to the discrepancy in regimens being tested in RCTs versus regimens used in practice by the treating Oncologists. The results also demonstrate that researchers tend to compare experimental treatments to inferior regimens. That is, researchers do not compare the most active experimental treatments in head to head trials.

The results of our subgroup analyses show that since 1996 the MM treatment network has evolved in such a way that the novel agents of thalidomide and bortezomib have become very important in maintaining network cohesion. In 1996, Attal et al. [20] demonstrated that ASCT was superior to chemotherapy. This is considered to be the first important breakthrough in the treatment of MM. This subgroup analysis also indicates that chemotherapy and MP are of mostly historical importance.

We also found that the largest number of treatment regimens was studied in the decades of the 1990s and 2000s. The three

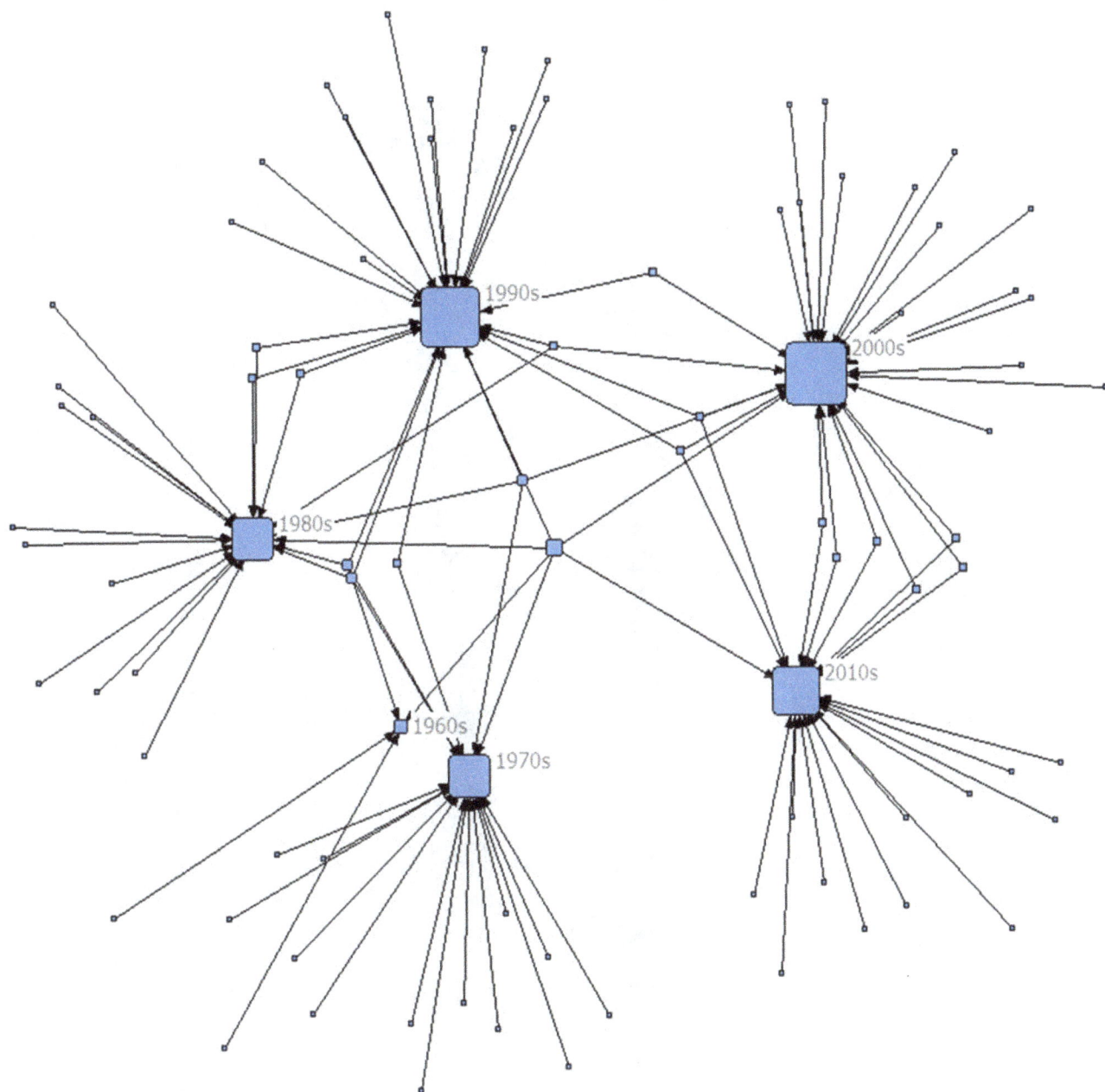

Figure 4. Decades in which treatments have been tested. Most treatment comparisons have been implemented in the decades of the 1990s and 2000s.

novel agents of *thalidomide*, *bortezomib*, and *lenalidomide* were developed in the late 1990s and early 2000s which may explain this increase in comparisons of treatment regimens during this time. Additionally, funding source has changed in recent years (since 1996) from being predominately publically funded to a mix of both private and public funding sources.

In this treatment network, designing trials which compare these treatment regimens to each other directly has been avoided by researchers and funders. As a result, better treatment regimens may not be discovered. The fastest rate of discovery occurs when a few hypotheses are tested sequentially. The lack of attention to the entire network is likely the reason that there is current confusion in the field and as a result guideline panels [23] are not able to

provide conclusive recommendations on the best first-line treatment from a list of 83 regimens.

Our analysis has some limitations. The main limitation is that we are inferring reasons from published trials on why researchers and funders choose which treatment to study. Since we only included trials examining treatment regimens used in induction or transplant setting, we cannot decipher how this treatment network fits into the larger network of all MM trials. Future research should focus on conducting a SNA on other areas of MM treatment such as supportive, maintenance, and salvage therapies. Nevertheless, our network analysis focuses on giving insight into first-line treatment, which is the practitioner's best attempt to slow down the progression of disease.

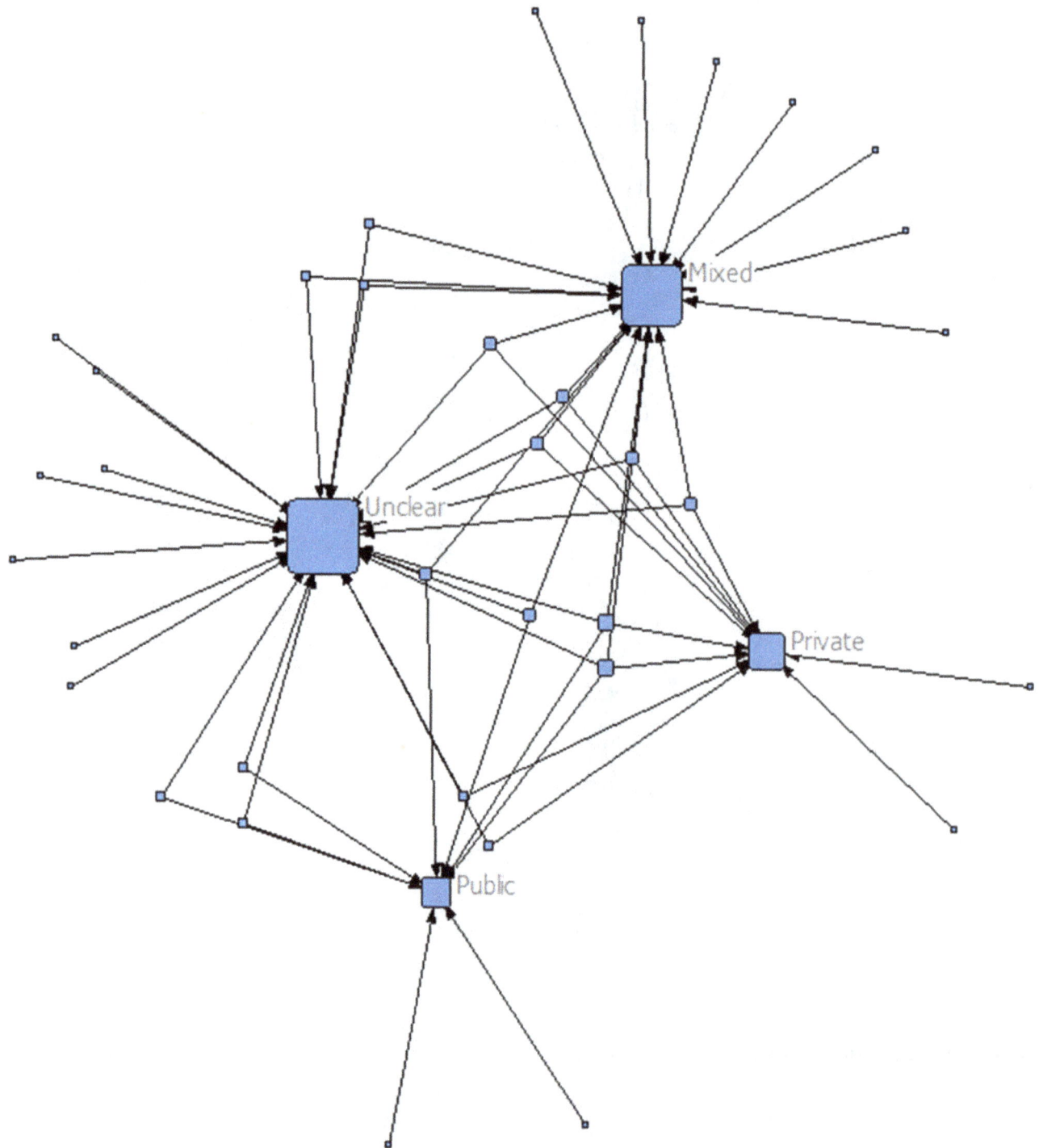

Figure 5. Funding type of trials published in the period 1996–2012. Most treatment comparisons have been funded by a mix of public and private entities. Even though the evidence is missing, we believe that the trials within the unclear funding node have been funded by private entities.

Furthermore, the current design does not allow for analysis of single arm RCTs, which may provide valuable information regarding a regimen's efficacy in MM, and does not include phase I or phase II trials. Finally, since this is the first SNA study on RCT treatments, it is impossible to compare our findings with similar networks in different diseases, which forced us to use random networks for comparison.

Performing SNA in RCTs may provide both funders and researchers with the overall assessment of existing evidence in a given field within the totality of research efforts that may help avoid isolation and duplication. Once performed, researchers may visualize the overall research network and determine the relevance of their hypotheses and if necessary derive future research directions such as those suggested in this study (e.g. MP to

Network statistics over time

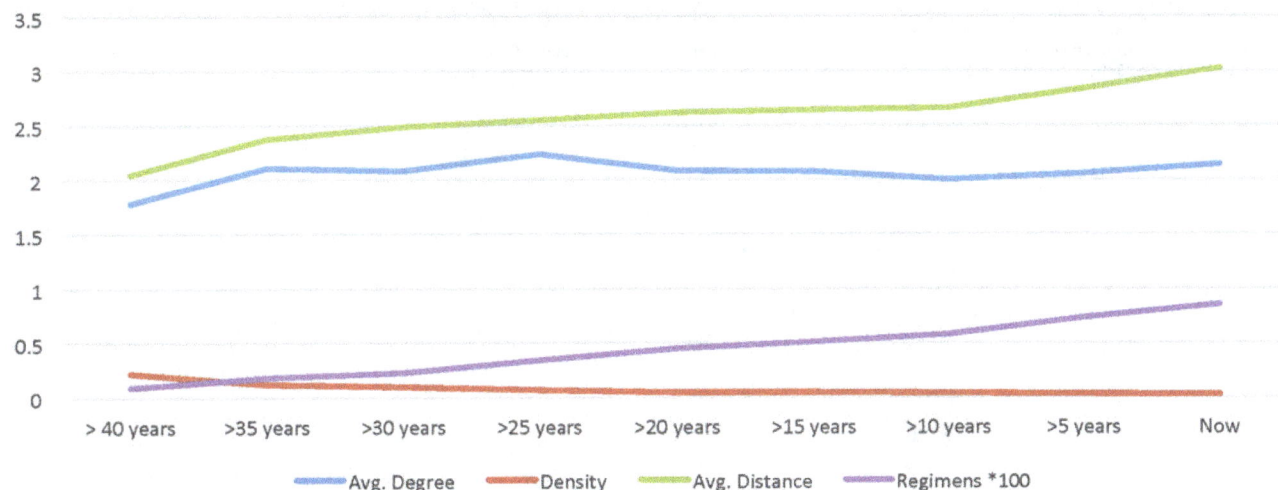

Figure 6. Evolution of centrality measures over time. There is little change in the network's centrality which stresses the fact that there is no coordinated research effort in MM.

combination chemotherapy; MPT to MPB; MPT to MPLen; MPB to MPLen; and MPB to single ASCT).

We conclude that research programs in myeloma are decentralized with a lack of connectivity among various research pathways. This results in lack of head-to-head RCTs of novel agents compared to each other or single ASCT. We have demonstrated that by using SNA to visually and analytically examine treatment networks prior to designing a clinical trial, researchers can better design studies to address more relevant clinical and research questions.

Supporting Information

File S1 Contains the following files: **Figure S1.** Entire treatment network. Each node is associated with a treatment participating in an RCT and each tie denotes a comparison between two treatments. The width of the ties among treatments denotes the number of times two treatments have been tested in RCTs. The network is comprised of 165 treatment comparisons. **Figure S2.** Connected component of network of RCTs published

between1996–2012. The width of the ties among treatments denotes the number of times two treatments have been tested in RCTs. **Figure S3.** Evolution of the treatment network over time. The figure presents the network's topology 40, 30, 20 and 1 year ago. **3a.** RCT network that includes trials performed more than 40 years ago; **3b.** RCT network that includes trials performed more than 30 years ago; **3c.** RCT network that includes trials performed more than 20 years ago; **3d.** RCT network that includes trials performed more than 1 year ago. **Figure S4** Funding type of all trials. Most treatment comparisons have been funded by the public sector.

Author Contributions

Conceived and designed the experiments: BD HM AT. Performed the experiments: HM AT. Analyzed the data: HM AT BD. Contributed reagents/materials/analysis tools: HM AT BD AK. Contributed to the writing of the manuscript: HM AT BD AK.

References

1. Breitkreutz I, Lokhorst HM, Raab MS, Holt B, Cremer FW, et al. (2007) Thalidomide in newly diagnosed multiple myeloma: influence of thalidomide treatment on peripheral blood stem cell collection yield. Leukemia 21: 1294–1299.
2. Holland JF, Hosley H, Scharlau C (1966) A Controlled Trial of Urethane Treatment in Multiple Myeloma. Blood 27: 328–342.
3. Mahony H, Kumar A, Berndt D, Chemudu S, Djulbegovic B (2012) Database of Randomized Trials in Myeloma (DRAM). University of South Florida and Millennium Pharmaceuticals, Inc., The Takeda Oncology Company.
4. Djulbegovic B, Kumar A (2008) Multiple myeloma: detecting the effects of new treatments. The Lancet 371: 1642–1644.
5. Kumar A, Hozo I, Wheatley K, Djulbegovic B (2011) Thalidomide versus bortezomib based regimens as first-line therapy for patients with multiple myeloma: A systematic review. American journal of hematology 86: 18–24.
6. Kumar A, Kharfan-Dabaja MA, Glasmacher A, Djulbegovic B (2009) Tandem versus single autologous hematopoietic cell transplantation for the treatment of multiple myeloma: a systematic review and meta-analysis. Journal of the National Cancer Institute 101: 100–106.
7. Kumar A, Loughran T, Alsina M, Durie BGM, Djulbegovic B (2003) Management of multiple myeloma: a systematic review and critical appraisal of published studies. The lancet oncology 4: 293–304.

8. Georgiev H, Tsalatsanis A, Kumar A, Djulbegovic B (2011) Social Network Analysis (SNA) of Research Programs in Multiple Myeloma (MM) American Society of Hematology Annual Meeting and Exposition. San Diego.
9. Haynes RB, McKibbon KA, Wilczynski NL, Walter SD, Werre SR (2005) Optimal search strategies for retrieving scientifically strong studies of treatment from Medline: analytical survey. Bmj 330: 1179.
10. Valente T (2010) Social networks and health: models, methods, and applications. New York Oxford University Press.
11. Wasserman S, Faust K (1994) Social Network Analysis. Cambridge: Cambridge University Press.
12. Newman MEJ (2001) The structure of scientific collaboration networks. Proceedings of the National Academy of Sciences 98: 404.
13. Friedkin NE (1982) Information flow through strong and weak ties in intraorganizational social networks. Social networks 3: 273–285.
14. Tsalatsanis A, Hozo I, Djulbegovic B (2010) Small world networks and treatment discovery process in cancer. pp. 6086.
15. Skvoretz J (2011) Workshop on Basic Network Methods. pp. 1–84.
16. Jackson M (2008) Social and Economic Networks. Princeton, New Jersey: Princeton University Press.
17. Freeman LC (1979) Centrality in social networks conceptual clarification. Social networks 1: 215–239.

18. Girvan M, Newman ME (2002) Community structure in social and biological networks. Proceedings of the National Academy of Sciences 99: 7821–7826.

19. Borgatti S (2003) KeyPlayer 1.44 ed. Boston, MA: Analytic Technologies.

20. Attal M, Harousseau JL, Stoppa AM, Sotto JJ, Fuzibet JG, et al. (1996) A prospective, randomized trial of autologous bone marrow transplantation and chemotherapy in multiple myeloma. Intergroupe Francais du Myelome. N Engl J Med 335: 91–97.

21. Borgatti SP (2002) Netdraw Network Visualization. 2.119 ed. Harvard, MA: Analytic Technologies.

22. Begg C, Cho M, Eastwood S, Horton R, Moher D, et al. (1996) Improving the quality of reporting of randomized controlled trials. The CONSORT statement. Jama 276: 637–639.

23. National Comprehensive Cancer Network (2013) Multiple Myeloma. version 1.2013 version 1.2013.

11

Risk Factors for Cisplatin-Induced Nephrotoxicity and Potential of Magnesium Supplementation for Renal Protection

Yasuhiro Kidera[1,2☉], Hisato Kawakami[3☉*], Tsutomu Sakiyama[3], Kunio Okamoto[3], Kaoru Tanaka[3], Masayuki Takeda[3], Hiroyasu Kaneda[3], Shin-ichi Nishina[3], Junji Tsurutani[3], Kimiko Fujiwara[2], Morihiro Nomura[2], Yuzuru Yamazoe[2], Yasutaka Chiba[4], Shozo Nishida[1], Takao Tamura[3], Kazuhiko Nakagawa[3]

1 Division of Pharmacotherapy, Kinki University Faculty of Pharmacy, Higashi-Osaka, Osaka, Japan, 2 Department of Pharmacy, Kinki University Faculty of Medicine, Osaka-Sayama, Osaka, Japan, 3 Department of Medical Oncology, Kinki University Faculty of Medicine, Osaka-Sayama, Osaka, Japan, 4 Division of Biostatistics, Clinical Research Center, Kinki University Faculty of Medicine, Osaka-Sayama, Osaka, Japan

Abstract

Background: Nephrotoxicity remains a problem for patients who receive cisplatin chemotherapy. We retrospectively evaluated potential risk factors for cisplatin-induced nephrotoxicity as well as the potential impact of intravenous magnesium supplementation on such toxicity.

Patients and Methods: We reviewed clinical data for 401 patients who underwent chemotherapy including a high dose ($\geq$ 60 mg/m^2) of cisplatin in the first-line setting. Nephrotoxicity was defined as an increase in the serum creatinine concentration of at least grade 2 during the first course of cisplatin chemotherapy, as assessed on the basis of National Cancer Institute Common Terminology Criteria for Adverse Events version 4.0. The severity of nephrotoxicity was evaluated on the basis of the mean change in the serum creatinine level. Magnesium was administered intravenously to 67 patients (17%).

Results: Cisplatin-induced nephrotoxicity was observed in 127 patients (32%). Multivariable analysis revealed that an Eastern Cooperative Oncology Group performance status of 2 (risk ratio, 1.876; P = 0.004) and the regular use of nonsteroidal anti-inflammatory drugs (NSAIDs) (risk ratio, 1.357; P = 0.047) were significantly associated with an increased risk for cisplatin nephrotoxicity, whereas intravenous magnesium supplementation was associated with a significantly reduced risk for such toxicity (risk ratio, 0.175; P = 0.0004). The development of hypomagnesemia during cisplatin treatment was significantly associated with a greater increase in serum creatinine level (P = 0.0025). Magnesium supplementation therapy was also associated with a significantly reduced severity of renal toxicity (P = 0.012).

Conclusions: A relatively poor performance status and the regular use of NSAIDs were significantly associated with cisplatin-induced nephrotoxicity, although the latter association was marginal. Our findings also suggest that the ability of magnesium supplementation to protect against the renal toxicity of cisplatin warrants further investigation in a prospective trial.

Editor: Ji-Hyun Lee, H. Lee Moffitt Cancer Center & Research Institute, United States of America

Funding: The authors have no support or funding to report.

Competing Interests: The authors have declared that no competing interests exist.

* Email: kawakami_h@dotd.med.kindai.ac.jp

☉ These authors contributed equally to this work.

Introduction

Cisplatin (*cis*-diammine-dichloroplatinum), an inorganic platinum chemotherapeutic drug, has been widely administered either alone or in combination with other agents for the clinical treatment of various solid tumors [1]. The efficacy of cisplatin is limited, however, by severe side effects such as nephrotoxicity, neurotoxicity, ototoxicity, and emetogenicity [2,3]. In particular, the nephrotoxicity of cisplatin is dose dependent and therefore limits the amount of drug that can be administered [4]. Procedures

to reduce such toxicity include aggressive hydration with saline and simultaneous administration of mannitol, which is now accepted as the standard of care for individuals treated with regimens containing a high dose ($\geq$60 mg/m^2) of cisplatin [5]. Unfortunately, renal toxicity still occurs even with such hydration, highlighting the need for more effective preventive strategies.

Another approach to limiting the nephrotoxicity of cisplatin is intravenous magnesium supplementation. Cisplatin-induced nephrotoxicity is accompanied by disturbance of the renal handling of electrolytes. In particular, depletion of magnesium has emerged as a common event associated with the acute renal toxicity induced by the drug [6]. Whereas several studies have demonstrated the efficacy of magnesium supplementation for prevention of hypomagnesemia during cisplatin treatment [7–10], only two prospective studies, each featuring a relatively small number of patients, have evaluated its efficacy in terms of protection against cisplatin-induced nephrotoxicity [11,12]. Despite the dearth of evidence in support of a beneficial effect of magnesium supplementation therapy on the renal toxicity of cisplatin, intravenous administration of magnesium is currently recommended for outpatients receiving high-dose cisplatin with a short hydration regimen [13]. We have therefore recently applied this procedure to all patients who receive such chemotherapy. However, given that magnesium supplementation has not been accepted as the standard of care, at least in Japan, most patients who receive high-dose cisplatin are treated with aggressive hydration in the inpatient setting.

We have now assessed a large group of unselected consecutive patients in an attempt to identify potential biological or pharmacological parameters that might predispose individuals to cisplatin-induced nephrotoxicity. We also retrospectively evaluated the potential impact of intravenous magnesium supplementation on this side effect of cisplatin treatment.

Patients and Methods

Eligibility criteria

We reviewed the cases in our database and retrospectively examined the clinical data of patients who received therapy including a high dose (≥ 60 mg/m^2) of cisplatin in the first-line setting at the Department of Medical Oncology, Kinki University Hospital, between January 2008 and August 2012. Patients were eligible if they had pathologically confirmed malignancies and an Eastern Cooperative Oncology Group performance status (PS) of 0 to 2. Patients were excluded from the study if they had a history of cisplatin treatment or had more than one cancer. The study protocol was approved by the ethics committee of Kinki University Hospital with the condition that all data be processed and analyzed anonymously, and written informed consent was provided by all patients. The study also conforms with the provisions of the Declaration of Helsinki.

Cisplatin administration

All regimens containing high-dose cisplatin were administered in the inpatient setting. Cisplatin was administered in 500 mL of 0.9% normal saline over 1 h. Most patients were prehydrated with 500 mL of one-quarter isotonic saline containing 5% glucose and 20 mEq of KCl, and they were posthydrated with 500 mL of 0.9% normal saline mixed with 500 mL of one-quarter isotonic saline containing 5% glucose, 20 mEq of KCl, and 10 mEq of sodium L-lactate, which was administered over 1 to 2 h and followed by 60 g of mannitol over 1 h and 20 mg of furosemide in 50 mL of 0.9% normal saline over 15 min. Antiemetic prophylaxis with 5-HT$_3$ serotonin receptor antagonists plus dexamethasone was administered 15 min before the onset of chemotherapy in all cases. A neurokinin 1 (NK1) receptor antagonist was added to the antiemetic cocktail from October 2010 in response to the approval of this drug in Japan. Magnesium sulfate (20 mEq) was administered with 500 mL of one-quarter isotonic saline over 1 h after cisplatin administration as magnesium supplementation therapy to all patients from July 2011.

Nephrotoxicity evaluation

According to a previous study [14], we adopted an increase in the serum concentration of creatinine as a measure of nephrotoxicity. The serum creatinine concentration was determined before the first course of cisplatin chemotherapy (baseline value) and weekly during chemotherapy. For evaluation of nephrotoxicity, the increase in the serum creatinine concentration was calculated as the maximum value during the first course of chemotherapy minus the baseline value. Given that the serum creatinine level is a denominator of the Cockcroft-Gault equation, changes in creatinine clearance over a short period are solely dependent on those in serum creatinine concentration. Nephrotoxicity was defined as an increase in the serum creatinine concentration of grade 2 or higher, according to the National Cancer Institute Common Terminology Criteria for Adverse Events (NCI CTCAE, version 4.0), during the first course of cisplatin chemotherapy.

Statistical analysis

To identify risk factors potentially associated with the occurrence of a nephrotoxicity event, each factor was compared by the unpaired Student's t test or Fisher's exact test. Factors in the analysis included age (≥ 70 vs. <70 years) and PS (2 vs. 0 or 1), given that chemotherapy might be expected to result in excessive toxicity in patients with an age of ≥ 70 years or a PS of 2 [15]. The other factors were sex (male vs. female), tumor type, concurrent radiation treatment, hypoalbuminemia (serum albumin concentration of <3.0 g/dL), enteral or total parenteral nutrition, type 2 diabetes, hydration (≤ 2000 mL), intravenous magnesium supplementation, oral intake of magnesium oxide as a laxative agent, use of antihypertensive medication, treatment with an NK1 receptor antagonist, and regular use of nonsteroidal anti-inflammatory drugs (NSAIDs). The risk factors were also evaluated in multivariable analysis with the Poisson regression model. The risk ratio with 95% confidence interval (CI) was calculated for the independent prognostic factors. The mean change in serum creatinine concentration was compared between groups with the use of box-and-whisker plots showing the range (maximum and minimum), median, and quartile range (75 and 25 percentiles) and was evaluated with the unpaired Student's t test. Statistical analysis was performed with the use of SAS software version 9.4 (SAS Institute, Cary, NC). A P value of <0.05 was considered statistically significant.

Results

Patient characteristics

A total of 401 patients who received chemotherapy including high-dose cisplatin were eligible for the analysis. Baseline characteristics of the eligible patients are summarized in Table 1. The median age was 65 years (range, 28–80), and most patients were male (77%) and had a good PS of 0 or 1 (94%). The most common malignancies were lung cancer (36%), head and neck cancer (23%), gastric cancer (19%), and esophageal cancer (16%). Median age, sex, PS, median serum creatinine concentration at baseline, median body surface area, median body mass index, and the median dose of cisplatin in the first course of chemotherapy did not differ significantly among the types of malignancy. The various chemotherapy regimens administered to the patients are shown in Table S1.

Table 1. Baseline characteristics of the 401 study patients.

Characteristic			All patients (n=401)	Lung cancer (n=144)	Head and neck cancer (n=92)	Gastric cancer (n=78)	Esophageal cancer (n=65)	Other malignancies (n=22)
Sex								
	Male	n (%)	308 (77)	107	74	57	54	16
	Female	n (%)	93 (23)	37	18	21	11	6
PS								
	0–1	n (%)	375 (94)	139	89	67	61	19
	2	n (%)	26 (6)	5	3	11	4	3
Baseline Cr (mg/dL)								
	Median		0.69	0.67	0.68	0.73	0.72	0.71
	(range)		(0.23–1.31)	(0.39–1.11)	(0.24–1.15)	(0.23–1.31)	(0.40–1.10)	(0.49–1.08)
BSA (m^2)								
	Median		1.61	1.62	1.56	1.60	1.60	1.60
	(range)		(1.15–2.21)	(1.29–2.21)	(1.29–1.96)	(1.22–1.90)	(1.15–1.87)	(1.28–1.92)
BMI (kg/m^2)								
	Median (range)		21.1 (11.6–35.3)	22.2 (14.9–35.3)	20.9 (11.6–34.0)	20.9 (15.2–33.5)	20.5 (13.4–28.1)	20.6 (16.4–28.8)
Cisplatin dose (mg/m^2)								
	Median		78.0	78.7	80.0	60.0	70.0	79.8
	(range)		(60.0–105)	(60.0–80.3)	(60.0–105)	(60.0–84.0)	(60.0–80.0)	(60.0–100)
Age (years)								
	Median		65	64	62	67	67	64
	(range)		(28–80)	(33–80)	(30–79)	(28–80)	(51–78)	(37–75)
	≥70	n (%)	97 (24)	30	21	25	18	3
	<70	n (%)	304 (76)	114	71	53	47	19
Concurrent radiation								
	Yes	n (%)	167 (42)	45	60	1	50	11
	No	n (%)	234 (58)	99	32	77	15	11
Hypoalbuminemia (serum albumin, <3.0 g/dL)								
	Yes	n (%)	43 (11)	14	3	18	8	0
	No	n (%)	358 (89)	130	89	60	57	22
Enteral nutrition or TPN								
	Yes	n (%)	42 (10)	2	20	2	16	2
	No	n (%)	359 (90)	142	72	76	49	20
Type 2 diabetes								
	Yes	n (%)	99 (25)	39	30	15	11	4

Table 1. Cont.

Characteristic		All patients	Lung cancer	Head and neck cancer	Gastric cancer	Esophageal cancer	Other malignancies
		(n=401)	(n=144)	(n=92)	(n=78)	(n=65)	(n=22)
		n (%)					
	No	302 (75)	105	62	63	54	18
Hydration of ≦2000 mL							
	Yes	34 (8)	0	23	6	1	4
	No	367 (92)	144	69	72	64	18
Use of NK1 receptor antagonist							
	Yes	230 (57)	66	68	46	38	12
	No	171 (43)	78	24	32	27	10
Intravenous magnesium supplementation							
	Yes	67 (17)	13	23	16	11	4
	No	334 (83)	131	69	62	54	18
Oral intake of magnesium oxide as a laxative agent							
	Yes	164 (41)	56	39	33	28	8
	No	237 (59)	88	53	45	37	14
Regular use of antihypertensive							
	Yes	157 (39)	55	44	24	28	6
	No	244 (61)	89	48	54	37	16
Regular use of NSAIDs							
	Yes	117 (29)	51	30	18	11	7
	No	284 (71)	93	62	60	54	15

Drug administration variables refer to the first course of cisplatin chemotherapy. Abbreviations: PS, performance status; Cr, serum creatinine concentration; BSA, body surface area; BMI, body mass index; TPN, total parenteral nutrition; NK1, neurokinin 1; NSAIDs, nonselective nonsteroidal anti-inflammatory drugs.

Table 2. Comparison of clinicopathologic characteristics as risk factors for cisplatin-induced nephrotoxicity.

Characteristic		Cisplatin nephrotoxicity		P value
		Yes (n=127)	No (n=274)	
		n (%)	n (%)	
Age (years)				
	Median	65	65	0.524
	(range)	(37–80)	(28–80)	
	≥70	31 (32)	66 (68)	0.944
	<70	96 (32)	208 (68)	
Sex				
	Male	97 (31)	211 (69)	0.899
	Female	30 (32)	63 (68)	
PS				
	0 or 1	111 (30)	264 (70)	**0.002**
	2	16 (62)	10 (38)	
Tumor type				
	Lung	40 (28)	104 (72)	**0.045***
	Head and neck	28 (30)	64 (70)	
	Gastric	23 (29)	55 (71)	
	Esophageal	31 (48)	34 (52)	
	Other	5 (23)	17 (77)	
Concurrent radiation				
	Yes	56 (34)	111 (66)	0.515
	No	71 (30)	163 (70)	
Hypoalbuminemia (serum albumin, <3.0 g/dL)				
	Yes	15 (35)	28 (65)	0.608
	No	112 (31)	246 (69)	
Enteral nutrition or TPN				
	Yes	17 (40)	25 (60)	0.220
	No	110 (31)	249 (69)	
Type 2 diabetes				
	Yes	26 (26)	73 (74)	0.214
	No	101 (33)	201 (67)	
Hydration of ≤2000 mL				
	Yes	13 (38)	21 (62)	0.441
	No	114 (31)	253 (69)	
Use of NK1 receptor antagonist				
	Yes	61 (27)	169 (73)	**0.013**
	No	66 (39)	105 (61)	
Intravenous magnesium supplementation				
	Yes	4 (6)	63 (94)	**<0.0001**
	No	123 (37)	211 (63)	
Oral intake of magnesium oxide as a laxative agent				
	Yes	48 (29)	116 (71)	0.445
	No	79 (33)	158 (67)	
Regular use of antihypertensive				
	Yes	51 (32)	106 (68)	0.826
	No	76 (31)	168 (69)	

Table 2. Cont.

Characteristic		Cisplatin nephrotoxicity		P value
		Yes (n=127)	No (n=274)	
		n (%)	n (%)	
Regular use of NSAIDs				
	Yes	44 (38)	73 (62)	0.125
	No	83 (29)	201 (71)	

Drug administration variables refer to the first course of cisplatin chemotherapy. Abbreviations: PS, performance status. TPN, total parenteral nutrition; NK1, neurokinin 1; NSAIDs, nonselective nonsteroidal anti-inflammatory drugs.
*P value for heterogeneity for the occurrence of nephrotoxicity among tumor types. P values of <0.05 are shown in bold.

Clinicopathologic analysis of risk factors for cisplatin nephrotoxicity

Cisplatin-induced nephrotoxicity was observed in 127 (32%) of the 401 enrolled patients, including 108, 16, and 3 patients with nephrotoxicity of grade 2, 3, and 4, respectively. Among these patients, 55 individuals developed irreversible renal failure. Fisher's exact test revealed that a PS of 2 ($P=0.002$), the absence of intravenous magnesium supplementation ($P<0.0001$), and the lack of treatment with an NK1 receptor antagonist ($P=0.013$) were significantly associated with cisplatin nephrotoxicity (Table 2). We also detected significant heterogeneity in the occurrence of nephrotoxicity among tumor types ($P=0.045$). Examination of the possible impact of concurrent chemotherapy agents on the prevalence of nephrotoxicity (Table S2) revealed no significant association between the use of these agents and such toxicity ($P=0.373$).

Multivariable analysis of risk factors for cisplatin nephrotoxicity

To assess the contribution of each individual risk factor to cisplatin-induced nephrotoxicity, we performed multivariable analysis (Table 3). A PS of 2 (risk ratio, 1.876; 95% CI, 1.229–2.864; $P=0.004$) and regular use of NSAIDs (risk ratio, 1.357; 95% CI, 1.004–1.835; $P=0.047$) were significantly associated with an increased risk for cisplatin nephrotoxicity, whereas intravenous magnesium supplementation (risk ratio, 0.175; 95% CI, 0.066–0.462; $P=0.0004$) was associated with a significantly reduced risk. We also found that esophageal cancer was an independent risk factor for nephrotoxicity compared with lung cancer (risk ratio,

Table 3. Risk ratio in multivariable analysis of potential predisposing factors for cisplatin-induced nephrotoxicity ($n=401$).

Factor		Risk ratio	95% CI	P value
Age (≥70 vs. <70 years)		1.006	0.990–1.023	0.475
Sex (male vs. female)		0.947	0.683–1.314	0.745
PS (2 vs. 0 or 1)		1.876	1.229–2.864	**0.004**
Concurrent radiation		1.071	0.769–1.491	0.684
Serum albumin (≥3.0 vs. <3.0 g/dL)		0.897	0.693–1.165	0.419
Enteral nutrition or TPN		0.989	0.643–1.520	0.959
Type 2 diabetes		0.872	0.599–1.270	0.476
Hydration (≤2000 or >2000 mL)		0.801	0.536–1.200	0.283
Use of NK1 receptor antagonist		0.878	0.663–1.163	0.363
Intravenous magnesium supplementation		0.175	0.066–0.462	**0.0004**
Oral intake of magnesium oxide as a laxative agent		0.933	0.703–1.240	0.634
Regular use of antihypertensive		1.010	0.810–1.485	0.553
Regular use of NSAIDs		1.357	1.004–1.835	**0.047**
Tumor type				
	Lung	1.000		
	Head and neck[a]	1.301	0.845–2.010	0.232
	Gastric[a]	1.071	0.678–1.692	0.770
	Esophageal[a]	1.937	1.277–2.940	**0.002**
	Other[a]	0.810	0.360–1.823	0.610

Drug administration variables refer to the first course of cisplatin chemotherapy. Abbreviations: CI, confidence interval; PS, performance status; TPN, total parenteral nutrition; NK1, neurokinin 1; NSAIDs, nonselective nonsteroidal anti-inflammatory drugs.
[a]These risk factors were compared with lung cancer.

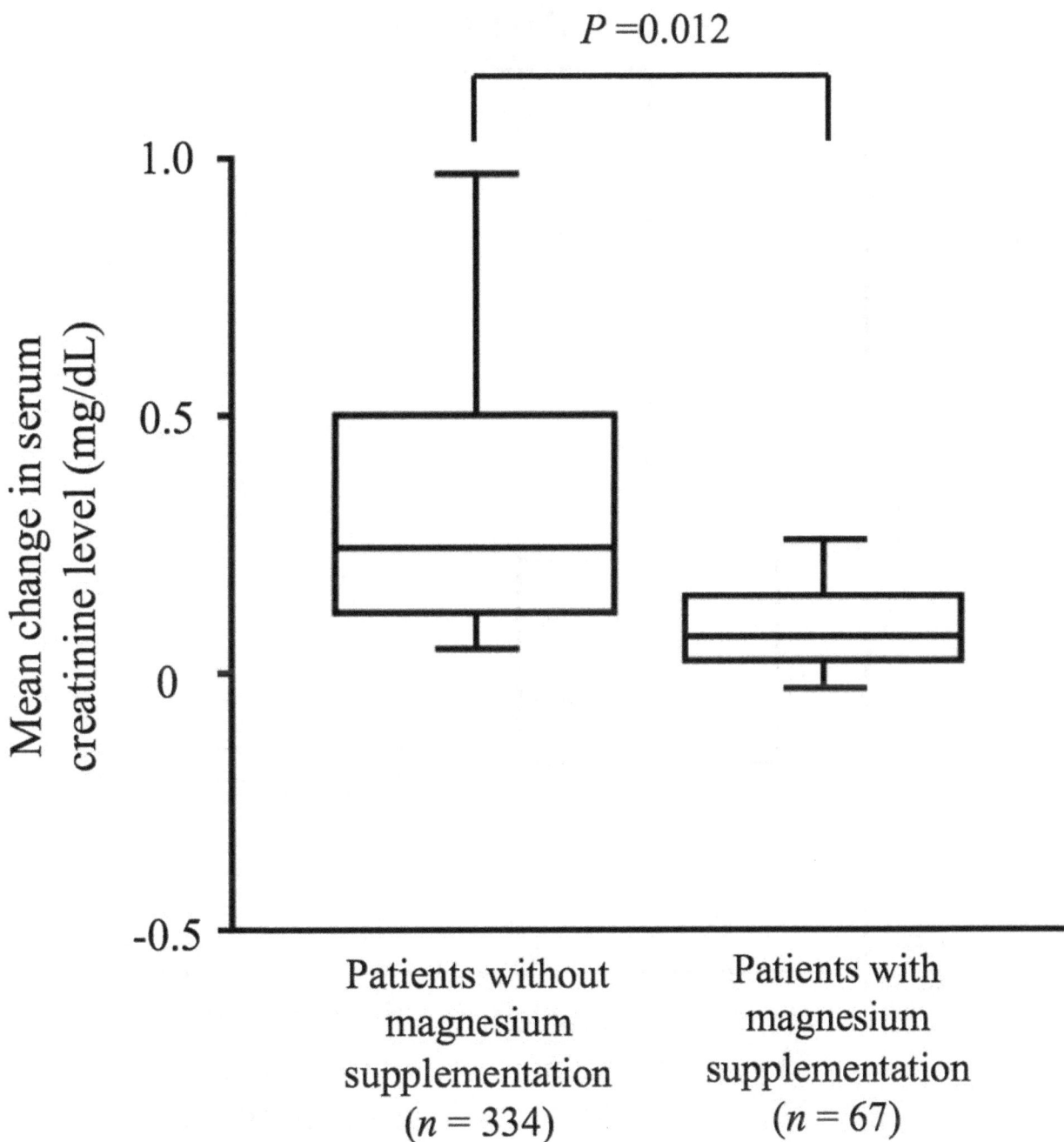

Figure 1. Box-and-whisker plot for the relation between intravenous magnesium supplementation and the mean change in serum creatinine concentration during the first course of cisplatin chemotherapy. The difference between the two groups was analyzed with the unpaired Student's *t* test.

1.937; 95% CI, 1.277–2.940; $P = 0.002$). Exploratory analysis revealed no significant interaction between intravenous magnesium supplementation and other covariates (data not shown).

Effect of magnesium supplementation on serum creatinine levels

As shown in Table 2, we found that the prevalence of cisplatin-induced nephrotoxicity was substantially lower in patients who received intravenous magnesium supplementation than in those who did not (6% vs. 37%). To investigate the effect of magnesium supplementation on cisplatin-induced nephrotoxicity, we evaluat-ed the mean change from baseline in the serum creatinine concentration during the first course of high-dose cisplatin therapy. Patients who received magnesium supplementation therapy ($n = 67$) showed a mean change in serum creatinine level of 0.188±0.081 mg/dL (mean ± SE), whereas those who did not receive the treatment ($n = 334$) showed a mean change of 0.444±0.043 mg/dL ($P = 0.012$), suggesting that magnesium supplementation therapy limited the elevation of serum creatinine level induced by cisplatin (Figure 1). We further examined how magnesium supplementation might prevent cisplatin-induced nephrotoxicity. Data on the serum magnesium concentration

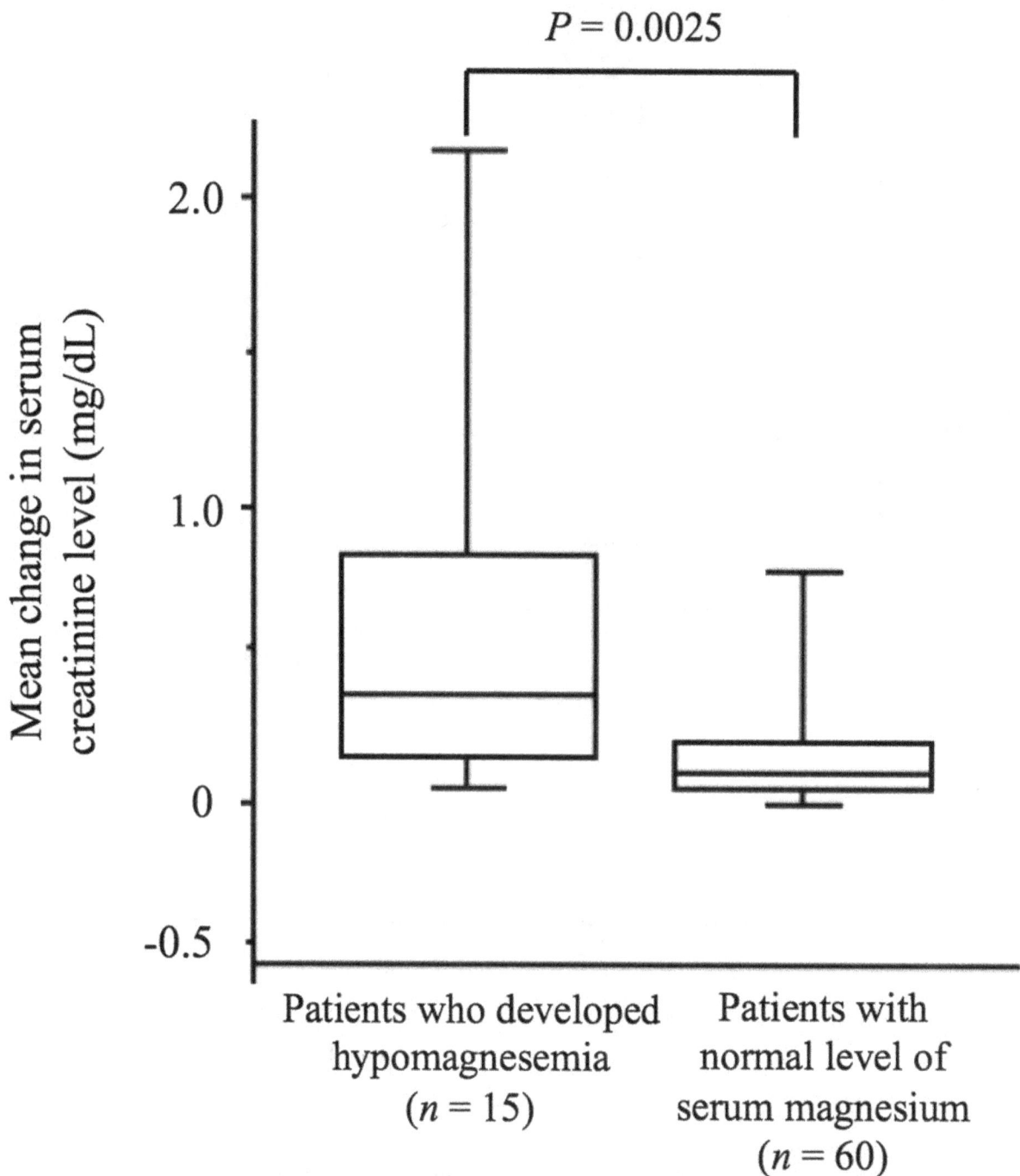

Figure 2. Box-and-whisker plot for the relation between the development of hypomagnesemia and the mean change in serum creatinine concentration during the first course of cisplatin chemotherapy. The difference between the two groups was analyzed with the unpaired Student's *t* test.

during the first course of cisplatin chemotherapy were available for 75 of the 401 study patients. No patient showed hypomagnesemia at baseline. Among the 52 patients who received magnesium supplementation, 6 individuals (12%) developed hypomagnesemia of grade 1 or worse, whereas 9 (39%) of the 23 patients who did not receive magnesium supplementation developed this condition ($P=0.040$), indicating that magnesium supplementation significantly reduced the proportion of patients who developed

hypomagnesemia. Furthermore, the 15 patients who developed hypomagnesemia during cisplatin treatment showed a significantly greater mean increase in the serum creatinine concentration from baseline compared with those who maintained a normal level of serum magnesium ($P=0.0025$) (Figure 2). These results suggest that intravenous magnesium supplementation protects against cisplatin-induced nephrotoxicity by preventing hypomagnesemia.

Discussion

Nephrotoxicity remains a clinical problem for 25 to 42% of patients treated with cisplatin [16–18]. In the present study, we found that 32% (127/401) of individuals who received cisplatin at a dose of at least 60 mg/m^2 developed acute nephrotoxicity despite the adoption of conventional measures of hydration and osmotic diuresis. Although the nephrotoxicity was transient and reversible in most cases, 43% (55/127) of the patients with acute nephrotoxicity went on to develop irreversible renal failure. These results indicate that the conventional prophylactic procedures were not sufficient to prevent cisplatin-induced nephrotoxicity in a subset of patients.

We found that magnesium supplementation therapy was significantly associated with both a reduced frequency and reduced severity of renal toxicity, consistent with previous observations [11,12]. Cisplatin treatment results in a substantial increase in magnesium excretion [19–21], with this effect being apparent even before the onset of overt renal toxicity [22], and hypomagnesemia is associated with cisplatin-induced nephrotoxicity [23]. In the present study, a decrease in the serum magnesium concentration was observed in 20% of patients and was significantly associated with renal toxicity during the first course of cisplatin treatment. Organic cation transporter 2 (OCT2) has been implicated in cisplatin nephrotoxicity in a study with isolated human proximal tubules [24], and hypomagnesemia results in up-regulation of OCT2 and thereby increases the renal accumulation of cisplatin and exacerbates acute kidney injury in an animal model [25]. These various findings suggest that magnesium supplementation protects against cisplatin-induced nephrotoxicity, likely by preventing hypomagnesemia, a notion that warrants validation in a prospective study. The dosage of magnesium sulfate for such supplementation therapy has varied widely in previous studies, ranging from 8 to 60 mEq [9–11,13,26,27], and it therefore remains to be standardized in future trials.

To assess the potential risk factors for cisplatin-induced nephrotoxicity, we performed multivariable analyses. Consistent with previous results [14,28], we found that a poor PS was associated with an increased risk for cisplatin nephrotoxicity. This finding underscores the notion that patients with a PS of 2, which is characterized by an increased risk for severe toxicity in general, need special attention with regard to the potential development of nephrotoxicity during high-dose cisplatin chemotherapy, especially given that such treatment in these patients is controversial [29]. We also found that the regular use of NSAIDs was associated with cisplatin-induced nephrotoxicity. Nonselective inhibition of cyclooxygenases 1 and 2 by NSAIDs attenuates prostaglandin-dependent renal function, including modulation of renal vascular tone and electrolyte and water excretion, in particular during renal stress, as manifested by a reduction in the rate of renal perfusion [30,31]. Such effects of NSAIDs might thus enhance cisplatin-induced nephrotoxicity. Although the significance of the association between the regular use of NSAIDs and cisplatin-induced nephrotoxicity was marginal ($P=0.047$) in our analysis, it is of concern because NSAIDs are commonly administered to manage cancer-related pain [32]. Further investigations are thus warranted to evaluate the potential risk of regular NSAID use during high-dose cisplatin chemotherapy.

With regard to tumor type, we found that individuals with esophageal cancer were at a significantly higher risk for cisplatin-induced nephrotoxicity than were those with lung cancer. To our knowledge, such an association has not previously been described. The median dosage of cisplatin in patients with esophageal cancer was 70 mg/m^2, which was not higher than that overall (78 mg/m^2). Moreover, whereas most patients with esophageal cancer in our analysis were treated with cisplatin together with 5-fluorouracil as the standard care, this regimen was also administered to patients with gastric or head and neck cancer. A difference in dosage or in the combination of chemotherapeutic agents thus could not account for the difference in nephrotoxicity among the malignancies. Caution is necessary in the interpretation of this finding, however, with further study being warranted to determine the mechanism of renal toxicity apparent selectively in patients with esophageal cancer.

Limitations of the present study include possible selection bias of treatment, which is inevitable in a retrospective analysis, and a small sample size for patients with a known serum magnesium concentration and for those who received intravenous magnesium supplementation. Even though all patients treated after July 2011 received magnesium sulfate regardless of their characteristics, cohort effects may still be present that influence the association between magnesium supplementation and nephrotoxicity. In addition, we could not fully assess the incidence and intensity of nonhematologic toxicities in our study as a result of its retrospective nature. Such toxicities, including nausea, vomiting, and diarrhea, might be associated with an increased risk for cisplatin-induced nephrotoxicity. Furthermore, comorbidities relevant to inherent nephrotoxicity, such as proteinuria, hypocalcemia, and renal tubular acidosis, were not assessed in the present study.

In conclusion, our data have revealed a significant association of cisplatin-induced nephrotoxicity with a relatively poor PS and, to a lesser extent, with the regular use of NSAIDs. Our findings also suggest that magnesium supplementation might be effective for protection against the renal toxicity of cisplatin, a conclusion that should be further addressed in a prospective trial.

Supporting Information

Table S1 Chemotherapy regimens according to tumor type.

Table S2 Association between concurrent chemotherapy agents and the occurrence of nephrotoxicity.

Author Contributions

Conceived and designed the experiments: H. Kawakami. Contributed reagents/materials/analysis tools: H. Kawakami YC. Wrote the paper: YK H. Kawakami JT YC. Collected the data: YK. Contributed study materials or patients: YK H. Kawakami TS KO KT MT S. Nishina JT KF MN YY S. Nishida TT KN. Analyzed and interpreted the data: YK H. Kawakami YC. Administrative support: S. Nishina TT KN. Contributed in critical revision of the manuscript for important intellectual content: YK H. Kawakami TS KO KT MT H. Kaneda S. Nishina JT KF MN YY YC S. Nishida TT KN.

References

1. Rozencweig M, von Hoff DD, Slavik M, Muggia FM (1977) Cis-diamminedichloroplatinum (II). A new anticancer drug. Ann Intern Med 86: 803–812.
2. Wang D, Lippard SJ (2005) Cellular processing of platinum anticancer drugs. Nat Rev Drug Discov 4: 307–320.
3. Pabla N, Dong Z (2008) Cisplatin nephrotoxicity: mechanisms and renoprotective strategies. Kidney Int 73: 994–1007.
4. Arany I, Safirstein RL (2003) Cisplatin nephrotoxicity. Semin Nephrol 23: 460–464.

5. dos Santos NA, Carvalho Rodrigues MA, Martins NM, dos Santos AC (2012) Cisplatin-induced nephrotoxicity and targets of nephroprotection: an update. Arch Toxicol 86: 1233–1250.

6. Lajer H, Daugaard G (1999) Cisplatin and hypomagnesemia. Cancer Treat Rev 25: 47–58.

7. Netten PM, de Mulder PH, Theeuwes AG, Willems JL, Kohler BE, et al. (1990) Intravenous magnesium supplementation during cisdiammine-dichloroplatinum administration prevents hypomagnesemia. Ann Oncol 1: 369–372.

8. Martin M, Diaz-Rubio E, Casado A, Lopez Vega JM, Sastre J, et al. (1992) Intravenous and oral magnesium supplementations in the prophylaxis of cisplatin-induced hypomagnesemia. Results of a controlled trial. Am J Clin Oncol 15: 348–351.

9. Evans TR, Harper CL, Beveridge IG, Wastnage R, Mansi JL (1995) A randomised study to determine whether routine intravenous magnesium supplements are necessary in patients receiving cisplatin chemotherapy with continuous infusion 5-fluorouracil. Eur J Cancer 31A: 174–178.

10. Vokes EE, Mick R, Vogelzang NJ, Geiser R, Douglas F (1990) A randomised study comparing intermittent to continuous administration of magnesium aspartate hydrochloride in cisplatin-induced hypomagnesaemia. Br J Cancer 62: 1015–1017.

11. Bodnar L, Wcislo G, Gasowska-Bodnar A, Synowiec A, Szarlej-Wcislo K, et al. (2008) Renal protection with magnesium subcarbonate and magnesium sulphate in patients with epithelial ovarian cancer after cisplatin and paclitaxel chemotherapy: a randomised phase II study. Eur J Cancer 44: 2608–2614.

12. Willox JC, McAllister EJ, Sangster G, Kaye SB (1986) Effects of magnesium supplementation in testicular cancer patients receiving cis-platin: a randomised trial. Br J Cancer 54: 19–23.

13. National Comprehensive Cancer Network (2013) NCCN chemotherapy order templates. Available: http://www.nccn.org/ordertemplates. Accessed: 2013 Nov 11.

14. Stewart DJ, Dulberg CS, Mikhael NZ, Redmond MD, Montpetit VA, et al. (1997) Association of cisplatin nephrotoxicity with patient characteristics and cisplatin administration methods. Cancer Chemother Pharmacol 40: 293–308.

15. Hesketh PJ, Chansky K, Lau DH, Doroshow JH, Moinpour CM, et al. (2006) Sequential vinorelbine and docetaxel in advanced non-small cell lung cancer patients age 70 and older and/or with a performance status of 2: a phase II trial of the Southwest Oncology Group (S0027). J Thorac Oncol 1: 537–544.

16. Ries F, Klastersky J (1986) Nephrotoxicity induced by cancer chemotherapy with special emphasis on cisplatin toxicity. Am J Kidney Dis 8: 368–379.

17. Kovach JS, Moertel CG, Schutt AJ, Reitemeier RG, Hahn RG (1973) Phase II study of cis-diamminedichloroplatinum (NSC-119875) in advanced carcinoma of the large bowel. Cancer Chemother Rep 57: 357–359.

18. de Jongh FE, van Veen RN, Veltman SJ, de Wit R, van der Burg ME, et al. (2003) Weekly high-dose cisplatin is a feasible treatment option: analysis on prognostic factors for toxicity in 400 patients. Br J Cancer 88: 1199–1206.

19. Mavichak V, Wong NL, Quamme GA, Magil AB, Sutton RA, et al. (1985) Studies on the pathogenesis of cisplatin-induced hypomagnesemia in rats. Kidney Int 28: 914–921.

20. Stewart AF, Keating T, Schwartz PE (1985) Magnesium homeostasis following chemotherapy with cisplatin: a prospective study. Am J Obstetr Gynecol 153: 660–665.

21. Ariceta G, Rodriguez-Soriano J, Vallo A, Navajas A (1997) Acute and chronic effects of cisplatin therapy on renal magnesium homeostasis. Med Pediatr Oncol 28: 35–40.

22. Daugaard G, Abildgaard U, Holstein-Rathlou NH, Bruunshuus I, Bucher D, et al. (1988) Renal tubular function in patients treated with high-dose cisplatin. Clin Pharmacol Ther 44: 164–172.

23. Lajer H, Kristensen M, Hansen HH, Nielsen S, Frokiaer J, et al. (2005) Magnesium depletion enhances cisplatin-induced nephrotoxicity. Cancer Chemother Pharmacol 56: 535–542.

24. Ciarimboli G, Ludwig T, Lang D, Pavenstadt H, Koepsell H, et al. (2005) Cisplatin nephrotoxicity is critically mediated via the human organic cation transporter 2. Am J Pathol 167: 1477–1484.

25. Yokoo K, Murakami R, Matsuzaki T, Yoshitome K, Hamada A, et al. (2009) Enhanced renal accumulation of cisplatin via renal organic cation transporter deteriorates acute kidney injury in hypomagnesemic rats. Clin Exp Nephrol 13: 578–584.

26. Tiseo M, Martelli O, Mancuso A, Sormani MP, Bruzzi P, et al. (2007) Short hydration regimen and nephrotoxicity of intermediate to high-dose cisplatin-based chemotherapy for outpatient treatment in lung cancer and mesothelioma. Tumori 93: 138–144.

27. Al Bahrani BJ, Moylan EJ, Forouzesh B, Della-Fiorentina SA, Goldrick AJ (2009) A short outpatient hydration schedule for cisplatin administration. Gulf J Oncol 5: 30–36.

28. Sweeney CJ, Zhu J, Sandler AB, Schiller J, Belani CP, et al. (2001) Outcome of patients with a performance status of 2 in Eastern Cooperative Oncology Group Study E1594: a phase II trial in patients with metastatic nonsmall cell lung carcinoma. Cancer 92: 2639–2647.

29. Gridelli C, Maione P, Rossi A, Guerriero C, Ferrara C, et al. (2006) Chemotherapy of advanced NSCLC in special patient population. Ann Oncol 17 (suppl 5): v72–v78.

30. Whelton A, Maurath CJ, Verburg KM, Geis GS (2000) Renal safety and tolerability of celecoxib, a novel cyclooxygenase-2 inhibitor. Am J Ther 7: 159–175.

31. Pope JE, Anderson JJ, Felson DT (1993) A meta-analysis of the effects of nonsteroidal anti-inflammatory drugs on blood pressure. Arch Intern Med 153: 477–484.

32. Ripamonti CI, Bandieri E, Roila F (2011) Management of cancer pain: ESMO Clinical Practice Guidelines. Ann Oncol 22 (suppl 6): vi69–vi77.

12

HIF-1α Inhibition Reverses Multidrug Resistance in Colon Cancer Cells via Downregulation of MDR1/P-Glycoprotein

Jianfang Chen[1⊚], **Zhenyu Ding**[1,2⊚], **Yonghai Peng**[1], **Feng Pan**[1], **Jianjun Li**[1], **Lan Zou**[1], **Yanling Zhang**[1], **Houjie Liang**[1]*

1 Department of Oncology and Southwest Cancer Center, Southwest Hospital, Third Military Medical University, Chongqing, China, **2** Department of Oncology, General Hospital of Shenyang Military Region, Shenyang, Liaoning, China

Abstract

Background: Multidrug resistance (MDR) is one of the major reasons chemotherapy-based treatments fail. Hypoxia is generally associated with tumor chemoresistance. However, the correlation between the heterodimeric hypoxia-inducible factor-1 (HIF-1) and the multidrug resistance (MDR1) gene/transporter P-glycoprotein (P-gp) remains unclear. This study aims to explore the molecular mechanisms of reversing colon cancer MDR by focusing on the target gene HIF-1α.

Methods: A chemotherapeutic sensitivity assay was used to observe the efficiency of MDR reversal in LoVo multicellular spheroids (MCS). The apoptotic level induced by different drugs was examined by flow cytometry (FCM). Binding of HIF-1α to the MDR1 gene promoter was evaluated by Chromatin immunoprecipitation (ChIP). The relationship between HIF-1α/P-gp expression and sensitivity to chemotherapy was analyzed.

Results: The sensitivity of LoVo MCS to all four chemotherapy drugs was decreased to varying degrees under hypoxic conditions. After silencing the HIF-1α gene, the sensitivities of LoVo MCS to all four chemotherapy drugs were restored. The apoptotic levels that all the drugs induced were all decreased to various extents in the hypoxic group. After silencing HIF-1α, the apoptosis level induced by all four chemotherapy drugs increased. The expression of HIF-1α and P-gp was significantly enhanced in LoVo MCS after treatment with hypoxia. Inhibiting HIF-1α significantly decreased the expression of MDR1/P-gp mRNA or protein in both the LoVo monolayers and LoVo MCS. The ChIP assay showed that HIF-1α was bound to the MDR1 gene promoter. Advanced colon carcinoma patients with expression of both HIF-1α and P-gp were more resistant to chemotherapy than that with non expression.

Conclusions: HIF-1α inhibition reverses multidrug resistance in colon cancer cells via downregulation of MDR1/P-gp. The expression of HIF-1α and MDR1/P-gp can be used as a predictive marker for chemotherapy resistance in colon cancer.

Editor: Michal Zmijewski, Medical University of Gdańsk, Poland

Funding: This work was supported by the National Natural Science Foundation of China (No.30973430 and No.81101629).(http://isisn.nsfc.gov.cn/egrantweb/). The funders had no role in study design, data collection and analysis, decision to publish, or preparation of the manuscript.

Competing Interests: The authors have declared that no competing interests exist.

* E-mail: lianghoujie@sina.com

⊚ These authors contributed equally to this work.

Introduction

Colon cancer is one of the most common malignant tumors throughout the world, and chemotherapy plays an important role in its treatment. However, the sensitivity to different chemotherapeutic regimens varies widely from individual to individual. Many cancer patients develop drug resistance, leading to poor treatment outcomes. Moreover, drug resistance mostly occurs in solid tumors in vivo but not in monolayers in vitro [1]. The tumor microenvironment plays a pivotal role in chemotherapy failure and drug resistance [2–4].

Hypoxia is a common feature of many malignant tumors, including colon cancer. A hypoxic tumor microenvironment is increasingly considered a critical component in determining drug resistance [5,6]. Hypoxia-inducible factor-1 (HIF-1) is a key factor in altering the biological characteristics of tumors. HIF-1α protein is overexpressed in multiple types of human cancer and is associated with worse prognosis in many cancers. Although many studies have indicated that hypoxia potentiates tumor resistance to chemotherapy and radiotherapy [7,8], how the hypoxic microenvironment contributes to anticancer drug resistance has not yet been established.

Multidrug resistance (MDR) is one of the major reasons why chemotherapy-based treatment failure occurs. Of the many mechanisms of MDR, the high expression of the human MDR1 gene and the P-glycoprotein (P-gp) transporter encoded by MDR1 is an important focus of research [9]. Tumor cells that overexpress MDR1/P-gp usually show resistance to various chemotherapeutics

[10,11]. Our previous study showed that HIF-1α protein expression is correlated with MDR1/P-gp expression in colon carcinoma tissue and a colon cancer cell line, and mRNA expression levels of HIF-1α and MDR1 are significantly higher in the same type of cells in hypoxic conditions than in normoxic conditions [12]. It remains unclear whether and how HIF-1α is involved in MDR in colon cancer via the interaction of MDR1/P-gp.

Exploring the influence of hypoxia on colon cancer MDR will help improve the effect of chemotherapy. In hypoxic microenvironment, we assume that HIF-1α may directly induce the expression of MDR1/P-gp which leads to MDR, and the reversal of colon cancer MDR can be achieved when HIF-1α expression is specifically inhibited. In the present study, we aim to explore the potential molecular mechanisms and feasibility of reversing colon cancer MDR by focusing on the target gene HIF-1α. We expect to provide a theoretical basis and experimental evidence for later related applications in clinical treatment.

Materials and Methods

Cell Culture

The human colon cancer cell line LoVo was obtained from the American Type Culture Collection (Manassas, VA, USA) and cultured in high-glucose Dulbecco's modified Eagle's medium (DMEM, Gibco, USA), supplemented with 10% fetal bovine serum (HyClone, USA) and antibiotics (1% penicillin and 1% streptomycin). For hypoxia exposure, cells were cultured for 24 hours in a modulator incubator chamber at 37°C with 1% O_2, 5% CO_2, and 94% N_2. Multicellular spheroids (MCS) were obtained by using the liquid overlay technique [13]. In brief, exponentially growing LoVo cells were added to culture medium plates that were previously coated with 2% agarose. The plates were gently and horizontally swirled for 10–15 minutes per 2–3 hours in the first 24 hours, and then for 10 minutes every 4 hours. Appropriate medium was refreshed every other day. For hypoxia experiments, appropriate MCS were established in normoxia for 48 hours and then cultured in hypoxia for another 24 hours.

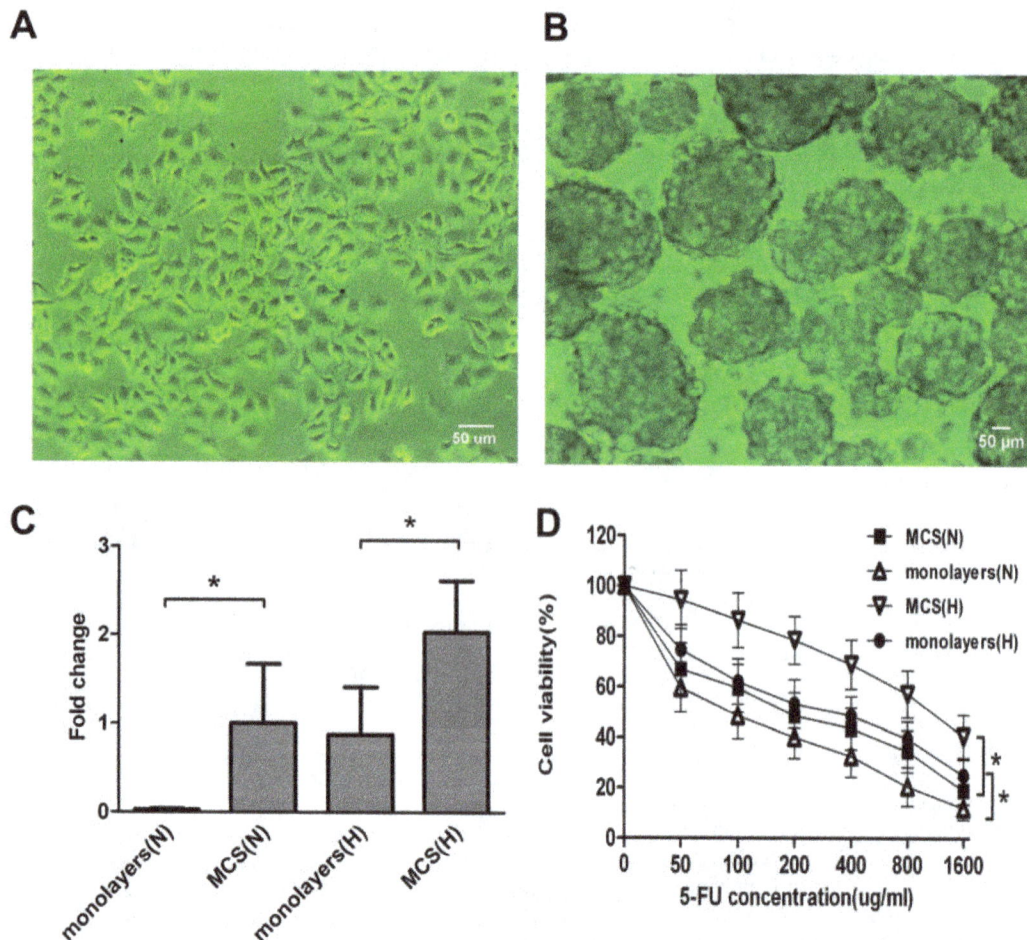

Figure 1. LoVo MCS show more resistance to chemotherapy than monolayers in hypoxia. (A) The morphology of LoVo monolayers. Scale bar = 50 μm. (B) The morphology of LoVo MCS. Scale bar = 50 μm. (C) Quantitative real-time PCR detected HIF-1α mRNA expression in LoVo MCS and in monolayers under normoxic and hypoxic conditions. The 18sRNA levels were used as internal control and the fold changes were calculated by the delta–delta Ct method. The experiments were performed in three biological replicates and PCR for each gene was done in duplicates (*$p < 0.05$). (D) Drug sensitivities (mean ± SD, n = 3) of LoVo MCS and LoVo monolayers to 5-FU in hypoxia or normoxia (*$p < 0.05$, N: normoxia, H: hypoxia).

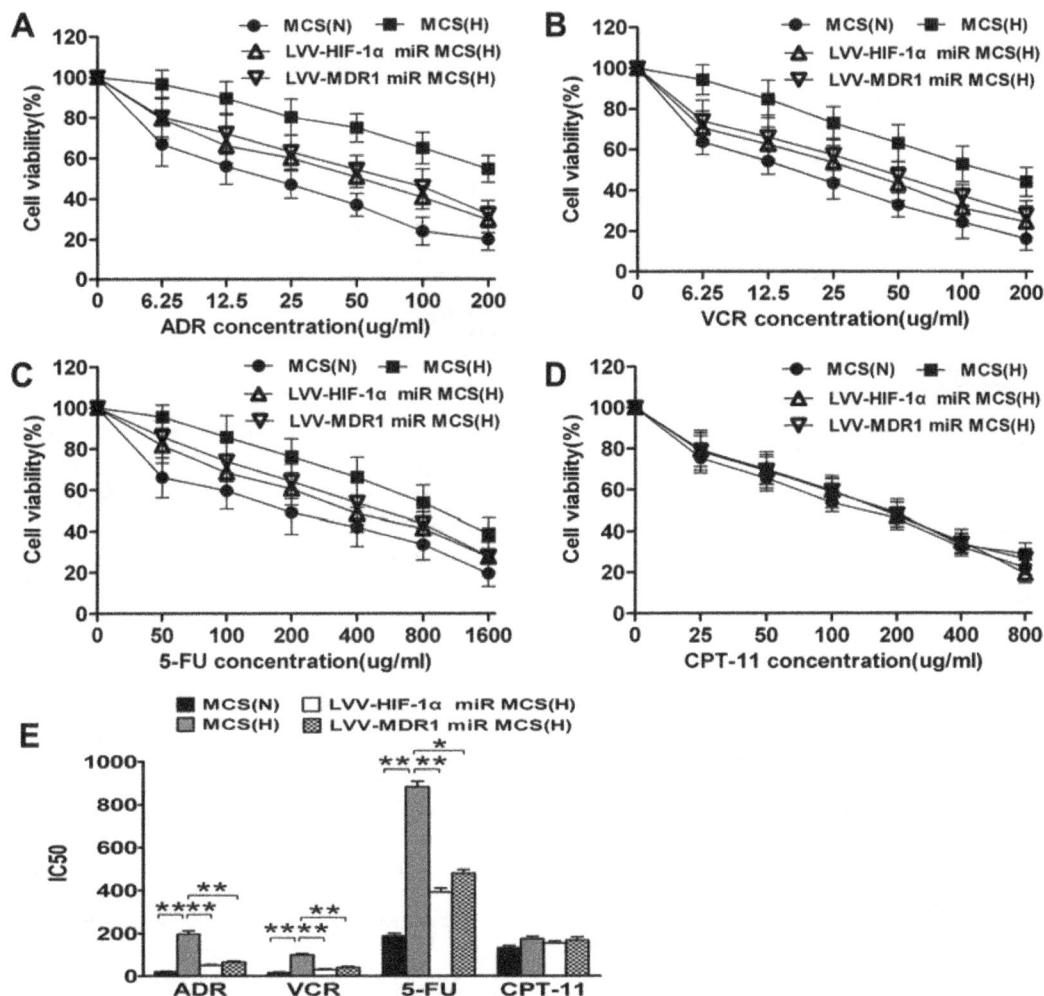

Figure 2. The sensitivity of different LoVo MCS groups to chemotherapy drugs was examined by MTT assay under normoxic and hypoxic conditions. (A) ADR. (B) VCR. (C) 5-FU. (D) CPT-11. (E) IC50 of different LoVo MCS groups to chemotherapeutics (mean ± SD, n = 3, **$p<$ 0.01, *$p<$0.05, N: normoxia, H: hypoxia).

Chemicals

Adriamycin (ADR, Hisun Pharmaceutica, China), vincristine (VCR, Hisun Pharmaceutica, China), 5-fluorouracil (5-FU, Sigma, MO, USA), or irinotecan (CPT-11, Hengrui Medicine, China) were all freshly prepared on the day of use by dissolving the required concentration in DMEM with 10% fetal bovine serum.

Chemotherapeutic Sensitivity Assay

LoVo cells were trypsinized, resuspended and counted, and 1000 cells were seeded into 96-well plates previously coated with 2% agarose to obtain MCS in normoxia. For hypoxia experiments, appropriate MSC were transferred into hypoxia for 24 hours and then incubated with gradient concentrations of drugs for another 24 hours in hypoxia. Cell viability was measured by the 3-(4, 5-dimethylthiazol-z-yl)-3, 5-diphenyltetrazolium bromide (MTT, BD Biosciences, NJ, USA) assay. Plates were incubated with MTT at 37°C for 4 hours, and the absorbance at 490 nm was measured by Model 550 Microplate Reader (Bio-Rad, CA, USA).

Quantitative Real-time PCR

Total RNA was extracted with TRIZOL reagent (Invitrogen, CA, USA) according to the manufacturer's instructions. The primers used were: 5′-GTTTGATTTTACTCATCCAT-3′ and 5′-TTCATAGTTCTTCCTCGG-3′ for HIF-1α; 5′-CTTGGCAGCAATTAGAAC-3′ and 5′-TCAGCAGGAAAG-CAGCAC-3′ for MDR1; 5′-CCTGGATACCGCAGCTAGGA -3′ and 5′-GCGGCGCAATACGAATGCCCC -3′ for 18sRNA. The first-strand cDNA synthesis was performed with cDNA synthesis kit (TaKaRa, Dalian, China). Quantitative real-time PCR was performed using the SYBR Green real-time PCR kit (TaKaRa). All normalizations were done using 18sRNA levels and the fold changes were calculated by the delta–delta Ct method. All experiments were performed in three biological replicates.

Western Blot Analysis

Total protein (50 μg) was separated by sodium dodecyl sulfate–polyacrylamide gel electrophoresis. After protein transfer to polyvinylidene fluoride microporous membranes (Bio-Rad), the membranes were blocked with 5% nonfat dry milk and incubated sequentially with the primary antibodies (HIF-1α 1:500; P-gp 1:200; β-actin 1:5000), followed by incubation with the fluorescein-linked anti-mouse (anti-rabbit) IgG (1:1000) and then incubation with anti-fluorescein alkaline phosphatase-conjugated antibody (1:5000). All antibodies were bought from Santa Cruz,

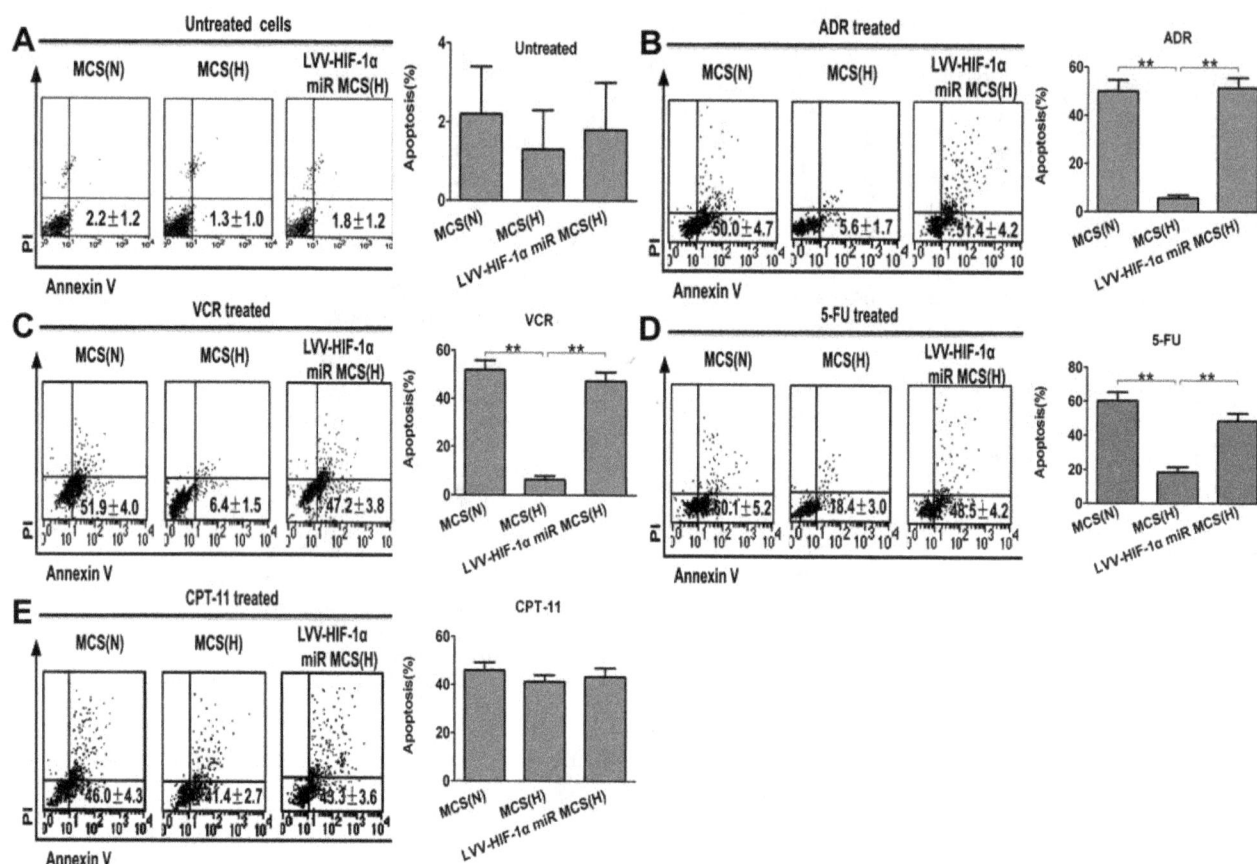

Figure 3. The change in the proportion of annexin V-positive apoptotic cells under normoxic and hypoxic conditions after treatment with chemotherapy drugs. The proportion of annexin V-positive apoptotic cells(lower right quadrant) was evaluated by flow cytometry using annexin V allophycocyanin (APC) and propidium iodide (PI) staining of LoVo MCS after treatment with (B) ADR (25 µg/ml), (C) VCR (25 µg/ml), (D) 5-FU (200 µg/ml) and (E) CPT-11 (200 µg/ml). Untreated cells were used as negative control. Data of each statistical graph of Annexin V-APC/PI staining is expressed in % of cells in the lower right quadrant and represent the mean ± SD of three independent experiments. The bar charts at the bottom of the flow cytometry scatterplots represent the % of cells undergoing apoptosis in the lower right quadrant (**$p<0.01$, N: normoxia, H: hypoxia).

CA, USA. The immune complexes were detected with the enhanced chemiluminescence reagent (Pierce, USA). For quantification, signals were densitometrically normalized to β-actin by Quantity One image analysis software (Bio-Rad).

HIF-1α siRNA Construction and Transfection

Pre-miRNA RNAi sequences for the target genes HIF-1α and MDR1 were designed and synthesized. After the two specific miRNA RNAi expression vectors with the reporter gene EmGFP targeting the human HIF-1α and MDR1 genes, respectively, were constructed and identified by restriction enzyme digestion and sequencing, the RNAi plasmids of HIF-1α and MDR1 were transfected into LoVo cells using the liposome Lipofectamine 2000 (Invitrogen, CA, USA). Stable positive clones were selected using blasticidin. The degrees of knockdown of HIF-1α and MDR1 were identified by PCR. The RNAi plasmids with better suppression effects were selected for subsequent construction of miRNA lentivirus expression clones. Two miRNA lentivirus expression clones, pLenti6/V5-GW/EmGFP-miR-HIF-1α and pLenti6/V5-GW/EmGFP-miR-MDR1, were constructed using Gateway recombination techniques (Invitrogen) and co-transfected into 293FT cells with the ViraPower packaging mix (Invitrogen). The titer was examined after infecting NIH/3T3 cells with

virus supernatant. Then, LoVo cells were infected with the two lentiviral vector-mediated miRNA RNAi systems and stably selected by blasticidin.

Chromatin Immunoprecipitation (ChIP)

Cells were plated into 100-mm-diameter dishes and, after 24 hours, incubated with 1% formaldehyde for 10 minutes at 37°C to cross-link proteins to DNA. The cross-linking reaction was quenched by the addition of one-tenth volume of 1.25 mol/L glycine. Cells were washed twice with ice-cold 1×PBS; resuspended in radioimmunoprecipitation assay buffer and kept on ice for 30 minutes. Then, cell lysates were sonicated on ice with a Hielscher UP200S ultrasound sonicator (Hielscher Ultrasonics GmbH, Germany) until the crosslinked chromatins were sheared to yield DNA fragments between 200 and 1000 bp. Supernatants were incubated with salmon sperm DNA/protein-50% agarose slurry to reduce non-specific background. Immunoprecipitation was then performed overnight at 4°C with 5 µg of anti-HIF-1α antibody (Santa Cruz, CA, USA). These supernatants were supplemented with 5 Mol/L NaCl and heated overnight at 65°C to reverse protein-DNA cross-links. The immunocomplexes were further treated with DNase-free and RNase-free proteinase K, and the DNA was purified by phenol/chloroform extraction

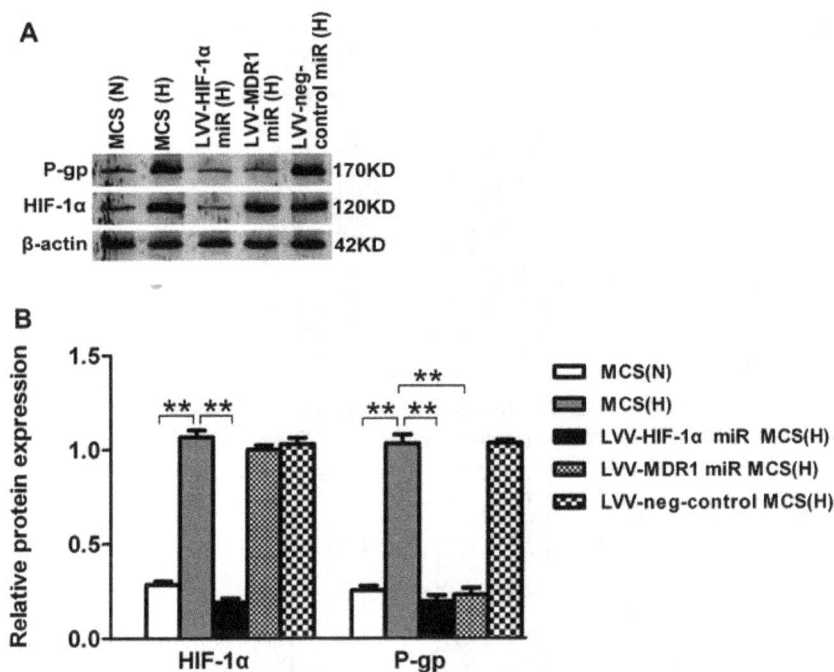

Figure 4. Expression levels of HIF-1α and P-gp in LoVo MCS with LVV-HIF-1α (or MDR1) miR stably transduced. (A) Western blot analyses were performed. β-actin was used as internal control. (B) Relative protein levels (mean ± SD, n = 3) of HIF-1α and P-gp were determined in each groups (**$p<0.01$, N: normoxia, H: hypoxia).

and ethanol precipitation. PCR was performed with primers specific for region which contains the hypoxia responsive enhancer site (5′-GCGTG-3′) of the MDR1 promoter [14]. The primers used were as follows: 5′-GGAGCAGTCATCTGTGGTGA-3′ and 5′-CTCGAATGAGCTCAGGCTTC-3′. As reported previously [24], human vascular endothelial growth factor (VEGF, an established HIF-1 target gene) was used as a positive control and primers flanking the hypoxia responsive enhancer of the VEGF promoter were 5′-GCCTCTGTCTGCCCAGCTGC-3′ and 5′-GTGGAGCTGAGAACGGGAAGC-3′. Immunoprecipitation with non-specific IgG (Santa Cruz) was performed as negative control. A sample representing linear amplification of the total input DNA was used as input control.

Detection of Apoptosis by Flow Cytometry (FCM)

Cells were prepared and treated as described above and then stained with allophycocyanin (APC)-conjugated annexin V and propidium iodide (PI) for 10 minutes at room temperature, according to the manufacturer's instructions (Annexin V-APC/PI Apoptosis Detection Kit; Jingmei Biotech, China). The population of annexin V-negative viable and annexin V-positive apoptotic cells was evaluated by FCM. Data were collected in a FACSCalibur instrument (BD Biosciences) and analyzed using CellQuest software (BD Biosciences).

Patients and Tumor Specimens

One hundred twenty patients with histologically confirmed advanced colon carcinoma and who underwent 5-FU-based chemotherapy at the Southwest Hospital, Third Military Medical University, Chongqing, China, between 2004 and 2008 were eligible for this study. This study was reviewed and approved by the Ethical and Protocol Review Committee of the Southwest Hospital, Third Military Medical University and all patients provided written consent form. The patients ranged in age from 30

to 79 years (mean age, 54 years); 73 were male, and 47 were female. Chemotherapy response was evaluated by CT scan or other radiographic means after two cycles of treatment, adopting the Response Evaluation Criteria in Solid Tumors Group criteria. Based on their chemotherapy response, patients were classified as responders or non-responders. Tissue specimens were fixed in 10% formalin, embedded in paraffin, and cut into 4-μm serial sections. The expression of HIF-1α and P-gp was examined by immunohistochemistry as previously described [12]. Clear brown-yellow staining restricted to the nuclei, cytoplasm, or cell membrane indicated positive expression of HIF-1α or P-gp. Positive expression was recorded as (+) and negative expression as (−).

Statistical Analysis

All data are provided as the mean ± SD. The results were analyzed by the chi-square test, Student's t test, and one-way analysis of variance (ANOVA). $p<0.05$ was considered significant. Statistical analyses were carried out using SPSS Version 13.0 for Windows (SPSS Inc., Chicago, IL, USA).

Results

LoVo MCS are more Resistant to Chemotherapy than Monolayers in Hypoxic Conditions

To mimic the hypoxic microenvironment of a tumor in vivo [15,16], LoVo MCS were obtained by using the liquid overlay technique. LoVo cells agglomerated with each other and proliferated rapidly. After being cultured for 48 hours, LoVo MCS were composed of a number of agglomerated cells (Figure 1B). Quantitative real-time PCR showed that the expression of HIF-1α was significantly higher in LoVo MCS than in LoVo monolayers, not only in hypoxic conditions but also in normoxia ($p<0.05$) (Figure 1C). Drug sensitivities to 5-FU were

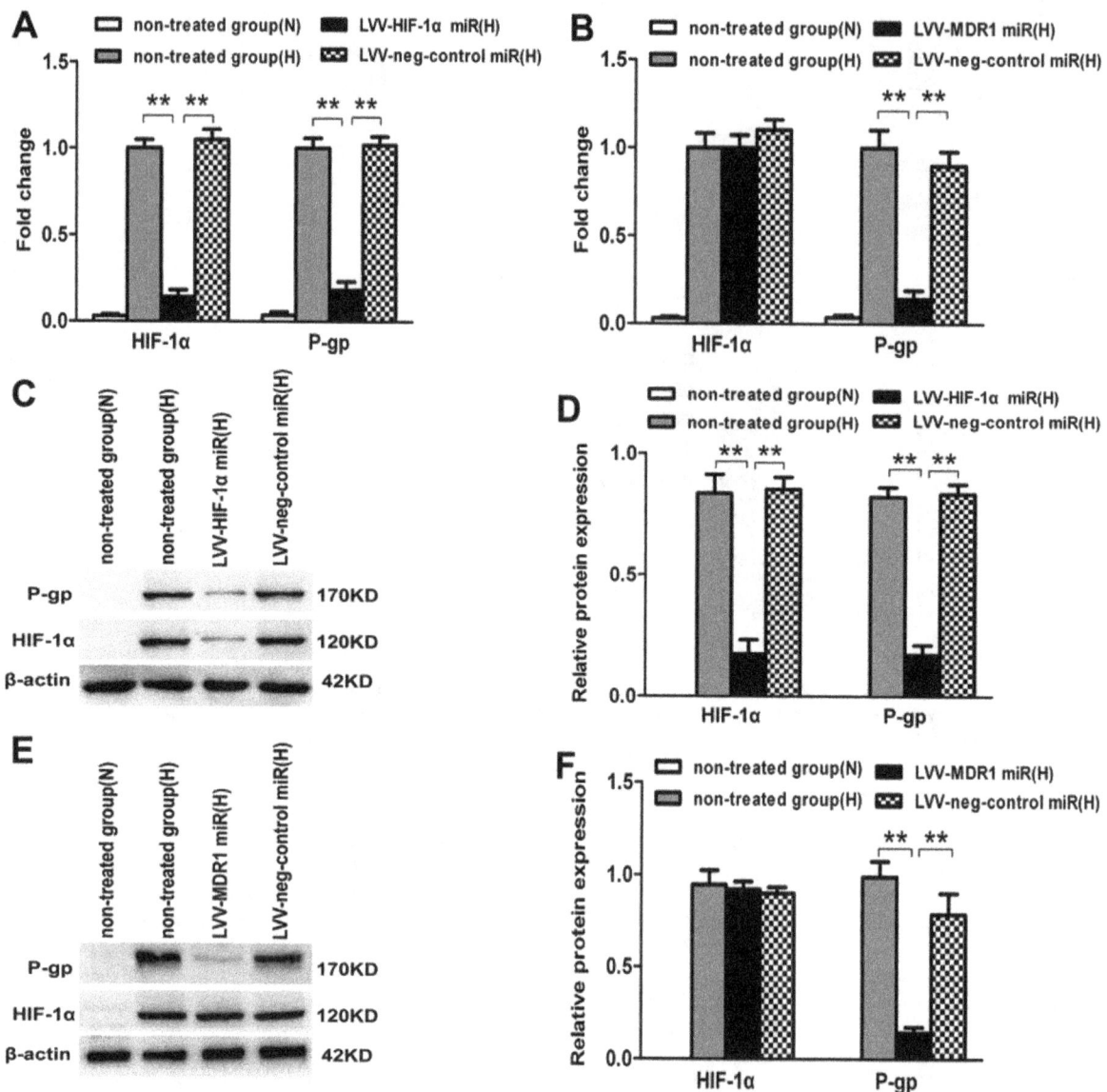

Figure 5. Expression levels of HIF-1α and MDR1/P-gp mRNA and protein in LoVo monolayers with LVV-HIF-1α miR stably transduced. (A, B) Quantitative real-time PCR detected HIF-1αor MDR1 mRNA expression in LoVo monolayers (hypoxia) with LVV-HIF-1α miR (A) or LVV-MDR1 miR (B) stably transduced. Non-treated monolayers in normoxia were used as normoxic control. The 18sRNA levels were used as internal control and the fold changes were calculated by the delta–delta Ct method. The experiments were performed in three biological replicates and PCR for each gene was done in duplicates (**$p<0.01$). (C–F) Western blot detected HIF-1α and P-gp protein expression in LoVo monolayers (hypoxia)with LVV-HIF-1α miR (C) or LVV-MDR1 miR (E) stably transduced. Non-treated monolayers in normoxia were used as normoxic control. (D, F) Comparison of expression levels (mean ± SD, n = 3) of HIF-1α and MDR1 protein of each group (**$p<0.01$).

evaluated, and the results showed that LoVo MCS were more resistant to 5-FU than were monolayers in hypoxia ($p<0.05$). Moreover, both LoVo MCS and monolayers were more resistant to 5-FU in hypoxic conditions than in normoxia (Figure 1D).

HIF-1α Inhibition Reverses Multidrug Resistance in LoVo MCS

Because LoVo MCS showed more resistance to chemotherapy than monolayers did in hypoxia, we wanted to investigate whether drug resistance changed when HIF-1α expression was specifically inhibited. We successfully established a LoVo MCS model and stable LVV-HIF-1α and LVV-MDR1 miR-infected groups. In hypoxic conditions, the sensitivity of LoVo MCS to chemotherapy

with each of the four drugs decreased to varying degrees. The 50%-inhibiting concentration (IC_{50}) values in the hypoxic group were all higher than those in the normoxic group (ADR, VCR, and 5-FU, $p<0.01$; CPT-11, $p>0.05$) (Figure 2). After silencing the HIF-1α gene, the sensitivities of LoVo MCS to all four chemotherapy drugs were restored to different extents. The relative reversal ratio between LVV-HIF-1α miR-infected group (hypoxia) and the MCS (hypoxia) for each drug was as follows: ADR, 82.8% ($p<0.01$); VCR, 83.8% ($p<0.01$); 5-FU, 70.7% ($p<0.01$); and CPT-11, 48.5% ($p>0.05$). After silencing the MDR1 gene, the relative reversal ratio between LVV-MDR1 miR-infected group (hypoxia) and the MCS (hypoxia) for each drug was

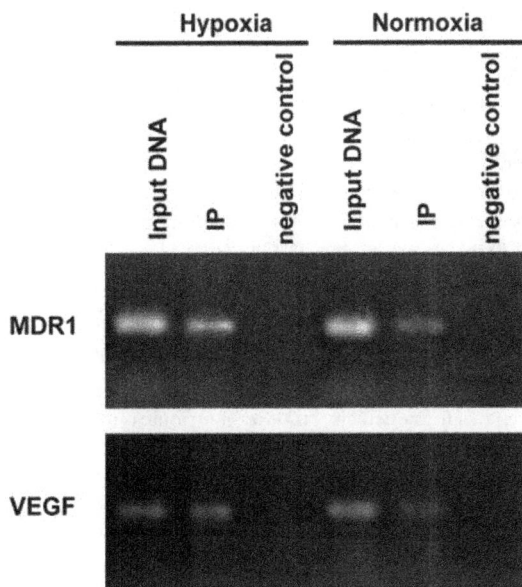

Figure 6. HIF-1α binds to the MDR1 and VEGF gene promoters in LoVo MCS. The binding of HIF-1α on the MDR1 and VEGF gene promoters was measured by ChIP. PCR analysis for the MDR1 gene promoter region was performed on immunoprecipitation samples (IP) with anti-HIF-1α antibody and with purified total input DNA from the LoVo MCS (normoxia and hypoxia). The VEGF gene promoter (an established HIF-1 target gene) was used as a positive control. Immunoprecipitation with non-specific IgG was performed as negative control. A sample representing linear amplification of the total input DNA was used as input control.

as follows: ADR, 74.2% ($p<0.01$); VCR, 70.9% ($p<0.01$); 5-FU, 58.1% ($p<0.05$); and CPT-11, 15.2% ($p>0.05$).

HIF-1α Inhibition Enhances the Apoptosis Induced by Chemotherapy Drugs in LoVo MCS

We then observed the apoptosis induced by chemotherapy drugs in LoVo MCS when HIF-1α expression was specifically inhibited. The analysis of apoptosis by FCM demonstrated that (Figure 3), compared with LoVo MCS under normoxic conditions, the apoptotic levels induced by the four drugs were all lower to varying degrees in the hypoxic group (ADR, VCR, and 5-FU, $p<0.01$; CPT-11, $p>0.05$). After efficiently silencing the target gene HIF-1α, the induced apoptosis level by ADR, VCR and 5-Fu was remarkably increased ($p<0.01$) and was 9.2-fold, 7.4-fold, and 2.6-fold respectively in contrast to that of LoVo MCS (hypoxia group). Nevertheless, the apoptosis level induced by CPT-11 was only 1.1-fold to hypoxia group, with no statistical significance ($p>0.05$).

MDR1/P-gp Protein Expression is Reduced in LoVo MCS after LVV-HIF-1α miR Transfection in Hypoxia

To explore the potential molecular mechanisms of reversing MDR by focusing on the target gene HIF-1α, we detected the expression of MDR-related genes in LoVo MCS when HIF-1α expression was specifically inhibited. Western blot showed that the expression of HIF-1α and P-gp in LoVo MCS was significantly enhanced after treatment for 24 hours in hypoxia ($p<0.01$). When HIF-1α was knocked down in the LVV-HIF-1α miR infected MCS, both HIF-1α and P-gp protein expression was downregulated compared with the negative control group ($p<0.01$). And, in the LVV-MDR1 miR infected MCS, the protein expression level of HIF-1α showed no difference while P-gp was reduced significantly compared with the negative control group (Figure 4). The results indicated that MDR1 was the downstream gene of HIF-1α and MDR1/P-gp expression will be reduced in LoVo MCS while HIF-1α was inhibited.

MDR1/P-gp mRNA and Protein Expression are Reduced in LoVo Monolayers after LVV-HIF-1α miR Transfection in Hypoxia

Because MDR1/P-gp protein expression was reduced in LoVo MCS after LVV-HIF-1α miR transfection, we further detected the expression of MDR-related genes in the LoVo monolayers in hypoxia. After stably infecting LoVo monolayers with LVV-HIF-1α miR and LVV-MDR1 miR, Quantitative real-time PCR and Western blot (Figure 5) demonstrated that in hypoxia, the mRNA and protein expression levels of HIF-1α and MDR1 in the LVV-HIF-1α miR group were significantly lower than those of the non-treated and negative control miR groups ($p<0.01$). However, in the LVV-MDR1 miR group, only the mRNA and protein expression levels of the MDR1 gene were statistically lower than those of the non-treated and negative control miR groups in hypoxia ($p<0.01$), whereas no differences in HIF-1α mRNA and protein were noted ($p>0.05$).

Binding of HIF-1α to the MDR1 Gene Promoter

We then utilized a ChIP assay to evaluate in LoVo MCS (both in normoxia and hypoxia) whether HIF-1α bound to the promoter region of the MDR1 gene. After precipitation of cell lysates with a specific anti-HIF-1α antibody, the MDR1 gene promoter and VEGF gene promoter (an established HIF-1 target gene) were amplified by PCR with specific primers. The results (Figure 6) showed that HIF-1α was bound to the MDR1 gene promoter in LoVo MCS not only in hypoxic conditions but also in normoxic conditions.

Table 1. The correlation between HIF-1α and P-gp expression and chemotherapy sensitivity.

	N	non-responders N (%)	Responders N (%)	p value*
HIF-1α (−)/P-gp (−)	19	7 (36.8)	12 (63.2)	
HIF-1α (+)/P-gp (−)	20	11 (45.0)	9 (55.0)	0.256
HIF-1α (+)/P-gp (+)	73	56 (76.7)	17 (23.3)	0.001
HIF-1α (−)/P-gp (+)	8	4 (50.0)	4 (50.0)	0.675

N: Number of patients;
*chi-square test; positive expression was recorded as (+) and negative expression as (−).

Patients with HIF-1α (+)/P-gp (+) are more Resistant to Chemotherapy

Our previous study has shown that HIF-1α and MDR1/P-gp expression levels correlate in tumor tissues of colon carcinoma [12]. To determine whether the expression of HIF-1α and MDR1/P-gp in colon cancer patients differs, as well as the related sensitivity to chemotherapy, immunohistochemical techniques were employed to detect the expression of HIF-1α and P-gp in the tumor tissues of 120 patients with advanced colon carcinoma who received 5-FU-based chemotherapy. We found that 73 of 120 cases (60.8%) expressed both HIF-1α and P-gp, and this HIF-1α (+)/P-gp (+) patient population was more resistant to chemotherapy than was the HIF-1α (−)/P-gp (−) population ($p = 0.001$, OR 5.647, 95% CI 1.920–16.606) (Table 1).

Discussion

Our previous study showed that HIF-1α protein expression is correlated with P-gp expression in colon carcinoma tissues and colon cancer cell lines, and HIF-1α and MDR1 mRNAs were found to be significantly higher in the same cells under hypoxic conditions than under normoxic conditions [12]. In the present study, we show that HIF-1α may directly influence the expression of MDR1/P-gp in hypoxic microenvironment and then mediate chemotherapy resistance not only in cultured cell monolayers but also in multicellular spheroids, and HIF-1α inhibition may reverse multidrug resistance via downregulation of MDR1/P-gp. Much evidence has demonstrated that a hypoxic microenvironment is conducive to the development and maintenance of cancers [17]. Moreover, cancer cells in hypoxic conditions show more resistance to antineoplastic drugs [18,19]. Some studies that have tried to explain this phenomenon have found that cells in hypoxic conditions generally divide slower than those in normoxic conditions, rendering therapies that target rapidly growing cells less effective [17]. Meanwhile, a study demonstrated that hypoxia could induce a number of genes, including MDR1/P-gp, in multicellular spheroids [16]. In our study, we found that HIF-1α bound to the MDR1 gene promoter in LoVo MCS not only in hypoxic conditions but also in normoxic conditions.

We successfully established a LoVo MCS model to mimic the hypoxic microenvironment of tumors in vivo. The chemotherapy sensitivity and apoptotic changes of LoVo MCS to ADR, VCR, 5-FU, and CPT-11 were examined in normoxia and hypoxia. The results showed that the chemotherapy sensitivities and apoptosis of LoVo MCS in response to the four drugs were all decreased to different degrees in hypoxic conditions. Of the four cytotoxic drugs, 5-FU and CPT-11 are the most commonly used in colon cancer, whereas resistance to ADR and VCR is thought to be closely related to MDR1/P-gp [20]. Silencing the HIF-1α gene restored the sensitivities of LoVo MCS to ADR, VCR, and 5-FU and induced a marked increase in the apoptotic level of each corresponding drug ($P < 0.01$). These results indicate that drug resistance of LoVo MCS can be reversed with a combination of the LVV-HIF-1α miR system and the above drugs. This finding concurs with the previous findings that inhibiting HIF-1α can enhance the sensitivity to chemotherapeutic agents in cancer cells such as fibrosarcoma, gastric cancer, and breast carcinoma [21–23]. Since Unruh et al. [24] found that the antiproliferative efficacy of carboplatin and etoposide is significantly enhanced by the inactivation of HIF-1α in mouse embryonic fibroblasts, the contribution of HIF-1α to drug resistance has been observed in various types of neoplastic cells in recent years [21,25–29]. However, the available data on the relationship between HIF-1α and the chemoresistance of cancer cells are conflicting. For example, some studies have demonstrated that the inactivation of HIF-1α in normoxia has no effect on drug responses in neuroblastoma and lung adenocarcinoma cells [30,31]. Recent studies have also argued for a resistance-mediating effect of HIF-1α, at least in some human cancers [4]. Additionally, we found there was a trend toward more sensitivity after HIF-1α or MDR1 inhibition, but the chemotherapy sensitivities to CPT-11 were not significantly different in the LoVo MCS groups. The result indicated that the mechanism of chemoresistance to CPT-11 did not depend on P-gp but rather went through another pathway, such as the CPT-11 metabolic product SN-38 [32–34].

The mechanism by which HIF-1α contributes to MDR is complex and remained unclear. HIF-1α may mediate MDR by regulating drug efflux, altering cell proliferation and survival, inhibiting DNA damage, or reprogramming metabolism. As one of the main members of the ABC transporter family, MDR1/P-gp reduces the intracellular concentrations of cytotoxic drugs by actively pumping the drugs out of cells and thereby protecting cancer cells from their antitumor effects [35]. MDR1 is a target gene of HIF-1. In recent years, the contribution of HIF-1-mediated P-gp expression to hypoxia-induced drug resistance has been observed in many tumor cells, such as gastric cancer, gliomas, and breast carcinoma [14,21,26,36]. In this study, we showed that the expression of HIF-1α and P-gp was significantly enhanced in LoVo MCS after treatment in hypoxia. HIF-1α inhibition by transfecting cells with a specific siRNA for HIF-1α significantly decreased the expression of MDR1/P-gp mRNA and protein in both LoVo monolayers and LoVo MCS. Furthermore, HIF-1α was bound to the MDR1 gene promoter directly. We indicated that HIF-1α activation may directly induce the expression of MDR1/P-gp and then lead to MDR.

To determine whether the expression of HIF-1α and MDR1/P-gp in colon cancer patients differs, as well as the related sensitivity to chemotherapy, immunohistochemistry were employed to detect the expression of HIF-1α and P-gp in the tumor tissues of 120 patients with advanced colon carcinoma who received 5-FU-based chemotherapy. We found that 73 of 120 cases (60.8%) expressed both HIF-1α and P-gp, and this HIF-1α (+)/P-gp (+) patient population was more resistant to chemotherapy than was the HIF-1α (−)/P-gp (−) population. Therefore, HIF-1α/MDR1 may be a promising target in the colon cancer treatment, and the reversal of colon cancer MDR can be achieved when HIF-1α/MDR1 expression is specifically inhibited. We suggest that the expression of HIF-1α and MDR1/P-gp can be used as a predictive marker for chemotherapy resistance in colon cancer.

In conclusion, we report that HIF-1α inhibition reverses MDR in colon cancer cells, which is associated with downregulation of MDR1/P-gp. Our results may have broad clinical implications for colon patients with HIF-1α (+)/P-gp (+) expression patterns, and combination therapies aimed at modulating HIF-1α expression in concert with standard chemotherapy regimens may provide a strategy to overcome tumor resistance.

Author Contributions

Conceived and designed the experiments: JC ZD HL. Performed the experiments: JC ZD YP. Analyzed the data: JC ZD YP FP JL. Contributed reagents/materials/analysis tools: LZ YZ. Wrote the paper: JC ZD HL.

References

1. Desoize B, Jardillier J (2000) Multicellular resistance: a paradigm for clinical resistance? Crit Rev Oncol Hematol 36: 193–207.
2. Morin PJ (2003) Drug resistance and the microenvironment: nature and nurture. Drug Resist Updat 6: 169–172.
3. Westhoff MA, Fulda S (2009) Adhesion-mediated apoptosis resistance in cancer. Drug Resist Updat 12: 127–136.
4. Rohwer N, Cramer T(2011) Hypoxia-mediated drug resistance: novel insights on the functional interaction of HIFs and cell death pathways. Drug Resist Updat 14: 191–201.
5. Brown JM (2007) Tumor hypoxia in cancer therapy. Methods Enzymol 435: 297–321.
6. Liang S, Galluzzo P, Sobol A, Skucha S, Rambo B, et al. (2012) Multimodality Approaches to Treat Hypoxic Non-Small Cell Lung Cancer (NSCLC) Microenvironment. Genes Cancer 3: 141–151.
7. Ramaekers CH, van den Beucken T, Meng A, Kassam S, Thoms J, et al. (2011) Hypoxia disrupts the Fanconi anemia pathway and sensitizes cells to chemotherapy through regulation of UBE2T. Radiother Oncol 101: 190–197.
8. Owen MR, Stamper IJ, Muthana M, Richardson GW, Dobson J, et al. (2011) Mathematical modeling predicts synergistic antitumor effects of combining a macrophage-based, hypoxia-targeted gene therapy with chemotherapy. Cancer Res 71: 2826–2837.
9. Wu CP, Calcagno AM, Ambudkar SV (2008) Reversal of ABC drug transporter-mediated multidrug resistance in cancer cells: evaluation of current strategies. Curr Mol Pharmacol 1: 93–105.
10. He Q, Zhang G, Hou D, Leng A, Xu M, et al. (2011) Overexpression of sorcin results in multidrug resistance in gastric cancer cells with up-regulation of P-gp. Oncol Rep 25: 237–243.
11. Chen LM, Liang YJ, Ruan JW, Ding Y, Wang XW, et al. (2004) Reversal of P-gp mediated multidrug resistance in-vitro and in-vivo by FG020318. J Pharm Pharmacol 56: 1061–1066.
12. Ding Z, Yang L, Xie X, Xie F, Pan F, et al. (2010) Expression and significance of hypoxia-inducible factor-1 alpha and MDR1/P-glycoprotein in human colon carcinoma tissue and cells. J Cancer Res Clin Oncol 136: 1697–1707.
13. Oktem G, Bilir A, Selvi N, Yurtseven ME, Vatansever S, et al. (2006) Chemotherapy influences inducible nitric oxide synthase (iNOS) and endothelial nitric oxide synthase (eNOS) activity on 3D breast cancer cell line. Oncol Res 16: 195–203.
14. Comerford KM, Wallace TJ, Karhausen J, Louis NA, Montalto MC, et al. (2002) Hypoxia-inducible factor-1-dependent regulation of the multidrug resistance (MDR1) gene. Cancer Res 62: 3387–3394.
15. Ravizza R, Molteni R, Gariboldi MB, Marras E, Perletti G, et al. (2009) Effect of HIF-1 modulation on the response of two- and three-dimensional cultures of human colon cancer cells to 5-fluorouracil. European Journal of Cancer 45: 890–898.
16. Wartenberg M, Donmez F, Ling FC, Acker H, Hescheler J, et al. (2001) Tumor-induced angiogenesis studied in confrontation cultures of multicellular tumor spheroids and embryoid bodies grown from pluripotent embryonic stem cells. FASEB J 15: 995–1005.
17. Brown JM (2000) Exploiting the hypoxic cancer cell: mechanisms and therapeutic strategies. Mol Med Today 6: 157–162.
18. Brown JM, Giaccia AJ (1998) The unique physiology of solid tumors: opportunities (and problems) for cancer therapy. Cancer Res 58: 1408–1416.
19. Cuvillier O, Ader I, Bouquerel P, Brizuela L, Gstalder C, et al. (2013) Hypoxia, therapeutic resistance, and sphingosine 1-phosphate. Adv Cancer Res 117: 117–141.
20. Kanagasabai R, Krishnamurthy K, Druhan LJ, Ilangovan G (2011) Forced expression of heat shock protein 27 (Hsp27) reverses P-glycoprotein (ABCB1)-mediated drug efflux and MDR1 gene expression in Adriamycin-resistant human breast cancer cells. J Biol Chem 286: 33289–33300.
21. Liu L, Ning X, Sun L, Zhang H, Shi Y, et al. (2008) Hypoxia-inducible factor-1 alpha contributes to hypoxia-induced chemoresistance in gastric cancer. Cancer Sci 99: 121–128.
22. Hao J, Song X, Song B, Liu Y, Wei L, et al. (2008) Effects of lentivirus-mediated HIF-1alpha knockdown on hypoxia-related cisplatin resistance and their dependence on p53 status in fibrosarcoma cells. Cancer Gene Ther 15: 449–455.
23. Dong XL, Xu PF, Miao C, Fu ZY, Li QP, et al. (2012) Hypoxia decreased chemosensitivity of breast cancer cell line MCF-7 to paclitaxel through cyclin B1. Biomed Pharmacother 66: 70–75.
24. Unruh A, Ressel A, Mohamed HG, Johnson RS, Nadrowitz R, et al. (2003) The hypoxia-inducible factor-1 alpha is a negative factor for tumor therapy. Oncogene 22: 3213–3220.
25. Brown LM, Cowen RL, Debray C, Eustace A, Erler JT, et al. (2006) Reversing hypoxic cell chemoresistance in vitro using genetic and small molecule approaches targeting hypoxia inducible factor-1. Mol Pharmacol 69: 411–418.
26. Nardinocchi L, Puca R, Sacchi A, D'Orazi G (2009) Inhibition of HIF-1alpha activity by homeodomain-interacting protein kinase-2 correlates with sensitization of chemoresistant cells to undergo apoptosis. Mol Cancer 8: 1.
27. Sasabe E, Zhou X, Li D, Oku N, Yamamoto T, et al. (2007) The involvement of hypoxia-inducible factor-1alpha in the susceptibility to gamma-rays and chemotherapeutic drugs of oral squamous cell carcinoma cells. Int J Cancer 120: 268–277.
28. Sullivan R, Pare GC, Frederiksen LJ, Semenza GL, Graham CH (2008) Hypoxia-induced resistance to anticancer drugs is associated with decreased senescence and requires hypoxia-inducible factor-1 activity. Mol Cancer Ther 7: 1961–1973.
29. Chen M, Huang SL, Zhang XQ, Zhang B, Zhu H, et al. (2012) Reversal effects of pantoprazole on multidrug resistance in human gastric adenocarcinoma cells by down-regulating the V-ATPases/mTOR/HIF-1alpha/P-gp and MRP1 signaling pathway in vitro and in vivo. J Cell Biochem 113: 2474–2487.
30. Hussein D, Estlin EJ, Dive C, Makin GW (2006) Chronic hypoxia promotes hypoxia-inducible factor-1alpha-dependent resistance to etoposide and vincristine in neuroblastoma cells. Mol Cancer Ther 5: 2241–2250.
31. Chang Q, Qin R, Huang T, Gao J, Feng Y (2006) Effect of antisense hypoxia-inducible factor 1alpha on progression, metastasis, and chemosensitivity of pancreatic cancer. Pancreas 32: 297–305.
32. Yeo EJ, Chun YS, Cho YS, Kim J, Lee JC, et al. (2003) YC-1: a potential anticancer drug targeting hypoxia-inducible factor 1. J Natl Cancer Inst 95: 516–525.
33. Sapra P, Kraft P, Pastorino F, Ribatti D, Dumble M, et al. (2011) Potent and sustained inhibition of HIF-1alpha and downstream genes by a polyethylene-glycol-SN38 conjugate, EZN-2208, results in anti-angiogenic effects. Angiogenesis 14: 245–253.
34. Kamiyama H, Takano S, Tsuboi K, Matsumura A (2005) Anti-angiogenic effects of SN38 (active metabolite of irinotecan): inhibition of hypoxia-inducible factor 1 alpha (HIF-1alpha)/vascular endothelial growth factor (VEGF) expression of glioma and growth of endothelial cells. J Cancer Res Clin Oncol 131: 205–213.
35. Tiwari AK, Sodani K, Dai CL, Ashby CR Jr, Chen ZS (2011) Revisiting the ABCs of multidrug resistance in cancer chemotherapy. Curr Pharm Biotechnol 12: 570–594.
36. Li J, Shi M, Cao Y, Yuan W, Pang T, et al. (2006) Knockdown of hypoxia-inducible factor-1alpha in breast carcinoma MCF-7 cells results in reduced tumor growth and increased sensitivity to methotrexate. Biochem Biophys Res Commun 342: 1341–1351.

13

Anti-VEGF-A Affects the Angiogenic Properties of Tumor-Derived Microparticles

Michal Munster[1]9, Ella Fremder[1]9, Valeria Miller[1], Neta Ben-Tsedek[1], Shiri Davidi[1], Stefan J. Scherer[2], Yuval Shaked[1]*

1 Department of Molecular pharmacology, Rappaport Faculty of Medicine, Technion, Haifa, Israel, 2 Hoffmann La Roche, Basel, Switzerland

Abstract

Tumor derived microparticles (TMPs) have recently been shown to contribute to tumor re-growth partially by inducing the mobilization and tumor homing of specific bone marrow derived pro-angiogenic cells (BMDCs). Since antiangiogenic drugs block proangiogenic BMDC mobilization and tumor homing, we asked whether TMPs from cells exposed to an antiangiogenic drug may affect BMDC activity and trafficking. Here we show that the level of VEGF-A is reduced in TMPs from EMT/6 breast carcinoma cells exposed to the anti-VEGF-A antibody, B20. Consequently, these TMPs exhibit reduced angiogenic potential as evaluated by a Matrigel plug and Boyden chamber assays. Consistently, BMDC mobilization, tumor angiogenesis, microvessel density and BMDC-colonization in growing tumors are reduced in mice inoculated with TMPs from B20-exposed cells as compared to mice inoculated with control TMPs. Collectively, our results suggest that the neutralization of VEGF-A in cultured tumor cells can block TMP-induced BMDC mobilization and colonization of tumors and hence provide another mechanism of action by which antiangiogenic drugs act to inhibit tumor growth and angiogenesis.

Editor: Francesco Bertolini, European Institute of Oncology, Italy

Funding: This work was supported by research grants from the Israel Cancer Research Fund, European Research Council under FP7 program, and a sponsored research agreement with Hoffmann La Roche. The funder, Roche, provided support in the form of a salary for author SJS, but did not have any additional role in the study design, data collection and analysis, decision to publish, or preparation of the manuscript. The specific roles of the authors are articulated in the 'author contributions' section.

Competing Interests: YS was a consultant for Roche and SJS was an employee of Roche. There are no patents, products in development or marketed products to declare.

* E-mail: yshaked@tx.technion.ac.il

9 These authors contributed equally to this work.

Introduction

Tumors undergo an angiogenic switch when the balance between pro-angiogenic and anti-angiogenic factors is perturbed, leading to tumor outgrowth and expansion [1,2,3]. Endothelial cells, which either rapidly divide from pre-existing vessels or home from the circulation to the tumor, actively participate in the tumor angiogenic process [4]. Endothelial progenitor cells (EPCs) constitute the major cell type to incorporate into the blood vessel wall in a systemic angiogenesis process, also called vasculogenesis [5]. In addition, other bone marrow derived cell (BMDC) types, such as myeloid derived suppressor cells (MDSCs), hemangiocytes, and Tie-2 expressing monocytes (TEMs) were also found to contribute to systemic tumor angiogenesis by supporting blood vessel growth and function via different paracrine mechanisms [6].

The contribution of EPCs to tumor blood vessel growth is controversial [7,8,9]. We recently demonstrated that the level of EPCs in the peripheral blood of mice rises rapidly in response to various cytotoxic agents, including chemotherapy and vascular disrupting agents (VDAs). Subsequently, these cells home to the treated tumor site, induce angiogenesis and thus aid in tumor cell repopulation leading to tumor re-growth [10,11]. TEMs and tumor associated macrophages (TAMs) have also been found to colonize treated tumors, and promote revascularization following therapy [12,13,14]. Importantly, the addition of an antiangiogenic drug to chemotherapy substantially reduces EPC mobilization and

homing to the treated tumor site, leading to enhanced treatment efficacy in part by blocking rebound angiogenesis [10,11]. Importantly, studies have demonstrated that it is the response of the host, rather than the tumor cells themselves, to such anti-cancer therapies, that facilitates systemic angiogenesis [15,16].

Tumor cells shed microparticles (MPs) which are a subset of microvesicles (MVs) along with exosomes. MPs vary in size (0.1–1 μm) and primarily contain cell membrane proteins and phospholipids representative of the cells they originate from [17,18]. Levels of circulating MPs in the blood increase significantly in a variety of disease states, including cancer [19]. Recent findings suggest that tumor-derived MPs (TMPs) may act as messengers and mediators of tumor growth. TMPs containing the oncogenic form of the endothelial growth factor receptor (EGFRvIII) expressed on glioma tumor cells were found to be fused with tumor cells lacking this oncogene [20,21]. Thus, a new way of communication between tumor cells in the tumor bed or at distant sites could be mediated by TMPs [21]. In a recent study we demonstrated that TMPs from cells exposed to paclitaxel chemotherapy induced BMDC mobilization and colonization of tumors, thereby contributing to angiogenesis and tumor re-growth [22]. However, the impact of antiangiogenic therapy in this context has not been elucidated.

Here we studied the effect of the anti-VEGF-A antibody, B20, on the angiogenic potential of TMPs collected from EMT/6 breast carcinoma cells. We show that the angiogenic properties of TMPs from cells exposed to anti-VEGF-A antibody are reduced due to a reduction in the VEGF-A content, when compared to TMPs from control cells. We demonstrate that TMPs from cells exposed to antiangiogenic therapy do not promote BMDC mobilization and endothelial cell homing to the tumor site. Overall, our results suggest that in addition to the antiangiogenic activity of anti-VEGF-A on endothelial cells, this treatment strategy may also inhibit the angiogenic properties of MPs shed from tumor cells in an anti-VEGF-A microenvironment.

Materials and Methods

Cell Culture

EMT-6 and 4T1 murine breast carcinoma and MDA-MB-231 human breast carcinoma cell lines were purchased from the American Type Culture Collection (ATCC, Manassas, VA, USA). Cell lines were grown in Dulbecco's modified Eagle's medium (DMEM) supplemented with 10% fetal calf serum, 1% L-glutamine, 1% sodium-pyruvate and 1% streptomycin. Human umbilical vein endothelial cells (HUVECs) (Lonza, Switzerland) were cultured in plates covered with 10% fibronectin (1 mg/ml Biological Industries, Beit HaEmek, Isreal) following 37°C incubation for 30 min. HUVECs were cultured in M199 medium (Sigma-Aldrich, Rehovot, Israel) supplemented with 20% heat inactivated fetal calf serum (FCS), 50 mg/ml endothelial cell growth supplement (ECGS), 50 mg/ml heparin, 10 mM Hepes, 1% L-glutamine, 1% sodium-pyruvate and 1% streptomycin.

Microparticle Extraction and Quantification

Cultured cells were grown in medium containing 10% fetal calf serum until they reached 80% confluency, at which point, the medium was replaced with serum free (SF) medium in the presence or absence of 2 μg/ml of B20, an antibody neutralizing both human and murine vascular endothelial growth factor (VEGF-A; kindly provided by Genentech Inc., San Francisco, CA, USA)[23,24]. In some experiments non-related IgG antibody was used as a control. After 48 hours, conditioned medium was collected and centrifuged at 1500 g/300 g for 20 minutes at 24°C to remove floating cells. The cell free supernatants were then centrifuged at 20,000 g for 1 hour at 4°C. The pellet was then washed with phosphate buffered saline (PBS), and the TMP-containing pellet was resuspended in PBS. TMPs were stored at −80°C until analyzed. Quantification of TMPs was performed using flow cytometry as previously described [22,25]. Briefly, 0.78 μm-sized beads (Calbiochem) were used to gate on TMP size. TMP number was obtained by calculating the ratio between 7.35 μm counting beads and the number of events collected at the TMP gate. A representative flow cytometry analysis of TMPs is presented in Figure 1A.

Quantification of the Expression Levels of VEGF-A

Half a million TMPs from MDA-MB231, 4T1 or EMT/6 cell cultures were applied to either human or murine VEGF-A enzyme-linked immunosorbent assay (ELISA) kits (R&D systems) in order to detect VEGF-A levels, in accordance with the manufacturer's instructions. Experiments were performed in triplicates.

Invasion and Migration of HUVECs Assessed by the Modified Boyden Chamber Assay

HUVEC invasion and migration properties were assessed using Matrigel- or fibronectin-coated Boyden chambers as previously described [26]. Briefly, serum-starved HUVEC cells (2×10^5 cells

per 0.2 ml medium) were added to the upper chamber that was coated with 50 μl Matrigel (BD Biosciences, San Jose, CA, USA) for assessing invasion, or with 50 μl fibronectin (10 μg/ml) for assessing migration. The lower compartment was filled with PBS that contained 5×10^6 TMPs from control cells or from cells exposed to 2 μg/ml B20 antibody, and subsequently lysed by 4 repeated freeze-thaw cycles. After 4 hours for migration, or 24 hours for invasion, HUVECs which migrated to the lower compartment of the chamber, were stained with crystal violet and images were captured using the Leica CTR 6000 microscope system (Leica Microsystems, Wetzlar, Germany) followed by cell counting. The experiments were carried out in triplicate, and results presented as means ± SD.

Microvessel Sprouting using Aortic Ring

One millimeter long aortic rings (n = 3/group) obtained from 8–10 week old BALB/c mice, were embedded in Matrigel (BD Bioscience) and overlaid with SF DMEM supplemented with 0.1×10^6 TMPs from control cells or from cells exposed to B20 antibodies. Plates were incubated at 37°C in a humidified 5% CO^2 atmosphere and the medium was replaced every other day. Images of the rings and microvessel sprouting were captured using Leica CTR 6000 microscope (Leica Microsystems).

Matrigel Plug Assay

Matrigel (0.5 ml; BD Biosciences) that contained TMPs from control cells or from cells exposed to B20 antibodies, was injected subcutaneously into each flank of 8–10 week old BALB/c mice (n = 4 mice/group). Plugs were removed 10 days later, and subsequently prepared for either histological assessment using hematoxylin and eosin (H&E) and endothelial cell staining, or flow cytometry for the evaluation of BMDCs. For flow cytometry, Matrigel plugs were prepared as a single cell suspension as previously described [27] and cells that infiltrated the plugs were identified as described below.

Animals and Tumor Model

Half a million EMT/6 cells were implanted subcutaneously in the flanks of 8–10 week old BALB/c mice (Harlan Biotech Israel, Rehovot, Israel). Tumor size was assessed regularly with Vernier calipers using the formula, width²×length×0.5. Mice were intravenously injected twice weekly with 0.5×10^6 TMPs collected from control cells or from cells exposed to B20 antibodies. Control mice were injected with PBS. Tumors were removed at end point (~1000–1500 mm³). All animal studies and experimental protocols were approved by the Animal Care and Use Committee of the Technion.

Evaluation of BMDCs by Flow Cytometry

BMDCs obtained from tumors, Matrigel plugs following single cell suspension, or whole blood following red blood cell lysis were analyzed by flow cytometry using the following antibody mixtures: CXCR4+/CD11+/VEGFR1+/CD45+ for identifying hemangio-cytes; CD11b+/Gr-1+ for identifying MDSCs; and VEGFR2+/7AAD/CD117+/CD45- for identifying viable CEPs as previously described [28]. All monoclonal antibodies were purchased from BD Biosciences, R&D systems, and Macs Militenyi Biotec (Bergisch Gladbach, Germany), and used according to the manufacturers' instructions. At least 100,000 events were acquired using a CyAn ADP flow cytometer and analyzed with Summit software (Beckman Coulter, Nyon, Switzerland).

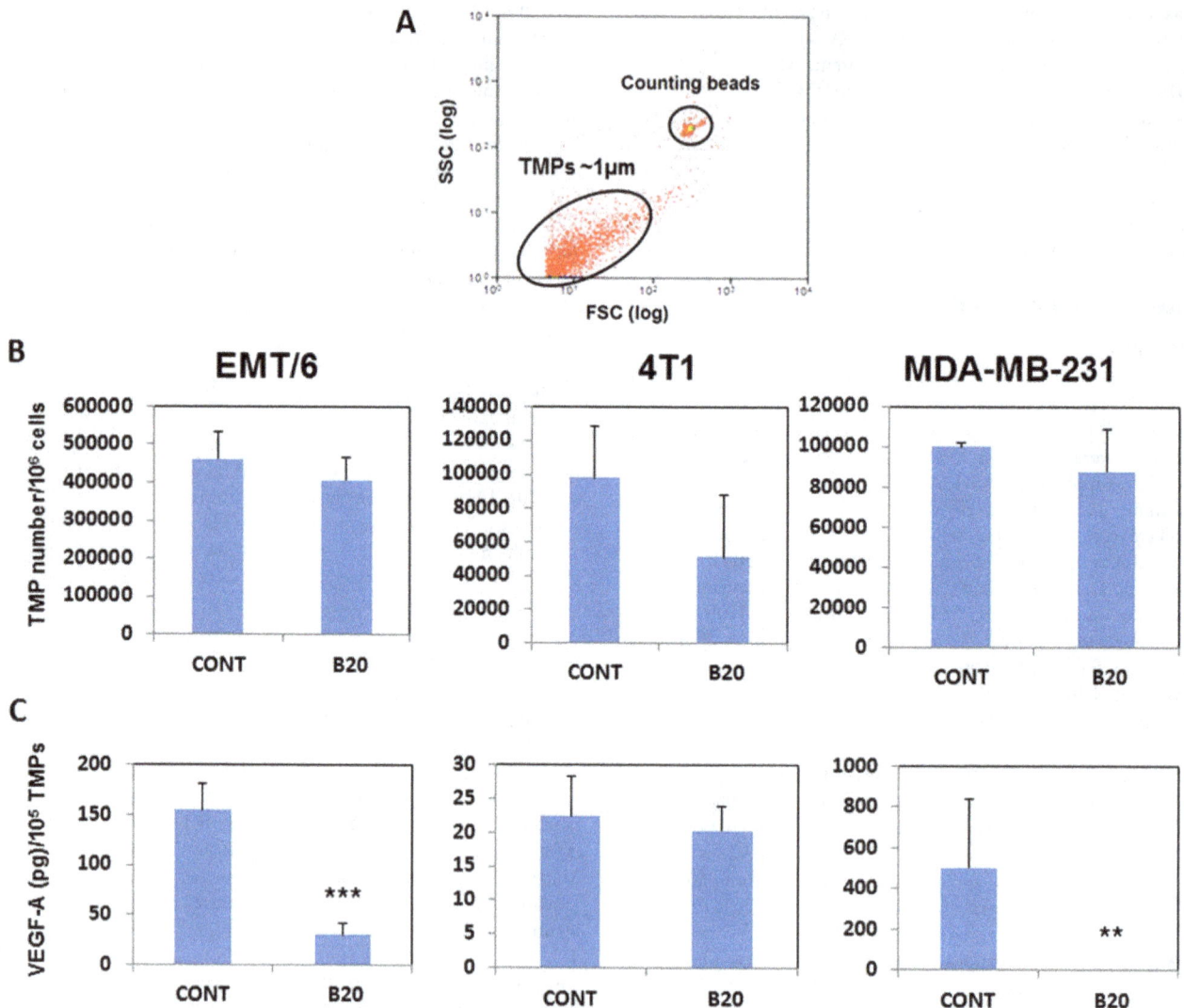

Figure 1. Exposing tumor cells to anti-VEGF-A antibodies reduces the level of VEGF-A in TMPs without affecting the number of TMPs. (A) A representative flow cytometry dotplot for TMP quantification. TMPs are approximately 1 μm, and counting beads are 7.35 μm. The number of TMPs per sample was calculated as the ratio between the number of events collected in the counting beads gate and the number of events collected in the TMPs gate over the total number of counting beads loaded in the sample. (B) EMT/6, 4T1 and MDA-MB231 breast carcinoma cells were either left untreated or exposed to 2 μg/ml B20 antibody for 48 h. TMPs were purified from conditioned medium and quantified by flow cytometry. Shown are the means ± S.D. of triplicates. (C) An equal number of TMPs (100,000) from untreated or B-20-exposed EMT/6, 4T1 and MDA-MB231 breast carcinoma cells were used to quantify the level of VEGF-A by ELISA. In some experiments control for B20 antibodies was used in a form of IgG in culture. Shown are the means ± S.D. of triplicates. **, 0.01>p>0.001.

Tissue Processing and Immunostaining

Tumors were embedded in OCT (Tissue-Tek, Sakura Finetek USA Inc., USA) and stored at −80°C. Matrigel plugs were embedded in 10% paraformaldehyde at room temperature (RT) for 24 hours. Subsequently, the plugs were embedded in OCT at 4°C for 48 hours and then stored at −80°C. Tumors or Matrigel plugs were cryosectioned (4–6 μm and 20–25 μm respectively), and then immunostained with an endothelial cell specific antibody (anti-mouse CD31, 1:200, BD Biosciences) and a secondary antibody conjugated with Cy3 (1:150, Jackson ImmunoResearch Laboratories Inc., West Grove, PA, USA), and with a pan-hematopoietic marker (anti-mouse CD45 conjugated with FITC, 1:150, BD Biosciences). Tumor cryosections were also used for analysis of blood vessel perfusion by Hoechst 33342 (40 mg/kg) (Sigma-Aldrich Israel Ltd., Rehovot, Israel), injected to mice

90 sec before mice were sacrificed, as previously described [10]. The number of vessel structures (positive for CD31 staining) and/or functional vessels (positive for Hoechst and CD31 staining) per field were counted and plotted (approximately 5 fields per tumor, n>20 fields/group). Tumor and Matrigel plugs sections were visualized under a Leica CTR 6000 microscope system (Lieca Microsystems).

Statistical Analysis

Data are presented as means ± standard deviation (SD). Statistically significant differences in mean values were assessed by one-way ANOVA, followed by Newman-Keuls ad hoc statistical test using GraphPad Prism 4 software (La Jolla, CA, USA). When applicable, statistical significance comparing only two groups was determined by two-tailed Student t-test. Significance was set at values of *P<.05, **P<.01, and ***P<.001.

Results

The Angiogenic Content but not Number of TMPs is Altered following anti-VEGF-A Drug Therapy

To investigate the effect of the anti-VEGF-A B20 antibody on TMPs, EMT/6, 4T1 and MDA-MB-231 breast carcinoma cells were exposed to B20 antibodies for 48 hours or left untreated. TMPs were then purified from the conditioned medium and quantified by flow cytometry as described [22,29]. A representative flow cytometry analysis of TMPs is shown in Figure 1A. The numbers of TMPs derived from the three cell lines treated with B20 antibodies were not significantly different to those from untreated control cells (Figure 1B). However, the VEGF-A content was substantially reduced in TMPs derived from EMT/6 and MDA-MB-231 but not 4T1 B20-exposed cells as compared to controls (Figure 1C).

TMPs from Cells Exposed to an Antiangiogenic Drug are Unable to Activate Endothelial Cells

To analyze the angiogenic properties of TMPs from cells exposed to B20 antibodies, equal numbers of TMPs derived from B20-exposed or control untreated EMT/6 cells were mixed with Matrigel and implanted in mice. As a negative control, mice were implanted with Matrigel containing PBS. After ten days, plugs were removed and stained with H&E or anti-CD31 antibodies to assess host cell colonization and angiogenesis. As expected, the number of colonizing host cells, among those endothelial cells, was greater in plugs containing TMPs from control cells as compared to control-PBS plugs, consistent with a previous study [22]. However, the number of host cells and endothelial cells (in red) in plugs containing TMPs from B20-exposed cells was significantly lower than their numbers in plugs containing TMPs from control cells (Figure 2A). In addition, microvessel density was significantly lower in the Matrigel plugs containing TMPs from cells exposed to B20 antibody when compared to plugs containing TMPs from control cells (p<0.05, Figure 2B).

Next, we evaluated the migration and invasion properties of endothelial cells in the presence of TMPs collected from untreated control or B20-exposed cells. Medium without added TMPs was used as a negative control. The medium containing TMPs from control cells induced invasion and migration of HUVECs through the Boyden chamber, similarly to a previous study [22], whereas medium containing TMPs from B20-exposed cells induced significantly lower numbers of migrating and invading HUVECs (p<0.01, Figure 2C and 2D). In addition, angiogenic activity, determined by microvessel sprouting in murine aortic rings, was not detected in the presence of TMPs collected from B20-exposed cells in contrast to control TMPs (Figure 2E). These results suggest that TMPs promote vessel sprouting and angiogenesis only when they originate from control cells; once tumor cells are exposed to anti-VEGF-A antibodies, their TMPs lose the ability to promote endothelial cell activity.

TMPs Derived from anti-VEGF-A-treated Cells Alter BMDC Mobilization

BMDCs, such as viable CEPs, hemangiocytes, and MDSCs, are known to promote tumor angiogenesis [30]. Therefore, to further understand the role of TMPs in angiogenesis, we investigated whether TMPs play a role in BMDC mobilization as well as the effect of anti-VEGF-A therapy on this process. To this end, half a

million TMPs collected from EMT/6 cells exposed to B20 antibody or their control counterparts were injected into the tail vein of 8–10 week old BALB/c mice. Mice injected with PBS were used as a negative control. One hour later, blood was drawn from the retro-orbital sinus and the levels of viable CEPs, hemangiocytes, and MDSCs were analyzed by flow cytometry. A representative flow cytometry analysis of the different BMDC types is shown in Figure 3. The results shown in Figure 4A demonstrate that the mobilization of all BMDC populations was substantially increased in mice injected with control TMPs as compared to PBS-injected mice, consistent with a previous study [22]. However, the mobilization of viable CEPs and hemangiocytes was not significantly different in mice injected with TMPs derived from B20-exposed and control cells although reduced viable CEP and hemangiocyte mobilization was observed. Interestingly, significantly higher levels of MDSCs were induced upon injection of TMPs from B20-exposed cells as compared to control cells (Figure 4A). It should be noted that the number of MDSCs colonizing tumors was found to substantially increase in antiangiogenic-treated tumors [31]. Overall, these results suggest that TMPs from B20-exposed cells do not affect systemic angiogenesis induced by viable CEPs and hemangiocyes, yet it can promote MDSC mobilization.

To assess whether TMPs bind directly to BMDCs and whether this binding is affected by anti-VEGF-A therapy, TMPs from control or B20-exposed cells were tagged with PKH26, a fluorescent dye which binds to membrane lipids, and incubated for one hour with BMDCs obtained from the femurs of BALB/c mice. One hour later, the BMDCs were immunostained for viable CEPs, hemangiocytes and MDSCs and subsequently analyzed by flow cytometry. TMPs from control and B20-exposed cells bound to hemangiocytes and MDSCs to similar extents. Binding of TMPs from B20-exposed cells to BMDCs was slightly but significantly increased, whereas binding to viable CEPs was dramatically decreased as compared to control TMPs (Figure 4B). Overall, these results suggest that TMPs bind directly to several types of BMDCs; however, once they are derived from B20-exposed cells, their binding properties to specific BMDCs are altered.

TMPs Derived from anti-VEGF-A-treated Cells do not Promote BMDC Colonization of Matrigel Plugs or Tumors

We next compared the profile of BMDCs that colonize Matrigel plugs in the presence of TMPs collected from B20-exposed and control EMT/6 cells. To this end, equal numbers of TMPs derived from B20-exposed or control untreated EMT/6 cells were mixed with Matrigel and implanted in mice. As a negative control, mice were implanted with Matrigel containing PBS. After ten days, plugs were removed, prepared as single cell suspensions and analyzed by flow cytometry for the presence of endothelial cells, hemangiocytes, and MDSCs. The number of all these cell types was lower in Matrigel plugs containing TMPs from B20-exposed cells when compared to control TMPs, although the number of hemangiocytes and MDSCs did not reach statistical significance. Of note, as previously demonstrated [22], Matrigel plugs containing PBS revealed minimal or no colonization of any of the BMDC types tested (Figure 5A). We next asked whether TMP-induced BMDC colonization has any effect on tumor growth. To test this, mice bearing EMT/6 tumors were injected twice weekly through the tail vein with 0.4×10^6 TMPs purified from control or B20-exposed EMT/6 cell cultures. PBS injections were used as a negative control. Tumor volumes were assessed by a caliper, and tumors were removed at endpoint in order to evaluate angiogenesis and BMDC colonization. Interestingly, no significant changes in tumor volumes and growth were observed between the groups

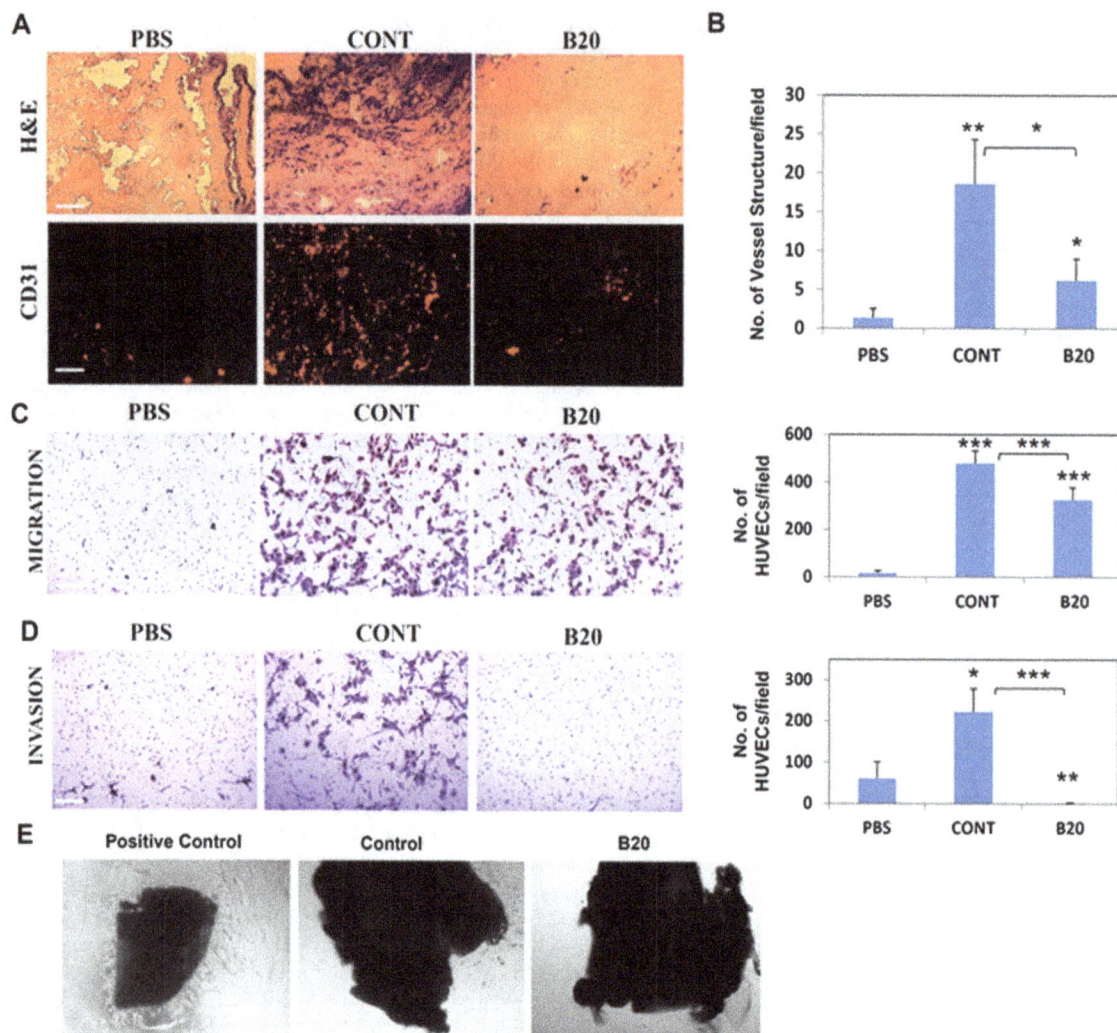

Figure 2. TMPs from cells exposed to anti-VEGF-A antibody exhibit reduced ability to promote endothelial cell activity. Matrigel plugs containing an equal number of TMPs (0.5×10^6) from untreated or B20-exposed EMT/6 cells were implanted into the flanks of 8–10 week old BALB/c mice. Matrigel plugs containing PBS were used as a negative control. Ten days later, plugs were removed and then sectioned. (A) Slides were stained with H&E or immunostained with the endothelial cell marker CD31 (designated in red) (scale bar = 100 μm). (B) Microvessel density in the plugs was calculated by counting vessel structures. (C–D) An equal number of TMPs (5×10^6) from untreated or B20-exposed EMT/6 cells were tested for HUVEC migration (C) and invasion (D) using the modified Boyden chamber assay. PBS was used as a negative control. Cells invading the membrane of the Boyden chamber were stained with Crystal Violet and images were captured using a Leica CTR 6000 microscope. The number of cells invading the membrane were counted and plotted (n>8/group). (E) Aortic rings from BALB/c mice (n = 4/group) were cultured in medium containing 0.1×106 TMPs from untreated or B20-exposed EMT/6 cells. Endothelial cell medium (ECGS) was used as a positive control. Images were captured using an inverted light microscope system (Leica CTR 6000 system) (Scale bar = 500 μm). *, $0.05 < p < 0.01$; **, $0.01 > p > 0.001$; ***, $p < 0.001$.

(Figure 5B). However, significant increases in microvessel density, functional vessels, and percentage of perfusion were observed in tumors of mice injected with TMPs from control cells compared with TMPs from B20-exposed cells or PBS control (Figure 5C and 5D). Again, no differences in hemangiocyte and MDSC colonization of tumors were observed between the groups (Figure 5E). Collectively, these results indicate that extrinsic addition of TMPs does not affect tumor growth, at least not at this tumor stage, but does alter the angiogenic properties in such tumors. TMPs from control cells exhibit a higher angiogenic potential than TMPs from cells treated with an antiangiogenic drug.

Discussion

Tumor cell repopulation and regrowth is often observed during the therapy-break periods between successive acute chemotherapies [15,16]. Our previous studies demonstrated that the induction of BMDC-mediated angiogenesis, particularly CEPs, can contribute to tumor re-growth, and it is partially mediated by SDF-1 and G-CSF [11,16,32]. Since some of these experiments were conducted in non-tumor bearing mice, we suggested that the host response to chemotherapy promotes angiogenesis therefore contributing to tumor re-growth [33]. In a subsequent study, we focused on the contribution of tumor cells to angiogenesis. TMPs from breast carcinoma cells exposed to paclitaxel chemotherapy induced BMDC mobilization and tumor homing, a process which was partially regulated by osteopontin [22]. Thus, chemotherapy

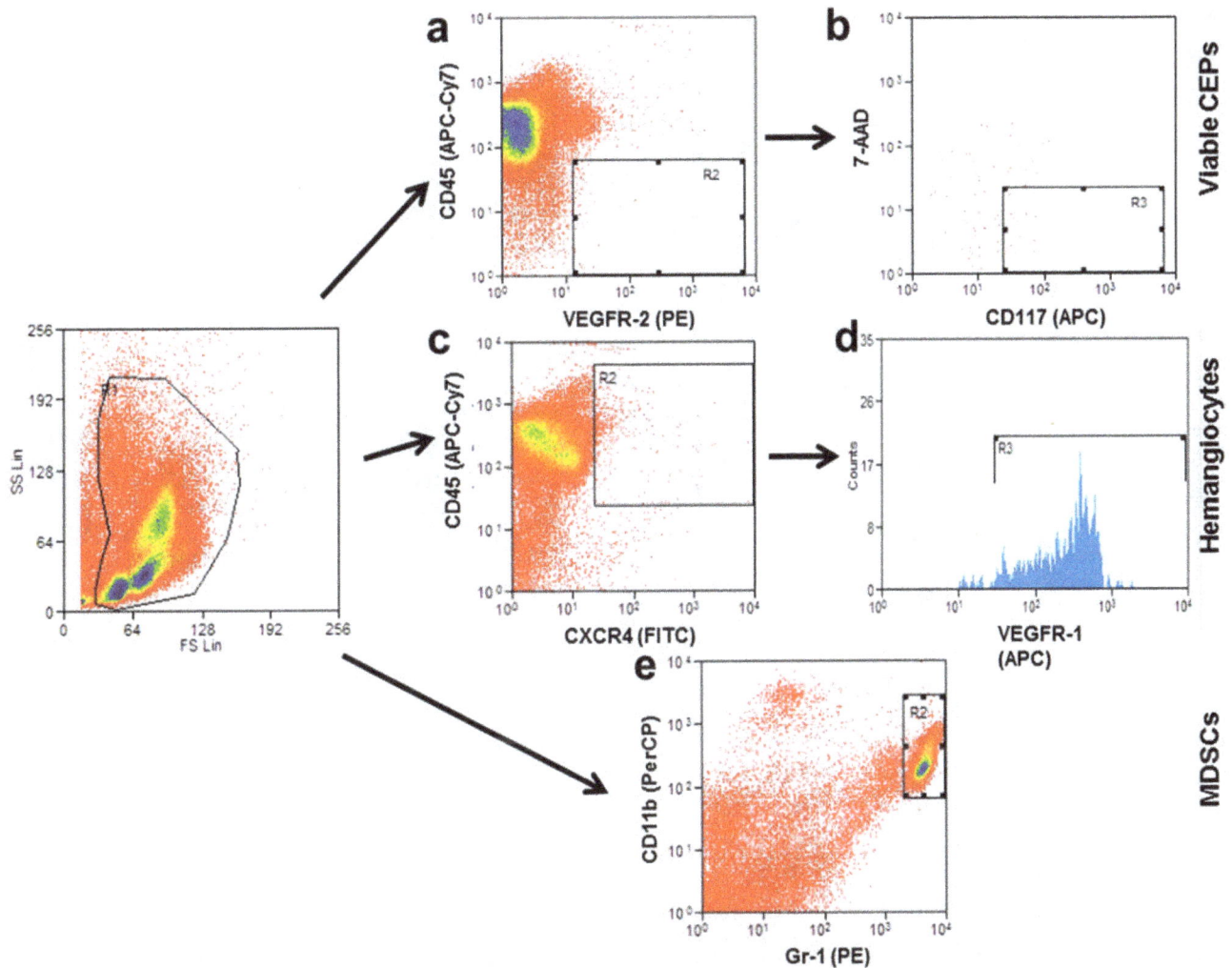

Figure 3. Representative flow cytometry plots of viable CEPs, hemangiocytes, and myeloid derived suppressor cells. An example of the analysis of flow cytometry data obtained from peripheral blood of BALB/c mice is presented. Viable CEPs are determined as (a) positive for VEGFR2 and negative for CD45 as well as (b) positive for CD117 and negative for 7-AAD. Hemangiocytes are determined as (c) positive for CD45 and CXCR4 as well as (d) positive for VEGFR1. Myeloid derived suppressor cells (MDSCs) are determined as positive for (e) both Gr-1 and CD11b.

affects tumor re-growth by two different processes. On the one hand, it stimulates production of various cytokines and growth factors in the host which in turn promote BMDC mobilization and tumor homing [32], and on the other hand, it promotes the production of TMPs from tumor cells which then can contribute to the same process [22]. It should be noted that increased number of TMPs has also been found in breast cancer patients undergo chemotherapy treatment [22], suggesting that the effects we observed in our in vitro tumor model could be recapitulated in vivo. In the current study, we report that the tumor proangiogenic effects induced by TMPs can be blocked by an antiangiogenic drug with the focus on anti-VEGF-A therapy. We show that TMPs from cells exposed to an anti-VEGF-A antibody have a reduced ability to stimulate BMDC mobilization and subsequent colonization of tumors.

The number of TMPs has been shown to substantially increased when tumor cells were exposed to paclitaxel chemotherapy when compared to untreated tumor cells [22]. In contrast, in the current study, we show that exposing cells to anti-VEGF-A neutralizing antibodies did not result in a significant change in the number of TMPs. The differences between the two scenarios could be related

to the fact that tumor cells undergo apoptosis in the presence of cytotoxic chemotherapy drug, while these apoptotic effects were absent when cells were exposed to a cytostatic drug which inhibits endothelial cells, and not tumor cells. We also demonstrated that TMPs from both untreated and B20-exposed cells bound directly to BMDCs with similar binding affinities, although the TMPs from cells exposed to anti-VEGF-A antibodies exhibited reduced angiogenic potential compared to TMPs from control cells by means of reduced HUVEC migration and invasion as well as BMDC colonization in Matrigel plugs. Consistently with the in vitro findings, also mice inoculated with TMPs from B20-exposed cells exhibited reduced microvessel density, functional vessels, and percentage of perfusion in tumors compared to mice inoculated with control TMPs. Thus TMPs from cells exposed to anti-VEGF-A antibodies inhibit the angiogenesis activities in growing tumors. It is yet to be determined whether other anti-angiogenic drugs such as small molecule tyrosine kinase inhibitors, e.g., sorfenib or sunitinib, would act in the same manner on TMPs by means of reducing their angiogenic content. It should be noted that the antiangiogenic content in microvessicles have been previously studied. For example, exosomes released from retinal

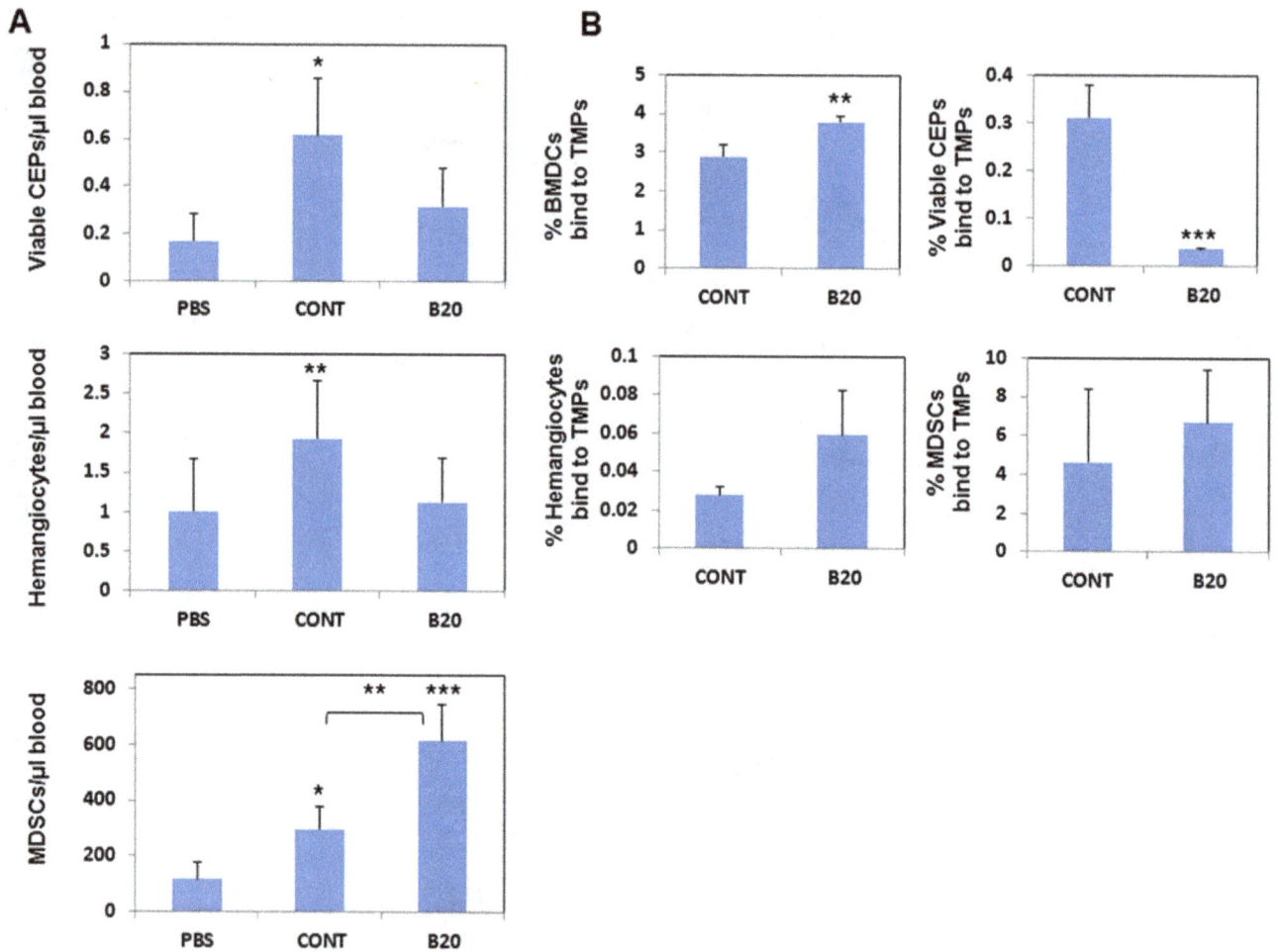

Figure 4. TMPs from cells exposed to anti-VEGF-A antibody do not induce viable CEP and hemangiocyte mobilization. (A) An equal number of TMPs (0.5×10^6) from untreated (CONT) or B20-exposed EMT/6 cells was injected into the tail vein of 8–10 week old non-tumor bearing BALB/c mice (n = 4 mice/group). Control mice were injected with PBS (PBS). One hour later, blood was drawn from the retro-orbital sinus for the evaluation of viable CEPs (CD45−/VEGFR2+/CD117+/7AAD−), MDSCs (Gr1+/CD11b+), and hemangiocytes (CD11b+/CXCR4+/VEGFR1+) using flow cytometry. (B) Half a million TMPs from untreated (CONT) or B20-exposed cells were tagged with PKH26, and subsequently injected into the tail vein of BALB/c mice (n = 4 mice/group). Control mice were injected with PBS. One hour later, blood was drawn by cardiac puncture and total BMDCs (CD45+), viable CEPs, hemagiocytes, and MDSCs were analyzed by flow cytometry. The percentage of the different cell types positive for tagged TMPs was plotted. **, 0.01>p>0.001; ***, p<0.001.

astroglial cells possess antiangiogenic content. Therefore, they inhibit the activity of neovascularization in the eye, hence promoting its protection from vascular dysfunction (such as age-related macular degeneration) [34]. Interestingly, in our study we demonstrated that tumor volume was not significantly different between the mice inoculated with TMPs from B20-exposed cells when compared to mice inoculated with TMPs from untreated control cells. Although the reasons for these findings were not uncovered, it is plausible that in a different tumor model in which tumor cells do not divide so rapidly, changes in tumor growth could have been observed, or when tumors would have left to grow for additional period of time.

The presence of B20 antibodies in culture altered the expression levels of VEGF-A and the angiogenic properties of TMPs. As such, it can explain the inhibition of viable CEP, hemangiocyte, and MDSC mobilization although the latter two did not reach statistical significance. Previous studies indicated that various proteins are enriched in MPs compared to their cell of origin [35,36]. As such, VEGF, similarly to other proangiogenic and antiangiogenic factors, may be enriched in TMPs in the same

manner. In a previous study, TMPs extracted from paclitaxel-exposed cells resulted in changes of various cytokines and growth factors as analyzed by a protein array. Among them, we found that SDF-1 was upregulated in TMPs from paclitaxel-exposed cells when compared to control TMPs [22]. Although in this study we solely focused on VEGF-A as we used an anti-VEGF-A antibody, it would be of interest to identify whether other pro-angiogenic and anti-angiogenic factors are affected by the lack of VEGF-A. Studying the properties of TMPs requires a more refined proteomic analysis. Nonetheless, we can speculate that the lack of VEGF-A in TMPs from cells exposed to anti-VEGF therapy could be due to the fact that B20 antibody interferes with the autocrine loop of VEGF-A in tumor cells [37]. Another possibility for the antiangiogenic activity of TMPs from cells exposed to anti-VEGF-A antibody could be due to the uptake of B20 antibodies either by tumor cells or by their TMPs, as recently was suggested that platelets can uptake bevacizumab, the humanized antibody against VEGF-A [38], and therefore it is plausible that such antibodies will be present in MPs. It should be noted that TMPs were undergo vigorous washes in order to minimize traces of B20

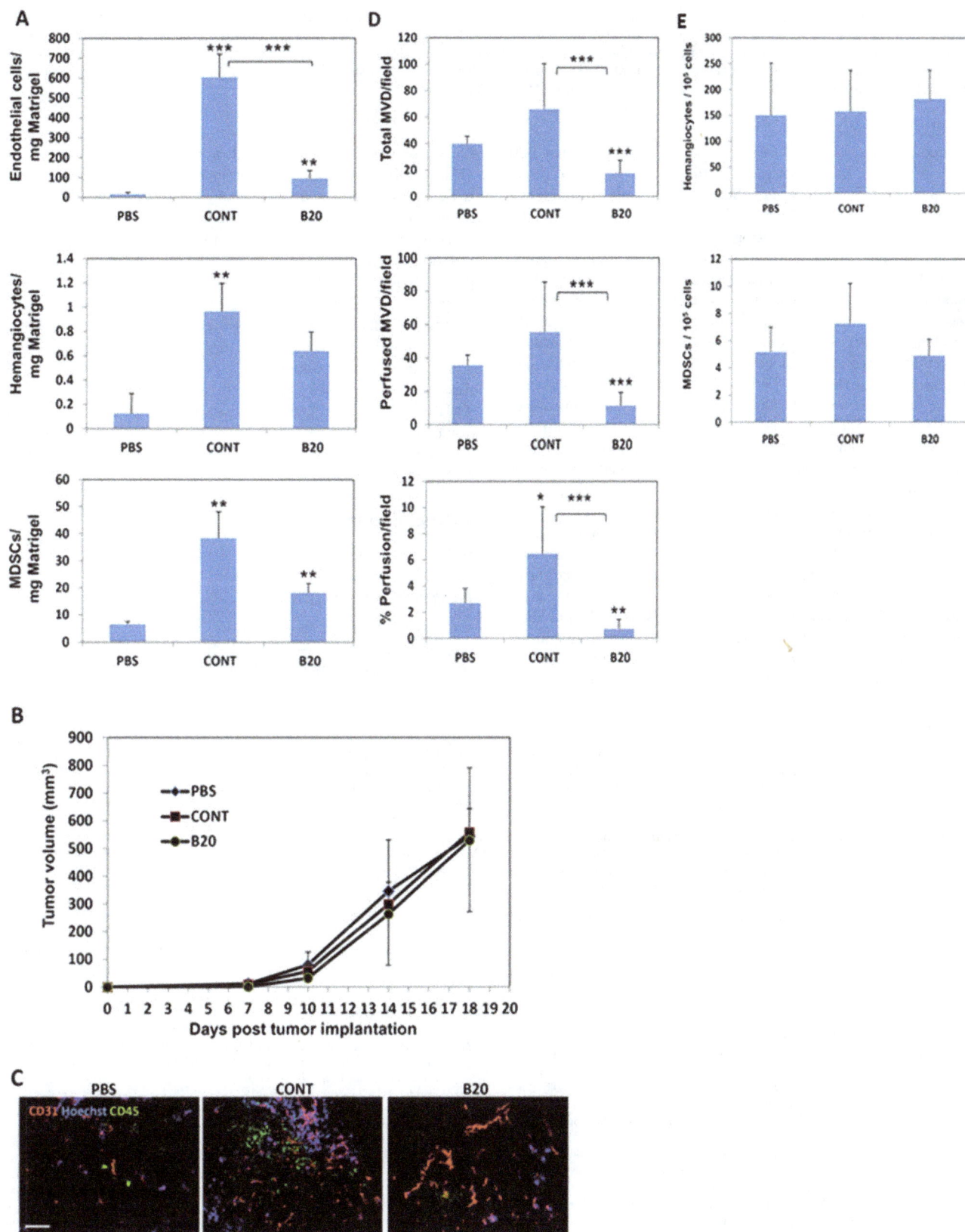

Figure 5. TMPs from cells exposed anti-VEGF-A antibody do not promote angiogenesis in tumors. (A) Matrigel plugs containing an equal number of TMPs (0.5×10^6) from untreated or B20-exposed EMT/6 cells were implanted into the flanks of 8–10 week old BALB/c mice. Matrigel plugs containing PBS were used as a negative control. Ten days later, plugs were removed and prepared as single cell suspensions. The extracted cells were immunostained for endothelial cells, hemangiocytes and MDSCs and analyzed by flow cytometry. Results are presented as the number of cells per 1 mg Matrigel. (B–E) Eight to ten week old BALB/c mice (n = 4 mice/group) were implanted with 0.5×10^6 EMT/6 cells into the flanks. When

tumors reached a size of approximately 50 mm^3, injections with 0.5×10^6 TMPs from untreated or B20-exposed EMT/6 cells were performed twice weekly. Control mice were injected with PBS. (B) Tumor growth was assessed by a Vernier caliper using the formula, width$^2 \times$length$\times 0.5$. Tumors were removed at endpoint, and subsequently were either (C) stained for CD31 (in red), CD45 (in green), and Hoechst (in blue) for the evaluation of (D) microvessel density and perfusion (scale bar = 100 μm), or (E) prepared as single cell suspensions for the evaluation of MDSCs and hemangiocytes colonization of tumors using flow cytometry. **, $0.01 > p > 0.001$; ***, $p < 0.001$.

antibodies in the culture. Overall, these results indicate that B20 may affect the tumor microenvironment not only via direct antiangiogenic activity on endothelial cells but also through the inhibition of specific BMDC colonization of tumors thereby preventing tumor systemic angiogenesis.

One of the major current obstacles in clinical oncology, especially in the case of antiangiogenic therapy, is the lack of suitable and reliable biomarkers to predict clinical outcome [39]. Several clinical and preclinical biomarkers such as levels of circulating endothelial cells in the peripheral blood, SNP-analysis of genes related to angiogenesis, among others, have been suggested (for review see [39]). More recently, the angiogenic profile of cancer stem cells (CSCs) has been shown preclinically to correlate with antiangiogenic treatment outcomes [40]. In this study, exposing cells to B20 antibodies resulted in reduced levels of VEGF-A in TMPs, suggesting that MPs should be further investigated as a surrogate biomarker for antiangiogenic activity. Indeed, MP-based technology is currently being tested in search of potential prognostic or predictive biomarkers for tumor growth [20]. It has been shown that platelets can take up bevacizumab [38], and as such platelets, as well as MPs found in plasma of bevacizumab-treated patients may serve as a biomarker for antiangiogenic therapy. In this regard, levels of MPs and their content in cancer patients have already been studied as diagnostic and prognostic biomarkers. For example, circulating levels of endothelial MPs and leukocyte MPs were found to correlate with

CEA and CA15-3 both of which are breast cancer biomarkers [17]. Furthermore, levels of plasma TMPs were elevated in patients with progressed gastric cancer [41]. As such, MPs could serve as potential diagnostic and/or prognostic biomarkers in the clinical settings. However, there are a few challenges in the isolation and purification of MPs as there are no standardized protocols for MPs' extraction and evaluation. In addition, MPs vary in size and type, and a greater distinction between the different populations of MPs is required, by using methods that are likely to provide accurate sizing of MPs compared with conventional flow cytometry [29]. Therefore, in the context of this study it would be of interest to evaluate levels of VEGF-A in TMPs or MPs, and correlate them with the clinical outcome of antiangiogenic drug treatments, with the notion that extensive efforts should be made to translate these pre-clinical results into standardized clinical testing.

Acknowledgments

B20 antibody was kindly provided by Genentech Inc.

Author Contributions

Conceived and designed the experiments: YS EF MM SS. Performed the experiments: MM EF VM NBT SD. Analyzed the data: MM EF YS. Contributed reagents/materials/analysis tools: SS. Wrote the paper: YS.

References

1. Weidner N, Folkman J, Pozza F, Bevilacqua P, Allred EN, et al. (1992) Tumor angiogenesis: A new significant and independent prognostic indicator in early-stage breast carcinoma. Journal National Cancer Institute 84: 1875–1887.

2. Folkman J (1985) Tumor angiogenesis. Advances in Cancer Research 43: 175–203.

3. Folkman J, Watson K, Ingber D, Hanahan D (1989) Induction of angiogenesis during transition from hyperplasia to neoplasia. Nature 339: 58–61.

4. Shaked Y, Voest EE (2009) Bone marrow derived cells in tumor angiogenesis and growth: are they the good, the bad or the evil? BiochimBiophysActa 1796: 1–4.

5. Asahara T, Murohara T, Sullivan A, Silver M, van der Zee R, et al. (1997) Isolation of putative progenitor endothelial cells for angiogenesis. Science 275: 964–967.

6. Kerbel RS (2008) Tumor angiogenesis. New England Journal of Medicine 358: 2039–2049.

7. Horrevoets AJ (2009) Angiogenic monocytes: another colorful blow to endothelial progenitors. AmJ Pathol 174: 1594–1596.

8. Gao D, Nolan D, McDonnell K, Vahdat L, Benezra R, et al. (2009) Bone marrow-derived endothelial progenitor cells contribute to the angiogenic switch in tumor growth and metastatic progression. BiochimBiophysActa 1796: 33–40.

9. Purhonen S, Palm J, Rossi D, Kaskenpaa N, Rajantie I, et al. (2008) Bone marrow-derived circulating endothelial precursors do not contribute to vascular endothelium and are not needed for tumor growth. ProcNatlAcadSciUSA 105: 6620–6625.

10. Shaked Y, Ciarrocchi A, Franco M, Lee CR, Man S, et al. (2006) Therapy-induced acute recruitment of circulating endothelial progenitor cells to tumors. Science 313: 1785–1787.

11. Shaked Y, Henke E, Roodhart JM, Mancuso P, Langenberg MH, et al. (2008) Rapid chemotherapy-induced acute endothelial progenitor cell mobilization: implications for antiangiogenic drugs as chemosensitizing agents. Cancer Cell 14: 263–273.

12. De Palma M, Lewis CE (2013) Macrophage regulation of tumor responses to anticancer therapies. Cancer Cell 23: 277–286.

13. Welford AF, Biziato D, Coffelt SB, Nucera S, Fisher M, et al. (2011) TIE2-expressing macrophages limit the therapeutic efficacy of the vascular-disrupting agent combretastatin A4 phosphate in mice. JClinInvest 121: 1969–1973.

14. DeNardo DG, Brennan DJ, Rexhepaj E, Ruffell B, Shiao SL, et al. (2011) Leukocyte complexity predicts breast cancer survival and functionally regulates response to chemotherapy. Cancer Discov 1: 54–67.

15. Kim JJ, Tannock IF (2005) Repopulation of cancer cells during therapy: an important cause of treatment failure. Nat Rev Cancer 5: 516–525.

16. Shaked Y, Kerbel RS (2007) Antiangiogenic strategies on defense: on the possibility of blocking rebounds by the tumor vasculature after chemotherapy. Cancer Res 67: 7055–7058.

17. Toth B, Liebhardt S, Steinig K, Ditsch N, Rank A, et al. (2008) Platelet-derived microparticles and coagulation activation in breast cancer patients. Thromb Haemost 100: 663–669.

18. Toth B, Lok CA, Boing A, Diamant M, van der Post JA, et al. (2007) Microparticles and exosomes: impact on normal and complicated pregnancy. Am J Reprod Immunol 58: 389–402.

19. Mostefai HA, Andriantsitohaina R, Martinez MC (2008) Plasma membrane microparticles in angiogenesis: role in ischemic diseases and in cancer. Physiol Res 57: 311–320.

20. Rak J (2010) Microparticles in cancer. SeminThrombHemost 36: 888–906.

21. Al-Nedawi K, Meehan B, Micallef J, Lhotak V, May L, et al. (2008) Intercellular transfer of the oncogenic receptor EGFRvIII by microvesicles derived from tumour cells. Nat Cell Biol 10: 619–624.

22. Fremder E, Munster M, Aharon A, Miller V, Gingis-Velitski S, et al. (2013) Tumor-derived microparticles induce bone marrow-derived cell mobilization and tumor homing: A process regulated by osteopontin. Int J Cancer.

23. Cahan MA, Walter KA, Colvin OM, Brem H (1994) Cytotoxicity of taxol in vitro against human and rat malignant brain tumors. Cancer Chemother-Pharmacol 33: 441–444.

24. Liang WC, Wu X, Peale FV, Lee CV, Meng YG, et al. (2006) Cross-species vascular endothelial growth factor (VEGF)-blocking antibodies completely inhibit the growth of human tumor xenografts and measure the contribution of stromal VEGF. J Biol Chem 281: 951–961.

25. Boilard E, Nigrovic PA, Larabee K, Watts GF, Coblyn JS, et al. (2010) Platelets amplify inflammation in arthritis via collagen-dependent microparticle production. Science 327: 580–583.

26. Gingis-Velitski S, Loven D, Benayoun L, Munster M, Bril R, et al. (2011) Host response to short-term, single-agent chemotherapy induces matrix metalloproteinase-9 expression and accelerates metastasis in mice. Cancer Res 71: 6986–6996.

27. Adini A, Fainaru O, Udagawa T, Connor KM, Folkman J, et al. (2009) Matrigel cytometry: a novel method for quantifying angiogenesis in vivo. J ImmunolMethods 342: 78–81.

28. Shaked Y, Bertolini F, Man S, Rogers MS, Cervi D, et al. (2005) Genetic heterogeneity of the vasculogenic phenotype parallels angiogenesis: implications for cellular surrogate marker analysis of antiangiogenesis. Cancer Cell 7 101–111.

29. van der Pol E, Hoekstra AG, Sturk A, Otto C, van Leeuwen TG, et al. (2010) Optical and non-optical methods for detection and characterization of microparticles and exosomes. J Thromb Haemost 8: 2596–2607.

30. Bertolini F, Shaked Y, Mancuso P, Kerbel RS (2006) The multifaceted circulating endothelial cell in cancer: from promiscuity to surrogate marker and target identification. Nature Rev Cancer 6: 835–845.

31. Shojaei F, Wu X, Malik AK, Zhong C, Baldwin ME, et al. (2007) Tumor refractoriness to anti-VEGF treatment is mediated by CD11b(+)Gr1(+) myeloid cells. Nat Biotechnol 25: 911–920.

32. Shaked Y, Tang T, Woloszynek J, Daenen LG, Man S, et al. (2009) Contribution of granulocyte colony-stimulating factor to the acute mobilization of endothelial precursor cells by vascular disrupting agents. Cancer Res 69: 7524–7528.

33. Voloshin T, Voest EE, Shaked Y (2013) The host immunological response to cancer therapy: An emerging concept in tumor biology. Experimental cell research.

34. Hajrasouliha AR, Jiang G, Lu Q, Lu H, Kaplan HJ, et al. (2013) Exosomes from retinal astrocytes contain antiangiogenic components that inhibit laser-induced choroidal neovascularization. J Biol Chem 288: 28058–28067.

35. Sinauridze EI, Kireev DA, Popenko NY, Pichugin AV, Panteleev MA, et al. (2007) Platelet microparticle membranes have 50- to 100-fold higher specific procoagulant activity than activated platelets. Thromb Haemost 97: 425–434.

36. Aharon A, Tamari T, Brenner B (2008) Monocyte-derived microparticles and exosomes induce procoagulant and apoptotic effects on endothelial cells. Thromb Haemost 100: 878–885.

37. Videira PA, Piteira AR, Cabral MG, Martins C, Correia M, et al. (2011) Effects of bevacizumab on autocrine VEGF stimulation in bladder cancer cell lines. UrolInt 86: 95–101.

38. Verheul HM, Lolkema MP, Qian DZ, Hilkes YH, Liapi E, et al. (2007) Platelets take up the monoclonal antibody bevacizumab. ClinCancer Res 13: 5341–5347.

39. Bertolini F, Marighetti P, Shaked Y (2010) Cellular and soluble markers of tumor angiogenesis: from patient selection to the identification of the most appropriate postresistance therapy. BiochimBiophysActa 1806: 131–137.

40. Benayoun L, Gingis-Velitski S, Voloshin T, Segal E, Segev R, et al. (2012) Tumor-initiating cells of various tumor types exhibit differential angiogenic properties and react differently to antiangiogenic drugs. Stem Cells 30: 1831–1841.

41. Baran J, Baj-Krzyworzeka M, Weglarczyk K, Szatanek R, Zembala M, et al. (2010) Circulating tumour-derived microvesicles in plasma of gastric cancer patients. Cancer Immunol Immunother 59: 841–850.

14

Biological Characteristics and Clinical Outcome of Triple Negative Primary Breast Cancer in Older Women – Comparison with Their Younger Counterparts

Binafsha M. Syed[1], Andrew R. Green[1], Christopher C. Nolan[1], David A. L. Morgan[2], Ian O. Ellis[1], Kwok-Leung Cheung[1]*

1 School of Medicine, University of Nottingham, Nottingham, United Kingdom, 2 Department of Oncology, Nottingham University Hospitals, Nottingham, United Kingdom

Abstract

Triple negative (ER, PgR and HER2 negative) breast cancers (TNBCs) are often considered as a poor prognostic phenotype. There is dearth of evidence showing the prevalence and biological behaviour of TNBCs in older women. This study aimed to analyse their biological characteristics in comparison with a well characterised younger series from a single centre with long term clinical follow-up. Over 37 years (1973–2010), 1,758 older (≥70 years) women with early operable (<5 cm) primary breast cancer were managed in a dedicated clinic and have complete clinical information available. Of these 813 patients underwent primary surgery and 575 had good quality tumour samples available for tissue microarray analysis using indirect immunohistochemistry. A total of 127 patients (22.1%) had TNBCs and full biological analysis of 15 biomarkers was performed. The results were compared with those of their younger (<70 years) counterparts 342 (18.9%) from a previously characterised, consecutive series of primary breast cancer treated in the same unit (1986–1998). The 127 older patients with TNBCs showed lower rates of Ki67 and CK 7/8 positivity and high rates of bcl2 and CK18 positivity when compared with their younger counterparts (p<0.05). There was no significant difference in the long term clinical outcome between the two age groups, despite the fact that 47% of the younger patients had adjuvant chemotherapy, while none in the older cohort received such treatment. EGFR, axillary stage and pathological size showed prognostic significance in older women with TNBCs on univariate analysis. Despite not having received adjuvant chemotherapy, the older series had clinical outcome similar to the younger patients almost half of whom had chemotherapy. This appears to be related to other biomarkers (in addition to ER/PgR/HER2) eg Ki67, bcl2 and cytokeratins which have different expression patterns influencing prognosis.

Editor: Domenico Coppola, H. Lee Moffitt Cancer Center & Research Institute, United States of America

Funding: The study is part of BM Syed's PhD project funded by her home institution Liaquat University of Medical & Health Sciences, Jamshoro/Higher Education Commission of Pakistan. The funders had no role in study design, data collection and analysis, decision to publish, or preparation of the manuscript.

Competing Interests: The authors have declared that no competing interests exist.

* Email: kl.cheung@nottingham.ac.uk

Introduction

The risk of breast cancer increases with advancing age. [1]. Oestrogen receptor (ER) positive tumours become more common in older women [2,3], suggesting a possible change in biology with age. Many studies have reported an inverse correlation between ER positivity and Human Epidermal Growth Factor Receptor-2 (HER2) expression [4,5,6,7]. Thus a small proportion of older women would be expected to have triple negative (ER, progesterone (PgR) and HER2 negative) breast cancers (TNBCs).

It is generally believed that TNBCs tend to have a poor prognosis. Given the lack of conventional therapeutic targets i.e. hormone receptors and HER2, patients with TNBCs are left with chemotherapy as the only systemic therapy option, if this is required as an adjuvant treatment. Conversely, owing to limited physiological reserve and increased number of co-morbidities, some older women may not be able to tolerate chemotherapy and also the Oxford Overview has not yet had sufficient number of older women from randomised trials to demonstrate a definite and

significant absolute benefit of chemotherapy in this age group [8]. Thus patients and clinicians both show reluctance to use chemotherapy, and its use in older women still remains debatable. A lot of research has recently been directed towards TNBCs but most of the studies are focused on younger patients with minimal or no representation of older women [9,10], while those focusing on older women showed inconsistency in defining the age cut-off for including patients in the older cohort [11] This study aimed to analyse the biology and clinical outcome of TNBCs in older (≥70 years) women and compare the results with their younger counterparts.

Methods

Over a period of 37 years (1973–2010) 1,758 older (≥70 years) women with early operable primary breast cancer were managed and followed up in a dedicated clinic, with availability of a complete set of clinical information from the date of diagnosis till death or last follow-up. Early operable primary breast cancer was defined clinically as tumour size of ≤5 cm, with no or palpable mobile ipsilateral axillary lymphadenopathy, without evidence of distant metastases (cT1-2, N0-1, M0). The patients were initially identified from the Histopathology archive of paper records (before 1987, N = 240) and a prospectively established computerised database (since 1987, N = 1,518). The clinical course of the disease was subsequently confirmed from the clinical notes. The dedicated clinic, which started off as a surgical clinic, had evolved into a combined surgical/oncology facility in the recent decade, following the same clinical guidelines at any time point. Although there has been a change in the management protocols over the period as previously described [12], most of the change was attributed to the use of endocrine therapy as far as systemic therapy was concerned. Therefore it would be unlikely that the changes had impacted on patients with TNBCs.

Among all these patients, 813 of them had surgery as their primary treatment. Of these, 575 had good quality tumour samples from their surgical specimens available for tissue microarray (TMA) construction. For the purpose of this study, the tumour samples were analysed using indirect immunohistochemistry (IHC) on TMAs for ER, PgR, HER2, p53, Cytokeratins (CK) 5/6, 7/8, 14, 17, 18, 19, Bcl2, E-Cadherin and Muc1. Assessment of Ki67 was done on whole tumour sections. Histological grade of the tumours was based on the original histology report, according to a uniform protocol using the Elston-Ellis modification of Scarff-Bloom Richardson (SBR) grading system after 1988 and SBR before 1988 [13].

Younger series

In order to compare with the younger (<70 years) patients, patients with stage matched (cT1-2,N0-1,M0) TNBCs were retrieved from a previously characterised institutional database (Nottingham/Tenovus series) along with the data of the above mentioned biomarkers [14,15,16]. The Nottingham Tenovus series consists of clinical and biological data of younger (<70 years) patients with early operable primary breast cancer established in 1980s and tumours were prospectively analysed using IHC on TMAs, constructed using surgical specimens (N = 1809). As it was planned at the outset of the project to compare the present older series with the younger patients, the variables collected for the older series were the same as those collected for the younger patients and the methods for tumour analyses were the same.

Tissue microarray construction

The TMAs were constructed following the previously described method [14,17], where the most representative part of the tumour was identified and a core of 0.6 mm thickness was obtained and implanted into the TMA block, by using a manual tissue microarrayer (MP06 Beecher Instruments Inc, USA).

Immunohistochemistry

Indirect IHC was performed using Streptavidin-Biotin Complex (ABC) method as previously described [14]. Briefly, TMA slides were incubated at 60° C for 10 minutes, followed by washing with two Xylene and three alcohol baths for 5 minutes and 10 seconds each respectively. The slides were treated with citrate buffer for 20 minutes to retrieve the antigen. Endogenous peroxidase activity was inhibited by 0.3% hydrogen peroxide. The slides were incubated for a specified time for the primary antibody at room temperature (details of the antibody dilution and incubation time are given in Table 1). The secondary antibody was applied for 45 minutes, followed by the treatment with diaminobenzidine and copper sulphate.

Immunohistochemical scoring

The IHC staining of the biomarkers was assessed by the percentage of cells stained as well as semi-quantitatively by McCarty's histochemical scoring (H-score) [18] method. For intra-observer reproducibility the cores were scored thrice (by BMS) and the average of the score was taken as the final score and for inter-observer concordance an expert pathologist blinded from the scores and the clinical data, scored 10% of cores. There was high inter and intra-observer concordance between the scorers (Kappa score ≥0.7).

Table 1 summarises the definitions of positivity of different biomarkers using pre-defined cut-offs.

Statistical methods

Comparison was made between the two age groups <70 and ≥ 70, using Chi-square test and time dependant variables were compared using Kaplan-Meier method with application of Log-rank and generalised Wilcoxon tests as appropriate for statistical significance. A p-value<0.05 was considered significant. Given the difference in length of follow-up of the two series, analysis was carried out according to time periods and comparison was done at five years from the date of diagnosis to avoid any potential bias. Breast cancer specific survival measures biological behaviour of the disease without being influenced by deaths due to causes other than breast cancer. As the older women are at higher chance of presenting with a number of co morbidities and a considerable proportion is life threatening [19], and lead to the higher rate of non breast cancer deaths [12,20], thus overall survival does not accurately measure virulence of tumours as it takes all causes of death into account. Therefore the two groups were compared in terms of breast cancer specific survival (defined as deaths due to breast cancer), local recurrence (defined as the re-appearance of the tumour in the same breast after wide local excision or in the mastectomy flap), regional recurrence (defined as appearance of the tumour in ipsilateral axilla) and metastases (defined as distant recurrence including bone, lung, liver, and also supraclavicular lymph nodes). Multivariate analysis was carried out using Cox-regression model. The Predictives Analytic Software (PASW 18, Chicago, Illinois) was used for data collection and analysis.

Ethical approval

The work presented in this manuscript was part of a study entitled 'Development of a molecular genetic classification of breast cancer' approved by the Nottingham Research Ethics Committee (approval number C1080301), who waived the need for written informed consent from the participants.

Results

Among all age groups 469 patients had TNBCs including 342 in women <70 years (342 out of 1809, 18.9%) and 127 in older (≥70 years) women (127 out of 575, 22.1%). Basic demographic characteristics of the two age groups are summarised in Table 2. Older women with TNBCs were significantly of larger pathological size and lower grade, but there were no significant differences in histological type and axillary stage.

Biological features

Comparison of the biomarkers between the two age groups showed that TNBCs in older women had significantly lower expression of Ki67, more normal p53 and higher expression of Bcl2 than younger women (Table 2). There was mixed luminal and basal cytokeratin expression with significantly higher expression of CK14 and CK18, but a reduction in the expression of

Table 1. A summary of the anti-bodies source, methods and cut-offs to define positivity of the markers used to analyse biology of early operable primary breast cancer in older women.

Biomarker	Antibody reference	Dilution	Incubation time	Antigen retrieval method	Cut –off to define positivity
ER	RM-9101-SP1/NeoMarkers	1:100	45 minutes	Citrate Buffer	0
PR	PgR 636/Dako	1:200	45 minutes	Citrate Buffer	0
HER2	Hercep test Kit- Dako	Pre-diluted	30 minutes	Not required	3+
Ki67	M 7240/Dako	1:100	45 minutes	Citrate Buffer	10
P53	DO-7/Novocastra	1:100	45 minutes	Citrate Buffer	5
CK5	M26/Thermo Scientific	1:100	45 minutes	Citrate Buffer	10
CK5/6	M7237/Dako	1:100	45 minutes	Citrate Buffer	10
CK7/8	34779/BioSciences	1:100	45 minutes	Citrate Buffer	10
CK14	LL002/Vector Laboratories	1:100	45 minutes	Citrate Buffer	10
CK17	E3/Vector Laboratories	1:100	45 minutes	Citrate Buffer	10
CK18	M7010/Dako	1:100	45 minutes	Citrate Buffer	10
CK19	CM 242A/Biocare Medical	1:100	45 minutes	Citrate Buffer	10
Bcl2	M0887/Dako	1:100	45 minutes	Citrate Buffer	10
E-Cadherin	M3612/Dako	1:100	45 minutes	Citrate Buffer	30
Muc1	NCL/Novocastra	1:300	45 minutes	Citrate Buffer	20
EGFR	31G7/Zymed	1:30	60 minutes	Proteinase K	0

CK7/8. There was no difference in the expression of CK17, CK5/6, CK 19 or Muc1.

Management pattern and clinical outcome

A considerable proportion (47%) of younger (<70 years) patients received adjuvant chemotherapy as compared to their older counterparts where none of them received chemotherapy (Table 2).

At a median follow-up of 46 (longest = 204) months in the older women and 119 (longest = 135) months in the younger patients, there was no significant difference in the clinical outcome of the disease, in terms of recurrence and survival (Table 3, Figure 1). However there was a trend of even better survival in the older women (5-years breast cancer specific survival in <70 = 73% versus 79% in older patients), though it did not reach statistical significance. The 5-year rates of local and regional recurrences in younger patients were 10% and 9% versus 14% and 14% respectively in older patients. The rates of metastases were 30% and 27% in younger and older groups respectively.

The clinical outcome remained similar (ie. no difference) when comparison was made with stratification according to histological grade (p-value>0.05) (Data not shown).

Prognostic factors

All the studied biomarkers were analysed for prognostic significance in the older series. Only EGFR showed prognostic significance in terms of breast cancer specific survival, along with stage and pathological size (Figure 2). Patients with EGFR positive tumours, axillary stage I or II disease, or pathological size <3 cm had significantly better breast cancer specific survival. However on multivariate analysis none of them showed any prognostic significance.

Discussion

The results of the study show that TNBCs in older women appear to have less aggressive biology as compared to their younger counterparts by having more low grade tumours, reduction of Ki67 expression, more frequent normal p53 and higher expression of Bcl2. There appears to be no significant difference in the clinical outcome in the two age groups despite the fact that a higher proportion of the younger patients received chemotherapy. Positive EGFR status, lower axillary stage (<4 positive nodes positive) and small pathological size (<3 cm) were associated with significantly better outcome in older women with TNBCs, on univariate analysis.

The age cut-offs defining the older population remain inconsistent across various studies eg 55, 60, 65, 70 or 75 years have all been used. We defined older population in our study as women ≥70 years of age. This age cut-off has been previously reported to have an association with the beginning of a rapid decline of physiological reserve [21]. Also this is the same age cut-off used by our unit when the Nottingham Prognostic Index was devised and in a few other randomised controlled trials comparing surgery and primary endocrine therapy in older women [22,23]. It would therefore appear to be reasonable to use such cut-off for the ease of comparability.

Overall TNBCs comprise 10–25% of the breast cancer population regardless of age [9,24,25,26]. There is dearth of knowledge regarding the pattern of TNBCs with advancing age. In our study the tumour analysis was carried out using surgical specimens where there was a natural selection of more ER negative tumours for primary surgery as those older women with ER positive tumours who presented with a number of co morbidities and/or refused to have surgery had an option of primary endocrine therapy. An audit of a recent consecutive series of older women (part of this larger series) where the status of ER, PR and HER2 was determined on needle core biopsies as part of standard pathology report at the time of their diagnosis showed 13.4% TNBCs [12]. Thus the higher number of TNBCs in older patients in this study (22.1%) probably reflects the higher ER negative tumours within the series.

This study has presented comparison of biology and clinical outcome of this apparently more aggressive phenotype of breast

Table 2. A summary of the general characteristics and biology and management pattern of triple negative breast cancer – young (<70 years) versus older (≥70 years).

Character	All N(%)	<70 years N(%)	≥70 years N(%)	p-value
Median age (range)	57.5 (25.91)	51(25–69)	75(70–91)	
Histological types				
Ductal carcinoma (no special type)	383(83.3)	276(82.4)	107(85.6)	0.12
Tubular carcinoma	12(2.6)	8(2.4)	4(3.2)	
Lobular carcinoma	8(1.7)	3(0.9)	5(4.0)	
Other types	57(12.4)	48(14.3)	9(7.2)	
Pathological size				0.002
≤2 cm	208 (45.4)	169(49.6)	39(33.3)	
>2 cm	250(54.6)	172(50.4)	78(66.7)	
Axillary lymph node status				0.61
No positive	263(62.2)	213(62.5)	50(61.0)	
1–3 positive	111(26.2)	91(26.7)	20(24.4)	
≥4 positive	49(11.6)	37(10.9)	12(14.6)	
Grade				0.007
1	8(1.8)	5(1.5)	3(2.8)	
2	45(10.0)	26(7.6)	19(17.4)	
3	396(88.2)	309(90.9)	87(79.8)	
Ki67 positive	303(75.4)	243(87.7)	60(48.0)	<0.001
p53 positive	242(52.7)	188(55.6)	54(44.6)	0.02
E-Cadherin positive	374(80.6)	284(84.0)	90(71.4)	0.002
Bcl2 positive	149(60.3)	57(43.5)	92(79.3)	<0.001
Muc1 positive	310(75.8)	215(75.2)	95(77.2)	0.37
CK5/6 positive	221(48.0)	160(46.8)	61(51.7)	0.20
CK7/8 positive	436(94.0)	328(95.9)	108(88.5)	0.005
CK14 positive	138(31.2)	97(28.7)	41(39.0)	0.03
CK17 positive	54(23.8)	25(22.5)	29(25.0)	0.38
CK18 positive	297(66.6)	195(60.2)	102(83.6)	<0.001
CK19 positive	401(86.6)	295(86.5)	106(86.9)	0.52
Management pattern				
Surgery without adjuvant chemotherapy	296(66.4)	169(53.0)	127(100)	
Surgery with adjuvant chemotherapy	150(33.6)	150(47.0)	0	

cancer from a large series in two age groups. Overall there was a higher rate of grade 3 tumours, high proliferative index, mutant p53, which is in keeping with the literature [25,26,27]. In this study, TNBCs in the younger patients showed aggressive biology with higher rate of grade 3 tumours, Ki67 expression and p53 mutations as seen in many other studies which included younger patients. However none of these studies compared the two age groups. There was a mixed picture of luminal (CK7/8 and 18) and basal (CK 14 and 17) markers. In the older women studied here, there was a high expression of luminal CK 18, which has never been reported in the literature and this may have an impact on the possible better clinical outcome as seen here. However the rate of CK7/8 positivity was higher in younger patients. The study showed a high expression of basal markers, in keeping with the literature [25,27] though it was even higher in older series which might be due to the higher representation of ER negative tumours

in older women where there is a frequent association with basal cytokeratins [28,29].

The overall outcome of the two age groups with TNBCs was poor with a 5-year breast cancer survival of 73% and 79% in <70 and ≥70 years age groups respectively, which is in keeping with the literature [30], as compared to that reported by us (5-year breast cancer survival being 91% and 90% respectively for the whole series of older women and in the ER positive subgroup) [12,20]. However, despite the fact that they did not receive any adjuvant chemotherapy, the older women did not do any worse than their younger counterparts. As described above, this could be explained biologically due to a preponderance of tumours with lower grade, low proliferation index, normal p53, high Bcl2 proteins and high expression of luminal cytokeratins which all have been shown to be associated with better clinical outcome. There is therefore an urgent need of further studies to investigate this so that clinicians would know how best to select older patients

Table 3. A summary of the clinical outcome of triple negative early operable primary breast cancer- younger (<70) versus older (≥ 70) patients.

Outcome measure	5-year rates in two age groups (%)		p-value
	<70 years	≥70 years	
Breast cancer specific survival	73	79	0.39
Local recurrence free survival	90	86	0.16
Regional recurrence free survival	91	86	0.40
Metastases free survival	70	73	0.56

for adjuvant chemotherapy. This is especially important in those older patients with poorer physiological reserve and significant co-morbidities. There could be a valid reason based on tumour biology for not recommending chemotherapy in some of these patients.

The expression of EGFR showed an association with better outcome. This has been reported in the literature where others have demonstrated better outcome of basal like tumours as compared to pure triple negative/quadruple negative (Quadruple negatives defined as the tumours negative for ER, PgR, HER2 and CK5/6 expression) tumours [9]. The risk of dying from breast cancer in the reported study was 43% higher in the group with negative CK5/6 and EGFR expression within triple negative

group as compared to the patients who had CK5/6 and EGFR positive expression [9]. In addition, studies have shown that EGFR when co-expressed with luminal cytokeratins tends to be associated with a better prognosis [31]. This might be a possible explanation of the better outcome associated with EGFR positivity seen in the present study, where a high expression of CK18 was present in most cases. The presence of EGFR overexpression is also a potential good news as anti-EGFR immunotherapy (e.g. cetuximab and eroltinib) could be exploited. There is a strong need of inclusion of older women in clinical trials with anti-EGFR therapies to assess their clinical effectiveness as well as safety profile.

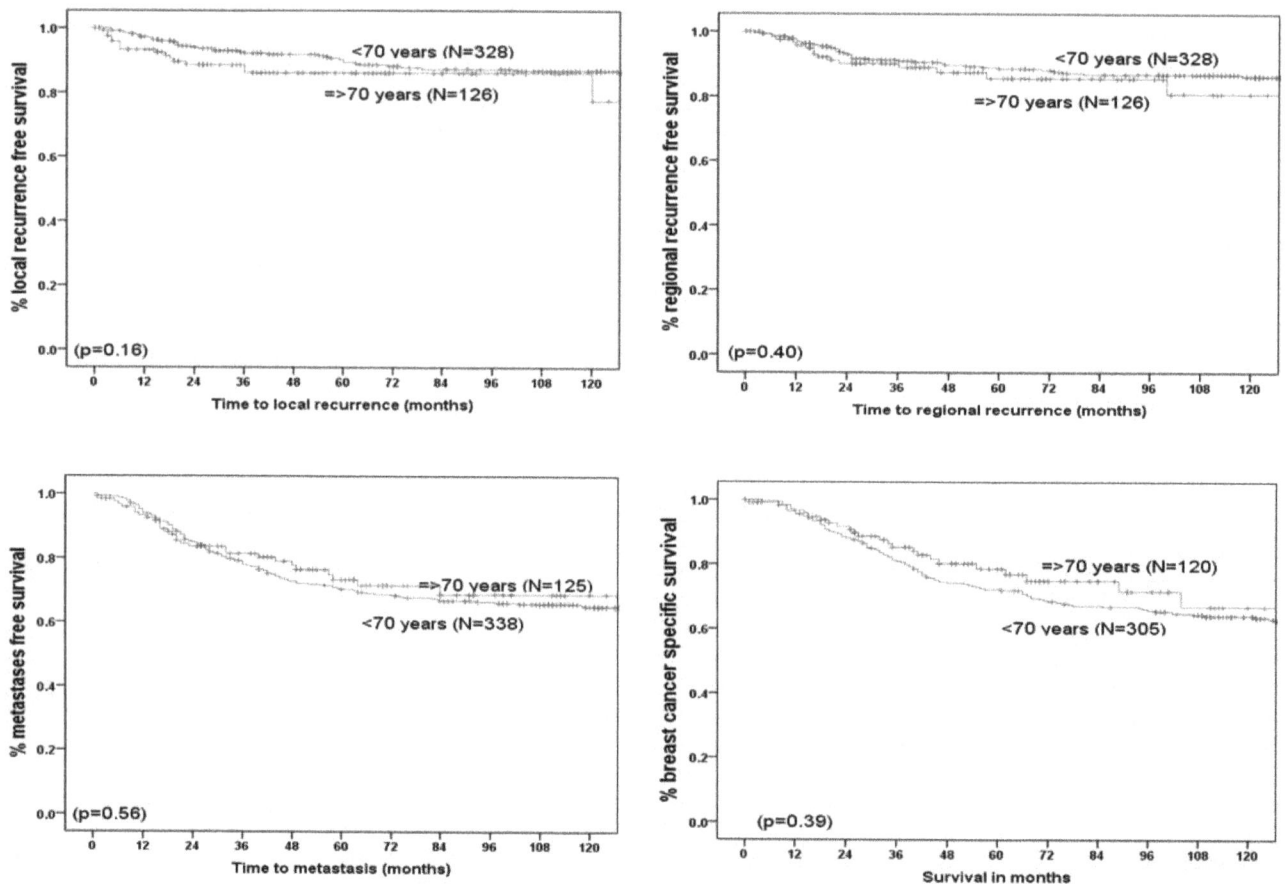

Figure 1. Pattern of clinical outcome of triple negative early operable primary breast cancer - Younger (<70 years) versus older (≥70 years).

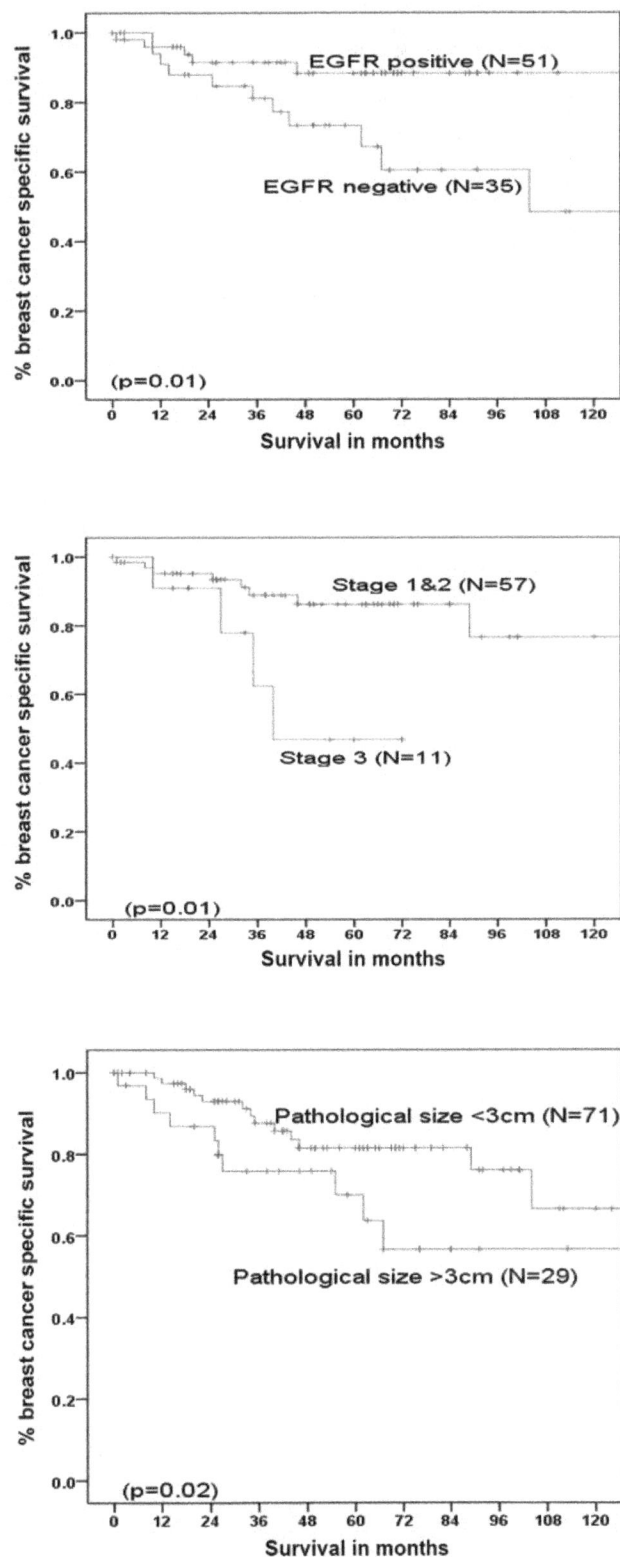

Figure 2. Prognostic factors showing significance influence on the breast cancer specific survival of older women with early operable triple negative breast cancer.

Conclusions

Despite not having received adjuvant chemotherapy, the older series had clinical outcome similar to the younger patients almost half of which had chemotherapy. This may be due to other biomarkers (in addition to ER/PR/HER2) which have different patterns in these age groups influencing prognosis. The place of adjuvant chemotherapy in the treatment of these patients has yet to be identified.

Author Contributions

Conceived and designed the experiments: BMS ARG DALM IOE KLC. Performed the experiments: BMS CCN. Analyzed the data: BMS. Contributed reagents/materials/analysis tools: BMS CCN ARG. Contributed to the writing of the manuscript: BMS ARG DALM IOE KLC.

References

1. Carol D, Melissa M, Siegel R, Jemal A (2010) Breast cancer facts & figures 2009–2010. American Cancer Society.
2. Diab S, Elledge R, Clark G (2000) Tumor characteristics and clinical outcome of elderly women with breast cancer. J Natl Cancer Inst 92: 550–556.
3. Cheung K, Wong A, Parker H, Li V, Winterbottom L, et al. (2008) Pathological Features of Primary Breast Cancer in The Elderly Based on Needle Core Biopsies-A Large Series From a Single Centre. Critical Review in Oncology Hematology 67: 263–267.
4. Haung H, Neven P, Drijkoningen M, Paridaens R, Wildiers H, et al. (2005) Hormone Receptors Do Not Predict The HER2/neu Status in All Age Groups of Women With An Operable Breast Cancer. Annals of Oncology 16: 1755–1761.
5. Al-Kuraya K, Schraml P, Torhorst J, Tapia C, Zaharieva B, et al. (2004) Prognostic relevance of gene amplifications and coamplifications in breast cancer. Cancer Res 64: 8534–8540.
6. Tsutsui S, Ohno S, Murakami S, Hachitanda Y, Oda S (2002) Prognostic value of c-erbB2 expression in breast cancer. J Surg Oncol 79: 216–223.
7. Knoop A, Bentzen S, Nielsen M, Rasmussen B, Rose C (2001) Value of epidermal growth factor receptor, HER2, p53, and steroid receptors in predicting the efficacy of tamoxifen in high-risk postmenopausal breast cancer patients. J Clin Oncol 19: 3376–3384.
8. Early Breast Cancer Trialists' Collaborative Group (EBCTCG) (2005) Effects of chemotherapy and hormonal therapy for early breast cancer on recurrence and 15-year survival: an overview of the randomised trials. Lancet 365: 1687–1717.
9. Choi Y, Oh E, Park S, Kim Y, Park Y, et al. (2010) Triple-negative, basal-like, and quintuple-negative breast cancers: better prediction model for survival. Biomed Central Cancer 10: 507.
10. Rakha E, El-Sayed M, Green A, Lee A, Robertson J, et al. (2007) Prognostic markers in triple-negative breast cancer. Cancer 109: 25–32.
11. Aapro M, Wildiers H (2012) Triple-negative breast cancer in the older population. Ann Oncol 23 Suppl 6: vi52–55.
12. Syed B, Johnston S, Wong D, Green A, Winterbottom L, et al. (2011) Long-term (37 years) clinical outcome of older women with early operable primary breast cancer managed in a dedicated clinic. Ann Oncol.
13. Elston C, Ellis I (1991) Pathological prognostic factors in breast cancer. I. The value of histological grade in breast cancer: experience from a large study with long-term follow-up. Histopathology 19: 403–410.
14. Abd El-Rehim D, Ball G, Pinder S, Rakha E, Paish C, et al. (2005) High-throughput protein expression analysis using tissue microarray technology of a large well-characterised series identifies biologically distinct classes of breast cancer confirming recent cDNA expression analyses. Int J Cancer: 340–350.
15. Aleskandarany M, Rakha E, Macmillan R, Powe D, Ellis I, et al. (2011) MIB1/Ki-67 labelling index can classify grade 2 breast cancer into two clinically distinct subgroups. Breast Cancer Res Treat 127: 591–599.
16. Rakha E, El-Sheikh S, Kandil M, El-Sayed M, Green A, et al. (2008) Expression of BRCAI protein in breast cancer and its prognostic significance. Hum Pathol: 857–865.
17. Camp R, Charette L, Rimm D (2000) Validation of tissue microarray technology in breast carcinoma. Lab Invest: 1943–1949.
18. Howell A, Barnes DM, Harland RN, Redford J, Bramwell VH, et al. (1984) Steroid-hormone receptors and survival after first relapse in breast cancer. Lancet 1: 588–591.
19. Fleming S, Rastogi A, Dmitrienko A, Johnson K (1999) A comprehensive prognostic index to predict survival based on multiple comorbidities: a focus on breast cancer. Med Care 37: 601–614.
20. Syed BM, Al-Khyatt W, Johnston SJ, Wong DW, Winterbottom L, et al. (2011) Long-term clinical outcome of oestrogen receptor-positive operable primary

breast cancer in older women: a large series from a single centre. Br J Cancer 104: 1393–1400.

21. Balducci L, Extermann M (2000) Management of cancer in the older person: a practical approach. Oncologist 5: 224–237.

22. Haybittle J, Blamey R, Elston C, Johnson J, Doyle P, et al. (1982) A prognostic index in primary breast cancer. Br J Cancer 45: 361–366.

23. Hind D, Wyld L, Reed M (2007) Surgery, with or without tamoxifen, vs tamoxifen alone for older women with operable breast cancer: cochrane review. Br J Cancer 96: 1025–1029.

24. Billar J, Dueck A, Stucky C, Gray R, Wasif N, et al. (2010) Triple-negative breast cancers: unique clinical presentations and outcomes. Ann Surg Oncol: S384–S390.

25. Kim J, Hwang T, Kang S, Lee S, Bae Y (2009) Prognostic significance of basal markers in triple-negative breast cancers. J Breast Cancer: 4–13.

26. Zhou X, Liu Q (2010) Clinicopathological characters of triple negative breast cancer. Chinese J Cancer Res: 17–20.

27. Tan D, Marchio C, Jones R, Savage K, Smith I, et al. (2008) Triple negative breast cancer: molecular profiling and prognostic impact in adjuvant anthracycline-treated patients. Breast Cancer Res Treat: 27–44.

28. Abd El-Rehim D, Pinder S, Paish C, Bell J, Blamey R, et al. (2004) Expression of luminal and basal cytokeratins in human breast carcinoma. J Pathol 203: 661–671.

29. Gusterson BA, Ross DT, Heath VJ, Stein T (2005) Basal cytokeratins and their relationship to the cellular origin and functional classification of breast cancer. Breast Cancer Res 7: 143–148.

30. Rakha E, Elsheikh S, Aleskandarany M, Habashi H, Green A, et al. (2009) Triple-Negative Breast Cancer: Distinguishing Between Basal and Nonbasal Subtypes. Clinical Cancer Research 15: 2302–2310.

31. Nogi H, Kobayashi T, Suzuki M, Tabei I, Kawase K, et al. (2009) EGFR as paradoxical predictor of chemosensitivity and outcome among triple-negative breast cancer. Oncol Rep 21: 413–417.

15

Is There a Benefit in Receiving Concurrent Chemoradiotherapy for Elderly Patients with Inoperable Thoracic Esophageal Squamous Cell Carcinoma?

Peng Zhang[1,9], Mian Xi[1,9], Lei Zhao[1], Jing-Xian Shen[2], Qiao-Qiao Li[1], Li-Ru He[1], Shi-Liang Liu[1], Meng-Zhong Liu[1]*

1 Sun Yat-sen University Cancer Center, State Key Laboratory of Oncology in South China, Collaborative Innovation Center for Cancer Medicine, Department of Radiation Oncology, Cancer Center, Sun Yat-sen University, Guangzhou, People's Republic of China, 2 Sun Yat-sen University Cancer Center, State Key Laboratory of Oncology in South China, Collaborative Innovation Center for Cancer Medicine, Imaging Diagnosis and Interventional Center, Cancer Center, Sun Yat-sen University, Guangzhou, People's Republic of China

Abstract

Background and purpose: The benefit of concurrent chemoradiotherapy (CCRT) in elderly patients with inoperable esophageal squamous cell carcinoma (SCC) is controversial. This study aimed to assess the efficiency and safety of CCRT in elderly thoracic esophageal cancer patients.

Methods and materials: Between January 2002 and December 2011, 128 patients aged 65 years or older treated with CCRT or radiotherapy (RT) alone for inoperable thoracic esophageal SCC were analyzed retrospectively (RT alone, n = 55; CCRT, n = 73).

Results: No treatment-related deaths occurred and no patients experienced any acute grade 4 non-hematologic toxicities. Patients treated with CCRT developed more severe acute toxicities than patients who received RT alone. The 3-year overall survival (OS) rate was 36.1% for CCRT compared with 28.5% following RT alone (p = 0.008). Multivariate analysis identified T stage and treatment modality as independent prognostic factors for survival. Further analysis revealed that survival was significantly better in the CCRT group than in the RT alone group for patients ≤ 72 years. Nevertheless, the CCRT group had a similar OS to the RT group for patients > 72 years.

Conclusion: Our results suggest that elderly patients with inoperable thoracic esophageal SCC could benefit from CCRT, without major toxicities. However, for patients older than 72 years, CCRT is not superior to RT alone in terms of survival benefit.

Editor: Andreas-Claudius Hoffmann, West German Cancer Center, Germany

Funding: This work was supported by the grant from the Sci-Tech Project Foundation of Guangdong Province (No.42012B031800287). Website: http://www.gdstc.gov.cn. PZ and MX received the funding. The funders provided help in data collection and analysis.

Competing Interests: The authors have declared that no competing interests exist.

* Email: liumengzhong@126.com

9 These authors contributed equally to this work.

Introduction

Esophageal cancer is remains a virulent disease, with a 5-year survival rate of only 17% [1]. The risk of esophageal cancer increases with age, with a mean age at diagnosis of 67 years [2]. The number of elderly patients with esophageal cancers is expected to increase in the near future as the number of elderly people increases.

Surgical resection is the preferred treatment for localized esophageal cancer patients. However, a recent population-based study showed that older patients have less intensive treatment of esophageal cancer including surgery [3]. In addition, the literature states that patients over the age of 70 have relatively high rates of

postoperative morbidity and mortality, and 75 years of age is often considered the age limit for surgery [4,5].

For the medically or technically inoperable patients, concurrent chemoradiotherapy (CCRT) is the mainstay of treatment for locally advanced esophageal cancer. The Radiation Therapy Oncology Group (RTOG) trial 85-01 established the superiority of CCRT compared with radiotherapy (RT) alone in esophageal cancer patients. However, the acute toxicity of this regimen was substantial: sixty-four percent of patients treated with CCRT experienced severe or life threatening side effects and only 23% of patients enrolled were aged over 70 [6].

Few studies have focused on elderly patients; therefore, no standard treatment modality has been established for inoperable

Table 1. Patient characteristics.

Characteristic	All patients (n = 128)	Patients with CCRT (n = 73)	Patients with RT alone (n = 55)
Age (years)			
> 72	57 (44.5%)	25 (34.2%)	32 (58.2%)
≤ 72	71 (55.5%)	48 (65.8%)	23 (41.8%)
Sex			
Male	89 (69.5%)	57 (78.1%)	32 (58.2%)
Female	39 (30.5%)	16 (21.9%)	23 (41.8%)
Charlson score			
≥ 1	42 (32.8%)	23(31.5%)	19 (34.5%)
< 1	86 (67.2%)	50 (68.5%)	36 (65.5%)
Pathological grade			
Well differentiated	10 (7.8%)	6 (8.2%)	4 (7.3%)
Moderately differentiated	47 (36.7%)	28 (38.3%)	19 (34.6%)
Poorly/undifferentiated	45 (35.2%)	21 (28.8%)	24 (43.6%)
Unknown	26 (20.3%)	18 (24.7%)	8 (14.5%)
Location			
Upper third	38 (29.7%)	24 (32.9%)	14 (25.4%)
Middle third	69 (53.9%)	38 (52.1%)	31 (56.4%)
Lower third	21 (16.4%)	11 (15.0%)	10 (18.2%)
Primary tumor length			
≤ 5 cm	78 (60.9%)	42 (57.5%)	35 (63.6%)
> 5 cm	50 (39.1%)	31 (42.5%)	20 (36.4%)
T stage			
T1-T2	25 (19.5%)	18 (24.7%)	10 (18.2%)
T3-T4	103 (80.5%)	55 (75.3%)	45 (81.8%)
N stage			
N0	26 (20.3%)	14 (19.2%)	15 (27.3%)
N1	102 (79.7%)	59 (80.8%)	40 (72.7%)
M stage			
M0	78 (60.9%)	40 (54.8%)	38 (69.1%)
M1	50 (39.1%)	33 (45.2%)	17 (30.9%)
Radiation dose (Gy)			
< 60	49 (38.3%)	23 (31.5%)	26 (47.3%)
≥ 60	79 (61.7%)	50 (68.5%)	29 (52.7%)

Abbreviations: CCRT, concurrent chemoradiotherapy; RT, radiotherapy.

esophageal cancer in elderly patients. Several studies have reported the efficacy and toxicity of CCRT in elderly patients with inoperable esophageal cancer, but the results were controversial [7–10]. In addition, the published reports are mainly on small series of patients, making it difficult to carry out reliable analysis. Therefore, we reviewed our institutional experience to evaluate the efficiency and safety of CCRT compared with RT alone in elderly thoracic esophageal cancer patients. We defined an elderly population according to Social Security and Medicare regulations as persons aged 65 years or older.

Patients and Methods

Ethics statement

This study was approved by the institutional review board (IRBs) of Cancer Center, Sun Yat-sen University. Written informed consent was obtained from all the patients in accordance with the regulations of the IRBs.

Patient's inclusion

Esophageal cancer patients treated with RT at Sun Yat-Sen University Cancer Center between January 2002 and December 2011 were retrospectively reviewed. The inclusion criteria were (1) aged 65 years or older at the time of diagnosis; (2) Eastern Cooperative Oncology Group performance status of ≤ 2; (3) histologically conformed as thoracic esophageal squamous carcinoma (SCC); (4) unable or refusing to undergo surgical resection; (5) no prior therapy; (6) no history of concomitant or previous malignancy; (7) complete and retrievable clinical records.

Among 795 esophageal cancer patients treated with RT from 2002 to 2011, 128 patients who fulfilled the criteria were included.

Table 2. Acute toxicity.

CTC Grade	Patients with CCRT (n=73)					Patients with RT alone (n=55)				
	0	1	2	3	4	0	1	2	3	4
Anemia	15	26	27	5	0	12	23	19	1	0
Leukocytopenia	9	18	29	12	5	8	24	16	7	0
Thrombopenia	27	23	16	7	0	26	23	6	0	0
Gastrointestinal	26	16	16	15	0	13	19	20	3	0
Skin toxicity	16	26	28	3	0	17	24	13	1	0
Esophagitis	12	30	27	4	0	16	23	14	2	0
Pneumonitis	50	16	5	2	0	39	13	2	1	0

Abbreviations: CCRT, concurrent chemoradiotherapy; RT, radiotherapy.

Patient pretreatment characteristics

The pretreatment work-up included complete history collection, physical examination, computed tomography (CT) scans of the chest and abdomen, barium esophagography, endoscopy, endoscopic ultrasonography, and pulmonary function test. Bone scans were performed if clinically indicated. The 6th edition (2002) of the American Joint Committee on Cancer TNM staging system was used to classify tumors. The Charlson comorbidity index was used to perform analysis of this cohort's comorbidity burden [11].

Treatment details

The majority of patients (102 of 128) received three-dimensional conformal radiotherapy (3DCRT) and other 26 patients were treated with intensity-modulated radiotherapy (IMRT). Gross tumor volume (GTV) was defined as any visible primary tumor on the computerized imaging or endoscopy and included metastatic lymph nodes. Clinical target volume (CTV) was defined as the GTV with superoinferior 3-cm and lateral 2-cm margins. The planning target volume (PTV) was created by adding 1-cm in the superoinferior dimension and 0.8-cm radically to the CTV. Radiotherapy was delivered with 6–8 MV photons using a 1.8–2.0 Gy daily fraction and five fractions per week. The median prescription dose was 60 Gy (range, 46–70 Gy) to PTV in 25–35 fractions administered over 5–7 weeks.

Application of concurrent chemotherapy was performed after careful evaluation of organ function, performance status, and severity of comorbidities. Platinum-based chemotherapy combined with 5-fluorouracil (5-FU) or docetaxel was administered to 73 patients and the remaining 55 patients received RT alone. In the CCRT group, 33 patients received two cycles of docetaxel 60 mg/m^2 and cisplatin 75 mg/m^2 delivered on day 1 and 22 of RT with standard premedication [12]. Forty patients were treated with two cycles of 60 mg/m^2 of cisplatin administered on days 1 and 29 and 1000 mg/m^2 of 5-FU administered as a continuous intravenous infusion for 96 hours on days 1–4 and 29–32 [13]. Dose reduction of chemotherapy was considered if any grade 4 hematological toxicities occurred.

Evaluation of response and toxicity

Patients were followed up every three months by physical examination, chest and abdominal CT, barium esophagography, and endoscopy or endoscopic ultrasonography. The clinical tumor response was evaluated 6–8 weeks after completion of RT according to the Response Evaluation Criteria in Solid Tumors (RECIST ver. 1.1). A complete response (CR) was defined as no remnant disease on CT image and pathological CR on endoscopy. The National Cancer Institute Common Toxicity Criteria (version 3.0) was used to score treatment toxicity.

Statistical analysis

The cutoff date of the last follow-up was April 30, 2013 for the censored data analysis. The Kaplan–Meier method was used to calculate overall survival (OS) and progression-free survival (PFS) for each potential prognostic factor, which were measured from the time of diagnosis. The log-rank test was used to test the differences between groups. The χ^2 test was used to compare patients' treatment-related toxicities between subgroups. Cox regression was used to perform multivariate analyses. All statistical analysis was performed using SPSS 16.0 software (SPSS Inc., Chicago, IL, USA). A p value of <0.05 was considered statistically significant.

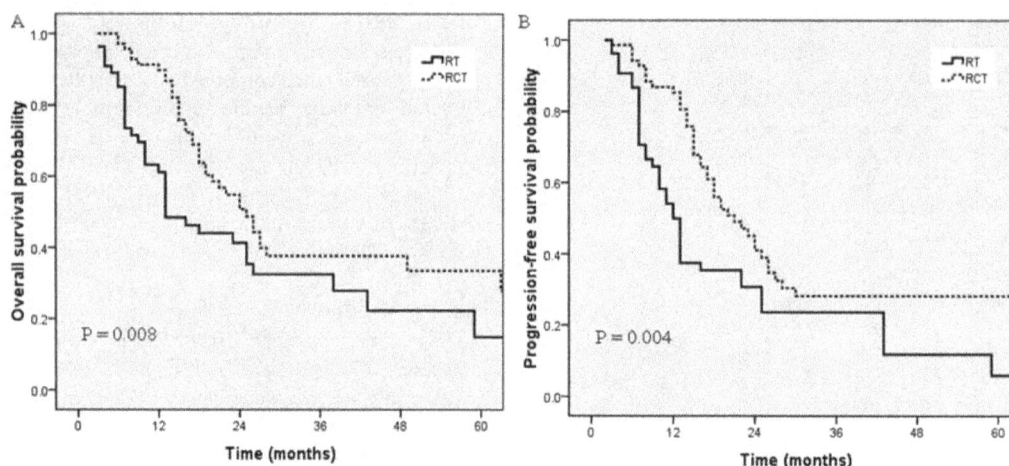

Figure 1. Overall survival (A) and progression-free survival (B) for the CCRT group and the RT alone group in the whole group of patients.

Results

Patients' characteristics

Clinical baseline characteristics are detailed in Table 1. The median age of the 128 patients was 72 years, ranging from 65 to 89 years. Twenty-eight patients (21.9%) had stage I/II disease and forty-nine patients (38.3%) had stage of III disease. Sixteen patients (12.5%) were diagnosed with stage IVa and the remaining 34 (26.6%) were diagnosed with stage IVb. Of the 34 stage IVb patients, except for one patient with liver metastasis and one with sacral bone metastasis, 32 had non-regional lymph nodal metastases. The Charlson score for the majority of patients was 0. Thirty patients (23.4%) had a Charlson score of 1, and 12 patients (9.4%) had a Charlson score $\geq$ 2. Twenty-three patients (18.0%) had chronic cardiovascular disease, 10 patients (7.8%) had chronic obstructive pulmonary disease, 17 patients (13.3%) had diabetes, and four patients (3.1%) had liver cirrhosis.

Tumor response and toxicity

All patients were evaluated for clinical tumor response. In the CCRT group (n = 73), CR was achieved in 17 (23.3%); partial response (PR) in 34 (46.6%); stable disease (SD) in 19 (26.0%); and progressive disease (PD) in 3 patients (4.1%), yielding an objective response rate of 67.1%. However, in the RT alone group (n = 55), the objective response rate declined to 47.3% (CR = 6 and PR = 20) and eight patients (14.5%) exhibited PD. A significant difference in response rate was observed between the two groups (p = 0.032).

All patients were evaluable for toxicity. As shown in Table 2, most treatment-related and documented acute toxicities were grade 1 and 2. No treatment-related deaths occurred and no patients experienced any acute grade 4 non-hematological toxicity. Most common grade 3 and 4 toxicities were leukopenia and gastrointestinal toxicity. Charlson score > 1 versus $\leq$ 1 did not influence the adverse events of grade 3–4 (p = 0.474). Acute grade 3–4 hematological toxicity was identified in 36.9% of the CCRT patients and 14.5% of the RT alone patients (p = 0.001). Patients treated with CCRT developed more grade $\geq$ 2 esophagitis and pneumonitis than patients who received RT alone (52.1% vs. 34.5%, p = 0.005).

Survival and prognostic analysis

The median follow-up period was 18.0 months (range, 3.0 to 89.0 months). During follow-up, 66 of the 128 patients (51.6%) relapsed and distant metastasis occurred in 33 patients (25.8%). Cancer was the cause of death in 64 patients (84.2%) among the patients who had died at the time of the current analysis (n = 76).

The 3-year OS and PFS rates for the whole group were 33.2% and 24.1%, respectively. The median OS of all patients was 16.0 months and the median PFS was 15.0 months. As shown in Fig.1, patients who received CCRT had a better OS compared with patients treated with RT alone (36.1% vs. 28.5% after 3 years, p = 0.008). The 3-year PFS rate of the CCRT group was also significantly higher than that for the RT alone group (27.2% vs. 16.3%, p = 0.004).

Sex, age, Charlson score, pathological grade, primary esophageal tumor location, tumor length, clinical T stage, clinical N stage, M stage, radiation dose and treatment modality were subjected to univariate analysis (Table 3). The results suggested that several variables were significantly associated with the OS: T stage (p<0.001), M stage (p = 0.012), tumor length (p = 0.039) and treatment modality (p = 0.008). The variables significantly associated with the PFS were: T stage (p = 0.007), M stage (p = 0.031) and treatment modality (p = 0.006).

To identify independent prognostic factors, the factors that were found to be significant on univariate analysis were subjected to multivariate analysis. Multivariate analysis revealed that clinical T stage (p = 0.002) and treatment modality (p = 0.002) were independent factors affecting OS and PFS in elderly esophageal SCC patients (Table 4).

Subgroup analysis

As the median age of the whole group was 72 years, we subdivided the elderly patients into two groups: > 72 years and $\leq$ 72 years. As shown in Fig. 2, for patients $\leq$ 72 years, OS and PFS were significantly better in the CCRT group than in the RT alone group (p = 0.003, 0.042). Median OS was 22.0 months in the CCRT group versus 13.0 months in the RT alone group. Nevertheless, for patients > 72 years, OS and PFS were similar in the two groups (p = 0.337, 0.363; Fig. 3).

Among patients who received CCRT, we further evaluated the efficacy of different chemotherapy regimens. Patients in the CCRT group were divided into two groups: those who received a

Table 3. Univariate analysis demonstrating factors associated with OS and PFS.

Factor	No.	OS p-value	PFS p-value
Sex		0.149	0.774
Male	89		
Female	39		
Age (years)		0.865	0.103
> 72	57		
≤ 72	71		
Charlson score		0.947	0.314
≥ 1	42		
< 1	86		
Pathological grade		0.847	0.683
Well differentiated	10		
Moderately differentiated	47		
Poorly/undifferentiated	45		
Unknown	26		
Location		0.325	0.634
Upper third	38		
Middle third	69		
Lower third	21		
Primary tumor length		0.039	0.169
≤ 5 cm	78		
> 5 cm	50		
T stage		0.000	0.007
T1-T2	25		
T3-T4	103		
N stage		0.804	0.359
N0	26		
N1	102		
M stage		0.012	0.041
M0	78		
M1	50		
Radiation dose (Gy)		0.056	0.226
< 60	49		
≥ 60	79		
Treatment modality		0.008	0.004
CCRT	73		
RT alone	55		

Abbreviations: OS, overall survival; PFS, progression-free survival; CCRT, concurrent chemoradiotherapy; RT, radiotherapy.

docetaxel combined regimen (n = 33) and those who received a 5-FU combined regimen (n = 40). The median OS periods were 21.0 and 17.0 months ($p = 0.013$), and the median PFS periods were 20.0 and 15.0 months ($p = 0.061$), respectively.

Discussion

Based on several clinical trials, CCRT has been the standard treatment for locally advanced esophageal cancer and is superior to RT alone [6]. However, very few studies have investigated CCRT in elderly patients [7–10]. The efficacy and toxicity of CCRT compared with RT alone for elderly patients have not been well documented previously. To clarify this issue, in the present study we compared the efficiency and safety of CCRT with RT alone in elderly patients with advanced thoracic esophageal SCC.

The surgical approach in elderly esophageal cancer patients remains a topic of debate because of the potentially higher rate of post-operative complications [14,15]. Several studies reported that CCRT was an effective treatment with no significant toxicity in elderly esophageal cancer patients [7–10,16–19]. However, Takeuchi et al. reported that an elderly patient group showed a significantly inferior median survival time compared with the nonelderly patient group (14.7 months $vs.$ 35.1 months, $P = 0.01$)

Table 4. Multivariate analysis of prognostic factors for patients with elderly esophageal SCC.

Endpoint	Variable	P^a	HR	95% CI for HR
OS	Tumor length	0.220	1.355	0.833–2.204
	T stage	0.002	3.139	1.546–6.371
	M stage	0.073	1.615	0.957–2.727
	Treatment modality	0.002	0.468	0.292–0.750
PFS	T stage	0.014	2.117	1.166–3.844
	M stage	0.032	1.668	1.044–2.665
	Treatment modality	0.001	0.480	0.308–0.747

Abbreviations: CI, confidence interval; HR, hazards ratio; OS, overall survival; PFS, progression-free survival; SCC, squamous cell carcinoma.
^{a}P values were calculated using an adjusted Cox proportional hazards model.

[20]. In the current study, patients who received CCRT had a 3-year OS of 37.6%, suggesting that CCRT is an effective treatment modality with a low incidence of severe toxicity for elderly patients.

Up to now, only two studies compared CCRT with RT alone in elderly esophageal cancer patients. Semrau et al. reported 51 patients aged ≥ 70 with inoperable esophageal cancer undergoing RT or CCRT, and revealed that patients treated with CCRT had a 2-year OS rate of 53.3% compared with 16.7% for RT patients ($P = 0.039$) [17]. In the study by Xu et al. [20], median OS for the CCRT group was 17 months, while it was 8 months in the RT group ($P = 0.013$). Consistent with previous reports, our study also revealed that CCRT had a higher response rate and an obvious survival benefit compared with RT alone, without a major increase in adverse events.

In the present study, 24 of 57 (42.1%) of patients aged older than72 years received CCRT, whereas 49 of 71 (69.0%) of patients between 65 and 72 years received CCRT. Given this difference in treatment, we consider our analysis to be a comparison of the treatment outcomes between relatively none-lderly patients (65–72 years old) and elderly patients (> 72 years). In the subgroup analysis, CCRT has a survival benefit compared with RT alone in patients between 65 and 72 years. Nevertheless, for patients > 72 years, OS and PFS were similar in the two groups. This may be partially explained by the poor life expectancy of patients older than 72 years. According to the Life Tables in 2010 in China, the average life expectancy was 74.8 years. The late toxicity of CCRT may be another reason. Marota et al reported that the 2-year cumulative incidence of late cardiopulmonary toxicities of Grade 3 or greater for patients 75 years or older was 29%, compared with 3% for younger patients, thus CCRT was not tolerated by patients older than 75 years [21].

Data on elderly patients who received RT alone are limited. Hishikawa et al. reported the survival within different age groups of esophageal cancer receiving external beam RT and brachytherapy boost, and revealed that the 2-year OS rate of patients aged 70–79 years was 17.2%, which is similar to the patients aged 43–69 years (16.7%). Therefore, the study suggested that RT should be the first choice of treatment for patients > 80 years old [22]. Yamakava et al, reported on 40 cases aged ≥ 80 years treated with RT alone and concluded that RT is a safe and effective treatment for esophageal cancer in patients over 80 years old [23]. In our study, in terms of the limited survival benefit of CCRT over RT, treatment modality should be evaluated on an

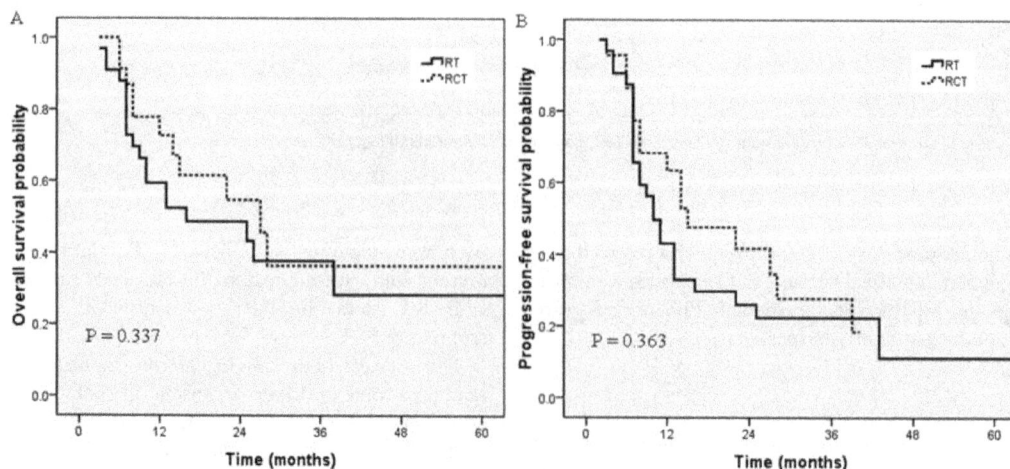

Figure 2. Overall survival (A) and progression-free survival (B) for the CCRT group and the RT alone group in patients older than 72 years.

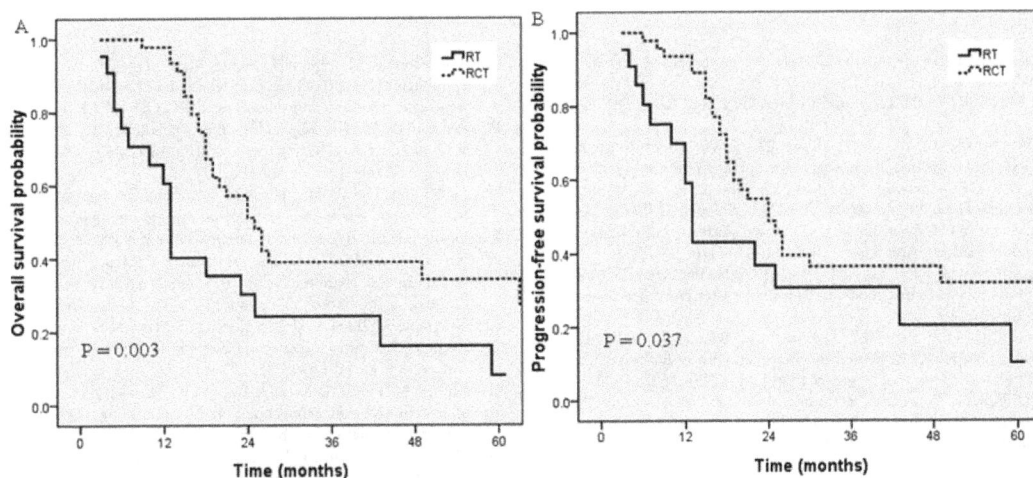

Figure 3. Overall survival (A) and progression-free survival (B) for the CCRT group and the RT alone group in patients between 65 and 72 years old.

individual basis in such cases and RT alone should be a reasonable option for patients in higher age groups.

Numerous studies on patients with advanced esophagogastric cancer suggested that cisplatin-based chemotherapy toxicities did not increase with age [24]. With regard to $\leq$ grade 3 side effects, it was possible to minimize and make tolerable such adverse events using previously described methods and careful close monitoring. Tougeron et al. reported that 4.6% of elderly patients who received combined chemoradiation experienced a grade 4 hematological toxicity [7]. In the CCRT group of our study, grade 4 hematological toxicities were observed in five patients (6.8%) only, suggesting that documented toxicities were not severe and supportive treatment was manageable. In addition, no treatment-related deaths occurred and no patients experienced any acute grade 4 non-hematologic toxicities. The incidence of severe acute toxicity in our cohort was lower than that reported in previous studies for non-elderly esophageal cancer patients [6,12]. Therefore, cisplatin-based CCRT is a safe treatment option for elderly esophageal SCC patients.

To improve survival for locally advanced esophageal cancer, taxane-based preoperative chemoradiotherapy schedules have been investigated in some exploratory trials. Wu et al compared the efficacy and feasibility of neoadjuvant chemoradiotherapy with docetaxel plus cisplatin or with cisplatin plus 5-FU for local advanced esophageal SCC, and showed that docetaxel plus cisplatin can be well tolerated and achieved a higher pathological complete response rate than cisplatin plus 5-FU (35.1% *vs.* 20.8%, $P = 0.048$) [25]. However, there has been no prospective randomized trial to validate the benefit of different concurrent chemotherapy regimens for definitive RT. Hsu et al retrospectively analyzed the effects of paclitaxel-based chemoradiation for esophageal SCC and showed improved local disease compared with the regimen of 5-FU and cisplatin [26]. In the CCRT group in our study, there was a survival advantage for patients who received the docetaxel combined regimen compared with those who received the 5-FU combined regimen; thus, a prospective study addressing this regimen is warranted.

Age as a prognostic factor is still debated and several studies did not show any prognostic significance for age [27,28]. Semrau et al. compared 152 patients aged < 70 years treated with the definitive CCRT protocol and 51 patients aged $\geq$ 70 with esophageal

cancer, and concluded that there was no significant difference in OS in the two groups; however, PFS showed a significant difference in favor of the $\geq$ 70 years group [17]. However, Takeuchi et al. demonstrated inferior survival in the elderly patient group compared with the non-elderly group. He attributed this to a lower response, a higher mortality from complications, and a lower compliance in the elderly group [20]. Our results showed that age has no bearing on the survival of elderly patients. This may be partially because our study did not include patients treated with best supportive care or endo-esophageal stenting only. The selected population may represent a favorable group of patients suffering from advanced esophageal cancer.

The prognostic value of comorbidity is far from conclusive. Tougeron et al. reported that a Charlson score $\leq$ 2 is an independent prognostic factor associated with better survival for elderly patients [16]. However, several studies showed that moderate to severe comorbidity are not predictive of survival [8,18]. In our study, a Charlson score $\geq$ 1 vs. <1 did not influence the incidence of adverse events. No significant association was found between the Charlson comorbidity index and OS or PFS; this may be attributed to the patients' selection bias.

The current study is limited by its retrospective design and the heterogeneity of the concurrent chemotherapy regimens. Considering all the aspects in the study, large-scale prospective clinical trials for elderly esophageal cancer patients are required in the future.

Conclusions

Elderly patients older than 65 years with inoperable thoracic esophageal SCC could benefit from CCRT without major toxicities. However, for patients older than 72 years, CCRT is not superior to RT alone in terms of survival benefit. Further prospective studies are warranted to confirm the results.

Author Contributions

Conceived and designed the experiments: PZ MX MZL. Performed the experiments: PZ MX LZ JXS QQL. Analyzed the data: QQL LRH SLL. Contributed reagents/materials/analysis tools: PZ MX QQL SLL. Contributed to the writing of the manuscript: PZ MX MZL.

References

1. Siegel R, Naishadham D, Jemal A (2013) Cancer Statistics, 2013. CA Cancer J Clin 63: 11–30.
2. Enzinger PC, Mayer RJ (2003) Esophageal cancer. N Engl J Med 349: 2241–2252.
3. Steyerberg EW, Neville B, Weeks JC, Earle CC (2007) Referral patterns, treatment choices, and outcomes in locoregional esophageal cancer: population-based analysis of elderly patients. J Clin Oncol 25: 2389–2396.
4. Kinugasa S, Tachibana M, Yoshimura H, Dhar DK, Shibakita M, et al. (2001) Esophageal resection in elderly esophageal carcinoma patients: improvement in postoperative complications. Ann Thorac Surg 71: 414–418.
5. Law S, Wong KH, Kwok KF, Chu KM, Wong J (2004) Predictive factors for postoperative pulmonary complications and mortality after esophagectomy for cancer. Ann Surg 240: 791–800.
6. Herskovic A, Martz K, al-Sarraf M, Leichman L, Brindle J, et al. (1992) Combined chemotherapy and radiotherapy compared with radiotherapy alone in patients with cancer of the esophagus. N Engl J Med 326: 1593–1598.
7. Tougeron D, Di Fiore F, Thureau S, Berbera N, Iwanicki-Caron I, et al. (2008) Safety and outcome of definitive chemoradiotherapy in elderly patients with oesophageal cancer. Br J Cancer 99: 1586–1592.
8. Anderson SE, Minsky BD, Bains M, Hummer A, Kelsen D, et al. (2007) Combined modality chemoradiation in elderly oesophageal cancer patients. Br J Cancer 96: 1823–1827.
9. Nallapareddy S, Wilding GE, Yang G, Iyer R, Javle M (2005) Chemoradiation is a tolerable therapy for older adults with esophageal cancer. Anticancer Res 25: 3055–3060.
10. Mak RH, Mamon HJ, Ryan DP, Miyamoto DT, Ancukiewicz M, et al. (2010) Toxicity and outcomes after chemoradiation for esophageal cancer in patients age 75 or older. Dis Esophagus 23: 316–323.
11. Reid BC, Alberg AJ, Klassen AC, Samet JM, Rozier RG, et al. (2001) Comorbidity and survival of elderly head and neck carcinoma patients. Cancer 92: 2109–2116.
12. Li QQ, Liu MZ, Hu YH, Liu H, He ZY, et al. (2010) Definitive concomitant chemoradiotherapy with docetaxel and cisplatin in squamous esophageal carcinoma. Dis Esophagus 23: 253–259.
13. Liu H, Lu L, Zhu Q, Hao Y, Mo Y, et al. (2011) Cervical nodal metastases of unresectable thoracic esophageal squamous cell carcinoma Characteristics of long-term survivors after concurrent chemoradiotherapy. Radiother Oncol 99: 181–186.
14. Sabel MS, Smith JL, Nava HR, Mollen K, Douglass HO, et al. (2002) Esophageal resection for carcinoma in patients older than 70 years. Ann Surg Oncol 9: 210–214.
15. Gockel I, Sultanov FS, Domeyer M, Goenner U, Junginger T (2007) Developments in esophageal surgery for adenocarcinoma: a comparison of two decades. BMC Cancer 7: 114.
16. Tougeron D, Hamidou H, Scotté M, Di Fiore F, Antonietti M, et al. (2010) Esophageal cancer in the elderly: an analysis of the factors associated with treatment decisions and outcomes. BMC Cancer 10: 510.
17. Semrau R, Herzog SL, Vallböhmer D, Kocher M, Hölscher A, et al. (2012) Radiotherapy in elderly patients with inoperable esophageal cancer. Is there a benefit? Strahlenther Onkol 188: 226–232.
18. Go SI, Sup Lee W, Hee Kang M, Song HN, Jin Kim M, et al. (2012) Response to concurrent chemoradiotherapy as a prognostic marker in elderly patients with locally advanced esophageal cancer. Tumori 98: 225–232.
19. Xu HY, Du ZD, Zhou L, Yu M, Ding ZY, et al. (2014) Safety and efficacy of radiation and chemoradiation in patients over 70 years old with inoperable esophageal squamous cell carcinoma. Oncol Lett 7: 260–266.
20. Takeuchi S, Ohtsu A, Doi T, Kojima T, Minashi K, et al. (2007) A retrospective study of definitive chemoradiotherapy for elderly patients with esophageal cancer. Am J Clin Oncol 30: 607–611.
21. Morota M, Gomi K, Kozuka T, Chin K, Matsuura M, et al. (2009) Late toxicity after definitive concurrent chemoradiotherapy for thoracic esophageal carcinoma. Int J Radiat Oncol Biol Phys 75: 122–128.
22. Hishikawa Y, Kurisu K, Taniguchi M, Kamikonya N, Miura T (1991) Radiotherapy for carcinoma of the esophagus in patients aged eighty or older. Int J Radiat Oncol Biol Phys 20: 685–688.
23. Yamakawa M, Shiojima K, Takahashi M, Saito Y, Matsumoto H, et al. (1994) Radiation therapy for esophageal cancer in patients over 80 years old. Int J Radiat Oncol Biol Phys 30: 1225–1232.
24. Trumper M, Ross PJ, Cunningham D, Norman AR, Hawkins R, et al. (2006) Efficacy and tolerability of chemotherapy in elderly patients with advanced oesophago-gastric cancer: A pooled analysis of three clinical trials. Eur J Cancer 42: 827–834.
25. Wu S, Chen MY, Luo JC, Wei L, Chen Z (2012) Comparison between docetaxel plus cisplatin and cisplatin plus fluorouracil in the neoadjuvant chemoradiotherapy for local advanced esophageal squamous cell carcinoma. Zhonghua Zhong Liu Za Zhi 34: 873–876.
26. Hsu FM, Lin CC, Lee JM, Chang YL, Hsu CH, et al. (2008) Improved local control by surgery and paclitaxel-based chemoradiation for esophageal squamous cell carcinoma: results of a retrospective non-randomized study. J Surg Oncol 98: 34–41.
27. Lagarde SM, ten Kate FJ, Reitsma JB, Busch OR, van Lanschot JJ (2006) Prognostic factors in adenocarcinoma of the esophagus or gastroesophageal junction. J Clin Oncol 24: 4347–4355.
28. Eloubeidi MA, Desmond R, Arguedas MR, Reed CE, Wilcox CM (2002) Prognostic factors for the survival of patients with esophageal carcinoma in the U.S.: the importance of tumor length and lymph node status. Cancer 95: 1434–1443.

16

Upregulation of Autophagy-Related Gene-5 (ATG-5) Is Associated with Chemoresistance in Human Gastric Cancer

Jie Ge[1], Zihua Chen[1], Jin Huang[2], Jinxiang Chen[2], Weijie Yuan[2], Zhenghao Deng[3], Zhikang Chen[1]*

1 Department of Gastrointestinal Surgery, Xiangya Hospital, Central South University, Changsha, Hunan, P. R. China, 2 Department of Oncology, Xiangya Hospital, Central South University, Changsha, Hunan, P. R. China, 3 Department of Pathology, Xiangya Hospital, Central South University, Changsha, Hunan, P. R. China

Abstract

Autophagy-related gene-5 (ATG-5) is one of the key regulators of autophagic cell death. It has been widely regarded as a protective molecular mechanism for tumor cells during the course of chemotherapy. In the present study, we investigated the expression pattern of ATG-5 and multidrug resistance-associated protein-1 (MRP-1) in 135 gastric cancers (GC) patients who were treated with epirubicin, cisplatin and 5-FU adjuvant chemotherapy (ECF) following surgical resection and explored their potential clinical significance. We found that both ATG-5 (77.78%) and MRP-1 (79.26%) were highly expressed in GC patients. ATG-5 expression was significantly associated with depth of wall invasion, TNM stages and distant metastasis of GC ($P<0.05$), whereas MRP-1 expression was significantly linked with tumor size, depth of wall invasion, lymph node metastasis, TNM stages and differentiation status ($P<0.05$). ATG-5 expression was positively correlated with MRP-1 ($rp = 0.616$, $P<0.01$). Increased expression of ATG-5 and MPR-1 was significantly correlated with poor overall survival (OS; $P<0.01$) and disease free survival (DFS; $P<0.01$) of our GC cohort. Furthermore, we demonstrated that ATG-5 was involved in drug resistant of GC cells, which was mainly through regulating autophagy. Our data suggest that upregulated expression of ATG-5, an important molecular feature of protective autophagy, is associated with chemoresistance in GC. Expression of ATG-5 and MRP-1 may be independent prognostic markers for GC treatment.

Editor: Pankaj K. Singh, University of Nebraska Medical Center, United States of America

Funding: This work was supported by National Natural Science Foundation of Hunan Province, China (No. 2012FJ6088). The funders had no role in study design, data collection and analysis, decision to publish, or preparation of the manuscript.

Competing Interests: The authors have declared that no competing interests exist.

* Email: 4059653@qq.com

Introduction

Despite a considerable decline in its incidence rate in many developed countries, gastric cancer (GC) remains the fourth most commonly diagnosed malignancy, and the second leading cause of cancer-related deaths worldwide [1]. Over the past decades, standard multimodal treatment strategies together with other recommended options (e.g. D2 dissection and adjuvant chemotherapy) have failed to cure a large proportion of patients affected with GC, especially for those with advanced and metastatic diseases, with worse survival rates being seen probably due to the presence of chemoresistance during treatment [2]. Hence, identification of novel molecular events underlying the development of this malignancy and its poor prognosis as well as understanding the mechanisms of GC chemoresistance are urgently required for more effective clinical intervention and better management of patients.

Under physiological conditions, autophagy is a lysosome-dependent self-digesting system primarily responsible for removal and recycling of long-lived proteins and damaged/obsolete intracellularorganelles in order to maintain cell homeostasis [3]. The proteins and organelles destined for destruction are sequestered within "double-membrane" vacuoles (autophagosomes),

followed by fusion with lysosomes to build complexes known as autophagosomes, where the contents are degraded by lysosomal hydrolases [4]. It has been documented that autophagy could be induced in response to many unfavorable conditions including nutrient deprivation, oxidative stress or DNA damages and serves as an adaptive cell mechanism, eventually allowing cells to survive and proliferate, while extensive or persistent autophagy results in cell death [5]. Impairments in physiological activation, assembly and function of the autophagic pathway have been increasingly observed in a wide variety of human cancers, although the exact role played by autophagy in cancer genesis and progression is still under controversy. Some data favor the idea that autophagy suppresses tumorigenesis, whereas other evidence suggest that autophagy is able to trigger tumor initiation and protects tumor cells from undergoing apoptosis [6]. Interestingly, inhibition of autophagy was recently found to enhance the anti-tumor activity of several cytotoxic agents. Li and colleagues reported that autophagy was activated as a protective mechanism against the cellular effects of 5-FU-treatment and inhibition of autophagy by 3-methyladenine augmented 5-FU-induced apoptosis in colon cancer cells [7,8]. On the other hand, some anticancer drugs (e.g. cetuximab and dasatinib) were demonstrated to induce autophagic cell death through different mechanisms in some cancer cells [9–

13]. The molecular machinery by which autophagy regulates survival or death of neoplastic cells remains largely obscure hitherto. The autophagy pathway is a highly-modulated dynamic process predominantly executed by the autophagy-related (ATG) family of genes, which is governed by several key kinases including mTOR, PI3k/Akt, AMPK and MAPK [14,15]. ATG-5 is a central regulator necessary for autophagy in terms of its involvement in autophagosome elongation [16]. Enforced expression of ATG-5 sensitized tumor cells to anticancer drug treatment both *in vitro* and *in vivo*; in contrast siRNA-mediated inhibition of ATG-5 led to partial resistance to chemotherapy [17].

Postoperative adjuvant chemotherapy is presently a major treatment for GC; however, the overall efficacy of chemotherapy remains poor possibly as a consequence of the presence of multidrug resistance (MDR) phenotype. Unlike other tumor entities, expression of the classical MDR-mediating molecules such as glutathione S-transferase and multidrug resistance gene 1 is not very prevalent in GC tissues, indicating that there might exist a complicated mechanism for the development of MDR in this malignant disease [18]. As one of the classical drug-resistant mechanisms, multidrug resistance-associated protein 1 (MRP1/ABCC1) has been found to be strongly expressed in GC and thus may exert pivotal roles in mediating MDR in GC [19,20]. However, it remains unknown whether MRP-1 expression is associated with ATG-5 expression. And also whether autophagy is involved in chemoresistence in GC patients is unclear.

In the present study, we first employed immunohistochemistry to investigate the expression profile of ATG-5 and MRP1 in a sum of 135 GC patients who received ECF (epirubicin, cisplatin and 5-FU) adjuvant chemotherapy following surgical resection. The correlations between ATG-5 and MRP-1 expression as well as their expression with various clinicopathological features of GC and clinical outcomes were also assessed.

Materials and Methods

Patients and tissue samples

A total of 135 GC patients consisting of 91 males and 44 females who underwent surgery at the Department of Gastrointestinal Surgery, Xiangya Hospital, Central South University (C.S.U), China, between January 1st 2007 and December 31st 2008 were enrolled in this study. The average age of the cohort was 53.62 ± 9.73 years, with a range of 26 to 72. Theprimary GC tumor tissuesand matched non-cancerous(NC) tissues located at least 5 cm away from the tumor core were obtained after surgical resection and immediately processed and stored until further use. None of the recruited patients had chemotherapy or radiotherapy prior to surgical operation. The histopathological diagnosis was carried out preoperatively and confirmed by surgery. All participants with stage IB to IV tumors received ECF chemotherapy after surgery (Dose: epirubicin 50 mg/m^2 on day 1, cisplatin 60 mg/m^2 on day 1 and continuous intravenous infusion of 5-FU 500 mg/m^2/d for 4 days, repeated every 3 weeks up to 24 weeks). The clinical characteristics of these patients were listed in Table 1.

All cases in this study were reviewed and all specimens were histopathologically re-examined in October, 2012. The depth of wall invasion, regional lymph node metastasis, and histological grade were confirmed by the same group of two experienced senior pathologists. The patients were categorized based on the differentiation status of cancer cells into three histological grades: well, moderate and poor. Based on a combination of loco-regional tumor involvement and the presence of metastasis, all cases were staged according to the TNM Classification of Malignant Tumours (TNM) stage grouping [21]. For the analysis of survival,

the date of operation was used to represent the start point of the follow-up visit. Patients who died of other diseases rather than GC or other unexpected events were excluded from the case collection. The cause of death recruited in this study was aggravation of GC. The overall survival (OS) was calculated as a period starting from the date of the initial surgery to the date of death, or the date of the last follow-up as the end point. The disease free survival (DFS) was defined as the time interval from surgery until the date of local relapse or first distant organ metastasis. Informed written consent was obtained from each patient before surgery and this study was approved by the Research Ethics Committee of Central South University, China. All specimens were handled and made anonymous according to the ethical and legal guidelines.

Immunohistochemistry

The fresh specimens were fixed in 10% neutral buffered formalin and subsequently embedded with paraffin. The paraffin-embedded tissues were cut at 4 μm and then deparaffinized with xylene and rehydrated for further H&E or peroxidase immunohistochemistry staining by using the DAKO EnVision System. In brief, following proteolytic digestion and blocking with endogenous peroxidase, tissue slides were incubated with the primary antibodies (ATG5: ab54033; MRP1: ab32574; Abcam Inc., Cambridge, UK) against respective target proteins at a dilution of 1:500 overnight at 4°C. After washing with PBS, peroxidase labeled polymer and substrate-chromogen were then employed in order to visualize the immnohistochemical staining. Finally, sections were counterstained with hematoxylin, cover-slipped with mounting medium, and examined by light microscopy. All the procedures were performed at the Department of Pathology, Xiangya Hospital, C.S.U. Slides were interpreted independently by two experienced pathologists, who were blind to patients' information. We quantified staining intensity and percentage of stained cells using a previously described approach [22,23]: the percentage of positively stained cells (0%−100%) was multiplied by the dominant intensity pattern of staining, considering 1 as negative or trace, 2 as weak, 3 as moderate and 4 as strong. Therefore, the overall score ranged from 0 to 400. Patients were subsequently categorized into four different subgroups: score 0−99, score 100−199, score 200−299 and score 300−400.

Western blot analysis

Whole cell extracts were prepared using 0.14 M NaCl, 0.2 M triethanolamine, 0.2% sodium deoxycholate, 0.5% Nonidet P-40 and supplemented with a protease inhibitor (all of the products were from Sigma, St. Louis, Missouri, USA). Then, protein sample was run through a 12% sodium dodecyl sulfate-polyacrylamide gel electrophoresis (SDS-PAGE) gel and transferred to a membrane. The transferred membranes were subsequently incubated overnight at 4°C with a primary antibody. After washing, the membrane was incubated with a horseradish peroxidase (HRP)-linked secondary antibody for 1 h at room temperature. The primary antibodies were anti-ATG-5 (Santa Cruz, CA, USA), anti-LC3A/B (abcam, Cambridge, UK) and anti-β-Actin (Santa Cruz, CA, USA). All reported results are the average ratios of three different independent experiments.

Cell proliferation assay

Cells were seeded onto 96 well plates (10000 cells/well) for 24 h before treatment. MTT assays were used to assess cell proliferation at different time point after treatment. The MTT assay was performed as follows: MTT was added to each well and the plates were incubated at 37°C for 4 h. The MTT medium mixture was then removed and 150 μL of dimethyl sulfoxide (DMSO) was

Table 1. Association between ATG-5 expression and clinicopathological characteristics of GC patients.

Factors	Patients (n = 135)	ATG-5 expression (%)				P
		0–99	100–199	200–299	300–400	
Gender						0.99
Male	91	21.98	14.29	46.15	17.58	
Female	44	22.73	15.91	45.45	15.91	
Age (years) Mean±SD	135	56.00±9.09	54.5±10.52	53.05±9.13	51.48±11.17	0.370▲
Tumor size (cm)						0.15
<5.0	80	25	18.75	43.75	12.5	
≥5.0	55	18.18	9.09	49.09	23.64	
Location of tumor						0.086
upper	21	19.05	33.33	38.1	9.52	
middle	35	11.43	12.5	54.29	22.86	
low	79	27.85	11.39	44.3	16.46	
H. pylori infection						0.961
Positive	73	23.29	15.07	43.84	17.81	
Negative	62	20.97	14.52	48.39	16.13	
Depth of wall invasion						<0.001
T1	10	50	20	30	0	
T2	15	66.67	13.33	13.33	6.67	
T3	32	25	12.5	43.75	18.75	
T4	78	8.97	15.38	55.13	20.51	
Lymph node metastasis						0.056
N0	18	22.22	33.33	38.89	5.56	
N1	36	33.33	5.56	50	11.11	
N2	44	22.73	9.09	47.73	20.45	
N3	37	10.81	21.62	43.24	24.32	
Distant metastasis						0.018
M0	131	22.9	15.27	46.56	15.27	
M1	4	0	0	25	75	
TNM stages						<0.001
IB	10	70	10	20	0	
II	31	45.16	32.26	22.58	0	
III	90	10	10	57.78	22.22	
IV	4	0	0	25	75	
Differentiation status						0.412
Well	17	41.18	17.65	23.53	17.65	
Moderate	60	20	16.67	48.33	15	
Poor	58	18.97	12.07	50	18.97	

▲Statistical analyses were carried out with the One-Way ANOVA test and others were carried out with the Pearson's χ^2 test.

added to each well. The absorbance was measured at 570 nm using a multiwall spectrophotometer.

RNA interference

siRNA duplexes targeting ATG-5 were synthesized as follows: siRNA-ATG5-486: GACGUUG GUAACUGACAAATT; siRNA-ATG5-695: GUCCAUCUAAGGAUGCAAUTT and siRNA-ATG5-938: GACCUUUCAUUCAGAAGCUTT. siRNA duplexes containing non-specific sequences were used as a negative control (NC): UUCUCCGAACGUGUCACGUTT. Different siRNAs were transfected separately into cells using the Lipofectamine 2000 reagent, and the medium was replaced 6 h after transfection.

Real-time RT-PCR

Total RNA from the cell lines and tissues were extracted using the Trizol reagent (Invitrogen, Carlsbad, USA), following the manufacturer's instructions. The concentration of RNA was measured using a spectrophotometer. A cDNA pool was synthesized using 1 μg of total RNA and TaqMan Reverse Transcription Reagents (Applied Biosystems, Foster City, USA) as described by the manufacturer. The expression of the target gene

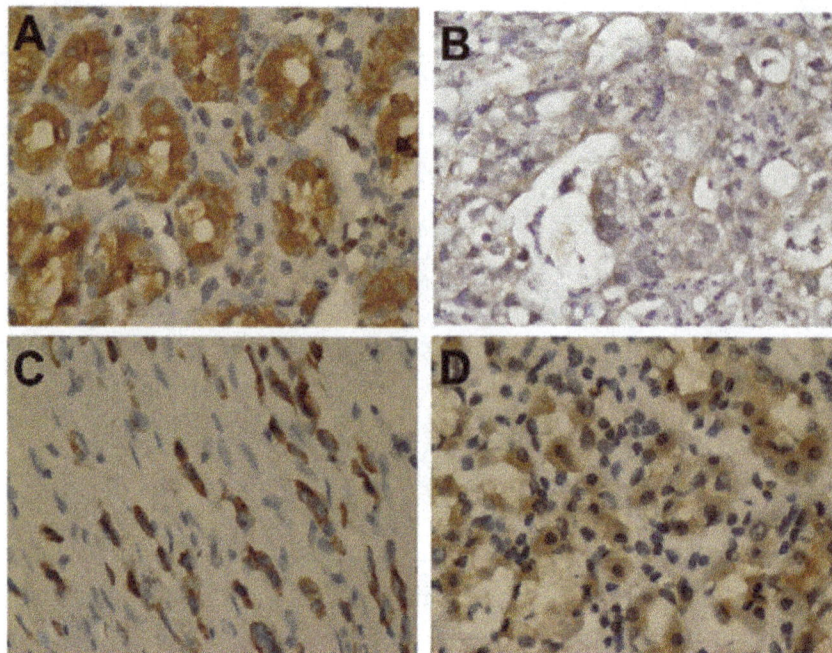

Figure 1. Representative images showing immunohistochemical staining for ATG-5 in non-tumorous and GC tumor tissues. (A) ATG-5 staining in non-cancerous gastric tissues scored 285(×200); (B) ATG-5 staining in GC tumor tissues scored 50(×400); (C) ATG-5 staining in GC tumor tissues scored 270(×400); (D) ATG-5 staining in GC tumor tissues scored 400(×200).

was evaluated using a relative quantification approach ($2^{-\Delta\Delta Ct}$ method) with β-actin as the internal reference.

Immunofluorescence assay

Cells were permeabilized with 0.3% Triton X-100 for 10 min followed by fixation with 2–4% Methanal for 15 min, and blocked with 3% sheep serum at room temperature for 60 min. Then, probed with primary antibodies anti-LC3B (Santa Cruz, CA, USA) overnight at room temperature, and cells were washed three times with PBS. Stained with Alexa Fluor 488 conjugated 488 rabbit anti-goat IgG for 1 h at room temperature, and then the cells were washed three times with PBS. Nuclei were visualized by staining with DAPI (Sigma, USA) for 2 min. The stained cells were observed with inverted fluorescence microscope.

Statistical analysis

All statistical analyses were performed with the SPSS software package 15.0 for Windows (SPSS Inc., Chicago, IL, USA). Quantitative data were presented as Mean ± SD. Pearson's χ^2 test was used to compare the difference among ranked data, while one-Way-ANOVA test was carried out to compare the difference among quantitative data. Survival analyses were carried out by using the Kaplan-Meier method and compared by the log-rank test. The Cox-regression model was performed to evaluate the independent hazard ratio of each variable in the multivariate analysis. The correlation between ATG5 and MRP1 expression was examined using Bivariate Correlation (Pearson) test. Differences were considered as statistically significant when P values were less than 0.05.

Results

Expression of ATG-5 and MRP-1 in GC

The expression pattern and location of ATG-5 and MRP-1 in our GC patients, who were treated with epirubicin, cisplatin and 5-FU adjuvant chemotherapy (ECF) following surgical resection, were examined using immunohistochemical analysis. Among the 135 GC specimens, 105(77.78%) were positive for ATG-5 immunoreactivity, and 107 (79.26%) were MRP-1 positive. As depicted in Figure 1, we found that ATG5 was predominantly expressed in the cytoplasm. Moreover, over-expression of ATG-5 was positively correlated with that of MRP-1 in GC. (r = 0.616, $P<0.001$), as revealed by the Bivariate Correlation test. The positive expression in adjacent non-cancerous tissues were 113(83.70%) for ATG-5 and 89(65.93%) for MRP-1. The data showed that both ATG-5 and MRP-1 were positively expressed in cancer and non-cancerous tissues, which suggest that ATG-5 and MRP-1 may be induced by chemotherapy in both tumor and non-tumor tissues. As all our patient samples were treated with ECF chemotherapy, and we found that both ATG-5 and MRP-1 were highly expressed and positively correlated in those samples. Meanwhile, previous study indicates that MRP-1 maybe associated with multi-drug resistance in GC. Together with previous finding, our results suggest that ATG-5 and MRP-1 may be involved in chemoresistance in GC patients.

Associations between expression of ATG-5 or MRP-1 and clinicopathological characteristics of GC

The associations of ATG-5 and MRP1 expression with various clinicopathological parameters of GC are shown in Table 1 and Table 2, respectively. Expression of ATG-5 was significantly associated with depth of wall invasion, distant metastasis and TNM stages of GC ($P<0.001$, $P = 0.018$, $P<0.001$ respectively). MRP-1 expression was significantly associated with increased tumor size, depth of wall invasion, regional lymph nodes metastasis, TNM stages ($P = 0.032$, $P<0.001$, P = 0.016, P< 0.001 respectively) and differentiation status ($P = 0.005$). To further determine the involvement o f ATG-5 and MRP-1 in the GC development, we performed survival analysis within our

Table 2. Association between MRP-1 expression and clinicopathological characteristics of GC patients.

Factors	Patients (n = 135)	ATG-5 expression (%)				P
		0–99	100–199	200–299	300–400	
Gender						0.675
Male	91	19.78	21.98	43.96	14.29	
Female	44	22.73	22.73	34.09	20.45	
Age (years) Mean±SD	135					0.084▲
Tumor size (cm)		54.61±10.31	56.23±8.97	53.31±9.56	49.45±9.61	0.032
<5.0	80					
≥5.0	55	22.5	30	33.75	13.75	
Location of tumor		18.18	10.91	50.91	20	0.15
upper	21					
middle	35	19.05	28.57	38.1	14.29	
low	79	22.86	11.43	40	25.71	
H. pylori infection		20.25	25.32	41.77	12.66	0.51
Positive	73					
Negative	62	16.44	23.29	41.1	19.18	
Depth of wall invasion		25.81	20.97	40.32	12.9	<0.001
T1	10					
T2	15	60	20	20	0	
T3	32	53.33	26.67	20	0	
T4	78	28.13	15.63	37.5	18.75	
Lymph node metastasis		6.41	24.36	48.72	20.51	0.016
N0	18					
N1	36	22.22	44.44	33.33	0	
N2	44	33.33	16.67	36.11	13.89	
N3	37	18.18	22.73	47.73	11.36	
Distant metastasis		10.81	16.22	40.54	32.43	0.193
M0	131	21.37	22.9	40.46	15.27	
M1	4	0	0	50	50	
TNM stages						<0.001
IB	10	70	20	10	0	
II	31	54.84	35.48	9.68	0	
III	90	4.44	18.89	54.44	22.22	
IV	4					
Differentiation status		0	0	50	50	0.005
Well	17	52.94	17.65	23.53	5.88	
Moderate	60	16.67	31.67	36.67	15	
Poor	58	15.52	13.79	50	20.69	

▲Statistical analyses were carried out with the One-Way ANOVA test and others were carried out with the Pearson's χ^2 test.

patient samples. Our survival analyses demonstrated that the total overall survival (OS) rate of our GC cohort was 43.70% with a mean survival of 39.849 months (95% CI, 35.636–44.061 months); whereas the disease free survival (DFS) rate was 34.07% with a mean survival of 35.802 months (95% CI, 31.618–39.986 months). We next classified the patients into four different subgroups according to the scores of immunohistochemistry staining. The Kaplan-Meier survival analysis revealed a higher ATG-5 expression was significantly associated with poorer OS ($P<0.001$) and DFS ($P = 0.003$). Pairwise comparisons indicated that patients carrying the highest ATG-5 expression (scores 300–400) had the poorest survival rates as compared to that of other subgroups

(Figure 2A and 2B). Consistently, upregulated MRP-1 expression was found to be significantly associated with poor OS ($P = 0.001$) and DFS ($P = 0.018$) of our GC patients. The subgroup with the highest MRP1 expression scores (0–99) appeared to have the worst prognosis (Figure 2C and 2D) in comparison with other subgroups. Our data also showed that there was a significant correlation between TNM stages and survival of GC patients. Patients with stage III and IV tumors displayed poorer prognosis as compared to those harboring stage IB and II tumors ($P<0.01$) (Figure 2E and 2F). More interestingly, the Cox's multivariate hazard regression model demonstrated that ATG-5 and MRP-1 expression levels and TNM stages were all independent and

Table 3. The multivariate Cox proportional hazard analysis of prognostic factors for OS and DFS rates of 135 GC patients.

Factors	OS				DFS			
	β	Wald	RR# (95.0% CI)	P	β	Wald	RR# (95.0% CI)	P
MRP-1(300-400)		13.035		0.005		11.843		0.008
MRP-1(0-99)	-1.797	9.388	0.166(0.052-0.523)	0.002	-1.785	10.408	0.168(0.0576-0.496)	0.001
MRP-1(100-199)	-1.121	7.799	0.326(0.148-0.716)	0.007	-0.938	6.578	0.391(0.191-0.802)	0.011
MRP-1(200-299)	-0.353	1.373	0.702(0.389-1.268)	0.216	-0.413	2.076	0.662(0.377-1.161)	0.146
ATG-5	0.379	5.538	1.460(1.065-2.002)	0.037	0.486	9.73	1.626 (1.198-2.207)	0.004
TNM stage	1.869	17.151	6.484(2.677-15.705)	<0.001	1.85	18.785	6.362(2.755-14.688)	<0.001
Tumor size	0.109	0.178	0.897(0.542-1.486)	0.673	0.091	0.146	0.913(0.573-1.456)	0.702
Differentiation status	0.177	0.821	1.194(0.814-1.752)	0.365	0.192	1.141	1.212(0.852-1.726)	0.285
Hp infection	-0.115	0.238	0.891(0.560-1.417)	0.626	-0.122	0.307	0.885(0.574-1.364)	0.579
Location	-0.021	0.017	0.979(0.710-1.350)	0.898	-0.091	0.356	0.913(0.677-1.231)	0.551
Gender	0.108	0.44	0.897(0.652-1.236)	0.507	0.187	0.579	0.829(0.512-1.343)	0.447

#Relative Risk; CI: confidence interval.

significant prognostic indicators for predicting the OS ($P = 0.037$, $P = 0.005$, $P < 0.001$ respectively) and DFS ($P = 0.004$, $P = 0.008$, $P < 0.001$ respectively) of GC (Table 3). Our data indicated the ATG-5 and MRP-1 were closely related with the GC development and may serve as poor prognosis markers in GC treatment.

ATG-5 was significantly upregulated in chemoresistant cells

To further explore the role of ATG-5 in the tumorigenesis and drug resistant. We detected the protein expression in several gastric cancer cell lines (AGS, BGC-832, SGC7901, SGC7901/DPP and MKN45) and in an immortalized human gastric epithelial mucosa cell line (GES). Interestingly, we found that ATG-5 was dramatically overexpressed in DPP resistant cell line, SGC7901/DPP cells, compared with all the other cell lines which include DPP sensitive SGC7901 cells (Figure 3A). We further confirmed that SGC7901/DPP cells are resistant to DPP treatment. The IC 25, IC50 and IC75 were 15.4 μM, 38.7 μM and 93.53 μM in SGC7901 cells. In contrast, The IC 25, IC50 and IC75 were 120.03 μM, 271.9 μM and 423.7 μM in SGC7901/DPP (Figure 3B). It is about 5 to 9 times higher than that in non-drug resistant cells. Our finding strongly suggests that ATG-5 contributes to drug resistant of the GC cells.

Inhibition of ATG-5 sensitized chemoresistant cells to drug treatment

To further prove that ATG-5 contributes to the drug resistant of the GC cells, we used small interfering RNAs (siRNAs) to knockdown the expression of ATG-5. Three siRNAs were designed. Our real time PCR and western blot results showed that all three siRNAs inhibited the expression of ATG-5 at both mRNA and protein level (Figure 4A and 4B). We chose one, siRNA-ATG5-695, with highest knockdown efficiency to perform the following experiment. We knockdown ATG-5 expression and then treated the cells with DPP. Cell proliferation ability was examined at 0, 48 and 72 hours after treatment. Our result showed that knockdowning ATG-5 did not affect cell proliferation in SGC7901/DPP cells compared with control siRNA (siRNA NC). DPP treatment alone slightly inhibited the proliferation of the cells. Interestingly, when we knockdown the expression of ATG-5 and treated the cells with DPP at the same time, the cell proliferation ability was further suppressed compared with cells treated with DPP alone 48 and 72 hours after treatment (Figure 4 C). Our data further support that ATG-5 contributes to the drug resistant of GC cells.

Autophagy was involved in the drug resistant of DC cells

As ATG-5 is a central regulator of autophagy, we speculated that autophagy may be involved in the drug resistant of GC cells. So we used 3MA, which is an autophagy inhibitor, to treat the drug resistant cells. As expected, we found that 3MA together with DPP treatment had a similar effect with ATG-5 kncokdown together with DPP treatment (Figure 4C and 4D). The data demonstrate that autophagy contributes to the drug resistant. Then, we examined whether autophagy was changed during the treatment. We used Immunofluorescence assay to detect LC3B expression level, which is an autophagy marker in the cells. Our data showed that autophagy was suppressed after silencing ATG-5 or treating the cells with 3MA (Figure 5A). And western blot result further confirmed that LC3A/B protein expression was only affected in cells treated with siRNA-ATG5 or 3MA. Accordingly, cell proliferation was further inhibited only when autophagy was inhibited (Figure 4 and figure 5). Therefore, our data revealed that

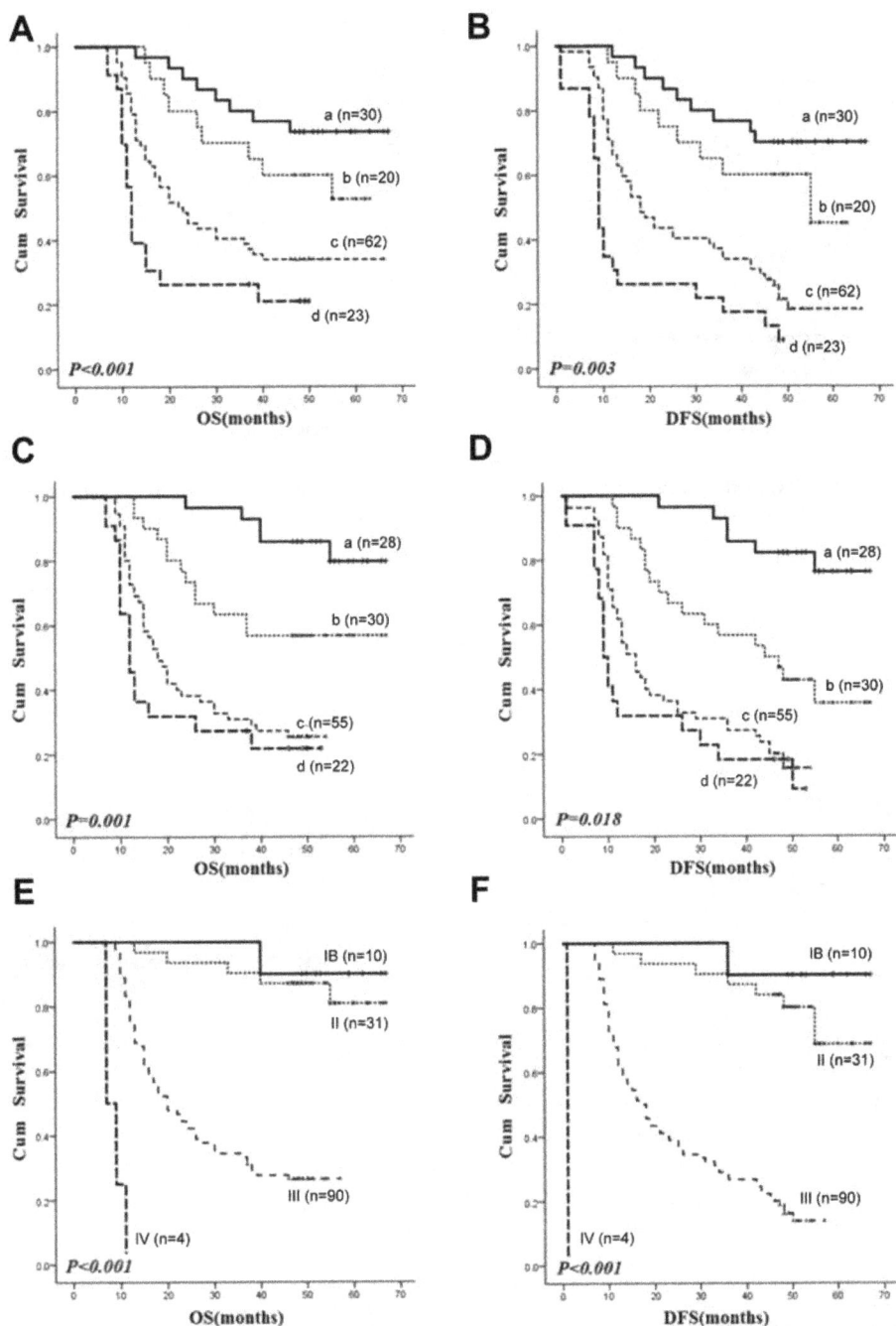

Figure 2. Kaplane-Meier statistical analyses showing OS and DFS in different subgroups of GC patients. (A and B) Patients were divided into four following subgroups based on ATG-5 immunostaining: scored 0–99 (curve a), scored 100–199 (curve b), scored 200–299 (curve c) and scored 300–400 (curve d). The difference among different subgroups was statistically significant as evaluated by overall Log-rank comparisons (OS: $P<0.001$, DFS: $P=0.003$). Pairwise Log-rank comparisons showed that the subgroup D exhibited the poorest survival rates as compared to other subgroups (OS: $P<0.05$, DFS: $P<0.01$). (C and D) Patients were divided into four following subgroups based on MRP-1 immunostaining: scored 0–99 (curve a), scored 100–199 (curve b), scored 200–299 (curve c) and scored 300–400 (curve d). The difference among various subgroups was statistically significant by overall Log-rank comparisons (OS: $P=0.001$, DFS: $P=0.018$). Pairwise Log-rank comparisons showed that the subgroup A had the most favorable prognosis among the four subgroups (OS: $P<0.05$, DFS: $P<0.001$). (E and F) Patients were divided into four subgroups according to different TNM stages. The difference among different subgroups was statistically significant by overall Log-rank comparisons (OS: $P<0.001$, DFS: $P<0.001$). Pairwise Log-rank comparisons showed that subgroups III or IV exhibited poorer survival rates than that of subgroups IB and II (OS: $P<0.01$, DFS: $P<0.001$).

ATG-5 was involved in the drug resistant of DC cells, which was mainly through affect the autophagy of the cancer cells.

Discussion

GC remains one of the most frequent malignant tumors on a global basis in spite of its declining incidence and the total number

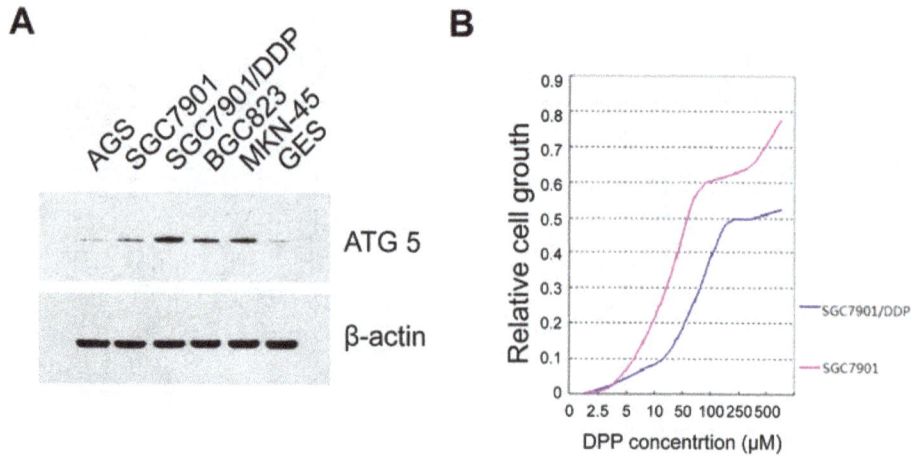

Figure 3. ATG-5 was upregulated in chemoresistant cells. (A) The level of ATG5 was detected in cell lines using western blot analysis. β -actin was used as internal controls.(B) The IC 25, IC50 and IC75 of SGC-7901 and SGC-7901/DDP cells were tested using the MTT assays after DPP treatment.

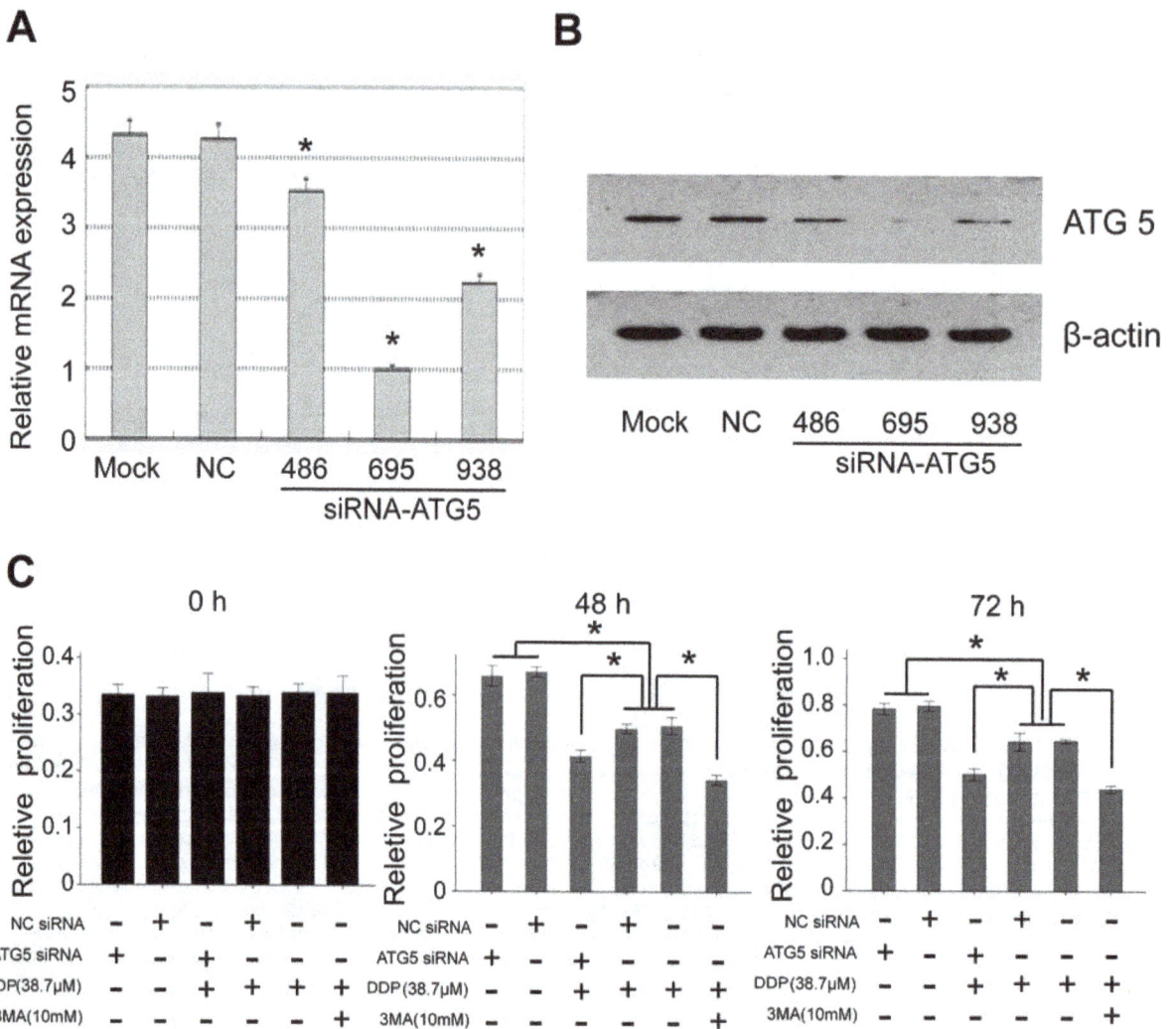

Figure 4. Silencing ATG-5 sensitized chemoresistant cells to drug treatment. (A) The mRNA level of ATG-5 was detected by real time PCR after treatment with siRNAs. GAPDH was used as internal controls. (B) The protein level of ATG-5 was detected by western blot after treatment with siRNAs. β -actin was used as internal controls. (C) The proliferation ability was tested using MTT assay 48 hours or 72 hours after different treatment.

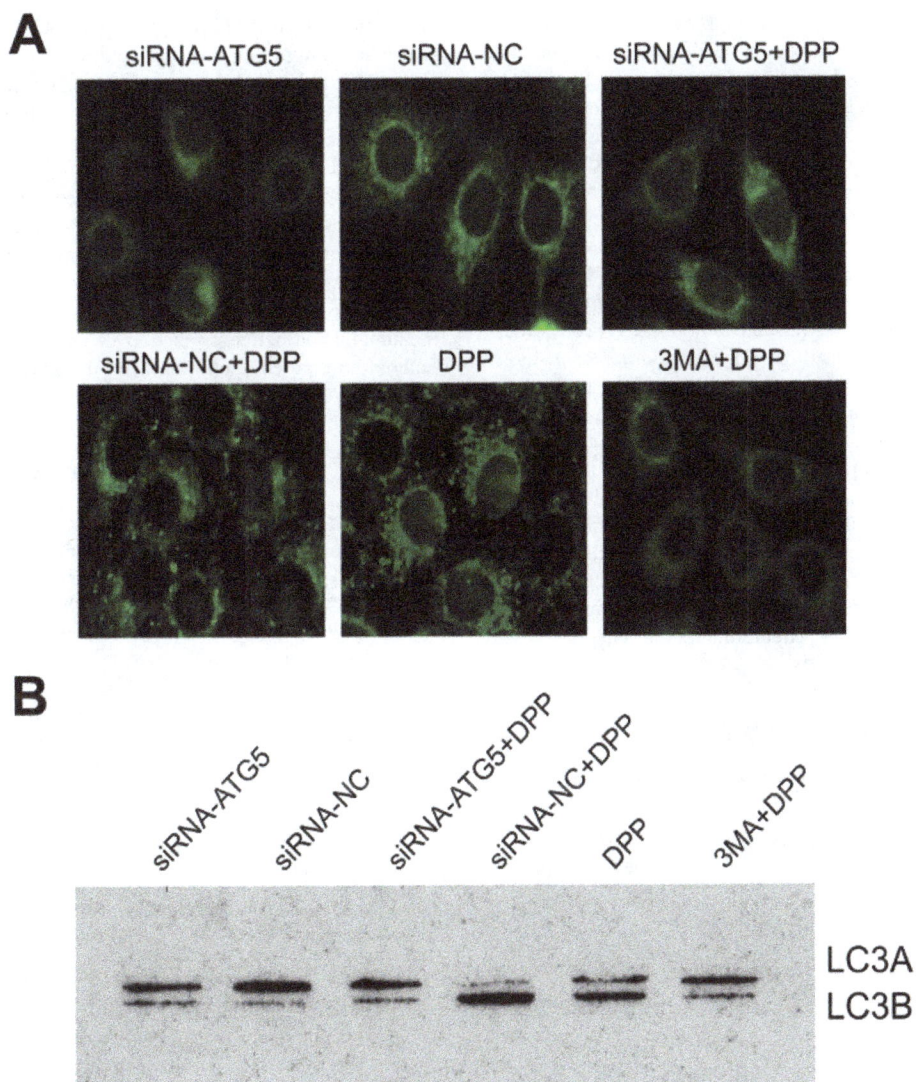

Figure 5. Autophagy was involved in the drug resistant of DC cells. (A) The autophagy was detected by immunofluorescence assay of LC3B in the cells 48 hours after different treatment. (B) The protein levels of LC3A and LC3B were tested by western blot. β-actin was used as internal controls.

is predicted to continuously climb as a result of population growth. In men, GC ranks the second in mortality rate; in women, it is the fourth in mortality [24,25]. The crude mortality rate of GC in China was 25.2 per 100 000 [26]. In our study, we examined the expression of ATG-5 and MRP-1 in a cohort of GC patient after chemotherapy. Then, we demonstrated that ATG-5 was upregulated in cisplatin (DDP) resistant cell line. Furthermore, after ATG-5 expression or aotophogy was inhibited, the cancer cells were sensitized to DPP treatment. Our results provide new insight into the mechanism of chemoresistant in GC progression.

We evaluated the exression profile of ATG-5 and MRP-1 in 135 Chinese GC patients. In an agreement with previous report [22], our results showed that a high percentage of GC tissues expressed ATG-5, and ATG-5 expression was statistically associated with depth of wall invasion, distant metastasis and TNM stages of GC. These findings support a notion that high expression level of ATG5 may contribute to, some extent, a more aggressive and malignant phenotype in GC. This viewpoint is further supported by our finding of the association between higher ATG5 expression

in GC and poorer prognosis of patients (see more discussion below). More importantly, we identified a positive correlation between ATG-5 and MRP1 expression in our GC cohort. Considering the fact that MRP1 is an ABC transmembrane transport protein well known to promote the MDR phenotype in GC, it is reasonable to propose that ATG-5 may be also implicated in conferring GC chemoresistance through certain unknown molecular mechanisms.

It is widely accepted that recurrence and metastasis are two major hurdles in our efforts to improve low OS and DFS survival rate of GC. Chemoresistance remains one of the most important reasons leading to tumor repopulation/recurrence following treatment. Appropriate option of individual treatment will be undoubtedly beneficial to improve the clinical outcome; nonetheless, current treatment decision is mostly dependent on the TNM stages [27,28]. Our survival analyses in the 135 GC patients with stage IB to IV tumors revealed that both ATG-5 and MRP-1 expression were able to independently predict the OS and DFS after treatment with adjuvant ECF chemotherapy, suggesting that monitoring their expression levels in combination of conventional prognostic markers may provide us with additional valuable information for a better evaluation of chemotherapy effect in GC patients. Interestingly, we found the ATG-5 was overexpressed in drug resistant GC cell lines. And silencing ATG-5 can sensitized the drug resistant cells to chemotherapy again. Our data suggest that ATG-5 may be a target for chemoresistant paitents.

Accumulating evidence has suggested that autophagy is capable to trigger both cell survival and cell death under different contexts. Liu et al reported that through inhibition of the PI3K/Akt/ mTOR pathway, β-elemene could induce protective autophagy to assist GC cells better adapt to stressful conditions and protect them from undergoing apoptosis death [29]. Furthermore, recent studies have shown that the PI3K/Akt/mTOR signaling pathway is frequently activated in human gastrointesti-nal malignancies [30]. The PI3K/Akt signaling also modulates MDR in GC cell through the regulation of p-glycoprotein, Bcl2 and Bax [31]. Likewise, some anticancer agents have been reported to inhibit mTOR signaling and induce autophagy in cancer cells by degrading many major components in the mTOR axis [14,32]. Overall, these data suggest that autophagy could be induced during chemotherapy, and suppression of autophagic pathways using autophagy inhibitor have potential to improve the chemotherapeutic effectiveness in GC patients with ATG-5 high expression. In support, we found that when autophagy was inhibited, the drug resistant cells were also sensitized to drug treatment again as silencing ATG-5 expression. So, our result support that autophagy contributes to chemoresistant in patient.

In summary, over-expression of ATG-5, a key molecular player of the autophagic pathway, is associated with chemoresistance in GC. Expression of ATG-5 and MRP-1 could be considered as independent prognostic markers for predicting OS and DFS of GC patients based on the currently obtained data. On the basis of TNM stages, detection of their expression levels may be clinically meaningful for better prediction of chemotherapeutic treatment outcomes in patients suffering from this malignant disease. Future studies involving assessment of a larger number of cases, ideally from a different ethnic background, are definitely warranted to confirm our findings in this study.

Author Contributions

Conceived and designed the experiments: JG Zihua Chen. Performed the experiments: JG WY JH. Analyzed the data: JG JC WY ZD Zhikang Chen. Contributed reagents/materials/analysis tools: Zihua Chen. Contributed to the writing of the manuscript: Zhikang Chen JG.

References

1. Jemal A, Bray F, Center MM, Ferlay J, Ward E, et al (2011) Global cancer statistics. CA Cancer J Clin 61: 69–90.
2. Zhang D, Fan D (2007) Multidrug resistance in gastric cancer: recent research advances and ongoing therapeutic challenges. Expert Rev Anticancer Ther 7: 1369–78.
3. Levine B (2007) Cell biology: autophagy and cancer. Nature 446: 745–7.
4. Maycotte P, Thorburn A (2011) Autophagy and cancer therapy. Cancer Biol Ther 11: 127–37.
5. Mizushima N (2007) Autophagy: process and function. Genes Dev 21: 2861–73.
6. Marx J (2006) Autophagy: is it cancer's friend or foe? Science 312: 1160–1.
7. Li J, Hou N, Faried A, Tsutsumi S, Kuwano H (2010) Inhibition of autophagy augments 5-fluorouracil chemotherapy in human colon cancer in vitro and in vivo model. Eur J Cancer 46: 1900–9.
8. Li J, Hou N, Faried A, Tsutsumi S, Takeuchi T, et al (2009) Inhibition of autophagy by 3-MA enhances the effect of 5-FU-induced apoptosis in colon cancer cells. Ann Surg Oncol 16: 761–71.
9. Li X, Fan Z (2010) The epidermal growth factor receptor antibody cetuximab induces autophagy in cancer cells by downregulating HIF-1alpha and Bcl-2 and activating the beclin 1/hVps34 complex. Cancer Res 70: 5942–52.
10. Sasaki K, Tsuno NH, Sunami E, Tsurita G, Kawai K, et al (2010) Chloroquine potentiates the anti-cancer effect of 5-fluorouracil on colon cancer cells. BMC Cancer 10: 370.
11. Amaravadi RK, Yu D, Lum JJ, Bui T, Christophorou MA, et al (2007) Autophagy inhibition enhances therapy-induced apoptosis in a Myc-induced model of lymphoma. J Clin Invest 117: 326–36.
12. Hwang MS, Baek WK (2010) Glucosamine induces autophagic cell death through the stimulation of ER stress in human glioma cancer cells. Biochem Biophys Res Commun 399: 111–6.
13. Le XF, Mao W, Lu Z, Carter BZ, Bast RC (2010) Dasatinib induces autophagic cell death in human ovarian cancer. Cancer 116: 4980–90.
14. Jung C, Ro S, Cao J, Otto N, Kim D (2010) mTOR regulation of autophagy. FEBS Lett 584: 1287–95.
15. Mirzoeva OK, Hann B, Hom YK, Debnath J, Aftab D, et al (2011) Autophagy suppression promotes apoptotic cell death in response to inhibition of the PI3K-mTOR pathway in pancreatic adenocarcinoma. J Mol Med (Berl) 89: 877–89.
16. Klionsky DJ (2007) Autophagy: from phenomenology to molecular understanding in less than a decade. Nat Rev Mol Cell Biol 8: 931–7.
17. Yousefi S, Perozzo R, Schmid I, Ziemiecki A, Schaffner T, et al (2006) Calpain-mediated cleavage of Atg5 switches autophagy to apoptosis. Nat Cell Biol 8: 1124–32.
18. Fan K, Fan D, Cheng LF, Li C (2000) Expression of multidrug resistance-related markers in gastric cancer. Anticancer Res 20: 4809–14.
19. Lacueva J, Perez-Ramos M, Soto J, Oliver I, Andrada E, et al (2005) Multidrug resistance-associated protein (MRP1) gene is strongly expressed in gastric carcinomas. Analysis by immunohistochemistry and real-time quantitative RT-PCR. Histopathology 46: 389–95.
20. Zhang D, Fan D (2010) New insights into the mechanisms of gastric cancer multidrug resistance and future perspectives. Future Oncol 6: 527–37.
21. Edge S, Byrd D, Compton C, Fritz A, Greene F, et al (2010) American Joint Committee on Cancer. AJCC cancer staging manual. 7th. New York: Springer.
22. An CH, Kim MS, Yoo NJ, Park SW, Lee SH (2011) Mutational and expressional analyses of ATG5, an autophagy-related gene, in gastrointestinal cancers. Pathol Res Pract 207: 433–7.
23. Ge J, Chen Z, Wu S, Chen J, Li X, et al (2009) Expression levels of insulin-like growth factor-1 and multidrug resistance-associated protein-1 indicate poor prognosis in patients with gastric cancer. Digestion 80: 148–58.
24. Black RJ, Bray F, Ferlay J, Parkin DM (1997) Cancer incidence and mortality in the European Union: cancer registry data and estimates of national incidence for 1990. Eur J Cancer 33: 1075–107.
25. Bray F, Sankila R, Ferlay J, Parkin DM (2002) Estimates of cancer incidence and mortality in Europe in 1995. Eur J Cancer 38: 99–166.
26. Sun XD, Mu R, Zhou YS, Dai XD, Zhang SW, et al (2004) [Analysis of mortality rate of stomach cancer and its trend in twenty years in China]. Zhonghua Zhong Liu Za Zhi 26: 4–9.
27. Cervantes A, Rosello S, Roda D, Rodriguez-Braun E (2008) The treatment of advanced gastric cancer: current strategies and future perspectives. Ann Oncol 19 Suppl 5: v103–7.
28. Suh YS, Lee HJ, Jung EJ, Kim MA, Nam KT, et al (2012) The combined expression of metaplasia biomarkers predicts the prognosis of gastric cancer. Ann Surg Oncol 19: 1240–9.
29. Liu J, Zhang Y, Qu J, Xu L, Hou K, et al (2011) beta-Elemene-induced autophagy protects human gastric cancer cells from undergoing apoptosis. BMC Cancer 11: 183.
30. Ko JK, Auyeung KK (2013) Target-oriented mechanisms of novel herbal therapeutics in the chemotherapy of gastrointestinal cancer and inflammation. Curr Pharm Des 19: 48–66.
31. Han Z, Hong L, Han Y, Wu K, Han S, et al (2007) Phospho Akt mediates multidrug resistance of gastric cancer cells through regulation of P-gp, Bcl-2 and Bax. J Exp Clin Cancer Res 26: 261–8.
32. Fu L, Kim Y, Wang X, Wu X, Yue P, et al (2009) Perifosine inhibits mammalian target of rapamycin signaling through facilitating degradation of major components in the mTOR axis and induces autophagy. Cancer Res 69: 8967–76.

17

Oxaliplatin-Based Adjuvant Chemotherapy without Radiotherapy Can Improve the Survival of Locally-Advanced Rectal Cancer

Jun Li[1,2], Yue Liu[2], Jian-Wei Wang[1,2], Yang Gao[2], Ye-Ting Hu[2], Jin-Jie He[1,2], Xiu-Yan Yu[1,2], Han-Guang Hu[2,3], Ying Yuan[2,3], Su-Zhan Zhang[1,2], Ke-Feng Ding[1,2]*

1 Department of Surgical Oncology, Second Affiliated Hospital, Zhejiang University School of Medicine, Hangzhou, Zhejiang Province, China, 2 The Key Laboratory of Cancer Prevention and Intervention, China National Ministry of Education, Hangzhou, Zhejiang Province, China, 3 Department of Medical Oncology, Second Affiliated Hospital, Zhejiang University School of Medicine, Hangzhou, Zhejiang Province, China

Abstract

Objective: To assess the impact of oxaliplatin-containing adjuvant chemotherapy on the survival of patients with locally-advanced rectal cancer.

Methods: Data on patients with pathologically-confirmed T3/4 or N1/2 rectal cancer who accepted radical surgery at our center from January 2002 to June 2009 were reviewed retrospectively. The patients' 5-year overall survival (OS), disease-specific survival (DSS), and recurrence-free survival (RFS) were analyzed by comparing those who accepted radical surgery only (Group S) with those who accepted radical surgery and oxaliplatin-containing adjuvant chemotherapy (Group SO).

Results: A total of 236 patients were analyzed (Group S 135; Group SO 101). Group S patients were older and had a higher proportion with stage II disease and more perioperative complications than those in Group SO ($P<0.05$). The OS and DSS of patients with stage III disease under 50 years of age or with mucinous adenocarcinoma were higher in Group SO than Group S ($P<0.05$). In addition, the OS of patients with stage N2b disease was higher in Group SO than Group S ($P=0.016$), and the OS of patients with stage N1a or N2b disease who received more than 8 weeks of oxaliplatin-containing chemotherapy was also higher in Group SO than Group S ($P<0.05$). Although the OS and DSS of patients with stage II disease in Group SO showed a tendency towards improvement, the differences between the groups were not statistically significant.

Conclusion: Adjuvant oxaliplatin-containing chemotherapy can improve the survival of patients with locally-advanced low and middle rectal cancers in comparison with observation. Randomized, prospective trials are warranted to confirm this benefit of oxaliplatin for rectal cancer.

Editor: Wenyu Lin, Harvard Medical School, United States of America

Funding: This work was supported by the National Natural Science Foundation of China (No. 81301890, http://www.nsfc.gov.cn/) and Zhejiang Provincial Natural Science Foundation of China (No. LY13H160010, http://www.zjnsf.gov.cn/index.aspx). The funders had no role in study design, data collection and analysis, decision to publish, or preparation of the manuscript.

Competing Interests: The authors have declared that no competing interests exist.

* Email: dingkefeng@zju.edu.cn

Introduction

There are obvious differences in adjuvant therapy schedules between colon cancer and rectal cancer. Chemotherapy regimens containing oxaliplatin, such as FOLFOX and XELOX, have been the standard adjuvant therapy for advanced colon cancer for some time [1–3]. For locally-advanced rectal cancer, preoperative 5-fluorouracil (5-FU) or capecitabine with radiotherapy is recognized as the standard therapy because of the decreased local recurrence rate and improved survival [4–6]. The postoperative use of oxaliplatin in rectal cancer resulted from an extrapolation of the available data in colon cancer. However, 2 phase III trials in patients with locally-advanced rectal cancer reported that the addition of oxaliplatin to the standard of 5-FU or capecitabine and radiation did not result in an increased tumor response but did cause greater toxicity [7,8]. Currently, no trials have assessed the

effect of single adjuvant chemotherapy regimens containing oxaliplatin for rectal cancer as the key role of radiotherapy was established 2 decades ago.

The first National Guideline for the Diagnosis and Treatment of Colorectal Cancer in China, which referred to the US National Comprehensive Cancer Network (NCCN) guideline, was published in 2010 [9]. Prior to 2010, the treatment scheme for locally-advanced low and middle rectal cancers in China was different to that in western countries [10]. Most surgeons in China accepted the concept of total mesorectal excision (TME) from the beginning of the 21st century. However, the role of radiotherapy had been underrated for some time. Consequently, Chinese surgeons preferred to perform surgery primarily and advised patients with T3/4 disease or with regional lymph node involvement to receive intensive postoperative combination chemotherapy containing oxaliplatin and 5-FU or capecitabine secondarily. Radiotherapy was used only for rectal cancer patients with unresectable tumors or uncertain resection margins. Obviously, this treatment scheme was similar to that used for colon cancer in western countries, even though there was a lack of supporting evidence from clinical trials. Although the scheme was subsequently abandoned, it provided the opportunity to study the effect of single adjuvant chemotherapy containing oxaliplatin without radiation for patients with rectal cancer.

In this retrospective study, we reviewed the available data on patients with locally-advanced rectal cancer who underwent surgery at our hospital prior to 2010. The efficacy of adjuvant chemotherapy containing oxaliplatin was analyzed by comparing survival differences between patients who had received surgery only (Group S) and those who had received surgery and adjuvant chemotherapy that included oxaliplatin (Group SO).

Patients and Methods

Patients

The colorectal cancer follow-up database at the Zhejiang University Cancer Institute (formerly the Key Laboratory of Cancer Prevention and Intervention, China National Ministry of Education) was reviewed. The follow-up deadline was April 1, 2013. Patients who underwent radical rectal cancer surgery from January 2002 to June 2009 were eligible for analysis. Inclusion criteria included: adenocarcinoma or mucinous adenocarcinoma ≤ 12 cm from the anal verge; pathologically-confirmed T3/4 or N1/2 disease in patients without a prior history of malignancy; neither transanal nor trans-sacral resection; single tumors or multiple tumors resectable by one operation; absence of distant metastases; and planned radical surgery, including non-R0 resection due to the presence of very large tumors. Exclusion criteria were: receipt of preoperative chemotherapy, single postoperative 5-FU/capecitabine chemotherapy regimens or other regimens that contained neither 5-FU/capecitabine nor oxaliplatin; receipt of perioperative radiotherapy; and death within a 3-month period postoperatively.

The study was approved by the Ethics Committee of the Second Affiliated Hospital, Zhejiang University School of Medicine. Written informed consent was not obtained by patients for their clinical records to be used in this study. However, the patients' information was made anonymous prior to analysis.

Statistical analysis

The following data were extracted: patients' demographic and cancer characteristics, surgical and perioperative complications, perioperative treatments, recurrences, and survival. The 7th edition of the TNM (tumor/node/metastasis) staging system was used. Data were analyzed with SPSS version 19.0. Survival was calculated from the date of operation. Gaussian distribution data were described by $\bar{\chi} \pm s$ and analyzed by t tests. Numeration data were analyzed by a χ^2 test or Fisher's exact probability test. Local recurrence-free survival (RFS) was defined as the time to local pelvic recurrences, disease-specific survival (DSS) as the time to death caused by rectal cancer, and overall survival (OS) as the time to death. Kaplan-Meier censored survival curves were used to present survival data with log-rank P values. A two-sided P value of 0.05 or less was considered to indicate statistical significance.

Results

Baseline characteristics

On the basis of the inclusion criteria, the number of patients eligible for analysis was 285. However, 49 patients were excluded as 6 had received preoperative chemotherapy, 20 had received single 5-FU/capecitabine postoperative chemotherapy regimens, 4 had received other chemotherapy regimens, and 19 had received radiotherapy preoperatively or postoperatively. Thus, the analysis was performed on 236 eligible patients (Group S 135; Group SO 101), 10 of whom were subsequently lost to follow-up. All of the patients in Group SO received chemotherapy, including not only oxaliplatin but also 5-FU/capecitabine. The median follow-up time was 53.5 months (range, 3 to 124 months).

Patients in Group S were older, had a higher proportion with stage II disease, and had more perioperative complications than patients in Group SO ($P<0.05$). However, other characteristics such as gender, distance from the anal verge, surgical method, and pathologic type were balanced between the 2 groups (Table 1). Three patients received R2 resection due to the presence of very large tumors. All of the longitudinal resection margins were pathologically clear. None of the patients' circumferential resection margins (CRMs) were reported.

Effect of oxaliplatin-containing adjuvant chemotherapy on 5-year survival

There were trends for the 5-year DSS and OS to be higher in patients with stage II and III disease who received oxaliplatin-containing adjuvant chemotherapy (Group OS) than in patients who received surgery only (Group OS) [Table 2], but the differences between the groups were not statistically significant ($P>0.05$). Subgroup analysis showed that both the DSS and OS of patients with stage III disease under 50 years age were higher in Group SO than in patients in Group S ($P<0.05$). Stratified analysis according to the N stage revealed a trend for patients with stage N2 disease in Group SO to have a better OS than those in Group S (52.2% vs 37.0%; $P = 0.064$). Further stratified analysis showed that the OS of patients with stage N2b disease in Group SO was increased in comparison with that of patients in Group S (45.8% vs 13.6%; $P = 0.016$). In addition, both the DSS and OS of patients with mucinous adenocarcinoma in Group SO were increased in comparison with patients in Group S ($P<0.05$) [Table 2; Figures 1 and 2].

Further analysis according to the duration of adjuvant chemotherapy revealed that patients with stage N1a disease who received more than 8 weeks of chemotherapy in Group SO had a better DSS (100% vs 75.0%; $P = 0.079$) and OS (100% vs 68.8%; $P = 0.032$) than patients in Group S. In addition, the OS of patients with stage N2b disease who received more than 8 weeks of chemotherapy was improved in comparison with patients in Group S (44.4% vs 18.2%, $P = 0.033$).

Although the RFS of patients with stage II disease in Group SO was higher than in Group S, the difference was not statistically significant; the 5-year local recurrence rates in the 2 groups were 0% and 8.3%, respectively ($P = 0.160$). Similarly, there was no difference in RFS between the 2 groups for patients with stage III disease; the 5-year local recurrence rates for these patients were 8.1% and 14.6%, respectively ($P = 0.419$) [Table 3]. No subgroups of patients who achieved a lower local recurrence rate following receipt of oxaliplatin-containing adjuvant chemotherapy were identified (Figure 1 and Table 3).

Table 1. Baseline demographic and cancer characteristics of the 236 patients who underwent radical surgery.

Characteristics	Group S (n = 135)	Group SO (n = 101)	P value
Gender, n (%):			0.131
Male	93 (68.89%)	60 (59.41%)	
Female	42 (31.11%)	41 (40.59%)	
Age, years (mean ± SD)	64.04±11.37	53.98±11.12	<0.001*
Distance to anal verge, cm (mean ± SD)	7.57±3.10	7.31±2.94	0.513
Surgical method, n (%):			0.944
AR	99 (73.88%)	76 (75.25%)	
APR	34 (25.37%)	24 (23.76%)	
Hartmann	1 (0.75%)	1 (0.99%)	
R0 resection, n (%):			1.000
Yes	133 (98.52%)	100 (99.01%)	
No	2 (1.48%)	1 (0.99%)	
Complications, n (%)			0.046*
Yes	15 (11.11%)	4 (3.96%)	
No	120 (88.89%)	97 (96.04%)	
Pathologic type, n (%):			0.380
Adenocarcinoma	127 (94.07%)	92 (91.09)	
Mucinous adenocarcinoma	8 (5.93%)	9 (8.91%)	
Differentiation, n (%):			0.074
Well-differentiated	64 (52.46%)	33 (35.87%)	
Moderately-differentiated	52 (42.62%)	52 (56.52%)	
Poorly-differentiated	6 (4.92%)	7 (7.61%)	
Lymph nodes (mean ± SD)	13.68±5.74	13.99±7.31	0.717
T stage, n (%):			0.336
1	0 (0%)	1 (0.99%)	
2	6 (4.44%)	9 (8.91%)	
3	66 (48.89%)	48 (47.52%)	
4	63 (46.67%)	43 (42.57%)	
N stage, n (%):			<0.001*
0	70 (51.85%)	27 (27.00%)	
1	44 (32.59%)	32 (32.00%)	
2	21 (15.56%)	41 (41.00%)	
TNM stage, n (%):			<0.001*
II	70 (51.85%)	27 (27.00%)	
III	65 (48.15%)	73 (73.00%)	

* Statistically significant difference between patient groups (P≤0.05).
AR, anterior resection; APR, abdominoperineal resection; Group S received surgery alone; Group SO received surgery and oxaliplatin-containing adjuvant chemotherapy.

Discussion

In the 1990s, a number of clinical trials demonstrated that postoperative radiotherapy reduced local recurrences in patients with locally-advanced rectal cancer [11,12]. Since then, radiotherapy has become the cornerstone of adjuvant therapy for advanced rectal cancer in western countries. During the first decade of the 21st century, preoperative radiochemotherapy with 5-FU became the standard adjuvant therapy for locally-advanced and resectable rectal cancer due to its efficacy in reducing local recurrences and improving survival [4–6]. At the same time, chemotherapy containing oxaliplatin also became the standard adjuvant therapy for resectable advanced colon cancer [1–3]. Therefore, several clinical trials tried to improve the treatment

effect of rectal cancer by adding oxaliplatin to preoperative radiochemotherapy. However, the results were disappointing because of both increased adverse events and no improvement in the tumor response [7,8]. As a result, there has been no evidence to support the use oxaliplatin as adjuvant therapy for locally-advanced rectal cancer. Nevertheless, it has become evident that there are still several issues regarding preoperative radiotherapy that remain to be clarified. For example, patients who receive preoperative radiotherapy suffer from sexual dysfunction, proctitis, enteritis and cystitis, especially females with a low body mass index [13,14]. Moreover, radiotherapy for patients with T3N0 rectal cancer has also been questioned [15,16]. Whether intensive chemotherapy without radiotherapy can

Table 2. Five-year survival of the patients after rectal cancer resection.

Characteristics	5-Year DSS			5-Year OS		
	Group S n (%)	Group SO n (%)	Log-rank P value	Group S n (%)	Group SO n (%)	Log-rank P value
TNM stage:						
II	68 (84.6%)	26 (100%)	0.191	68 (76.6%)	26 (90.1%)	0.261
III	58 (58.9%)	73 (63.7%)	0.523	58 (54.4%)	73 (61.2%)	0.195
Age:						
<50 years	14 (73.8%)	31 (84.9%)	0.373	14 (62.9%)	31 (79.0%)	0.205
Stage II	6 (100%)	9 (100%)	NA	6 (100%)	9 (88.9%)	0.414
Stage III	8 (42.9%)	22 (80.7%)	0.022*	8 (31.3%)	22 (76.7%)	0.002*
≥50 years	112 (72.8%)	69 (66.6%)	0.449	112 (67%)	69 (62.9%)	0.947
Stage II	62 (82.9%)	17 (100%)	0.299	62 (74.2%)	17 (90.9%)	0.240
Stage III	50 (61.0%)	51 (54.0%)	0.705	50 (58.2%)	51 (52.2%)	0.994
T stage:						
2	6 (83.3%)	9 (100%)	0.317	6 (83.3%)	9 (100%)	0.317
3	64 (72.5%)	48 (70.5%)	0.760	64 (67.6%)	48 (64.0%)	0.627
4	56 (72.2%)	42 (70.1%)	0.388	56 (63.1%)	42 (68.4%)	0.974
N stage:						
N1	40 (64.3%)	32 (78.8%)	0.280	40 (62.5%)	32 (72.4%)	0.314
N1a	16 (67.5%)	16 (85.9%)	0.313	16 (67.5%)	16 (85.9%)	0.146
N1b+c	24 (61.9%)	16 (71.1%)	0.704	24 (59.2%)	16 (59.1%)	0.932
N2	18 (46.1%)	41 (52.2%)	0.333	18 (37.0%)	41 (52.2%)	0.064
N2a	7 (71.4%)	16 (52.5%)	0.609	7 (71.4%)	16 (52.5%)	0.609
N2b	11 (20.2%)	25 (45.8%)	0.161	11 (13.6%)	25 (45.8%)	0.016*
Pathologic type:						
Adenocarcinoma	119 (75.0%)	91 (70.9%)	0.578	119 (68.8%)	91 (66.4%)	0.930
Well-differentiated	60 (72.4%)	32 (70.8%)	0.830	60 (67.9%)	32 (64.2%)	0.650
Moderately- differentiated	49 (79.2%)	52 (75.8%)	0.765	49 (70.7%)	52 (72.4%)	0.902
Poorly-differentiated	5 (66.7%)	7 (42.9%)	0.551	5 (53.3%)	7 (42.9%)	0.949
Mucinous adenocarcinoma	7 (35.7%)	9 (88.9%)	0.034*	7 (28.6%)	9 (88.9%)	0.013*

* Statistically significant difference between patient groups (P≤0.05).
DSS, disease-specific survival; Group S received surgery alone; Group SO received surgery and oxaliplatin-containing adjuvant chemotherapy; NA, not available; OS, overall survival.

improve the prognosis of locally-advanced rectal cancer remains unknown.

In this retrospective study, we observed survival differences between patients with locally-advanced curable rectal cancer who received surgery alone and those who received surgery and oxaliplatin-containing adjuvant chemotherapy. Our findings showed that some patients with stage III rectal cancer can benefit from oxaliplatin-containing adjuvant chemotherapy, including: (1) patients with stage III disease less than 50 years of age; (2) patients with stage N2 disease, especially those with stage N2b disease; and (3) patients with stage N1a disease who received more than 8 weeks of chemotherapy. The DSS and OS of patients with stage II disease also showed a trend towards improvement, but the differences versus Group S did not reach statistical significance. It was of interest that no specific subgroup of patients achieved a reduced local recurrence rate with oxaliplatin-containing adjuvant chemotherapy. This indicates that the survival benefit that was achieved might be the result of reduced distant metastases rather than decreased local recurrences.

At present, there is no direct evidence to support the use of oxaliplatin-based chemotherapy alone for middle and low rectal cancers. The key role of radiotherapy has been well established, and all trials that have studied oxaliplatin in combination with radiotherapy have failed, which, prior to this study, has made it ethically difficult to assess the effect of single oxaliplatin-containing adjuvant chemotherapy regimens for rectal cancer in clinical trials. In comparison with the reported results with standard preoperative radiochemotherapy, the findings of this study indicate that single oxaliplatin-containing adjuvant chemotherapy provides non-inferior overall survival. The 5-year overall survival rate of patients in Group SO was 68.8% (90.1% for stage II disease and 61.2% for stage III disease). In the NSABP R-03 trial, the 5-year OS rate was 74.5% for patients who received preoperative radiochemotherapy that contained 5-FU [5]. In the EORTC 22921 trial, patients with locally-advanced resectable rectal cancer were randomly assigned to receive preoperative radiotherapy, preoperative chemoradiotherapy, preoperative radiotherapy and postoperative chemotherapy, or preoperative chemoradiotherapy and postoperative chemotherapy. The combined 5-year OS rate

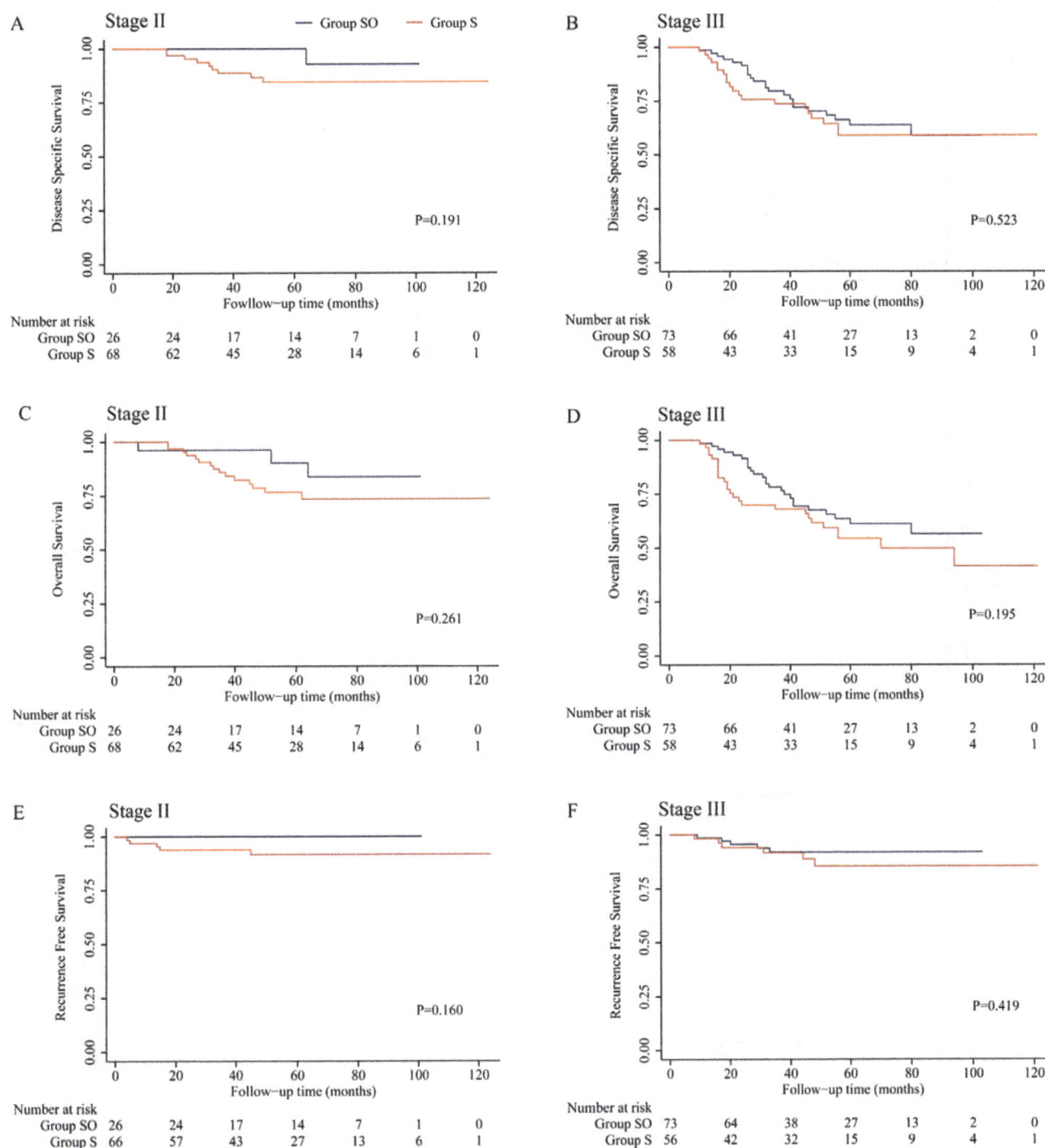

Figure 1. Kaplan-Meier curves for patients who received oxaliplatin-based adjuvant chemotherapy or surgery alone. A, C and E: patients with stage II disease. B, D and F: patients with stage III disease.

for all 4 groups was 65.2% [17]. Our results indicate that oxaliplatin-containing adjuvant chemotherapy may be as effective as the present standard of radiochemotherapy. In view of the non-inferior 5-year overall survival for patients in Group SO in this study (61.2% for patients with stage III disease and 76.7% for patients with stage III disease under 50 years of age), it seems reasonable to perform studies of oxaliplatin-containing chemotherapy instead of radiotherapy in some patients, e.g. young females because of concerns over ovarian dysfunction with

radiotherapy, and patients with contraindications to radiotherapy [5,6]. Moreover, patients with rectal cancers in which the surgical CRM is found to be clear by magnetic resonance imaging (MRI) might also be able to receive intensive adjuvant chemotherapy and thereby avoid radiotherapy [18]. The feasibility of this approach needs to be confirmed by prospective, randomized trials.

Recently, several studies have reported results with the application of oxaliplatin in rectal cancer instead of combining it with preoperative radiotherapy. The large multicenter, phase II

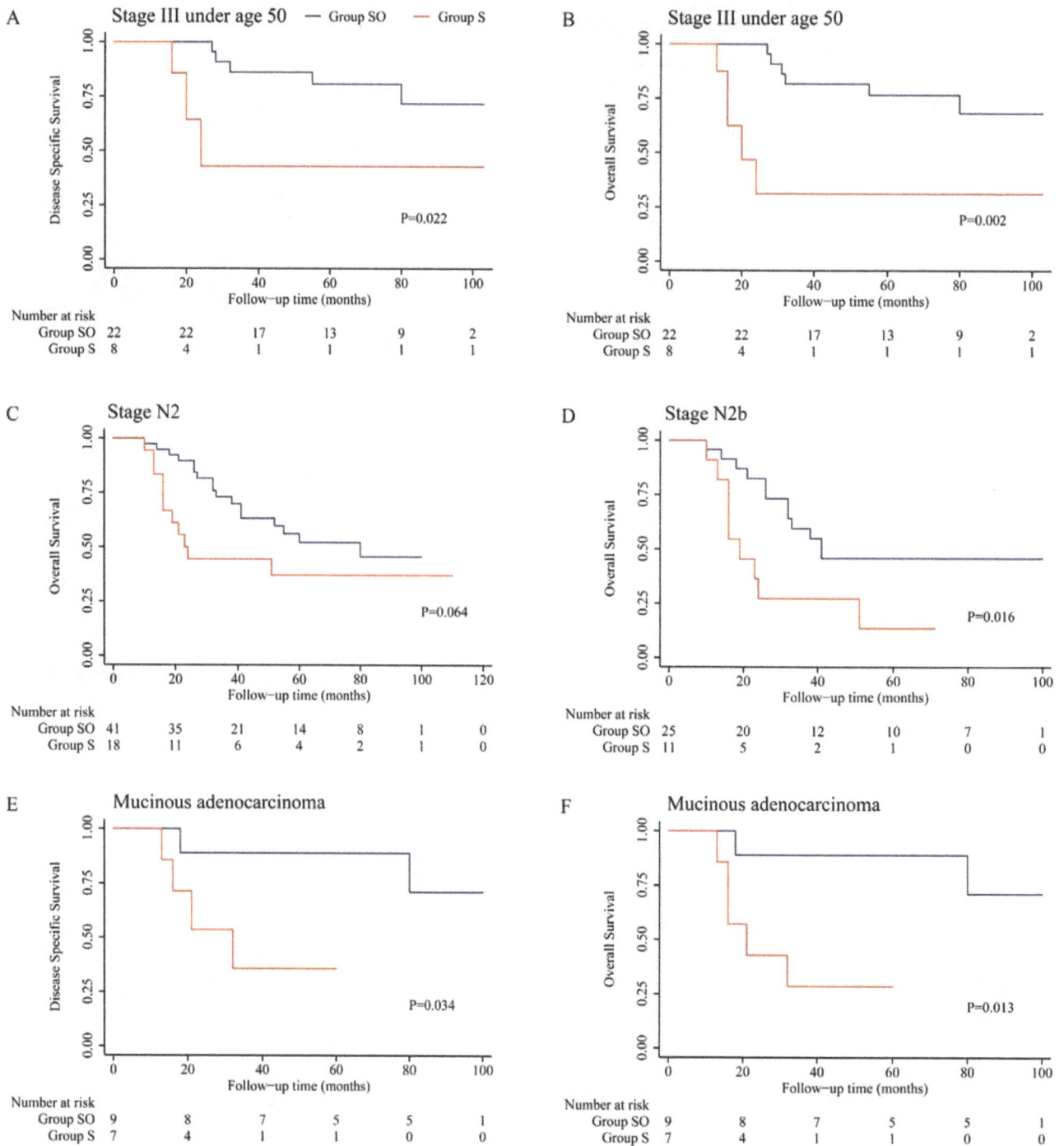

Figure 2. Kaplan-Meier curves for subgroups of patients who received oxaliplatin-based adjuvant chemotherapy or surgery alone. A and B: stage III patients under 50 years of age. C: patients with stage N2 disease. D: patients with stage N2b disease. E and F: patients with mucinous adenocarcinoma.

ADORE study used postoperative oxaliplatin-based adjuvant chemotherapy (FOLFOX) in patients who had received preoperative radiochemotherapy [19]. The 3-year disease-free survival was 71.6% in patients who received FOLFOX postoperative adjuvant chemotherapy, as compared with 62.9% in patients who received 5-FU/leucovorin ($P = 0.047$). In a subgroup analysis, patients with yp stage III, ypN1b, ypN2, and minimally-regressed tumors benefited more from FOLFOX than 5-FU/leucovorin.

Two other recent studies have explored the question of whether intensive chemotherapy containing oxaliplatin could replace preoperative radiotherapy. A small phase II study conducted in New York reported a pathologic complete response rate of 25% and a 4-year overall survival rate of 91% for patients with locally-advanced rectal cancer who received FOLFOX with bevacizumab as preoperative therapy without routine radiotherapy [20]. Another phase II study conducted in Japan reported that

Table 3. Five-year local recurrence-free survival of the patients after rectal cancer resection.

Characteristics	5-Year RFS		
	Group S n (%)	Group SO n (%)	Log-rank *P* value
TNM stage:			
II	66 (91.7%)	26 (100%)	0.160
III	56 (85.4%)	73 (91.9%)	0.419
Age:			
<50 years	13 (100%)	31 (95.8%)	0.564
Stage II	6 (100%)	9 (100%)	NA
Stage III	7 (100%)	22 (94.4%)	0.739
≥50 years	109 (88.0%)	69 (93.5%)	0.369
Stage II	60 (90.8%)	17 (100%)	0.225
Stage III	49 (84.4%)	51 (90.9%)	0.567
T stage:			
2	6 (100%)	9 (100%)	NA
3	64 (86.7%)	48 (90.0%)	0.649
4	52 (90.4%)	42 (97.5%)	0.268
N stage:			
N1	40 (83.8%)	32 (96.7%)	0.166
N1a	16 (100%)	16 (100%)	NA
N1b+c	24 (73.3%)	16 (92.9%)	0.321
N2	18 (92.3%)	41 (87.8%)	0.800
N2a	7 (83.3%)	16 (85.9%)	0.799
N2b	11 (100%)	25 (89.7%)	0.448
Pathologic type:			
Adenocarcinoma	116 (89.6%)	91 (94.8%)	0.270
Well-differentiated	59 (90.1%)	32 (92.6%)	0.679
Moderately-differentiated	47 (86.8%)	52 (97.8%)	0.097
Poorly-differentiated	5 (100%)	7 (85.7%)	0.398
Mucinous adenocarcinoma	6 (80.0%)	9 (87.5%)	0.572

Group S received surgery alone; Group SO received surgery and oxaliplatin-containing adjuvant chemotherapy; NA, not available; RFS, local recurrence-free survival.

neoadjuvant therapy using mFOLFOX6 instead of radiotherapy was a safe and efficacious treatment option for rectal cancer, with a pathologic complete response rate of 10.3% and an R0 resection rate of 91.0% [21]. All of these findings indicate that oxaliplatin-containing adjuvant chemotherapy may be effective in rectal cancer when synchronous use of preoperative radiotherapy is to be avoided.

This study had several limitations. Firstly, as it was a retrospective study with only a small sample, there was selection bias in the patients included. As described above, patients in Group S were older, contained a higher proportion with stage II disease, and had more perioperative complications than patients in Group SO ($P<0.05$). Therefore, patients who were young with a good physical status and a higher risk of recurrences were more liable to receive adjuvant chemotherapy. Consequently, to eliminate the effects of selection bias, we used a stratification analysis.

Secondly, no CRM status was reported. As we reported in 2009 [10], this is a serious shortcoming of the treatment of rectal cancer in China, even in university-affiliated hospitals. However, for patients in Group S, the high number of lymph nodes harvested (mean 13.68), the non-inferior 5-year local recurrence rate (8.3%

in stage II disease and 14.6% in stage III disease), and the disease-specific survival rate (84.6% in stage II disease and 58.9% in stage III disease) were comparable to the results reported by Heald et al. [22], indicating the good quality of surgery at our center. Thirdly, it was not feasible to compare outcome differences between patients who received oxaliplatin-containing adjuvant chemotherapy and those who received perioperative radiotherapy in this study, as only 19 patients who had very large tumors or obvious lymph node metastases received radiotherapy.

In conclusion, we found that adjuvant chemotherapy containing oxaliplatin without radiotherapy can improve the survival of patients with locally-advanced low and middle rectal cancers in comparison with observation. Randomized, prospective trials are warranted to confirm this benefit of oxaliplatin for rectal cancer.

Acknowledgments

Preliminary results from this study were submitted to the ASCO 2012 Annual Congress as an abstract [J Clin Oncol 30 (suppl): abstract e14024, 2012]. We gratefully thank Content Ed Net, Shanghai Co. Ltd for editorial assistance with the manuscript.

Author Contributions

Conceived and designed the experiments: JL KFD. Performed the experiments: JL YL YG YTH JJH XYY HGH. Analyzed the data: JL JWW YY SZZ KFD. Contributed reagents/materials/analysis tools: JL YL KFD. Wrote the paper: JL YL JWW YG YTH JJH XYY HGH YY SZZ KFD.

References

1. Andre T, Boni C, Navarro M, Tabernero J, Hickish T, et al. (2009) Improved overall survival with oxaliplatin, fluorouracil, and leucovorin as adjuvant treatment in stage II or III colon cancer in the MOSAIC trial. J Clin Oncol 27: 3109–3116.

2. Haller DG, Tabernero J, Maroun J, de Braud F, Price T, et al. (2011) Capecitabine plus oxaliplatin compared with fluorouracil and folinic acid as adjuvant therapy for stage III colon cancer. J Clin Oncol 29: 1465–1471.

3. Yothers G, O'Connell MJ, Allegra CJ, Kuebler JP, Colangelo LH, et al. (2011) Oxaliplatin as adjuvant therapy for colon cancer: updated results of NSABP C-07 trial, including survival and subset analyses. J Clin Oncol 29: 3768–3774.

4. Folkesson J, Birgisson H, Pahlman L, Cedermark B, Glimelius B, et al. (2005) Swedish Rectal Cancer Trial: long lasting benefits from radiotherapy on survival and local recurrence rate. J Clin Oncol 23: 5644–5650.

5. Roh MS, Colangelo LH, O'Connell MJ, Yothers G, Deutsch M, et al. (2009) Preoperative multimodality therapy improves disease-free survival in patients with carcinoma of the rectum: NSABP R-03. J Clin Oncol 27: 5124–5130.

6. van Gijn W, Marijnen CA, Nagtegaal ID, Kranenbarg EM, Putter H, et al. (2011) Preoperative radiotherapy combined with total mesorectal excision for resectable rectal cancer: 12-year follow-up of the multicentre, randomised controlled TME trial. Lancet Oncol 12: 575–582.

7. Aschele C, Cionini L, Lonardi S, Pinto C, Cordio S, et al. (2011) Primary tumor response to preoperative chemoradiation with or without oxaliplatin in locally advanced rectal cancer: pathologic results of the STAR-01 randomized phase III trial. J Clin Oncol 29: 2773–2780.

8. Gerard JP, Azria D, Gourgou-Bourgade S, Martel-Lafay I, Hennequin C, et al. (2012) Clinical outcome of the ACCORD 12/0405 PRODIGE 2 randomized trial in rectal cancer. J Clin Oncol 30: 4558–4565.

9. China Ministry of Health (2010) National Guideline of Diagnosis and Treatment for Colorectal Cancer (2010 edition). Available: http://www.gov.cn/gzdt/2010-10/25/content_1729651.htm. Accessed 22 January, 2014.

10. Ding KF, Chen R, Zhang JL, Li J, Xu YQ, et al. (2009) Laparoscopic surgery for the curative treatment of rectal cancer: results of a Chinese three-center case-control study. Surg Endosc 23: 854–861.

11. Medical Research Council Rectal Cancer Working Party (1996) Randomised trial of surgery alone versus surgery followed by radiotherapy for mobile cancer of the rectum. Lancet 348: 1610–1614.

12. Colorectal Cancer Collaborative Group (2001) Adjuvant radiotherapy for rectal cancer: a systematic overview of 8,507 patients from 22 randomised trials. Lancet 358: 1291–1304.

13. Stephens RJ, Thompson LC, Quirke P, Steele R, Grieve R, et al. (2010) Impact of short-course preoperative radiotherapy for rectal cancer on patients' quality of life: data from the Medical Research Council CR07/National Cancer Institute of Canada Clinical Trials Group C016 randomized clinical trial. J Clin Oncol 28: 4233–4239.

14. Wolff HA, Conradi LC, Schirmer M, Beissbarth T, Sprenger T, et al. (2011) Gender-specific acute organ toxicity during intensified preoperative radio-chemotherapy for rectal cancer. Oncologist 16: 621–631.

15. Kachnic LA, Hong TS, Ryan DP (2008) Rectal cancer at the crossroads: the dilemma of clinically staged T3, N0, M0 disease. J Clin Oncol 26: 350–351.

16. Wo JY, Mamon HJ, Ryan DP, Hong TS (2011) T3N0 rectal cancer: radiation for all? Semin Radiat Oncol 21: 212–219.

17. Bosset JF, Collette L, Calais G, Mineur L, Maingon P, et al. (2006) Chemotherapy with preoperative radiotherapy in rectal cancer. N Engl J Med 355: 1114–1123.

18. Daniels IR, Moran BJ, Heald RJ (2004) Surgery alone: is total mesorectal excision sufficient for rectal cancer? Front Radiat Ther Oncol 38: 28–36.

19. Yong SH BN, KP Kim, JL Lee, JO Park, et al. (2014) Adjuvant chemotherapy with oxaliplatin/5-fluorouracil/leucovorin (FOLFOX) versus 5-fluorouracil/leucovorin (FL) for rectal cancer patients whose postoperative yp stage 2 or 3 after preoperative chemoradiotherapy: updated results of 3-year disease-free survival from a randomized phase II study (The ADORE). J Clin Oncol 32 (suppl): abstr 3502. Available: http://meetinglibrary.asco.org/content/131515-144. Accessed 21 August 2014.

20. Schrag D, Weiser MR, Goodman KA, Gonen M, Hollywood E, et al. (2014) Neoadjuvant chemotherapy without routine use of radiation therapy for patients with locally advanced rectal cancer: a pilot trial. J Clin Oncol 32: 513–518.

21. Junichi K KF, Kazuhiko Y, Hajime Y, Hayato K, et al. (2014) Neoadjuvant mFOLFOX6 for stage II/III rectal cancer patients with a T3/T4 tumor. J Clin Oncol 32 (suppl): abstr 3554. Available: http://meetinglibrary.asco.org/content/127855-144. Accessed 21 August 2014.

22. Heald RJ, Moran BJ, Ryall RD, Sexton R, MacFarlane JK (1998) Rectal cancer: the Basingstoke experience of total mesorectal excision, 1978–1997. Arch Surg 133: 894–899.

18

A Bayesian Meta-Analysis of Multiple Treatment Comparisons of Systemic Regimens for Advanced Pancreatic Cancer

Kelvin Chan[1,2]*, Keya Shah[1], Kelly Lien[1], Doug Coyle[3], Henry Lam[1], Yoo-Joung Ko[1]

1 Sunnybrook Odette Cancer Centre, University of Toronto, Toronto, ON, Canada, **2** Division of Biostatistics, Dalla Lana School of Public Health, University of Toronto, Toronto, ON, Canada, **3** University of Ottawa, Ottawa, ON, Canada

Abstract

Background: For advanced pancreatic cancer, many regimens have been compared with gemcitabine (G) as the standard arm in randomized controlled trials. Few regimens have been directly compared with each other in randomized controlled trials and the relative efficacy and safety among them remains unclear.

Methods: A systematic review was performed through MEDLINE, EMBASE, Cochrane Central Register of Controlled Trials, and ASCO meeting abstracts up to May 2013 to identify randomized controlled trials that included advanced pancreatic cancer comparing the following regimens: G, G+5-fluorouracil, G+ capecitabine, G+S1, G+ cisplatin, G+ oxaliplatin, G+ erlotinib, G+ nab-paclitaxel, and FOLFIRINOX. Overall survival and progression-free survival with 95% credible regions were extracted using the Parmar method. A Bayesian multiple treatment comparisons was performed to compare all regimens simultaneously.

Results: Twenty-two studies were identified and 16 were included in the meta-analysis. Median overall survival, progression free survival, and response rates for G arms from all trials were similar, suggesting no significant clinical heterogeneity. For overall survival, the mixed treatment comparisons found that the probability that FOLFIRINOX was the best regimen was 83%, while it was 11% for G+ nab-paclitaxel and 3% for G+ S1 and G+ erlotinib, respectively. The overall survival hazard ratio for FOLFIRINOX versus G+ nab-paclitaxel was 0.79 [0.50–1.24], with no obvious difference in toxicities. The hazard ratios from direct pairwise comparisons were consistent with the mixed treatment comparisons results.

Conclusions: FOLFIRINOX appeared to be the best regimen for advanced pancreatic cancer probabilistically, with a trend towards improvement in survival when compared with other regimens by indirect comparisons.

Editor: Jonathan R. Brody, Thomas Jefferson University, United States of America

Funding: The authors have no support or funding to report.

Competing Interests: Keya Shah has read the journal's policy and the authors of this manuscript have the following competing interests: Yoo-Joung Ko declared that he received research support and honoraria from Sanofi-Aventis, and Celgene; however, he has no stock ownership. The remaining authors have no competing interests to declare.

* Email: kelvin.chan@sunnybrook.ca

Introduction

Pancreatic cancer is the 4th leading cause of cancer death in the United States and 5th in the United Kingdom [1,2] with most cases being categorized as either metastatic or locally advanced at first presentation [3]. As potentially curative surgical resection can be performed in only 15–20% of pancreatic cancer patients [4], the treatment goal for the majority of these patients is palliative in nature. For more than 15 years, the current standard of care for advanced disease has been chemotherapy with gemcitabine alone (G), after it was shown in a phase III randomized control trial (RCT) to offer greater symptom relief with a modest 1-year survival advantage (18% versus 2%) when compared to 5-fluorouracil [5]. Since then, a number of phase II and III RCTs have attempted to improve the gemcitabine anti-tumour activity

through gemcitabine-based combinations with cytotoxic and/or targeted agents such as capecitabine, oxaliplatin, erlotinib, and cisplatin [6–10]. Recent trials have also compared gemcitabine alone to gemcitabine plus nab-paclitaxel (GnP), and a combination regimen without gemcitabine consisting of folinic acid, fluorouracil, irinotecan hydrochloride and oxaliplatin (FOLFIRINOX) [11,12]. The trial of G versus GnP found statistically significant hazard ratios (HRs) for overall survival (OS) in favour of the GnP combination. The safety analysis found that serious life-threatening toxicity was not increased with GnP and that adverse events were acceptable and manageable. Thus, the authors concluded that GnP may be considered as a new standard of treatment for advanced pancreatic cancer [11]. In the FOLFIRINOX trial, survival was significantly better in the FOLFIRINOX group, but with an increased occurrence of adverse events. The study concluded that FOLFIRINOX should also be considered as a first-line option for advanced pancreatic cancer patients; however, due to safety concerns, it should be reserved for patients younger than 75 years of age and with a good performance status [12]. No currently ongoing trials directly compare GnP and FOLFIRI-NOX. While the addition of these two chemotherapy regimens and their improvement in survival represent significant recent progress over gemcitabine monotherapy, the most effective chemotherapy strategy in clinical practice remains to be determined.

As direct comparison of combination therapies has been tested mostly against single agent gemcitabine as the control arm in most clinical trials, the relative effectiveness of the various regimens remains unclear. In these instances, multiple treatment comparisons (MTC) can be used to synthesize evidence from RCTs using both direct (head-to-head) and indirect (using a common comparator) comparisons [13]. MTC are valuable tools that are frequently employed by healthcare decision makers such as the National Institute for Health and Clinical Excellence and the Canadian Agency for Drugs and Technologies in Health, where their usage is gaining widespread acceptance [14,15].

The aim of this study was to perform Bayesian MTC in order to determine the most effective treatment for advanced pancreatic cancer, taking into account the efficacy and safety profiles of each regimen. Through our analysis, we were able to achieve this goal.

Methods

Literature Search

We conducted a systematic literature review through the MEDLINE, EMBASE, and Cochrane Centre Register of Controlled Trials databases, as well as ASCO meeting abstracts up to and including May 23, 2013. Trials were limited to first-line treatment in pancreatic cancer or adenocarcinoma patients. Studies were limited to randomized controlled trials (RCTs) that used one of the following chemotherapy regimens: G, G + fluorouracil (GF), G + capecitabine (GCap), G + S1 (GS), G + cisplatin (GCis), G + oxaliplatin (GOx), G + erlotinib (GE), GnP, and FOLFIRINOX. These regimens were determined a priori by the authors, as they are clinically the most commonly considered treatments for advanced pancreatic cancer with prior studies suggesting possible benefits to patients. The outcomes of interest included OS, progression-free survival (PFS), and grade 3/4 toxicities. RCTs that did not include patients with advanced pancreatic cancer were excluded. Non-randomized trials and those concerning other malignancies, such as neuroendocrine tumours or lymphoma, were excluded. Trials comparing radiotherapy, hormonal, or gene therapy, and those comparing chemotherapy to no treatment (best supportive care) were excluded. No language restrictions were imposed. The articles that were not freely available to us were requested from the authors.

Screening

Two independent authors reviewed the literature search results and included studies that met the prespecified eligibility criteria. When reports overlapped or were duplicated, we retained the study with the most recent data that could be used in the meta-analysis. Discrepancies were resolved by consensus or by a third author. Our review has been reported using the PRISMA reporting guidelines (Checklist S1).

Data Abstraction and Analysis

Data recorded included the following: first author, publication year, study location, regimens being compared, number of patients randomized to each treatment arm, median age of patients, percentage of patients with performance status of ECOG 0, 1, or 2 and the percentage of patients with locally advanced or advanced disease respectively was recorded (Appendix S1 and S2). The treatments were sorted into categories based on the regimen: G, GF, GCap, GS, GCis, GOx, GE, GnP, and FOLFIRINOX. Risk of bias assessment was performed using the Cochrane risk of bias tool [16].

The data extracted from each study included the following: OS, PFS, objective response rate (ObRR), and the occurrence of adverse events (febrile neutropenia, neuropathy, fatigue, and diarrhea) for all the chemotherapy regimens. If median values for PFS and OS were available, they were also recorded. If the HRs for OS and PFS were detailed in the publication, they were extracted directly, along with 95% confidence intervals (CIs) from Cox regression. Otherwise, HRs were calculated using the methods outlined by Parmar et al [17]. A two-tailed $p < 0.05$ value was recorded whenever available to determine whether a statistically significant difference was detected between the two regimens being compared. Two independent authors extracted data and discrepancies were reviewed by a third author to reach consensus.

Statistical Analysis

We first made pairwise comparisons of regimens from the trials based on direct evidence only. We then performed MTC in a Bayesian model. The MTC combined direct and indirect evidence for specific pairwise comparisons and allowed data across a range of regimens to be compared in a simple network. Bayesian methods combine likelihoods, as a function of the parameters with a prior probability distribution based on previous knowledge, to obtain a posterior probability distribution of the parameters [18]. The posterior probabilities provide a straightforward way to calculate the most effective treatment in the absence of head-to-head trials. By plotting the posterior densities of the direct, indirect, and network estimates, direct and indirect evidence can be combined to provide a network estimate and a single effect size. This effect size has increased precision than that of any one type of evidence alone. The Bayesian approach has undergone significant development in recent years and is able to monitor convergence in posterior distribution and reflect the uncertainty in estimating heterogeneity, offering significant improvements over the frequentist random-effects model, which cannot estimate that uncertainty. In more complex networks, especially those involving multi-armed trials, Bayesian approaches are more developed and more accessible than their frequentist counterparts [18,19].

Analyses were done using Bayesian Markov Chain Monte-Carlo (MCMC) sampling in WinBUGS, version 1.4.3 and reported according to the Quality of Reporting of Meta-analyses (QUOROM) and International Society for Pharmacoeconomics and Outcomes Research (ISPOR) guidelines. In WinBUGS, 3 chains were fit with 40,000 burn-ins and 40,000 iterations each. Assessment of convergence was done using model diagnostics, such as trace plots and the Brooks-Gelman-Rubin statistic [20]. Model fit was determined based on the residual deviance and deviance information criterion (DIC) for each outcome measure. The random effects model was used for OS, PFS, and ObRR because the residual deviance was less than the number of unconstrained data points and the deviance information criterion for each of these outcome measures favoured this model over the fixed effects model. Fixed effects were used in reporting toxicities

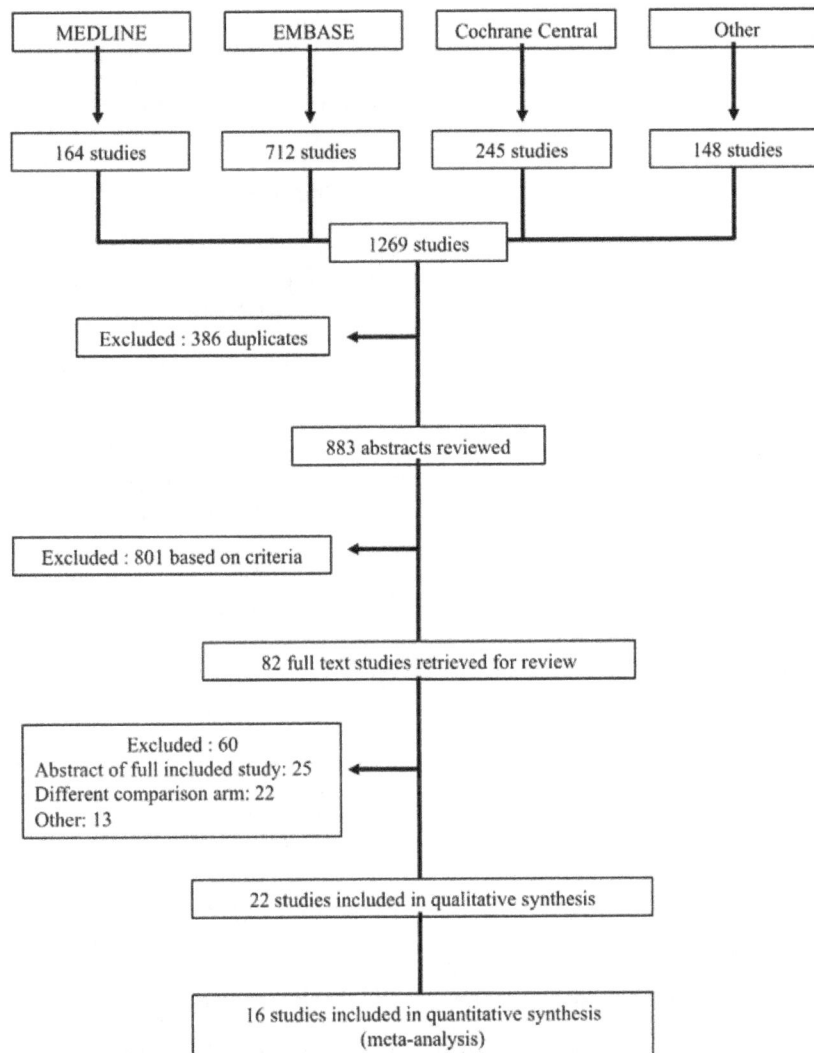

Figure 1. PRISMA Flow diagram of included and excluded trials identified from the literature search. There were 13 studies that were excluded after full text review for "other" reasons. The reasons are as follows: 4 were secondary analyses, 2 were quality of life studies, 2 were pooled analyses, 1 study was not randomized, 1 was a review, 1 was a tumour marker study, 1 was a safety analysis, and 1 study was excluded because it was retrospective.

because the residual deviance and DIC favoured this model. We used the following non-informative prior distributions: uniform (0,2) for standard deviation of the random effects model and normal (0, tau = 0.0001) for log[HR]s. Non-informative priors were used because this allowed the trial data to inform the results, rather than letting strong priors dictate the results.

The primary endpoint was OS and the secondary endpoints were PFS and ObRR. OS and PFS were summarized as log[HR], ObRR and toxicities were summarized as log[Odds Ratio]. Effect sizes are described with 95% credible regions (CRs), since "credible" is a more appropriate term than "confidence" when conducting Bayesian MTC. Consistency between direct and indirect evidence was assessed by comparing direct pairwise comparison estimates to the results generated in the MTC. Probability of each regimen being the best among all regimens were computed by ranking the relative efficacies of all regimens in each iteration and then calculating the proportion of each regimen being ranked first across all iterations [21]. In order to assess the comparability of included studies, between-study heterogeneity

was estimated and reported using the I^2 statistic; the value of I^2 lies between 0% and 100%, where 0% indicates no observed heterogeneity and larger values show increasing heterogeneity [17].

Based on the HR results of the MTC, we attempted to project the survival of patients receiving each of the regimens and compared the results to the median OS of G. Projected median OS was calculated using a median OS of 5.65 months for G as reported by Buris et al [5]. Survival was estimated based on the MTC results and the methods presented by Altman and Andersen [22].

Results

Literature Search Results

Figure 1 shows a flow diagram of the selection process for the studies included in our meta-analysis. 1269 studies were identified from the literature search, 386 studies were excluded because they were duplicates, and 801 were excluded after the abstracts were reviewed based on the prespecified criteria. Of the 82 studies that

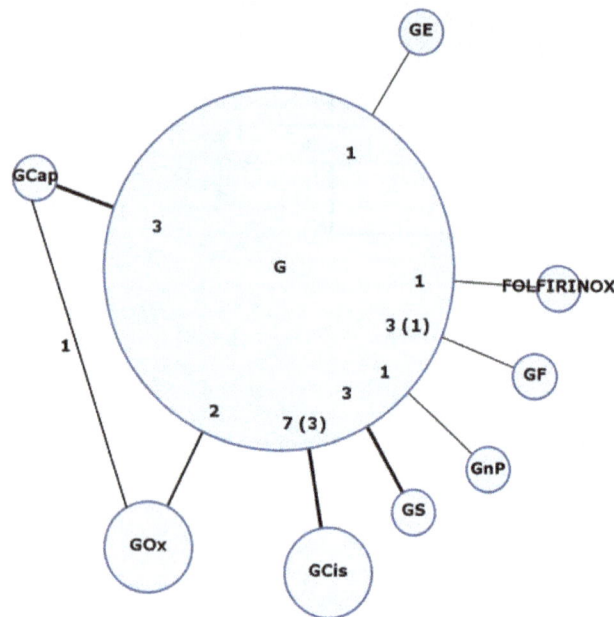

Figure 2. Treatment strategy network. Numbers represent the number of studies comparing the linked regimens; brackets represent the number included in the quantitative analysis.

underwent full text review, 25 were excluded because they were an abstract of a full-included study, 22 had a different comparison arm, 4 were secondary analyses, 2 were quality of life studies, 2 were pooled analyses, 1 study was not randomized, 1 was a review, 1 was a tumour marker study, 1 was a safety analysis, and 1 study was excluded because it was retrospective. Twenty-two studies were identified to be included in this review [6–12,23–38]. 16 studies, involving 5488 randomized patients contained sufficient data to be included in the quantitative synthesis (meta-analysis). The studies included in the meta-analysis consisted of 15 manuscripts and 1 ASCO meeting abstract, which was subsequently published as a full manuscript [38]. The subsequent publication was reviewed and the results were verified and found to be identical to the results reported in the original abstract [11,38].

Study Quality

A summary of the risk of bias for each included study can be found in Appendices S14 and S15. All included studies were randomized and 12 out of the 16 studies followed intention-to-treat analysis for the primary endpoint, thus minimizing selection bias and attrition bias, respectively. Only one study had blinding of patients or personnel. Although blinding of outcome assessors was not explicitly indicated, 13 studies had OS as the primary endpoint, which would not be influenced by the outcome assessor. Therefore there is a low risk of detection bias in these studies. Allocation concealment was not mentioned in any of the studies, so some potential selection bias may be present.

Trial Characteristics

The chemotherapy regimens used in the included studies were G vs. GF (three studies), G vs. GCap (three studies), G vs. GS (three studies), G vs. GCis (seven studies), G vs. GOx (two studies), G vs. GE (one study), G vs. FOLFIRINOX (one study), GCap + GOx (one study), and G + GnP (one study). The treatment strategy network is shown in Figure 2. All trials included in the

meta-analysis reported median PFS and OS. There was no significant clinical heterogeneity between the studies based on the patient characteristics and outcomes in the G reference arm (median PFS = 3 to 4 months, median OS = 6 to 7 months) (Appendix S3).

Comparison of Regimens

The outcomes assessed in all the trials were OS, PFS, ObRR, and number of toxicity-related adverse events. Of the 16 trials that compared different regimens, seven found statistically significant differences in OS based on direct evidence only (Figure 3). These seven studies compared G alone to a different treatment arm. Direct comparisons detected statistically significant improvements in OS with GnP versus G (HR = 0.72, [95% CR 0.62–0.84]), GCap versus G (HR = 0.86, [0.75–0.98]), GE versus G (HR = 0.82, [0.69–0.97]), FOLFIRINOX versus G (HR = 0.57, [0.45–0.72]), GOx versus G (HR = 0.87, [0.76–0.98]), and GS versus G (HR = 0.80, [0.66 to 0.96]). These results can be seen in Figure 3. Statistical heterogeneity ($I^2 > 35\%$) was found only for the comparisons of GCis versus G (seven studies, $I^2 = 64\%$) and GF versus G (three studies, $I^2 = 62\%$) for OS. The direct comparisons for PFS with I^2 values are shown in Appendix S4.

Through our Bayesian MTC, HR comparisons were made of OS (Figure 4) and PFS (Appendix S5) to compare all the regimens simultaneously. The results of the MTC were similar to the results seen in direct pairwise comparisons (Appendix S9). For OS, the results of the Bayesian MTC found that the probability that FOLFIRINOX was the best regimen was 83%, while it was 11% for GnP and 3% for GS and GE, respectively. For PFS, the Bayesian MTC found an 80% probability that FOLFIRINOX was the best regimen. Figure 5 shows the probabilities of each treatment regimen being the best in terms of OS. The probabilities for PFS can be seen in Appendix S6.

The next best regimens according to the calculated probabilities are GnP, GE, and GS. The OS HR for FOLFIRINOX versus GS was 0.72 [0.48–1.11], FOLFIRINOX versus GnP was 0.79 [0.50–1.24], and FOLFIRINOX versus GE was 0.70 [0.44–1.10], where HRs are given with 95% CRs. The PFS HR for FOLFIRINOX versus GS was 0.78 [0.47–1.40], FOLFIRINOX versus GnP was 0.68 [0.37–1.27], and FOLFIRINOX versus GE was 0.61 [0.33–1.15].

Projected survivals were estimated comparing each regimen to G. The projected median OS ranged from 5.8 months for GCis and 9.9 months for FOLFIRINOX (see Table 1). The number needed to treat (NNT) at 6 months and 1 year relative to G have been shown in Table 1. The NNT at 1 year ranges from 5 for FOLFIRINOX to 146 for GCis. These estimates will be helpful in clinical decision-making and providing information to patients.

Odds ratio (OR) comparisons were made of ObRR (Appendix S7) to compare all the regimens simultaneously. The Bayesian MTC found a 58% probability that FOLFIRINOX is the best regimen in terms of ObRR, while it was 33% and 8% for GnP and GS respectively. The ObRR HR [95% CR] for FOLFIRINOX versus GnP is 1.59 [0.74–2.94]. The probabilities that each treatment regimen is the best in terms of ObRR are shown in Appendix S8.

The toxicity-related adverse events assessed in this study were febrile neutropenia and grade 3/4 fatigue, neuropathy, and diarrhea, as these are the most clinically relevant treatment related toxicities. ORs with 95% CRs were reported for each comparison with sufficient direct evidence available to make network estimates (Appendices S10, S11, S12, and S13). Based on cross-trial comparisons, there was no obvious difference in toxicities for

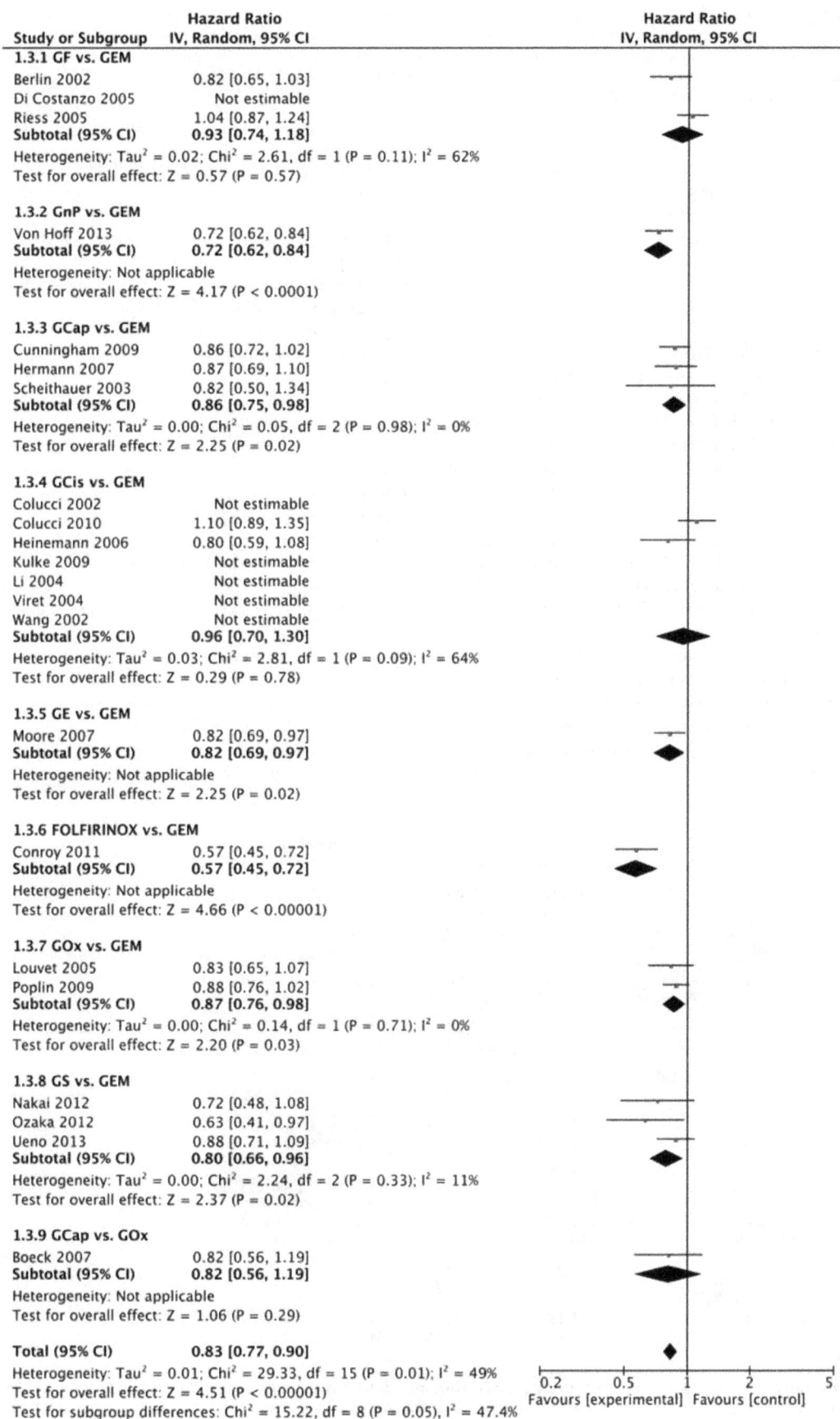

Study or Subgroup	Hazard Ratio IV, Random, 95% CI	Hazard Ratio IV, Random, 95% CI
1.3.1 GF vs. GEM		
Berlin 2002	0.82 [0.65, 1.03]	
Di Costanzo 2005	Not estimable	
Riess 2005	1.04 [0.87, 1.24]	
Subtotal (95% CI)	**0.93 [0.74, 1.18]**	

Heterogeneity: Tau^2 = 0.02; Chi^2 = 2.61, df = 1 (P = 0.11); I^2 = 62%
Test for overall effect: Z = 0.57 (P = 0.57)

1.3.2 GnP vs. GEM		
Von Hoff 2013	0.72 [0.62, 0.84]	
Subtotal (95% CI)	**0.72 [0.62, 0.84]**	

Heterogeneity: Not applicable
Test for overall effect: Z = 4.17 (P < 0.0001)

1.3.3 GCap vs. GEM		
Cunningham 2009	0.86 [0.72, 1.02]	
Hermann 2007	0.87 [0.69, 1.10]	
Scheithauer 2003	0.82 [0.50, 1.34]	
Subtotal (95% CI)	**0.86 [0.75, 0.98]**	

Heterogeneity: Tau^2 = 0.00; Chi^2 = 0.05, df = 2 (P = 0.98); I^2 = 0%
Test for overall effect: Z = 2.25 (P = 0.02)

1.3.4 GCis vs. GEM		
Colucci 2002	Not estimable	
Colucci 2010	1.10 [0.89, 1.35]	
Heinemann 2006	0.80 [0.59, 1.08]	
Kulke 2009	Not estimable	
Li 2004	Not estimable	
Viret 2004	Not estimable	
Wang 2002	Not estimable	
Subtotal (95% CI)	**0.96 [0.70, 1.30]**	

Heterogeneity: Tau^2 = 0.03; Chi^2 = 2.81, df = 1 (P = 0.09); I^2 = 64%
Test for overall effect: Z = 0.29 (P = 0.78)

1.3.5 GE vs. GEM		
Moore 2007	0.82 [0.69, 0.97]	
Subtotal (95% CI)	**0.82 [0.69, 0.97]**	

Heterogeneity: Not applicable
Test for overall effect: Z = 2.25 (P = 0.02)

1.3.6 FOLFIRINOX vs. GEM		
Conroy 2011	0.57 [0.45, 0.72]	
Subtotal (95% CI)	**0.57 [0.45, 0.72]**	

Heterogeneity: Not applicable
Test for overall effect: Z = 4.66 (P < 0.00001)

1.3.7 GOx vs. GEM		
Louvet 2005	0.83 [0.65, 1.07]	
Poplin 2009	0.88 [0.76, 1.02]	
Subtotal (95% CI)	**0.87 [0.76, 0.98]**	

Heterogeneity: Tau^2 = 0.00; Chi^2 = 0.14, df = 1 (P = 0.71); I^2 = 0%
Test for overall effect: Z = 2.20 (P = 0.03)

1.3.8 GS vs. GEM		
Nakai 2012	0.72 [0.48, 1.08]	
Ozaka 2012	0.63 [0.41, 0.97]	
Ueno 2013	0.88 [0.71, 1.09]	
Subtotal (95% CI)	**0.80 [0.66, 0.96]**	

Heterogeneity: Tau^2 = 0.00; Chi^2 = 2.24, df = 2 (P = 0.33); I^2 = 11%
Test for overall effect: Z = 2.37 (P = 0.02)

1.3.9 GCap vs. GOx		
Boeck 2007	0.82 [0.56, 1.19]	
Subtotal (95% CI)	**0.82 [0.56, 1.19]**	

Heterogeneity: Not applicable
Test for overall effect: Z = 1.06 (P = 0.29)

Total (95% CI)	**0.83 [0.77, 0.90]**	

Heterogeneity: Tau^2 = 0.01; Chi^2 = 29.33, df = 15 (P = 0.01); I^2 = 49%
Test for overall effect: Z = 4.51 (P < 0.00001)
Test for subgroup differences: Chi^2 = 15.22, df = 8 (P = 0.05), I^2 = 47.4%

0.2 0.5 1 2 5
Favours [experimental] Favours [control]

Figure 3. Forest plot of direct comparisons between the regimens. Forest plot showing hazard ratio comparisons with 95% CI for overall survival (OS) from meta-analyses of direct comparisons between different combinations of gemcitabine (GEM), gemcitabine + fluorouracil (GF), gemcitabine + nab-paclitaxel (GnP), gemcitabine + capecitabine (GCap), gemcitabine + cisplatin (GCis), gemcitabine + erlotinib (GE), FOLFIRINOX, gemcitabine + oxaliplatin (GOx), and G + S1 (GS). I^2 values indicate statistical heterogeneity, where 0% indicates no observed heterogeneity and larger values show increasing heterogeneity (17).

FOLFIRINOX and GnP. The raw numbers of toxicities from each included study can be found in Appendix S3.

When comparing the direct pairwise comparisons to the results generated from the MTC, we found that the results are consistent (Appendix S9).

Discussion

Key Findings and Implications

Based on the analysis of both the direct evidence and MTC, FOLFIRINOX had the highest probability of being the best regimen in terms of both OS (83%) and PFS (80%). In our study, selected comparisons of FOLFIRINOX with the regimens that had the next highest probabilities were also conducted. These results provide further evidence, albeit indirect, that FOLFIR-INOX may be the most effective regimen in the treatment of advanced pancreatic cancer. Although this meta-analysis allows for network comparisons of FOLFIRINOX with other chemotherapy regimens, further large prospective trials with FOLFIR-INOX and the other regimens, especially GnP, would ideally be performed to confirm these results.

For over the past 15 years, gemcitabine monotherapy has been the standard of care in many countries for the treatment of metastatic pancreatic cancer based on its modest clinical efficacy. Although the tumor response rate and survival benefit of gemcitabine is modest, its favorable toxicity profile and ease of administration has led to its wide spread and continued use. Many

studies have attempted to improve on the efficacy of gemcitabine by adding either another chemotherapeutic agent or a targeted agent. However, the vast majority of the phase III studies conducted in this setting have been remarkably negative with the exception of the addition of erlotinib and more recently, nab-paclitaxel [38,39]. Although the gemcitabine and erlotinib study demonstrated a statistically significant overall survival benefit in favour of the combination, the modest improvement in survival and higher toxicity likely influenced a more broad adoption of this regimen.

In addition, a population-based study conducted in 2012 examined the tolerance and effectiveness of FOLFIRINOX at three institutions [40]. The median PFS and OS reported in this study were 7.5 and 13.5 months respectively [40]. The PFS and OS from this study were actually higher than those from the pivotal randomized trial by Conroy et al [12]. However, this may be attributed to the fact that the population-based study included patients with all stages of pancreatic cancer, while the Conroy study enrolled only those with metastatic disease [12,40]. With respect to adverse events, the observed rate of febrile neutropenia in the population-based study was 4.9%, which is similar to the rate observed in the Conroy study (5.4%), which suggests that the results of the clinical trial may be generalizable to an uncontrolled setting. This population-based study concluded that FOLFIR-INOX was clinically effective in the treatment of advanced pancreatic adenocarcinoma and that the toxicity profile of the regimen does not outweigh the benefits in terms of ObRR and

Control									
					Experimental				
Treatment	**G**	**GF**	**GCap**	**GOx**	**GCis**	**FOLFIRINOX**	**GE**	**GS**	**GnP**
G		0.94 0.75 – 1.18	0.83 0.67 – 1.02	0.88 0.73 – 1.09	0.98 0.75 – 1.24	0.57 0.40 – 0.80	0.82 0.60 – 1.11	0.79 0.62 – 0.98	0.72 0.53 – 0.97
GF	1.06 0.85 – 1.34		0.88 0.65 – 1.20	0.94 0.70 – 1.30	1.04 0.73 – 1.44	0.60 0.40 – 0.92	0.87 0.60 – 1.28	0.84 0.60 – 1.14	0.76 0.54 – 1.12
GCap	1.20 0.98 – 1.48	1.14 0.83 – 1.54		1.07 0.83 – 1.39	1.18 0.85 – 1.60	0.69 0.46 – 1.03	0.99 0.69 – 1.43	0.96 0.69 – 1.27	0.87 0.61 – 1.25
GOx	1.13 0.92 – 1.38	1.07 0.77 – 1.43	0.94 0.72 – 1.20		1.10 0.78 – 1.50	0.64 0.43 – 0.95	0.93 0.64 – 1.33	0.90 0.64 – 1.19	0.82 0.56 – 1.16
GCis	1.03 0.81 – 1.33	0.97 0.70 – 1.36	0.85 0.63 – 1.18	0.91 0.67 – 1.28		0.58 0.39 – 0.90	0.84 0.57 – 1.27	0.81 0.58 – 1.12	0.74 0.51 – 1.10
FOLFIRINOX	1.75 1.24 – 2.48	1.66 1.09 – 2.48	1.45 0.97 – 2.16	1.55 1.05 – 2.33	1.71 1.11 – 2.59		1.44 0.91 – 2.28	1.39 0.90 – 2.07	1.27 0.80 – 1.99
GE	1.22 0.90 – 1.65	1.15 0.79 – 1.66	1.01 0.70 – 1.45	1.08 0.75 – 1.57	1.19 0.79 – 1.74	0.70 0.44 – 1.10		0.97 0.65 – 1.38	0.88 0.58 – 1.34
GS	1.26 1.02 – 1.62	1.19 0.87 – 1.66	1.05 0.79 – 1.44	1.11 0.84 – 1.55	1.23 0.89 – 1.73	0.72 0.48 – 1.11	1.27 0.78 – 2.24		0.91 0.64 – 1.35
GNP	1.39 1.03 – 1.87	1.31 0.89 – 1.89	1.15 0.80 – 1.64	1.23 0.87 – 1.77	1.35 0.91 – 1.96	0.79 0.50 – 1.24	1.12 0.61 – 2.05	0.88 0.50 – 1.41	

Figure 4. Hazard ratio comparisons of overall survival (OS) from mixed treatment comparisons. Median values given with 95% credible regions. Hazard ratios (HRs) expressed as experimental vs. control. G, gemcitabine; GF, gemcitabine + fluorouracil; GCap, gemcitabine + capecitabine; GOx, gemcitabine + oxaliplatin; GCis, gemcitabine + cisplatin; FOLFIRINOX; GE, gemcitabine + erlotinib; GS, gemcitabine + S1; GnP, gemcitabine + nab-paclitaxel.

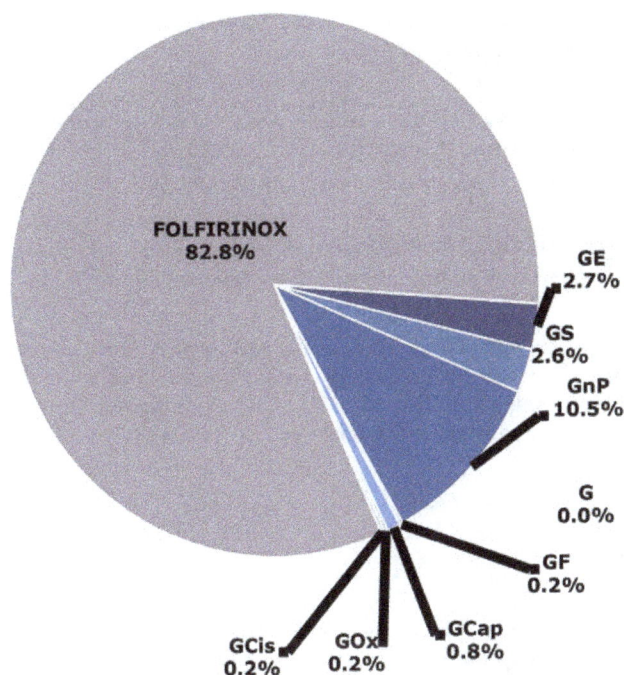

Figure 5. Probabilities that each treatment regimen is the best based on overall survival (OS). G, gemcitabine; GF, gemcitabine + fluorouracil; GCap, gemcitabine + capecitabine; GOx, gemcitabine + oxaliplatin; GCis, gemcitabine + cisplatin; FOLFIRINOX; GE, gemcitabine + erlotinib; GS, gemcitabine + S1; GnP, gemcitabine + nab-paclitaxel.

age and those with an ECOG performance status of 2. Therefore, FOLFIRINOX may be more challenging to prescribe in elderly or frail patients and caution should be taken in these cases. Ongoing prospective population-based studies are being performed to assess the efficacy and safety of FOLFIRINOX outside of clinical trials, which will provide further real life experience of the regimen. In addition, no population-based studies conducted to evaluate the survival benefit and toxicity of GnP so further research should be done in order to compare FOLFIRINOX with GnP in clinical practice.

Strengths and Limitations

There are a number of strengths of the current MTC. For example, a comprehensive and robust search strategy was used, with data being extracted by two authors independently to ensure accuracy. Although MTC allow indirect comparisons to be made, these indirect estimates may be influenced by potential biases and uncertainties. Multiple-treatment comparison meta-analysis should be interpreted with caution and specifically, the underlying assumptions of homogeneity and consistency of studies across the network should be carefully scrutinized. In our study, heterogeneity between studies was indeed assessed and reported using I^2 values. Although some heterogeneity was noted in the comparisons of GCis versus G and GF versus G, all studies in included in the meta-analysis were comparable in terms of patient characteristics and outcomes in the G reference arm (median PFS $= 3–4$ months, median OS $= 6–7$ months). The HRs from direct pairwise comparisons and the MTC were also compared and found to be consistent (Appendix S9). A limitation of our analysis was the small number of studies included which is a reflection of the landscape of the medical evidence. For many of the comparisons, data was extracted from only one trial so any biases or limitations from that study were more likely to affect the conclusions drawn from the MTC. Another limitation of this method is that it is based on published group data, rather than individual patient information. Individual patient data may allow for more patterns to be seen in terms of risk factors, however, it would still remain difficult to make strong inferences in such a complex network of treatments.

Both the FOLFIRINOX and nab-paclitaxel trials included only those patients with metastatic pancreatic cancer in contrast to the other gemcitabine combination studies, which enrolled both metastatic and locally advanced pancreatic patients. One of the

survival [12,40]. Although FOLFIRINOX demonstrates the best overall survival, progression-free survival, and objective response rate as per the large Phase III Trial [12], it is important to note that this regimen has a higher toxicity profile. When comparing the safety profiles of FOLFIRINOX and GnP from two separate clinical trials, the rate of febrile neutropenia in patients treated with FOLFIRINOX was 5.4% [12], while it was 3% in the GnP group [11]. G-CSF was administered in 42.5% of patients receiving FOLFIRINOX [11] and in 26% of patients receiving GnP [12]. In addition, it is important to note that the FOLFIRINOX study excluded patients older than 75 years of

Table 1. Comparisons of each regimen with Gemcitabine (G).

Regimen Name	OS Hazard Ratio when compared with G	Projected Median OS (months)*	NNT at 6 months when compared with G	NNT at 1 year when compared with G
FOLFIRINOX	0.57	9.9	6	5
G + nab-paclitaxel	0.72	7.8	9	9
G + S1	0.79	7.2	12	12
G + erlotinib	0.82	6.9	15	14
G + capecitabine	0.83	6.8	16	15
G + oxaliplatin	0.88	6.4	23	23
G + fluorouracil	0.94	6.0	46	47
G + cisplatin	0.98	5.8	141	146
G	—	5.65	—	—

Footnotes: Hazard ratios when comparing each regimen with Gemcitabine (G), projected median overall survival (OS), number needed to treat (NNT) at 6 months and 1 year when compared with G. Projected median OS was calculated using a median OS of 5.65 months as reported by Buris et al (5). Survival and NNT was estimated based on the mixed treatment comparisons results and the method by Altman and Andersen (22).

reasons behind this shift in patient profile of advanced pancreatic studies were the recommendations of a group of experts convened in 2009 by the National Cancer Institute in the United States based on the well described differences in survival between those with locally advanced and metastatic disease. Unfortunately, this difference in patient population across the trials included in our study could not be accounted for. However, given that the inclusion of locally advanced patients tends to magnify the overall and progression free survival, we do not expect this difference in the patients included in the studies to significantly influence our observed results.

As RCTs directly comparing FOLFIRINOX and GnP, or other existing regimens are unlikely to be conducted in advanced pancreatic cancer in the future due to both commercial and scientific reasons, indirect comparisons such as ours may represent the best possible level of evidence as to which regimen is best. Such indirect evidence may still in fact be informative in terms of both clinical and policy decision-making.

Conclusions

Our meta-analysis reviewed and analyzed the existing high-quality evidence for treating advanced pancreatic cancer in an MTC, which help synthesize evidence and may inform decision-making in the absence of direct pairwise comparisons. Based on our MTC, FOLFIRINOX appears to be the most effective regimen, however, direct pairwise comparisons are warranted to definitively address. Existing uncertainties of the relative effectiveness of FOLFIRINOX, as well as the potential toxicities and long-term effects suggest that further clinical trials and longitudinal studies are needed.

Supporting Information

Appendix S1 Summary table of trial characteristics included in systematic review and quantitative synthesis.

Appendix S2 Studies identified through the literature search. The geographic location of the institution of the primary investigator is described in the case where no study location was specified.

Appendix S3 Extracted data for PFS, OS, ObRR, and side effects (febrile neutropenia, neuropathy, fatigue, diarrhea) for each relevant reference arms from the studies included in this review.

Appendix S4 Forest plot showing hazard ratio comparisons with 95% CI for PFS from meta-analyses of direct comparisons between various systemic regimens for advanced pancreatic cancer.

Appendix S5 Hazard ratio comparisons of PFS from network meta-analysis. Median values given with 95% credible regions. HR expressed as experimental vs. control.

Appendix S6 Probabilities that each treatment regimen is the best based on PFS.

Appendix S7 Odds ratio comparisons of objective response rate. Median values given with 95% credible regions. HR expressed as experimental vs. control.

Appendix S8 Probabilities that each treatment regimen is the best in terms of objective response rate.

Appendix S9 Table comparing OS results from direct pairwise comparisons (HR with 95% CI) and network meta-analysis (HR with 95% CR) for various chemotherapy regimen comparisons.

Appendix S10 Odds ratio comparisons of febrile neutropenia rates. Median values given with 95% credible regions. HR expressed as experimental vs. control.

Appendix S11 Odds ratio comparisons of grade 3 or 4 neuropathy rates. Median values given with 95% credible regions. HR expressed as experimental vs. control.

Appendix S12 Odds ratio comparisons of grade 3 or 4 fatigue rates. Median values given with 95% credible regions. HR expressed as experimental vs. control.

Appendix S13 Odds ratio comparisons of grade 3 or 4 diarrhea rates. Median values given with 95% credible regions. HR expressed as experimental vs. control.

Appendix S14 Risk of bias graph for all included trials.

Appendix S15 Risk of bias summary for all included trials.

Checklist S1 Completed PRISMA Checklist for reporting a systematic review and/or meta-analysis.

Acknowledgments

Chris Cameron and Dr. Sharon Straus for their guidance on Bayesian statistical analysis and comments on the manuscript. **Previous Presentations of the Manuscript**: Presented in part in the poster discussion at the Annual Meeting of the American Society of Clinical Oncology 2013, Chicago, USA.

Author Contributions

Conceived and designed the experiments: KC YK DC. Performed the experiments: KC KL KS HL YK. Analyzed the data: KC KL KS. Wrote the paper: KC KS KL HL YK. Revised the manuscript: DC.

References

1. American Cancer Society (2013) Cancer facts and figures 2013. Available: http://www.cancer.org/acs/groups/content/@epidemiologysurveilance/documents/document/acspc-036845.pdf Accessed 2013 July 30.

2. Office for National Statistics (2011) Cancer Survival in England patients diagnosed 2005–2009 followed up to 2010. Available: http://www.ons.gov.uk/ons/rel/cancer-unit/cancer-survival/2005-2009-followed-up-to-2010/stb-cancer-survival-2005-09-and-followed-up-to-2010.html Accessed 2014 July 4.

3. Warsame R, Grothey A (2012) Treatment options for advanced pancreatic cancer: A review. Expert Rev Anticancer Ther 12: 1327–36.

4. Li D, Xie K, Wolff R, Abbruzzese JL (2004) Pancreatic cancer. Lancet 363: 1049–57.

5. Burris HA 3rd, Moore MJ, Andersen J, Green MR, Rothenberg ML, et al. (1997) Improvements in survival and clinical benefit with gemcitabine as first-line therapy for patients with advanced pancreas cancer: a randomized trial. J Clin Oncol 15: 2403–13.

6. Herrmann R, Bodoky G, Ruhstaller T, Glimelius B, Bajetta E, et al. (2007) Gemcitabine plus capecitabine compared with gemcitabine alone in advanced pancreatic cancer: a randomized, multicenter, phase III trial of the Swiss Group for Clinical Cancer Research and the Central European Cooperative Oncology Group. J Clin Oncol 25: 2212–7.

7. Cunningham D, Chau I, Stocken DD, Valle JW, Smith D, et al. (2009) Phase III randomized comparison of gemcitabine versus gemcitabine plus capecitabine in patients with advanced pancreatic cancer. J Clin Oncol 27: 5513–8.

8. Moore MJ, Goldstein D, Hamm J, Figer A, Hecht JR, et al. (2007) Erlotinib plus gemcitabine compared with gemcitabine alone in patients with advanced pancreatic cancer: a phase III trial of the National Cancer Institute of Canada Clinical Trials Group. J Clin Oncol 25: 1960–6.

9. Boeck S, Hoehler T, Seipelt G, Mahlberg R, Wein A, et al. (2008) Capecitabine plus oxaliplatin (CapOx) versus capecitabine plus gemcitabine (CapGem) versus gemcitabine plus oxaliplatin (mGemOx): final results of a multicenter randomized phase II trial in advanced pancreatic cancer. Ann Oncol 19: 340–7.

10. Heinemann V, Quietzsch D, Gieseler F, Gonnermann M, Schonekas H, et al. (2006) Randomized phase III trial of gemcitabine plus cisplatin compared with gemcitabine alone in advanced pancreatic cancer. J Clin Oncol 24: 3946–52.

11. Von Hoff DD, Ervin TJ, Arena FP, Chiorean EG, Infante JR, et al. (2012) Randomized phase III study of weekly nab-paclitaxel plus gemcitabine versus gemcitabine alone in patients with metastatic adenocarcinoma of the pancreas (MPACT). J Clin Oncol suppl 34: abstract LBA148.

12. Conroy T, Desseigne F, Ychou M, Bouche O, Guimbaud R, et al. (2011) FOLFIRINOX versus gemcitabine for metastatic pancreatic cancer. N Engl J Med 364: 1817–25.

13. Li T, Puhan MA, Vedula SS, Singh S, Dickersin K (2011) Network meta-analysis-highly attractive but more methodological research is needed. BMC Med 9: 79.

14. Wells GA, Sultan SA, Chen L, Khan M, Coyle D (2009) Indirect Evidence: indirect treatment comparisons in meta-analysis. Ottawa: Canadian Agency for Drugs and Technologies in Health. Available: http://www.cadth.ca/en/products/health-technology-assessment/publication/884 Accessed 2014 July 4.

15. (2008) Erlotinib for the treatment of non-small-cell lung cancer. London: National Institute for Health and Clinical Excellence. Available: http://www.nice.org.uk/Guidance/TA162 Accessed 2014 July 4.

16. Higgins JP, Altman DG (2008) Assessing risk of bias in included studies. In: Higgins JPT, Green S, editors. Cochrane handbook for systematic reviews of interventions. Wiley. pp. 187–241.

17. Parmar MK, Torri V, Stewart L (1998) Extracting summary statistics to perform meta-analyses of the published literature for survival endpoints. Stat Med 17: 2815–34.

18. Sutton AJ, Abrams KR (2001) Bayesian methods in meta-analysis and evidence synthesis. Stat Methods Med Res 10: 277–303.

19. Higgins JP, Thompson SG, Deeks JJ, Altman DG (2003) Measuring inconsistency in meta-analyses. BMJ 327: 557–60.

20. Ntzoufras I (2009) Bayesian modeling using WinBUGS. New York: Wiley. 220 p.

21. Hoglin DC, Hawkins N, Jansen JP, Scott DA, Itzler R, et al. (2011) Conducting Indirect-Treatment-Comparison and Network-Meta-Analysis Studies: Report of the ISPOR Task Force on Indirect Treatment Comparisons Good Research Practices –Part 2. Value Health 14: 429–437.

22. Altman DG, Andersen PK (1999) Calculating the number needed to treat for trials where the outcome is time to an event. BMJ 319: 1492–1495.

23. Berlin JD, Catalano P, Thomas JP, Kugler JW, Haller DG, et al. (2002) Phase III study of gemcitabine in combination with fluorouracil versus gemcitabine alone in patients with advanced pancreatic carcinoma: Eastern Cooperative Oncology Group Trial E2297. J Clin Oncol 20: 3270–5.

24. Colucci G, Giuliani F, Gebbia V, Biglietto M, Rabitti P, et al. (2002) Gemcitabine alone or with cisplatin for the treatment of patients with locally advanced and/or metastatic pancreatic carcinoma: a prospective, randomized phase III study of the Gruppo Oncologia dell'Italia Meridionale. Cancer 94: 902–10.

25. Colucci G, Labianca R, Di Costanzo F, Gebbia V, Carteni G, et al. (2010) Randomized phase III trial of gemcitabine plus cisplatin compared with single-agent gemcitabine as first-line treatment of patients with advanced pancreatic cancer: the GIP-1 study. J Clin Oncol 28: 1645–51.

26. Di Costanzo F, Carlini P, Doni L, Massidda B, Mattioli R, et al. (2005) Gemcitabine with or without continuous infusion 5-FU in advanced pancreatic cancer: a randomised phase II trial of the Italian oncology group for clinical research (GOIRC). Br J Cancer 93: 185–9.

27. Kulke MH, Tempero MA, Niedzwiecki D, Hollis DR, Kindler HL et al. (2009) Randomized phase II study of gemcitabine administered at a fixed dose rate or in combination with cisplatin, docetaxel, or irinotecan in patients with metastatic pancreatic cancer: CALGB 89904. J Clin Oncol 27: 5506–12.

28. Li CP, Chao Y (2004) A prospective randomized trial of gemcitabine alone or gemcitabine plus cisplatin in the treatment of metastatic pancreatic cancer. J Clin Oncol, 2004 ASCO Annual Meeting Proceedings (Post-Meeting Edition) 22: Abstract 4144.

29. Louvet C, Labianca R, Hammel P, Lledo G, Zampino MG, et al. (2005) Gemcitabine in combination with oxaliplatin compared with gemcitabine alone in locally advanced or metastatic pancreatic cancer: results of a GERCOR and GISCAD phase III trial. J Clin Oncol 23: 3509–16.

30. Nakai Y, Isayama H, Sasaki T, Sasahira N, Tsujino T, et al. (2012) A multicentre randomised phase II trial of gemcitabine alone vs gemcitabine and S-1 combination therapy in advanced pancreatic cancer: GEMSAP study. Br J Cancer 106: 1934–9.

31. Ozaka M, Matsumura Y, Ishii H, Omuro Y, Itoi T, et al. (2012) Randomized phase II study of gemcitabine and S-1 combination versus gemcitabine alone in the treatment of unresectable advanced pancreatic cancer (Japan Clinical Cancer Research Organization PC-01 study). Cancer Chemother Pharmacol 69: 1197–204.

32. Poplin E, Feng Y, Berlin J, Rothenberg ML, Hochster H, et al. (2009) Phase III, randomized study of gemcitabine and oxaliplatin versus gemcitabine (fixed-dose rate infusion) compared with gemcitabine (30-minute infusion) in patients with pancreatic carcinoma E6201: a trial of the Eastern Cooperative Oncology Group. J Clin Oncol 27: 3778–85.

33. Riess A, Niedergethmann HM, Molk ISM, Hammer C, Zippel K, et al. (2005) A Randomised, Prospective, Multicenter, Phase III trial of Gemcitabine, 5-Fluourouracil (5-FU), Folinic Acid vs. Gemcitabine alone in Patients with Advanced Pancreatic Cancer. J Clin Oncol, 2005 ASCO Annual Meeting Proceedings 23: Abstract 4009.

34. Scheithauer W, Schull B, Ulrich-Pur H, Schmid K, Raderer M, et al. (2003) Biweekly high-dose gemcitabine alone or in combination with capecitabine in patients with metastatic pancreatic adenocarcinoma: a randomized phase II trial. Ann Oncol 14: 97–104.

35. Ueno H, Ioka T, Ikeda M, Ohkawa S, Yanagimoto H, et al. (2013) Randomized phase III study of gemcitabine plus S-1, S-1 alone, or gemcitabine alone in patients with locally advanced and metastatic pancreatic cancer in Japan and Taiwan: GEST study. J Clin Oncol 31: 1640–8.

36. Viret F, Ychou M, Lepille D, Mineur L, Navarro F, et al. (2004) Gemcitabine in combination with cisplatin (GP) versus gemcitabine (G) alone in the treatment of locally advanced or metastatic pancreatic cancer: Final results of a multicenter randomized phase II study. J Clin Oncol, 2004 ASCO Annual Meeting Proceedings 22: Abstract 4118.

37. Wang X, Ni Q, Jin M, Li Z, Wu Y, et al. (2002) Gemcitabine or gemcitabine plus cisplatin for in 42 patients with locally advanced or metastatic pancreatic cancer. Zhonghua zhong liu za zhi. Chinese journal of oncology 24: 404–7.

38. Von Hoff DD, Ervin T, Arena FP, Chiorean EG, Infante J, et al. (2013) Increased survival in pancreatic cancer with nab-paclitaxel plus gemcitabine. N Engl J Med 369: 1691–703.

39. Philip PA, Mooney M, Jaffe D, Eckhardt G, Moore M, et al. (2009) Consensus Report of the National Cancer Institute Clinical Trials Planning Meeting on a Pancreas Cancer Treatment. J Clin Oncology 27: 5660–9.

40. Peddi PF, Lubner S, McWilliams R, Tan BR, Picus J, et al. (2012) Multi-institutional experience with FOLFIRINOX in pancreatic adenocarcinoma. JOP 13: 497–501.

19

Cellular Intrinsic Mechanism Affecting the Outcome of AML Treated with Ara-C in a Syngeneic Mouse Model

Wenjun Zhao[1]⑨, Lirong Wei[1]⑨, Dongming Tan[1], Guangsong Su[1], Yanwen Zheng[1], Chao He[1], Zhengwei J. Mao[2], Timothy P. Singleton[3], Bin Yin[1,4,5]*

1 Cyrus Tang Hematology Center, Jiangsu Institute of Hematology, the First Affiliated Hospital, Soochow University, Suzhou, Jiangsu Province, PR China, **2** Division of Hematopathology, Department of Laboratory Medicine and Pathology, University of Minnesota Medical Center-Fairview, Minneapolis, Minnesota, United States of America, **3** Department of Laboratory of Medicine and Pathology, University of Minnesota, Minneapolis, Minnesota, United States of America, **4** Thrombosis and Hemostasis Key Lab of the Ministry of Health, Soochow University, Suzhou, Jiangsu Province, PR China, **5** Collaborative Innovation Center of Hematology, Soochow University, Suzhou, Jiangsu Province, PR China

Abstract

The mechanisms underlying acute myeloid leukemia (AML) treatment failure are not clear. Here, we established a mouse model of AML by syngeneic transplantation of BXH-2 derived myeloid leukemic cells and developed an efficacious Ara-C-based regimen for treatment of these mice. We proved that leukemic cell load was correlated with survival. We also demonstrated that the susceptibility of leukemia cells to Ara-C could significantly affect the survival. To examine the molecular alterations in cells with different sensitivity, genome-wide expression of the leukemic cells was profiled, revealing that overall 366 and 212 genes became upregulated or downregulated, respectively, in the resistant cells. Many of these genes are involved in the regulation of cell cycle, cellular proliferation, and apoptosis. Some of them were further validated by quantitative PCR. Interestingly, the Ara-C resistant cells retained the sensitivity to ABT-737, an inhibitor of anti-apoptosis proteins, and treatment with ABT-737 prolonged the life span of mice engrafted with resistant cells. These results suggest that leukemic load and intrinsic cellular resistance can affect the outcome of AML treated with Ara-C. Incorporation of apoptosis inhibitors, such as ABT-737, into traditional cytotoxic regimens merits consideration for the treatment of AML in a subset of patients with resistance to Ara-C. This work provided direct in vivo evidence that leukemic load and intrinsic cellular resistance can affect the outcome of AML treated with Ara-C, suggesting that incorporation of apoptosis inhibitors into traditional cytotoxic regimens merits consideration for the treatment of AML in a subset of patients with resistance to Ara-C.

Editor: Linda Bendall, University of Sydney, Australia

Funding: This study is supported by the National Key Scientific Project of China ("973 Program", No. 2011CB933501), the NSFC Project (No. 81070417), and the Priority Academic Program Development of Jiangsu Higher Education Institutions (PAPD program). The funders had no role in study design, data collection and analysis, decision to publish, or preparation of the manuscript.

Competing Interests: The authors have declared that no competing interests exist.

* Email: yinbin@hotmail.com

⑨ These authors contributed equally to this work.

Introduction

Acute myeloid leukemia (AML) is an aggressive hematologic malignancy characterized by a clonal expansion of myeloid blasts in the marrow and other sites. Despite the progresses made in AML therapy, such as hematopoietic stem cell transplantation, all-trans retinoic acid [1] and arsenic trioxide [2], the outcomes of most AML patients remain poor. In fact, the 5-year survival for patients with AML diagnosed from 2006 to 2010 was reported to be around 20% [3]. Failures in treatment of AML can be largely attributed to the refractoriness of leukemic cells to current therapies. However, the biological mechanisms underlying leukemic resistance to treatment are unclear.

Mouse models of leukemia have been attractive because of their close mimicking of human diseases in many aspects [4]. The past few years have witnessed a large amount of effort in the search for and the assessment of novel anti-leukemia treatment strategies in these mouse models. Recently, Mulloy's group evaluated standard cytosine-arabinoside (Ara-C) and doxorubicin regimens in AML xenografts using an immunodeficient mouse model, and showed that this system is useful for evaluation of novel chemotherapy in combination with standard induction treatment [5]. Because the microenvironment plays an important role in leukemic progression and response to therapy [6] and because immune cells are part of the tumor microenvironment [6], we investigated the effects of chemotherapy in immunocompetent mice and attempted to explore the mechanisms for differential drug responses.

Although enormous effort has been put into the exploration of targeted treatment of AML in the recent years, Ara-C remains one of the most effective drugs in the treatment of myeloid malignancies and demands more attentions [7,8]. It is specific to the S-phase of the cell cycle and therefore exhibits more toxicity to neoplastic cells that are in active synthesis of DNA. However, the outcomes of Ara-C-based treatment vary among patients. Genetic factors of leukemic cells have been associated with their response to treatment. MLL translocations predict poor outcome, whereas other chromosomal abnormalities such as AML1-ETO and inv(16), are associated with better prognosis [9,10]. Our earlier work demonstrated that Nf1 deficiency conferred Ara-C resistance to AML cells and that leukemic cells with loss-of-function mutation in p53 were selected for and grew out during the acquirement of resistance to Ara-C, indicating these genetic changes affected chemotherapeutic responses of leukemia [11,12]. Recently, p53 status has also been reported to significantly affect tumor response to targeted therapy [13]. Other factors contributing to the chemotherapeutic response need to be investigated.

To investigate the cellular mechanisms responsible for poor treatment response, we established a syngeneic mouse model of AML by transplanting BXH-2 derived myeloid leukemic cells to immunocompetent mice. The BXH-2 strain of mice spontaneously develops AML at a high incidence, mainly through retrovirally insertional mutagenesis arising from infection by a murine leukemia virus (MuLV) [14] Using this AML mouse model treated with an efficacious Ara-C-based regimen that we developed, we found that leukemic cell load, and the sensitivity of leukemic cells to Ara-C determined the survival. Gene expression profiling was performed to reveal the molecular changes in Ara-C resistant leukemic cells. Of interest, we demonstrated that the Ara-C resistant leukemic cells could be suppressed in vitro and in vivo by inhibition of anti-apoptosis proteins.

Materials and Methods

1. Ethics Statement

The cell line used in this study, B117, was originally established from primary AML cells developed in BXH-2 strain of mice, and published in independent studies thereafter [15]. This cell line is available upon request. All animal work was done in accordance with protocols approved by the Soochow University Institutional Animal Care and Use Committee.

2. Cell culture, drug and chemical

B117P and its derived cells were grown as described previously [15]. All culture media and supplements, except noted individually, were obtained from Invitrogen (Carlsbad, CA, USA). Ara-C was purchased from Pfizer Italia S.R.L (Neriviano, Italy). ABT-737 was obtained from Biochempartner Co. (Shanghai, China).

3. Animals

C57BL/6J and C3H/HeJ strains of mouse were obtained from Model Animal Research Center of Nanjing, and maintained in a Special Pathogen Free environment in our university animal facility. Six- to eight-week-old B6C3F1 mice generated by mating C57BL/6 and C3H/HeJ were used for leukemia transplantation and drug treatment. Moribund animals were euthanized as the end point in the survival experiments. Since this is an acute leukemia mouse model, these animals did not show obviously detectable sickness until a few hours prior to being moribund. To minimize suffering and difficulty of the mice, the husbandry conditions and health status of mice were monitored on a daily basis for any signs of sickness and maintained from fighting or tail clipping. During the late stage of the experiments, wet food was put on the floor of the cages. Moribund mice were euthanized using a CO_2 chamber. The criteria for humane euthanasia of mice involved in this study were determined by observation of signs of illness including lethargy, hunched posture, rough coat, and significant body weight loss. For collection of peripheral blood to count cells, mice were bled quickly followed by an immediate application of antibiotic analgesics.

4. Cytotoxicity assays

The MTS (3-(4,5-dimethylthiazol-2-yl)-5-(3-carboxymethoxyphenyl)-2-(4-sulfophenyl)- 2H-tetrazolium, Amresco, USA) tetrazolium assay was used to determine cytotoxic response of AML cell lines, as described before [12]. 1×10^5 cells were plated into flat-bottom 96-well plates (Corning Inc., Corning, NY, USA) in 200 μL of ASM media with various concentrations of Ara-C. After three days of incubation, 20 μL of MTS solution was added to each well and incubated at 37°C for 2 hours. The optical density at 650 nm was recorded as a reference, and subtracted from OD490 readings to eliminate nonspecific absorbance. Data from individual experiments are presented as the mean percentage of corrected OD490 of triplicate cultures ± SD.

5. Histopathology

The various mouse organ specimens were processed for histological analysis according to standard procedure [16]. Briefly, tissues were fixed in 4% paraformaldehyde, paraffin embedded, sectioned, and stained with hematoxylin and eosin. Morphological examination of leukemic cells and peripheral blood from leukemic recipient mice or normal mice used Wright-Giemsa staining method. Images were captured using an Olympus FSX100 at 20X for hematoxylin and eosin stained tissue sections, and 200X for hematoxylin and eosin or 600X for slides stained by Wright-Giemsa, respectively.

6. Flow cytometry

B117 cells and bone marrow cells flushed from mouse femurs and tibias were blocked prior to incubation with antibodies staining for Mac-1 and Gr-1 (BD Pharmingen, New Jersey, USA). To detect apoptosis, cells were stained with Annexin V-FITC apoptosis detection kit (Biouniquer, Nanjing, China) following the manufacturer's protocol. After staining, cells were washed and analyzed on a FACScan (BD Biosciences, Franklin Lakes, USA) using FlowJo software (Tree-Star Inc, Ashland, USA).

7. Measurement of B117P cell load using a specific proviral insertion tag

Genomic DNA was extracted from B117P and mouse white blood cells using the TIANamp Genomic DNA Kit (TianGen Co., China), according to the manufacturer's instructions. B117P specific proviral insertion tags were isolated using APE-PCR, as recently reported [17]. One of the tags was chosen as a molecular marker for B117P cells whose abundance can be reflected by measuring this tag using quantitative real-time polymerase chain reaction (See the following description of qPCR for details). The primers used for amplification of B117 tag were 5′ CTGAGATGAGGCGCAACAT 3′ (forward) and 5′ CCTGTGGTTCAAGTGAAGC 3′ (reverse), and β-actin gene as the internal reference 5′ GATCATTGCTCCTCCTGAGC 3′ (forward) and 5′ GACTCATCGTACTCCTGCTTG 3′ (reverse).

8. Gene expression profiling

Total RNA was extracted with TRIzol reagent according to the protocol (Molecular Research Center, Cincinnati, OH, USA), followed by DNase I treatment to eliminate potential genomic DNA contamination. Three samples of B117P and B117HS were analyzed by Super Biotek Co. Briefly, RNA was amplified and labeled using the OneArray Amino Allyl aRNA Amplification Kit

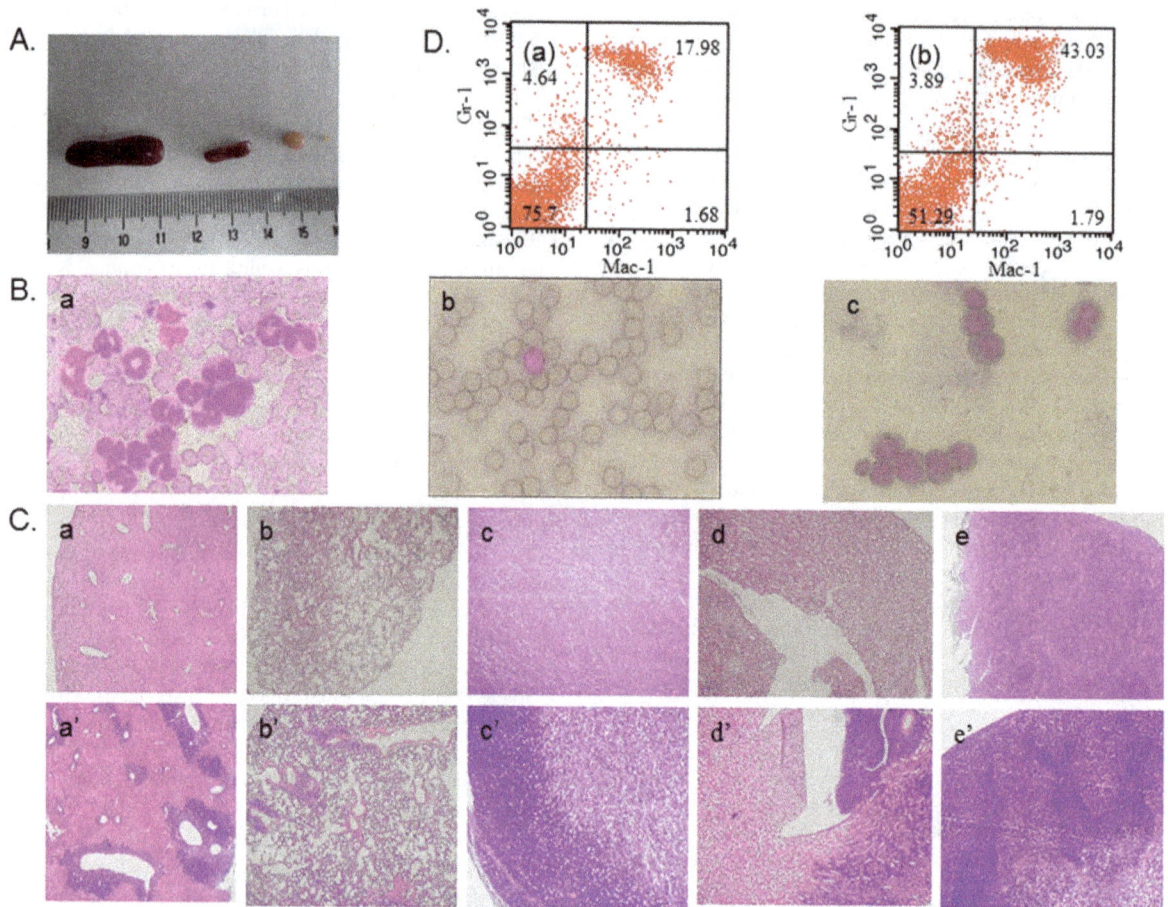

Figure 1. Establishment and characterization of an AML mouse model for evaluating treatment response by transplanting of BXH-2 derived myeloid leukemic cells into syngeneic mice (B6C3F1). Fig. 1A) Gross anatomic examination of spleen and lymph node collected from leukemic (left) or normal (right) mice. Fig. 1B) Morphological examination of peripheral blood smears from (a) recipient mice, (b) normal mice and (c) of B117 cells (Wright-Giemsa staining). Representative fields are shown here. Fig. 1C) Pathologic examination of organ sections, including liver (a & a'), lung (b & b'), lymph node (c & c'), kidney (d & d'), and spleen (e & e'), obtained from normal (a~e) versus leukemic (a'~e') mice (H & E staining). Fig. 1D) Immunophenotypic analysis of bone marrow cells recovered from normal (a) or leukemic (b) mice.

(Phalanx Biotech Group, Taiwan) and Cy5 dyes (Amersham Pharmacia, Piscataway, NJ, USA) and hybridized to Mouse Whole Genome OneArray with Phalanx hybridization buffer using Phalanx Hybridization System. Data was normalized using Rosetta Resolver System (Rosetta Biosoftware). A heat map of genes with $\log_2$ ratio ≥ 1 or $\log_2$ ratio ≤ -1 and p-value<0.05 was generated using Cluster 3.0 and TreeView and Gene set enrichment analysis was performed using ArrayTrack software (http://edkb.fda.gov/webstart/arraytrack/).

9. Quantitative real-time polymerase chain reaction (qPCR)

0.1 μg of total RNA was reverse transcribed with oligo(dT)n, using the SuperScript II First Strand cDNA Synthesis system (Invitrogen) according to the manual. qPCR was performed using SYBR Green method (Applied Biosystems, Foster city, CA, USA). Individual reaction contains diluted cDNA, 400 nM forward and reverse primers each, and 12.5 μL 2x PCR master mixes. PCR reaction was denatured at 95°C for 10 minutes, followed by 40 cycles of 95°C for 15 seconds and 60°C for 1 minute. The fold changes were calculated by the $2^{-\triangle\triangle Ct}$ method using ABI Prism 7500 SDS Software. The specific primers used for amplification of Dnmt3L were 5′ CTCTGGAAGAGCAATGGCTG 3′ (forward)

and 5′ GACTTCGTACCTGATCATCTC 3′ (reverse), Plau 5′ GTGGCAGTGTACTTGGAGCT 3′ (forward) and 5′ GCATC-TATCTCACAGTGCTC 3′ (reverse), CD72 5′ GAACAGCG-CATCTAACCATCT 3′ (forward) and 5′ GTCGCAGTTGGTTGCTCTG 3′ (reverse), Uba7 5′ GAGT-TATACTCCAGGCAGCT 3′ (forward) and 5′ CACTGAG-CAGCCAAGTCAG 3′ (reverse), Pdrg1 5′ GAGTGTCTCT-GAAGATGTGAT 3′ (forward) and 5′ GTTGACTCCGCAGCCTTTCT 3′ (reverse), and β-actin transcript levels for normalization 5′ CAAGCAGGAGTACGAT-GAGT 3′ (forward) and 5′ GCCATGCCAATGTTGTCTCT 3′ (reverse), respectively.

10. Statistical analysis

Two-tailed Student's t-tests were performed using Microsoft Excel. A p-value of <0.05 was considered statistically significant. Kaplan-Meier estimates were used to calculate survival, and log-rank was used to calculate the p-value. Survival was defined as from the day of injection of tumor cells.

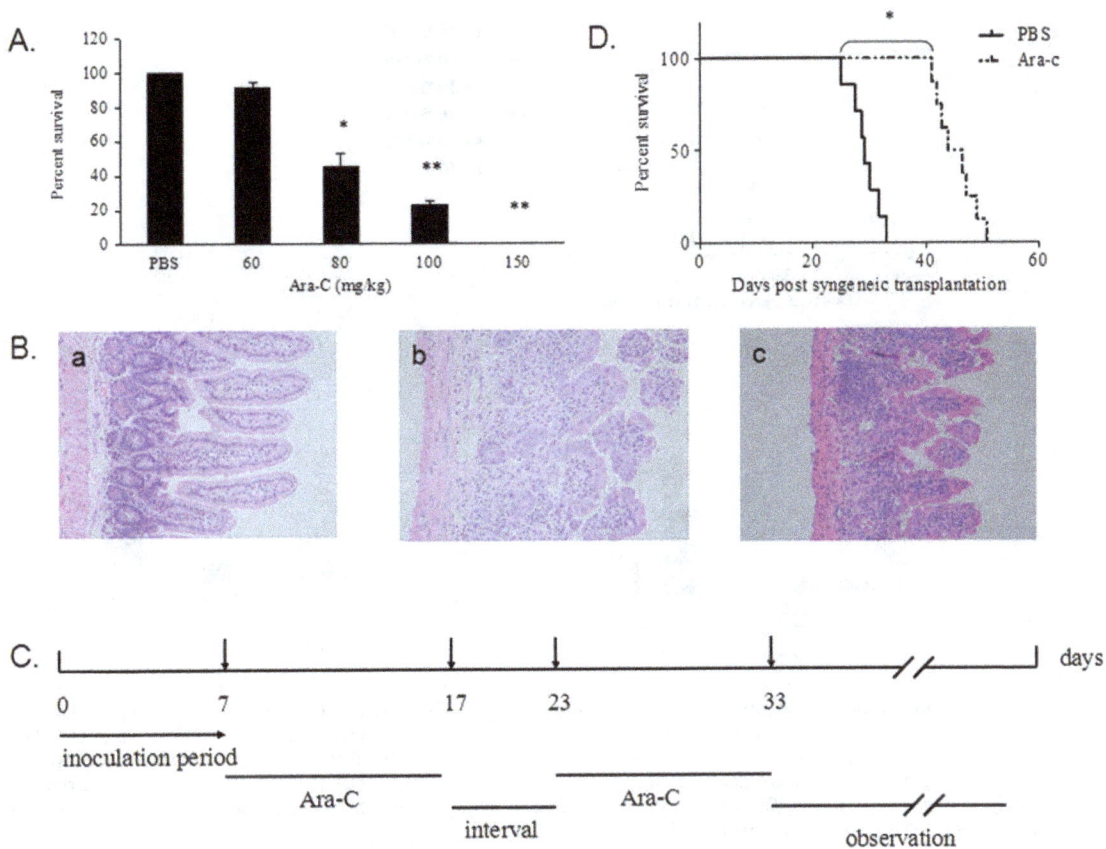

Figure 2. Development of an efficacious Ara-C-based regimen for the treatment of AML in mice. Fig. 2A) The survival rate of mice treated with Ara-C at various doses or with 100 µL of PBS control, in accordance with the treatment scheme described in the text. The mice were watched for a period of 50 days. The results shown here are representative of data obtained from 3 separate experiments. Fig. 2B) Histopathological examination of intestine affects Ara-C treatment. Fig. 2C) Treatment protocol for AML mice. The day of infusion of leukemic cells was considered as day 0. Fig. 2D) Suppression of leukemia using the treatment protocol. B6C3F1 mice transplanted with 2×10^5 B117P cells via tail vein were treated with either Ara-C (n = 12) or PBS (n = 12) as the control. *p<0.05.

Results

1. Establishment and characterization of a syngeneically transplanted AML mouse model for evaluation of treatment response

To establish an AML mouse model that is suitable for evaluation of chemotherapeutic response, we intravenously infused 2×10^5 B117 cells into a syngeneic B6C3F1 mouse. All recipient B6C3F1 mice (n = 12) reproducibly developed a hematologic disease resembling AML around a month following the transplantation, manifested by body weight loss, increased white blood cell counts, and being moribund. The necropsy showed enlarged spleen, lymph nodes and liver (Fig. 1A). Wright-Giemsa stained peripheral blood smears from diseased mice highlighted aggregates of heterogeneous blast cells with prominent nucleoli and nuclear indentations (Fig. 1B). Histopathological studies of liver, lung, lymph node, kidney and spleen revealed diffuse infiltration of the tissues with blast cells (Fig. 1C). Immunophenotypic staining of the bone marrow cells harvested from sick recipient mice showed an increased percentage of Mac-1$^+$Gr-1$^+$ cells (43%), compared with that for normal mice (18%) (Fig. 1D). These results indicated that an AML mouse model had been successfully created through a syngeneic transplantation of BXH-2 derived leukemia cells.

2. Development of an efficacious Ara-C based regimen for the treatment of AML in mice

One adverse effect of Ara-C treatment lies in its cause of damage to normal tissues. For the development of a protocol for Ara-C treatment of the mouse AML, it was important to determine the maximum tolerable dose (MTD) of Ara-C that could not only kill the tumor cells in vivo but also spare mice from the damage. To do so, we tested a range of doses of Ara-C on B6C3F1 mice that were intraperitoneally administered once a day for two courses of consecutive ten-day treatments with a five-day interval. We found that injection of 60 mg/kg of Ara-C gave rise to 5%~10% moribund animals which was further increased as the dose went up, till 100% reaching the end point mostly within the first course at 150 mg/kg (Fig. 2A). During the treatment, a significant body weight loss, a decrease in white blood cell counts, and frequent diarrhea were observed. Histopathological examination of intestine tissues of treated mice was indicative of a damage that became more severe with the increasing doses of Ara-C (Fig. 2B). These symptoms were consistent with the cytotoxicity of Ara-C. Therefore, the dose of 50 mg/kg of Ara-C was chosen for further studies.

Following several rounds of testings, we optimized the treatment scheme as illustrated in Fig. 2C. In order to examine its efficacy, AML mice created by intravenous infusion of 2×10^5 B117 cells were then treated with the protocol. Compared with the control

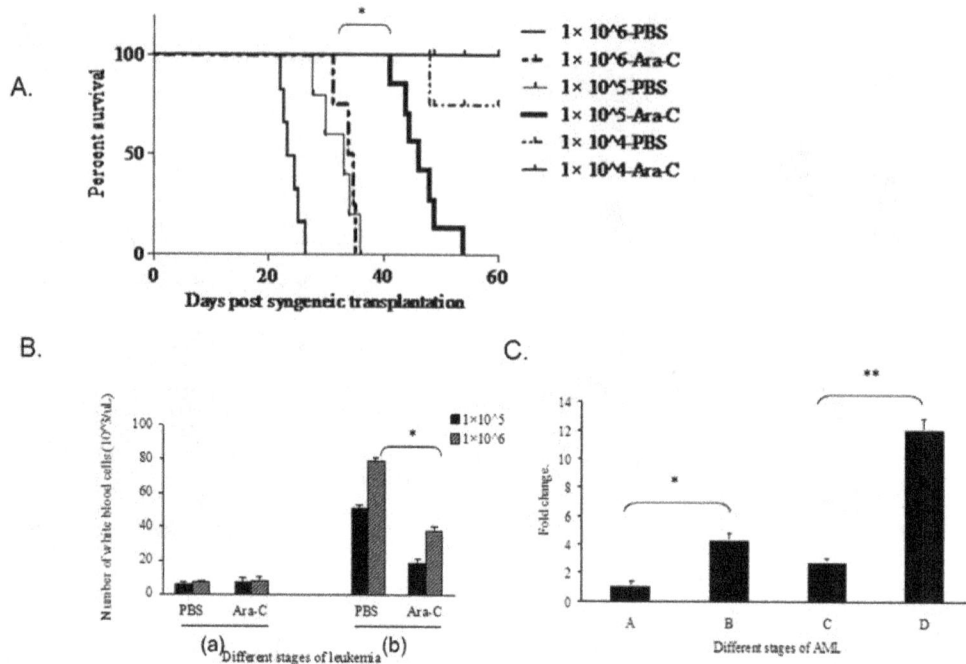

Figure 3. The effect of leukemic load on the survival of recipient mice. Fig. 3A) The survival of B6C3F1 mice receiving different dose of B117P cells and treated with either Ara-C or PBS. Each group included 12 mice. The mice were watched for 60 days. Fig. 3B) The white blood cell counts at different stages of transplanted leukemia in the mouse model. (a) before transplant, (b) after the first course of treatment. Fig. 3C) The abundance of B117 tag in the peripheral blood of recipient mice detected by q-PCR, taking β-actin as the reference, at different time points, (A) 2 days following the transplantation, (B) right before the treatment, (C) following the first course of treatment, (D) following the second course of treatment. *p<0.05, **p<0.01. The data were presented as mean +/− SD of triplicate.

(PBS) group, Ara-C treatment significantly prolonged the survival of mice for 12~14 days (Fig. 2D), suggesting that this Ara-C treatment protocol did not kill B6C3F1 mice but effectively suppressed leukemic cell growth in vivo.

3. The effect of leukemic load on the outcome of Ara-C treatment

To examine whether AML load had an impact on the treatment outcome, three different numbers of B117P cells were transplanted into B6C3F1 mice, followed by treatment either with PBS as control groups, or with Ara-C according to the above described protocol. As can be seen in Fig. 3A, infusion of 1×10^4 of B117P cells followed by Ara-C treatment did not cause moribund animal within the period of observation, whereas only 3 (25%) mice died in the PBS control group, indicative of an insufficient induction of reproducible leukemia at this cell dose. When the number of cells increased up to 1×10^5 and 1×10^6, the survival of recipient mice became shorter. Consistent with our previous observations, Ara-C treatment delayed the onset of disease, relative to the control groups. Notably, Ara-C treated mice infused with 1×10^5 B117P cells survived significantly longer than those with 1×10^6 cells, indicating that a higher level of blast cell load was associated with poor survival of Ara-C treated mice.

The recipient mice, when they became moribund, showed typical leukemic manifestations, with regard to their changed appearance and enlarged hematopoietic organs. The peripheral white blood cells of mice obtained at different stages of transplanted leukemia were counted, and the B117P tag quantified by qPCR. Following the first course of treatment, all four groups of mice displayed high counts of white blood cells, compared to normal B6C3F1 mice (Fig. 3B), consistent with moribund mice from transplanted leukemia and not from Ara-C toxicity. In PBS

control groups, mice initially receiving 1×10^6 B117P cells died gradually, and had a greater increase in the numbers of white blood cells than mice injected with 1×10^5 cells which were still normal (Fig. 3C). Interestingly, Ara-C treated mice transplanted with either 1×10^5 or 1×10^6 cells had decreased cell counts in comparison with respective PBS control mice (Fig. 3B). This is consistent with our observation of the prolonged survival of Ara-C treated recipient mice, indicating, again, that this Ara-C treatment protocol could effectively reduce the number of blast cells. In addition, Ara-C treated mice infused with 1×10^6 cells exhibited an increased cell counts relative to mice receiving 1×10^5 cells (Fig. 3B). When they became sick after surviving the second course of treatment, mice showed markedly increased white blood cells (data not shown).

The abundance of B117P cells present in peripheral blood was also monitored by measuring the B117P-specific proviral insertion tag that has previously been identified by APE-PCR [17]. As shown in Fig. 3C, the B117P tag was detected as early as 2 days following the transplantation, and found to be increased later. The levels of B117P tag were decreased following the first course of Ara-C treatment, but became high again when animals were moribund after the second course of treatment. This indicated that changes of the number of B117P cells in the peripheral blood of mice followed a pattern similar to those of white blood cell counts.

The differential survival of mice receiving between 1×10^5 and 1×10^6 leukemic cells shown here suggested that leukemic load affected the survival of untreated recipient mice and the outcome of Ara-C therapy for AML.

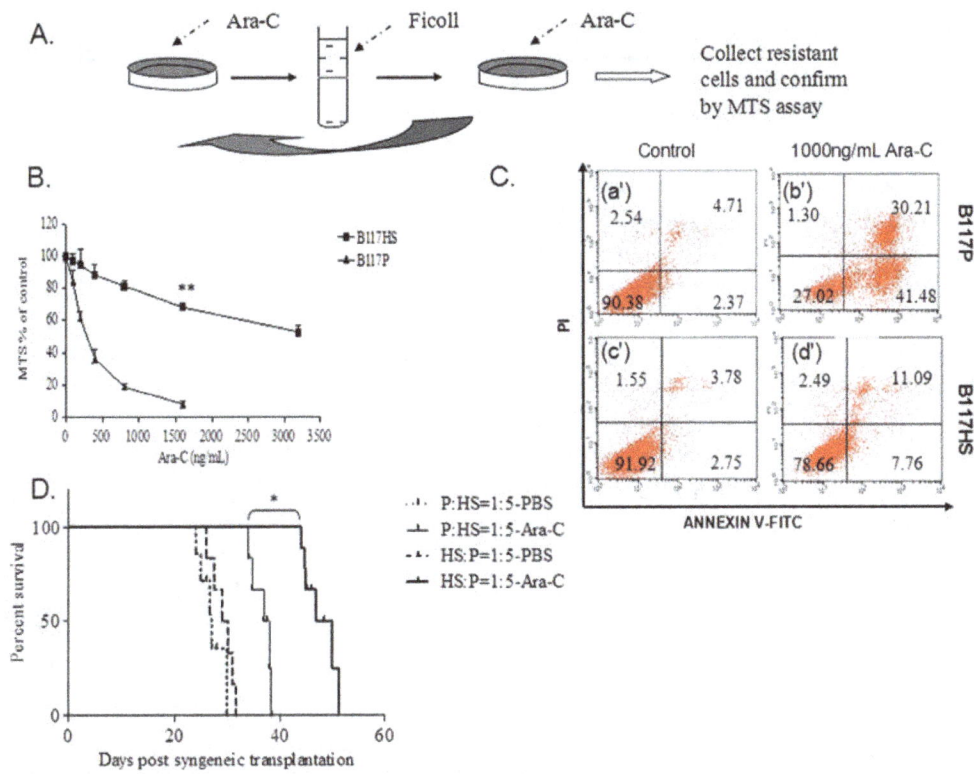

Figure 4. Sensitivity of leukemic cells to Ara-C determined the survival of treated AML mice. Fig. 4A) Selection scheme for generation of Ara-C resistant AML cells (B117HS). Fig. 4B) Comparision of B117P with B117HS in their sensitivities to Ara-C by MTS assay. **p<0.01. Fig. 4C) B117P or B117HS treated either with cell culture medium (a′ and c′) as control or with 1000 ng/mL Ara-C for 48 hours (b′ and d′) were subjected to flow cytometry analysis, according to the Methods. Fig. 4D) Survival of B6C3F1 mice transplanted with 2×10^5 leukemic cells containing different proportions of B117P and B117HS cells, followed by the treatment with Ara-C or PBS control. Each group included 12 B6C3F1 mice. *p<0.05.

4. Sensitivity of leukemia cells to Ara-C determined the survival of treated AML mice

We next asked whether the presence of drug-resistant cells in the leukemic population could impact the outcome of chemotherapy. Firstly, to generate isogenic leukemic cells with different drug sensitivity, we put B117P cells under selection against Ara-C at an initial concentration of 160 ng/mL. This concentration was chosen based on our previous observation that it could give rise to marked cytotoxicity but was no higher than the IC50 of B117P [12]. Thus, over 50% of treated cells could survive this initial treatment (data not shown). As depicted in Fig. 4A, a highly Ara-C resistant cell line, designated as B117HS, was derived from B117P by consecutive exposure to increasing concentrations of Ara-C, as described before [12]. It took about 10 weeks to produce B117HS. To verify the drug resistance of B117HS cells, we then performed MTS assay to determine their sensitivity to Ara-C. As shown in Fig. 4B, the IC50 of B117HS to Ara-C was about ten times higher than that of B117P. Flow cytometry analysis showed that treatment with 1000 ng/mL Ara-C induced apparent apoptosis of B117P and B117HS cells (Fig. 4C).

With the Ara-C resistant cells obtained, we next evaluated the effects of drug sensitivity of leukemic cells on the survival of transplanted animals. To better mimic the clinical context, we mixed B117P and B117HS at the ratio of 1:5 or 5:1, and transplanted the mixtures into B6C3F1 mice, prior to the drug treatment. All mice displayed similar signs of illness including lethargy, hunched posture, rough coat, and body weight loss, and eventually being moribund from AML. As shown in Fig. 4D, no obvious difference in the survival of mice between control groups

B117P:B117HS (1:5) and B117P:B117HS (5:1) was detected. However, Kaplan-Meier analysis showed that, among Ara-C treated mice, B117P:B117HS (5:1) group survived significantly (p<0.05) longer than B117P:B117HS (1:5) group, indicating that an increased proportion of B117HS cells resulted in a poor outcome of chemotherapy. These data suggested that the existence of drug-resistant cells in leukemic population could affect the outcome of Ara-C treatment in vivo.

5. Gene expression profiling of leukemic cells sensitive or resistant to Ara-C

In order to further explore the intrinsic mechanism determining response to chemotherapy at a molecular level, a comparison of gene expression profiles between Ara-C resistant B117HS cells and their parental B117P-derived passage control cells was performed by Super Biotek using Mouse OneArray Microarray. Fluorescent aRNA targets were prepared from 1 or 2.5 µg total RNA samples using OneArray Amino Allyl aRNA Amplification Kit (Phalanx Biotech Group, Taiwan) and Cy5 dyes (Amersham Pharmacia, Piscataway, NJ, USA). Fluorescent targets were hybridized to the Mouse Whole Genome OneArray with Phalanx hybridization buffer using Phalanx Hybridization System. After 16 hrs hybridization at 50°C, non-specific binding targets were washed away by three different washing steps (Wash I 42°C 5 min; Wash II 42°C 5 min, 25°C 5 min; Wash III rinse 20 times), and the slides were dried by centrifugation and scanned by Axon 4000B scanner (Molecular Devices, Sunnyvale, CA, USA). The intensities of each probe were obtained by GenePix 4.1 software (Molecular Devices). Genechip hybridization data were collected,

Table 1. Genes upregulated or downregulated in B117HS compared with B117P.

Gene name	Super biotek probe set ID	Gene description	n-fold
Upregulated			
Thbs1	PH_mM_0014241	thrombospondin 1	99.99
CD63	PH_mM_0009050	CD63 antigen	99.99
Dnmt3L	PH_mM_0000812	DNA (cytosine-5-)-methyltransferase 3-like	70.09
Plau	mMC007080	plasminogen activator, urokinase	47.5
Tgfb3	mMC024423	transforming growth factor, beta 3	33.15
Rbpms	mMC016216	RNA binding protein gene with multiple splicing	19.03
Zmat3	mMC026312	zinc finger matrin type 3	18.95
ABCB9	mMR028795	ATP-binding cassette, sub-family B (MDR/TAP), member 9	16.46
Vopp1	mMC008041	vesicular, overexpressed in cancer, prosurvival protein 1	12.89
Gdf5	mMC004863	growth differentiation factor 5	11.9
Vegfa	PH_mM_0001624	vascular endothelial growth factor A	10.43
Kdr	PH_mM_0001297	kinase insert domain protein receptor	9.51
Stim1	PH_mM_0014218	stromal interaction molecule 1	8.05
Bcl2	mMR026887	B cell leukemia/lymphoma 2	5.26
Downregulated			
CD72	PH_mM_0008460	CD72 antigen	68.63
Psmb9	mMC008677	proteasome (prosome, macropain) subunit, beta type 9 (large multifunc- tional peptidase 2)	46.48
Parp8	mMC009866	poly (ADP-ribose) polymerase famil- y, member 8	33.08
Ripk3	PH_mM_0001581	receptor-interacting serine-threonine kinase 3	23.91
Traf3ip2	mMC006086	TRAF3 interacting protein 2	17.8
SOX4	mMR027907	SRY-box containing gene 4	16.22
Uba7	mMC023220	ubiquitin-like modifier activating enzyme 7	15.13
Pdrg1	mMC022475	p53 and DNA damage regulated 1	14.69
Cmpk2	mMC005508	cytidine monophosphate (UMP-CMP) kinase 2, mitochondrial	9.9
Lgals1	mMC003871	lectin, galactose binding, soluble 1	9.85
Ttc3	mMR026668	tetratricopeptide repeat domain 3	9.04

corrected, normalized, and statistically analyzed using programs including statistical Analysis of Microarray, GeneData Analyst, Principal Components Analysis and Cluster. As shown in Fig. 5A, a list of 578 genes with t-test ($p < 0.01$) and fold-change (≥ 5.5) analysis was obtained, including 366 up-regulated and 266 down-regulated known genes in B117HS cells. Many of these genes were involved in resistance to chemotherapy or tumor formation and metastasis (Table 1). Expression changes for Dnmt3L, Plau, Bcl2, CD72, Uba7 and Pdrg1 genes were confirmed by quantitative real-time PCR analysis using the ABI7500 (Fig. 5B). Our microarray study revealed extensive changes in gene expression levels of Ara-C resistant cells, and some of these may influence chemotherapy response and warrant further exploration.

6. Sensitivity of Ara-C resistant leukemic cells to an inhibitor of anti-apoptosis proteins (ABT-737)

Because of the result of gene expression profiling including up-regulated Bcl-2, we were curious whether Ara-C resistant cells were responsive to inhibition of anti-apoptotic proteins. Previous studies have shown that ABT-737, a BH3 mimetic, inhibited the pro-survival function of Bcl-2, Bcl-xL and Bcl-w, and induced apoptosis in a variety of cancer cell types [18–21]. We first examined the response of B117HS to ABT-737 in vitro. As shown in Fig. 6A, ABT-737 treated B117HS cells exhibited considerable

apoptosis and/or necrosis compared to the control. To examine if B117P cells can be effectively treated by ABT-737, we performed MTS assay to measure the sensitivity of B117P to ABT-737. We found that B117P cells were sensitive to ABT-737 treatment, with an estimated IC50 of 2 μM (figure 6B(a)). Interestingly, B117HS exhibited a significantly lower IC50 compared with B117P ($p < 0.05$; figure 6B(a)), indicating that B117HS became even more sensitive to ABT-737 than B117P cells. Then, we determined the sensitivity of cultured B117HS to the combined treatment with Ara-C plus ABT-737 by MTS assay, and found that combined use of 0.4 μM of ABT-737 and an escalation of concentrations of Ara-C ranging from 200 ng/mL to 3200 ng/mL significantly reduced the viability of B117HS cells relative to the treatment with Ara-C alone (Fig. 6B(b)). These data indicated that ABT-737 had a suppressive effect on Ara-C resistant cells, and encouraged us to further examine the in vivo activity of ABT-737. As we observed previously, single agent Ara-C was effective in delaying the progression of leukemia in recipient mice. Excitingly, the combined treatment with Ara-C and ABT-737 suppressed leukemia and prolonged the survival to an even greater extent than the group treated with Ara-C alone (Fig. 6C(a)). However, mice transplanted with B117P-dervied leukaemia had no significantly different survival following the treatment with ABT-737 plus Ara-C compared with Ara-C treatment alone (Fig. 6C(b)).

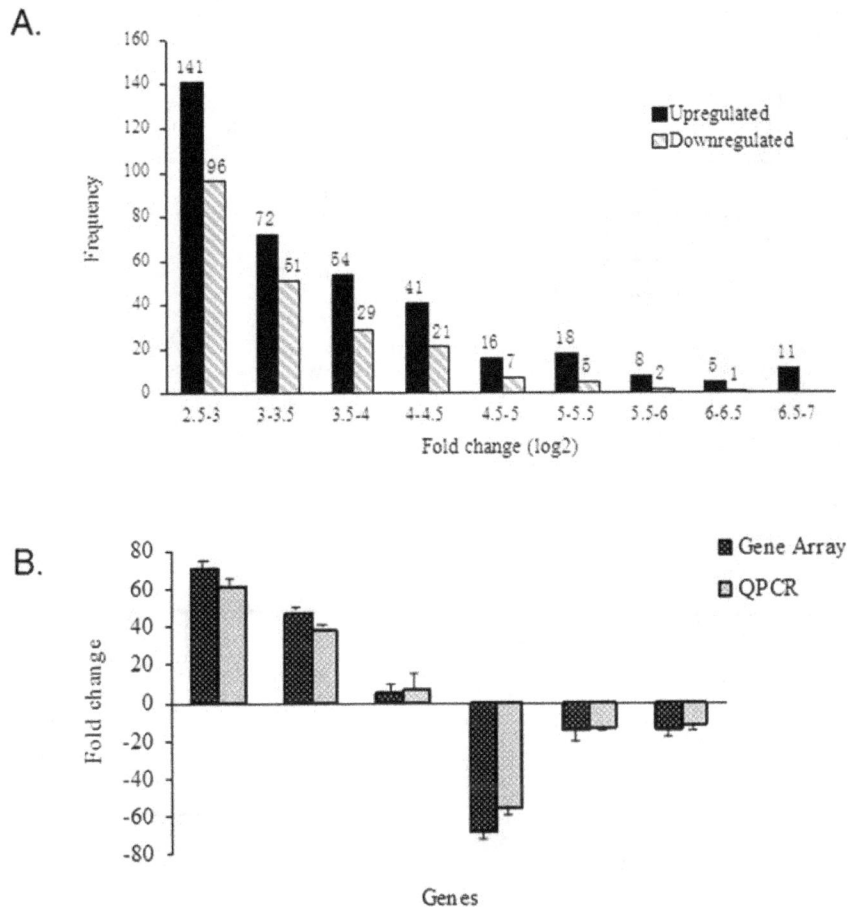

Figure 5. Gene expression profiling of leukemic cells sensitive or resistant to Ara-C. Fig. 5A) Histogram plot shows the distribution of genes with a fold change (log_2) over 2.5. Fold changes were calculated by Rosetta Resolver 7.2 with error model adjusted by Amersham Pairwise Ration Builder for signal comparison of samples. Fig. 5B) Validation of the differences in expression of Dnmt3L, Plau, Bcl-2, CD72, Uba7 and Pdrg1 genes by quantitative PCR. In order to verify the direction and magnitude of the changes in gene expression induced by resistance of Ara-C in the gene microarrays, q-PCR was performed using primers to the selected genes whose expression levels were significantly altered in the array analysis.

Ara-C resistance of AML cells could be partially reversed by the treatment with ABT-737. These results suggest that inhibition of anti-apoptosis may improve the outcome of Ara-C treatment of AML with intrinsic resistance.

Discussion

The cure of AML represents a clinical challenge. Although a large body of work has focused on the responses of leukemic cells to a variety of chemotherapeutics, most patients die from relapse. In this report, we investigated the cellular factors contributing to poor prognosis. We found that leukemic cell load within a certain range and intrinsic cellular chemosensitivity are important factors determining the outcome of in vivo treatment of AML.

Targeted therapy of AML with small molecules has been intensely pursued over the past decade. The small compounds act on certain genes or their encoded products that are specifically or preferentially critical to malignant cell survival or proliferation, and can effectively kill tumor cells while having minor side effects. However, the array of molecules that have been developed so far have not proven efficacious in patients, in general [22]. On the other hand, since the standard first line of chemotherapy includes Ara-C we focused on the investigation of AML response to this classic drug.

A variety of mouse models have been developed to study the initiation, progression, and maintenance of AML including chromosome translocation-associated leukemia [23,24], and mutant gene-induced myeloid malignancy [25]. Recently, by crossing PML-RARA transgenic mice with BXH-2 mice, Kogan's group has identified a new cooperating pathway to leukemogenesis: Sox4 overexpression accelerated PML-RARα initiated acute promyelocytic leukemia with increased penetrance and reduced latency of disease [26]. Most of the AML mouse models that have been reported are xenografts of human leukemic cells. In contrast to ALL, AML xenotransplantation models are hampered by the problems of inadequate engraftment and a short life span of the animals [27]. Importantly, these systems are usually immunocompromised to facilitate successful engraftment. In this study, we developed an immunocompetent AML mouse model to complement xenotransplant models and mirror the pathology and response to chemotherapy in patients because it is known that the microenvironment can significantly affect tumor response to therapeutics. Based on this mouse model, we developed an Ara-C treatment protocol that has a minimum toxicity but this confirms that suppressed the growth of transplanted AML cells and prolonged the survival of recipient mice. In our study, we found that the two courses of 10-day consecutive treatment scheme with 50 mg/kg of Ara-C worked well.

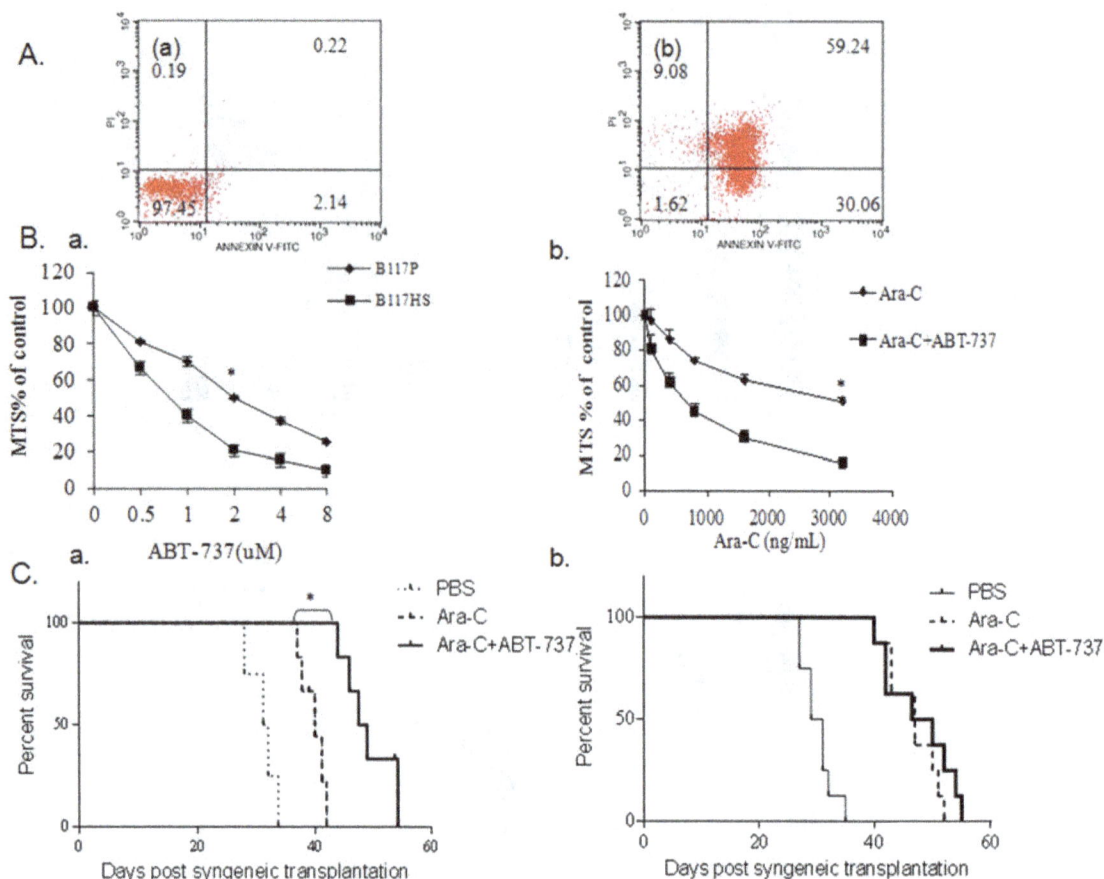

Figure 6. Sensitivity of Ara-C resistant leukemic cells to an inhibitor of anti-apoptosis proteins (ABT-737). Fig. 6A) In vitro induced apoptosis of B117HS cells by ABT-737. B117HS cells were treated with either DMEM medium as control (a) or with 2.0 μM of ABT-737 (b) for two days, followed by apoptosis analysis according to the Methods. Fig. 6B) Sensitivity of B117P and B117HS cells to ABT-737 (a). Cells were treated with 0.5 μM~8 μM of ABT-737 for three days prior to the MTS assay as described in the Methods. *p<0.05. Sensitivity of B117HS cells to Ara-C alone or in combination with ABT-737. (b). B117HS cells were treated with Ara-C alone or Ara-C combined with 0.4 μM of ABT-737 for three days prior to the MTS assay as described in the Methods. *p<0.05. Fig. 6C) Kaplan-Meier curves of recipient mice treated with Ara-C alone or in combination with ABT-737. B6C3F1 mice were infused with 2×10^5 B117HS cells (a) or B117P cells (b), followed by the treatment with PBS, Ara-C (50 mg/kg), or Ara-C (50 mg/kg) and ABT-737 (25 mg/kg), respectively. Each group contained 8 mice. *p<0.05.

In clinical practice, the number of leukemic blast cells is associated with the outcome of treatment. Measurement of leukemic load can be a useful tool in order to predict risk of relapse in patients [28]. Tumor load is also an important index for AML treatment by allogeneic bone marrow transplantation (BMT), and intermediate dose of Ara-C is suggested to be used to reduce leukemic load prior to allogeneic BMT [29]. In addition, it is helpful to monitor changes in tumor load following transplantation, since immunotherapy is known to be effective for low tumor burden. Some investigators have found an association between persistence of minimum residual disease and risk of relapse. Nevertheless, data from the literature remain contradictory and further correlations should be established [30]. Using a syngeneic transplantation mouse model, we showed that AML cell load of $1 \times 10^{5~6}$ were correlated with the survival of Ara-C treated recipient mice. In agreement, Mulloy observed that early treatment of transplanted AML cells before they expanded out could result in some cures, whereas mice with significant leukemic grafts were not cured using treatment by Ara-C plus doxorubicin [5]. Furthermore, Esteve et al. recently reported that patients with AML harboring a low burden of FLT3-ITD mutation and concomitant NPM1 mutation have a favorable

outcome [31]. It appears that heavy leukemic load disrupts normal hematopoiesis more severely or more frequently results in leukemic infiltration of extramedullary organs which is commonly seen in patients with AML. Indeed, we noticed the marked infiltration of transplanted leukemia cells into organs, such as liver, lung, kidney, gastrointestinal tract (data not shown).

It is well established that tumor microenvironment and chronic inflammation play an important role in malignant transformation and progression [6]. Furthermore, it has been found that microenvironment can provide protection from cell death induced by treatment with chemotherapeutics or targeted small molecules for various types of tumors, including solid tumors, multiple myeloma, CLL, CML, AML as well [32–34]. Paradoxically, chemotherapy induced damage to tumor niches promote the development of tumor therapy resistance in some instances [35,36]. Therefore, to evaluate the intrinsic cellular effect on treatment outcome, it would be more appropriate to have a model with a normal microenvironment. Instead of immunodeficient mice, we have established a mouse model with syngeneic transplantation of AML. By following an optimized Ara-C treatment protocol, we demonstrated that the portion of leukemic cells ($>1 \times 10^5$) with intrinsic drug resistance affected the survival of treated mice. The intrinsic sensitivity of AML cells affected the outcome of AML treatment with Ara-C. This may help explain the observations that AML cells from different patients showed differential sensitivity to chemotherapy in a xenograft model [5]. Furthermore, heavy tumor load may also give rise to an increased probability of having resistant cell clones or of deriving them during chemotherapy, and influencing leukemia treatment response. Interestingly, our molecular study found extensive changes between sensitive and resistant cells in the expression levels of many genes that are involved in the regulation of several important cellular properties, such as proliferation, survival, metabolism, etc. These results reinforce the idea of intrinsic cellular mechanisms contributing to the treatment outcome of AML. Whether the differentially expressed genes are directly involved in the regulation of leukemic drug response awaits further exploration.

When they become resistant to chemotherapeutics, leukemic cells may retain or even upregulate their intrinsic anti-apoptotic mechanisms. We found that the growth of both Ara-C sensitive and resistant leukemic cells could be inhibited by a Bcl-2-specific BH3 mimetic, called ABT-737. Interestingly, resistant B117HS cells were even more effectively treated by ABT-737 than B117P cells in vitro and in vivo, which may be at least in part explained by the so-called onco-addiction hypothesis. This was a surprise to us, initially, even it was within our conceptual assumptions beforehand, because, although the onco-addiction is an interesting concept which can be translated into efficacious therapy for tumors in some cases, this concept may not equally well suit into every cases. Therefore, based on these analyses, and given the fact that the Ara-C sensitive and resistant B117 cells have similar expression levels of BCL-XL but are different for BCL-2, it seems that the Ara-C resistant B117HS cells are now reliant on BCL-2 function, and that Ara-C resistant leukemic cells with increased BCL-2 expression can become more sensitive to BCL-2 inhibition. ABT-737 has previously been demonstrated to be effective against

AML and other forms of hematologic malignancies [18,19,21,37–39]. The inhibition of resistant cells by ABT-737 suggests that AML cells with intrinsic resistance to Ara-C remain sensitive to the suppression of anti-apoptotic pathway. There may be potential benefit from using this novel therapy in combination with standard induction Ara-C. In consistence, Jordan and collaborators found that BCL-2 was upregulated in leukemia stem cells enriched primary AML populations, and that BCL-2 inhibitors (ABT-263 or ABT-737) induced cell death by targeting leukemia stem cell mitochondrial energy generation and showed in vivo therapeutic effects against engrafted primary human AML cells [40]. Recently, Abbott Laboratories developed a new Bcl-2-specific BH3 mimetic, ABT-199, which was shown to be efficacious against aggressive Myc-driven murine lymphomas with significantly reduced adverse side effects [41]. Although it seems to be an improved version, whether the new Bcl-2 inhibitory compound can also have in vivo activities against AML cells, especially those with intrinsic chemoresistance, merits further investigations using animal models such as the one that we developed and described in this study.

We have described a syngeneic engraftment mouse model for AML, and showed that this immunocompetent mouse system is valuable for investigating the therapeutic response. The leukemic cell load above certain range and cellular intrinsic chemosensitivity are important factors contributing to the outcome of therapy for AML.

Acknowledgments

We would like to thank Dr. David A. Largaespada for his critical review.

Author Contributions

Conceived and designed the experiments: BY ZJM. Performed the experiments: WZ LW DT. Analyzed the data: BY ZJM GS. Contributed reagents/materials/analysis tools: BY TPS. Assisted with the experiments: YZ CH.

References

1. Ipek Y, Hulya D, Melih A (2012) Disseminated exfoliative dermatitis associated with all-transretinoic Acid in the treatment of acute promyelocytic leukemia. Case Rep Med 2012: 236174.

2. Liu P, Han ZC (2003) Treatment of acute promyelocytic leukemia and other hematologic malignancies with arsenic trioxide: review of clinical and basic studies. Int J Hematol 78: 32–39.

3. Pulte D, Gondos A, Brenner H (2010) Expected long-term survival of patients diagnosed with acute myeloblastic leukemia during 2006–2010. Ann Oncol 21: 335–341.

4. Bin Yin, Largaespada DA (2006) Models of acute myeloid leukemia: Prospects for drug development and testing. Drug Discovery Today 3: 137–142.

5. Wunderlich M, Mizukawa B, Chou FS, Sexton C, Shrestha M, et al. (2013) AML cells are differentially sensitive to chemotherapy treatment in a human xenograft model. Blood 121: e90–97.

6. Coussens LM, Zitvogel L, Palucka AK (2013) Neutralizing tumor-promoting chronic inflammation: a magic bullet? Science 339: 286–291.

7. Connelly P, Quinn BP (2011) Manufacturing decline yields drug shortages. Science 333: 156–157.

8. Kaiser J (2011) Shortages of cancer drugs put patients, trials at risk. Science 332: 523–523.

9. Coenen EA, Raimondi SC, Harbott J, Zimmermann M, Alonzo TA, et al. (2011) Prognostic significance of additional cytogenetic aberrations in 733 de novo pediatric 11q23/MLL-rearranged AML patients: results of an international study. Blood 117: 7102–7111.

10. Marcucci G, Mrozek K, Ruppert AS, Maharry K, Kolitz JE, et al. (2005) Prognostic factors and outcome of core binding factor acute myeloid leukemia patients with t(8;21) differ from those of patients with inv(16): a Cancer and Leukemia Group B study. J Clin Oncol 23: 5705–5717.

11. Yin B, Morgan K, Hasz DE, Mao Z, Largaespada DA (2006) Nf1 gene inactivation in acute myeloid leukemia cells confers cytarabine resistance through MAPK and mTOR pathways. Leukemia 20: 151–154.

12. Yin B, Kogan SC, Dickins RA, Lowe SW, Largaespada DA (2006) Trp53 loss during in vitro selection contributes to acquired Ara-C resistance in acute myeloid leukemia. Experimental hematology 34: 631–641.

13. Yu JL, Rak JW, Coomber BL, Hicklin DJ, Kerbel RS (2002) Effect of p53 status on tumor response to antiangiogenic therapy. Science 295: 1526–1528.

14. Jenkins NA, Copeland NG, Taylor BA, Bedigian HG, Lee BK (1982) Ecotropic murine leukemia virus DNA content of normal and lymphomatous tissues of BXH-2 recombinant inbred mice. Journal of virology 42: 379–388.

15. Largaespada DA, Shaughnessy JD Jr, Jenkins NA, Copeland NG (1995) Retroviral integration at the Evi-2 locus in BXH-2 myeloid leukemia cell lines disrupts Nf1 expression without changes in steady-state Ras-GTP levels. Journal of virology 69: 5095–5102.

16. Konoplev S, Huang X, Drabkin HA, Koeppen H, Jones D, et al. (2009) Cytoplasmic localization of nucleophosmin in bone marrow blasts of acute myeloid leukemia patients is not completely concordant with NPM1 mutation and is not predictive of prognosis. Cancer 115: 4737–4744.

17. Xu Z, Li Y, Mao ZJ, Yin B (2013) The development of APE-PCR for the cloning of genomic insertion sites of Biologia 68: 766–772.

18. Del Gaizo Moore V, Schlis KD, Sallan SE, Armstrong SA, Letai A (2008) BCL-2 dependence and ABT-737 sensitivity in acute lymphoblastic leukemia. Blood 111: 2300–2309.

19. Deng J, Carlson N, Takeyama K, Dal Cin P, Shipp M, et al. (2007) BH3 profiling identifies three distinct classes of apoptotic blocks to predict response to ABT-737 and conventional chemotherapeutic agents. Cancer cell 12: 171–185.

20. Kang MH, Kang YH, Szymanska B, Wilczynska-Kalak U, Sheard MA, et al. (2007) Activity of vincristine, L-ASP, and dexamethasone against acute lymphoblastic leukemia is enhanced by the BH3-mimetic ABT-737 in vitro and in vivo. Blood 110: 2057–2066.

21. High LM, Szymanska B, Wilczynska-Kalak U, Barber N, O'Brien R, et al. (2010) The Bcl-2 homology domain 3 mimetic ABT-737 targets the apoptotic machinery in acute lymphoblastic leukemia resulting in synergistic in vitro and in vivo interactions with established drugs. Molecular pharmacology 77: 483–494.

22. Gillies RJ, Verduzco D, Gatenby RA (2012) Evolutionary dynamics of carcinogenesis and why targeted therapy does not work. Nature reviews 12: 487–493.

23. Barabe F, Kennedy JA, Hope KJ, Dick JE (2007) Modeling the initiation and progression of human acute leukemia in mice. Science 316: 600–604.

24. Kumar AR, Sarver AL, Wu B, Kersey JH (2010) Meis1 maintains stemness signature in MLL-AF9 leukemia. Blood 115: 3642–3643.

25. Nardi V, Naveiras O, Azam M, Daley GQ (2009) ICSBP-mediated immune protection against BCR-ABL-induced leukemia requires the CCL6 and CCL9 chemokines. Blood 113: 3813–3820.

26. Omidvar N, Maunakea ML, Jones L, Sevcikova S, Yin B, et al. (2013) PML-RARalpha co-operates with Sox4 in acute myeloid leukemia development in mice. Haematologica 98: 424–427.

27. Malaise M, Neumeier M, Botteron C, Dohner K, Reinhardt D, et al. (2011) Stable and reproducible engraftment of primary adult and pediatric acute myeloid leukemia in NSG mice. Leukemia 25: 1635–1639.

28. Zhu H-H, Zhang X-H, Qin Y-Z, Liu D-H, Jiang H, et al. (2013) MRD-directed risk stratification treatment may improve outcomes of t (8; 21) AML in the first complete remission: results from the AML05 multicenter trial. Blood 121: 4056–4062.

29. Beran M (2000) Intensive chemotherapy for patients with high-risk myelodysplastic syndrome. Int J Hematol 72: 139–150.

30. Perez-Simon JA, Caballero D, Diez-Campelo M, Lopez-Perez R, Mateos G, et al. (2002) Chimerism and minimal residual disease monitoring after reduced intensity conditioning (RIC) allogeneic transplantation. Leukemia 16: 1423–1431.

31. Pratcorona M, Brunet S, Nomdedeu J, Ribera JM, Tormo M, et al. (2013) Favorable outcome of patients with acute myeloid leukemia harboring a low-allelic burden FLT3-ITD mutation and concomitant NPM1 mutation: relevance to post-remission therapy. Blood 121: 2734–2738.

32. Zhang B, Li M, McDonald T, Holyoake TL, Moon RT, et al. (2013) Microenvironmental protection of CML stem and progenitor cells from tyrosine kinase inhibitors through N-cadherin and Wnt-beta-catenin signaling. Blood 121: 1824–1838.

33. Straussman R, Morikawa T, Shee K, Barzily-Rokni M, Qian ZR, et al. (2012) Tumour micro-environment elicits innate resistance to RAF inhibitors through HGF secretion. Nature 487: 500–504.

34. Uy GL, Rettig MP, Motabi IH, McFarland K, Trinkaus KM, et al. (2012) A phase 1/2 study of chemosensitization with the CXCR4 antagonist plerixafor in relapsed or refractory acute myeloid leukemia. Blood 119: 3917–3924.

35. Sun Y, Campisi J, Higano C, Beer TM, Porter P, et al. (2012) Treatment-induced damage to the tumor microenvironment promotes prostate cancer therapy resistance through WNT16B. Nature medicine 18: 1359–1368.

36. Kessenbrock K, Plaks V, Werb Z (2010) Matrix metalloproteinases: regulators of the tumor microenvironment. Cell 141: 52–67.

37. Oltersdorf T, Elmore SW, Shoemaker AR, Armstrong RC, Augeri DJ, et al. (2005) An inhibitor of Bcl-2 family proteins induces regression of solid tumours. Nature 435: 677–681.

38. Szymanska B, Wilczynska-Kalak U, Kang MH, Liem NL, Carol H, et al. (2012) Pharmacokinetic modeling of an induction regimen for in vivo combined testing of novel drugs against pediatric acute lymphoblastic leukemia xenografts. PloS one 7: e33894.

39. Beurlet S, Omidvar N, Gorombei P, Krief P, Le Pogam C, et al. (2013) BCL-2 inhibition with ABT-737 prolongs survival in an NRAS/BCL-2 mouse model of AML by targeting primitive LSK and progenitor cells. Blood 122: 2864–2876.

40. Lagadinou ED, Sach A, Callahan K, Rossi RM, Neering SJ, et al. (2013) BCL-2 inhibition targets oxidative phosphorylation and selectively eradicates quiescent human leukemia stem cells. Cell stem cell 12: 329–341.

41. Vandenberg CJ, Cory S (2013) ABT-199, a new Bcl-2-specific BH3 mimetic, has in vivo efficacy against aggressive Myc-driven mouse lymphomas without provoking thrombocytopenia. Blood 121: 2285–2288.

20

Prognostic Nomograms for Predicting Survival and Distant Metastases in Locally Advanced Rectal Cancers

Junjie Peng[1,2♦], Ying Ding[3♦], Shanshan Tu[4], Debing Shi[1,2], Liang Sun[5], Xinxiang Li[1,2], Hongbin Wu[1,2], Sanjun Cai[1,2]*

1 Department of Colorectal Surgery, Fudan University Shanghai Cancer Center, Shanghai, China, 2 Department of Oncology, Shanghai Medical College, Fudan University, Shanghai, China, 3 Department of Biostatistics, University of Pittsburgh, Pittsburgh, Pennsylvania, United States of America, 4 Department of Statistics, University of Pittsburgh, Pittsburgh, Pennsylvania, United States of America, 5 School of Science and Technology, Georgia Gwinnett College, Atlanta, Georgia, United States of America

Abstract

Aim: To develop prognostic nomograms for predicting outcomes in patients with locally advanced rectal cancers who do not receive preoperative treatment.

Materials and Methods: A total of 883 patients with stage II–III rectal cancers were retrospectively collected from a single institution. Survival analyses were performed to assess each variable for overall survival (OS), local recurrence (LR) and distant metastases (DM). Cox models were performed to develop a predictive model for each endpoint. The performance of model prediction was validated by cross validation and on an independent group of patients.

Results: The 5-year LR, DM and OS rates were 22.3%, 32.7% and 63.8%, respectively. Two prognostic nomograms were successfully developed to predict 5-year OS and DM-free survival rates, with c-index of 0.70 (95% CI = [0.66, 0.73]) and 0.68 (95% CI = [0.64, 0.72]) on the original dataset, and 0.76 (95% CI = [0.67, 0.86]) and 0.73 (95% CI = [0.63, 0.83]) on the validation dataset, respectively. Factors in our models included age, gender, carcinoembryonic antigen value, tumor location, T stage, N stage, metastatic lymph nodes ratio, adjuvant chemotherapy and chemoradiotherapy. Predicted by our nomogram, substantial variability in terms of 5-year OS and DM-free survival was observed within each TNM stage category.

Conclusions: The prognostic nomograms integrated demographic and clinicopathological factors to account for tumor and patient heterogeneity, and thereby provided a more individualized outcome prognostication. Our individualized prediction nomograms could help patients with preoperatively under-staged rectal cancer about their postoperative treatment strategies and follow-up protocols.

Editor: Keping Xie, The University of Texas MD Anderson Cancer Center, United States of America

Funding: This work was supported by the grants from Shanghai Municipal Commission of Health and Family Planning Program KJ201204. The funders had no role in study design, data collection and analysis, decision to publish, or preparation of the manuscript.

Competing Interests: The authors have declared that no competing interests exist.

* Email: caisanjun@gmail.com

♦ These authors contributed equally to this work.

Background

Colorectal cancer is the most commonly diagnosed gastrointestinal malignancy in the world. As most of patients with rectal cancer present with locally advanced disease at diagnosis, neoajuvant chemoradiation is the standard recommendation to improve patients' outcomes including quality of life. Compared to colon cancer, treatment is more heterogeneous in rectal cancer. In real clinical practice, approximately 20–50% of patients with stage II–III rectal cancer in North America receive definitive surgery prior to adjuvant treatment [1,2], and the proportion is even higher in Asia [3]. The reasons for not giving neoadjuvant therapy may be multifarious. Although neoadjuvant chemoradiotherapy (CRT) has been confirmed to improve local control for locally advanced rectal cancer, its efficacy in preventing distant metastases and improving OS remains controversial [4]. Because preoperative CRT is associated with increased complications compared to surgery alone, we sought to characterize patients with locally advanced rectal cancer who were adequately treated with surgery followed by adjuvant chemotherapy[5–7].

Currently, the TNM stage system from the American Joint Commission on Cancer (AJCC) and the International Union Against Cancer [8,9] is the most reliable prognostic system for all stages of rectal cancer patients with or without preoperative treatment [10,11]. However, TNM staging does not integrate demographic features like age, or other pathological features like histopathology, perineural invasion, or tumor location, into a patient's outcome prediction. More individualized outcome prediction models could help physicians advise patients about personalized treatment strategies and follow-up protocols.

Developing a nomogram for prognosis or treatment prediction has been considered helpful in individualized medicine and successful applications have been utilized in many malignancies[12–15]. This statistically based tool provides a predicted probability of a specific outcome, using a combined set of proven or potential prognostic factors. Recently, a nomogram was developed to predict outcomes of locally advanced rectal cancers with preoperative radiotherapy or CRT [16]. However, due to changes in pathological features after preoperative treatment, this nomogram only applies to patients who receive preoperative treatment. Our study was designed to develop prognostic nomograms for patients with locally advanced rectal cancer who did not receive preoperative treatment.

Materials and Methods

Ethics

A retrospective study was conducted at the Fudan University Shanghai Cancer Center. This study was approved by the Fudan University Shanghai Cancer Center Institutional Ethics Committee. According to hospital routine, patients are asked to provide a written informed consent after their admission that their clinical and outcome information will be used in future scientific studies. Patients' records and follow-up information were anonymized and de-identified prior to analysis. The institutional Ethics Committee approved the exception of informed consent if informed consent could not be obtained due to patients' death or lost of follow-up in our institutional database.

Patient Population

All patients with AJCC stage II–III (restaged according to 7th Edition) [8] rectal cancers were collected from the institutional colorectal cancer database. The statistical analyses were performed for patients operated between 1986 and 2005 (N = 833), whose tumors were located within 15 cm from anal verge. Patients who met one of the following criteria were excluded: (1) received preoperative treatment, (2) synchronous distant metastases, (3) surgery without curative intent, and (4) complete loss of follow-up after surgery.

An independent group of patients with stage II–III rectal cancer (N = 84) who were operated between January 2006 and June 2007 were selected for validation (Table 1).

Follow-up

According to institutional follow-up protocol, all patients were asked to follow-up every 3–6 months after surgery in the first 3 years, and 6–12 months thereafter in the next two years. Follow-up information was recorded in the database. A minimum follow-up of 60 months was required for the patients who are alive in the validation dataset so that their 5-year survival status is known. The primary endpoint is the overall survival (OS) time. Local recurrence (LR) time and distant metastases (DM) time are the secondary endpoints. The LR time was calculated from the time of surgery to the time when cancer recurrence was determined in the pelvis or anastomosis by physical examination, colonoscopy, or imaging studies. The DM time was defined from the time of surgery to the identification of distant recurrence. There were three times of massive follow-up for all off-records patients via mail or telephone in1996, 2002, and 2007.

Statistical Model Creation

Kaplan-Meier plots and log-rank tests were performed for each potential predictive variable for the primary endpoint OS and the secondary endpoints LR and DM. Cox proportional hazards (PH) model was performed to develop the predictive model for OS. All decisions with respect to the grouping of the categorical variables and categorizing the continuous variables were made before modeling. These predictive models were the basis for the nomograms and the estimated probabilities of interest (e.g., 5-year OS) were calculated and presented in the nomograms.

Model Validation

Each nomogram went through two validation procedures: internal validation using the study patients for the model creation and external validation using the independent validation patients. For each outcome variable, the predicted probability from the nomogram was compared with the actual status (e.g., alive or dead 5 years from surgery) for these uncensored observations. In addition, the Harrell's concordance index (c-index) was calculated for each nomogram [17]. This index calculates the proportion of all usable patient pairs in which the predictions and the outcomes are concordant and has a similar interpretation to that of the AUC. All the above validation analyses were performed for the study patient data and the independent validation data.

All the statistical analyses were performed using R 3.0.1.

Results

Outcomes and survival analyses

Of the 833 patients with locally advanced rectal cancer in training group, 267 patients (32%) experienced local recurrence and/or distant metastases, and 263 patients (31.5%) died of cancer or other reasons up to our last follow-up. Of those alive, median follow-up time was 51 months. The 5-year LR, DM, OS probabilities (estimated using Kaplan-Meier method) for all patients were 22.3%, 32.7% and 63.8%, respectively.

Demographic and clinicopathologic variables that potentially predict OS, LR and DM were collected, including age, gender, tumor location, preoperative carcinoembryonic antigen level (CEA), tumor differentiation, tumor histopathology, number of metastatic lymph nodes, number of total sampled lymph nodes, lymphovascular invasion, perineural invasion, T classification, N classification and adjuvant treatment. For each outcome variable (LR, DM, and OS), univariate analysis identified statistically significant predictors in the demographic features, clinical features, pathological features and treatment modalities. 5-year local control, distant control and overall survival rates were provided for every category of each predictor with p-values obtained from the Log-rank tests (Table 1).

Nomograms

For the development of nomograms, all patients in the main dataset were included (N = 833), and the nomograms were validated using the external dataset (N = 84). Two nomograms for overall survival and distant metastases were successfully developed (Figure 1). The predictors included in the nomograms are gender, age ($<$ = 49, 50–69, $>$ = 70), tumor location ($<$5 cm, 5 cm-10 cm, $>$10 cm), adjuvant chemotherapy (No/Yes), adjuvant chemoradiotherapy (No/Yes), T classification (T1–T2, T3, T4), N classification (N0, N1a, N1b, N2a, N2b), CEA ($<$ = 5, $>$5) and ratio of metastatic lymph nodes. Table 2 presents the hazard ratio (HR) with 95% CI and the pvalue for each predictor, and the c-index for the main dataset and the external dataset respectively. For OS prediction, the c-index was 0.76 in external validation, with a 95% CI of 0.67 to 0.86. Similarly, for DM prediction, the c-index was 0.73 (95% CI, 0.63–0.84). However, the nomogram for local recurrence prediction was not developed because of the poor c-index value in external validation (c-index, 0.6; 95% CI, 0.45–0.75).

Table 1. Characteristics of all patients with locally advanced rectal cancer and outcomes for 833 patients in training group.

Variable	Training Group No. (%) (n = 833)	Local Control 5 Year	Local Control P-value	Distant Control 5 Year	Distant Control P-value	Overall Survival 5 Year	Overall Survival P-value	Validation Group No. (%) (n = 84)
Demographic Variables								
Gender								
Male	490 (58.8)	0.770	0.423	0.637	0.006	0.608	0.008	50 (59.5)
Female	343 (41.2)	0.787		0.725		0.682		34 (40.5)
Age, years								
<=49	262 (31.4)	0.738	0.354	0.649	0.191	0.609	0.097	29 (34.5)
50-69	432 (51.9)	0.802		0.699		0.668		50 (59.5)
>=70	139 (16.7)	0.772		0.637		0.604		5 (6.0)
Clinical Variables								
Tumor location								
Low (<5 cm)	181 (21.7)	0.656	<0.001	0.638	0.221	0.563	0.011	26 (31.0)
Mid (5cm, 10 cm)	570 (68.5)	0.806		0.677		0.651		54 (64.3)
High (>10 cm)	82 (9.8)	0.846		0.719		0.715		4 (4.8)
CEA								
<=5	406 (48.7)	0.817	0.005	0.696	0.073	0.660	0.062	67 (79.8)
>5	427 (51.3)	0.740		0.650		0.616		17 (20.2)
Pathological Variables								
Pathology								
Adenocarcinoma	683 (82.0)	0.773	0.947	0.683	0.184	0.653	0.128	79 (94.0)
MAC or SRC	150 (18.0)	0.792		0.625		0.574		5 (6.0)
Tumor grade								
Low-intermediate grade	708 (85.0)	0.788	0.119	0.681	0.272	0.643	0.356	65 (77.4)
High grade	125 (15.0)	0.713		0.630		0.612		19 (22.6)
pT classification								
T1	13 (1.6)	0.587	0.003	0.539	0.002	0.539	0.001	0 (0)
T2	93 (11.2)	0.83		0.711		0.676		3 (3.6)
T3	351 (42.1)	0.836		0.756		0.725		81 (86.4)
T4	376 (45.1)	0.714		0.589		0.550		0 (0)
pN classification								
N0	324 (38.9)	0.837	<0.001	0.774	<0.001	0.775	<0.001	14 (16.7)
N1a	142 (17.1)	0.753		0.699		0.683		13 (15.5)
N1b	152 (18.2)	0.793		0.638		0.539		24 (28.6)
N2a	112 (13.4)	0.734		0.581		0.548		18 (21.4)

Table 1. Cont.

Variable	Training Group							Validation Group
	No. (%)	Local Control		Distant Control		Overall Survival		No. (%)
	(n = 833)	5 Year	P-value	5 Year	P-value	5 Year	P-value	(n = 84)
N2b	103 (12.4)	0.619		0.451		0.396		15 (17.8)
Lymphovascular invasion								
Yes	178 (21.4)	0.780	0.956	0.610	0.139	0.547	0.019	42 (50.0)
No	655 (78.6)	0.776		0.691		0.666		42 (50.0)
Perineural invasion								
Yes	111 (13.3)	0.698	0.076	0.544	0.003	0.515	0.002	34 (41.5)
No	722 (86.7)	0.787		0.692		0.656		50 (58.5)
No. of metastatic lymph nodes								
= 0	324 (38.9)	0.775	<0.001	0.837	0.002	0.774	<0.001	14 (16.7)
>=1	509 (61.1)	0.552		0.735		0.606		70 (83.3)
Treatment Variables								
Surgery type								
AR	494 (59.3)	0.832	<0.001	0.689	0.087	0.660	0.012	51 (60.7)
APR	339 (40.7)	0.697		0.649		0.607		33 (39.3)
Adjuvant treatment								
No treatment	252 (30.3)	0.676	<0.001	0.662	0.332	0.633	0.670	16 (19.0)
CT only	277 (33.3)	0.781		0.698		0.663		25 (29.8)
CRT only	123 (14.8)	0.822		0.718		0.612		3 (3.6)
CRT plus CT	181 (21.7)	0.905		0.697		0.628		40 (47.6)

Note: Tumor location was determined the distance from anal verge by preoperative colonoscopy or digital examination.

Abreviations: pT stage, pathological T stage; pN stage, pathological N stage; CEA, carcinoembryonic antigen; MAC, mucinous adenocarcinoma; SRC, signet ring cell carcinoma; AR, anterior resection; APR, abdominoperineal resection; CT, chemotherapy; CRT, chemoradiotherapy.

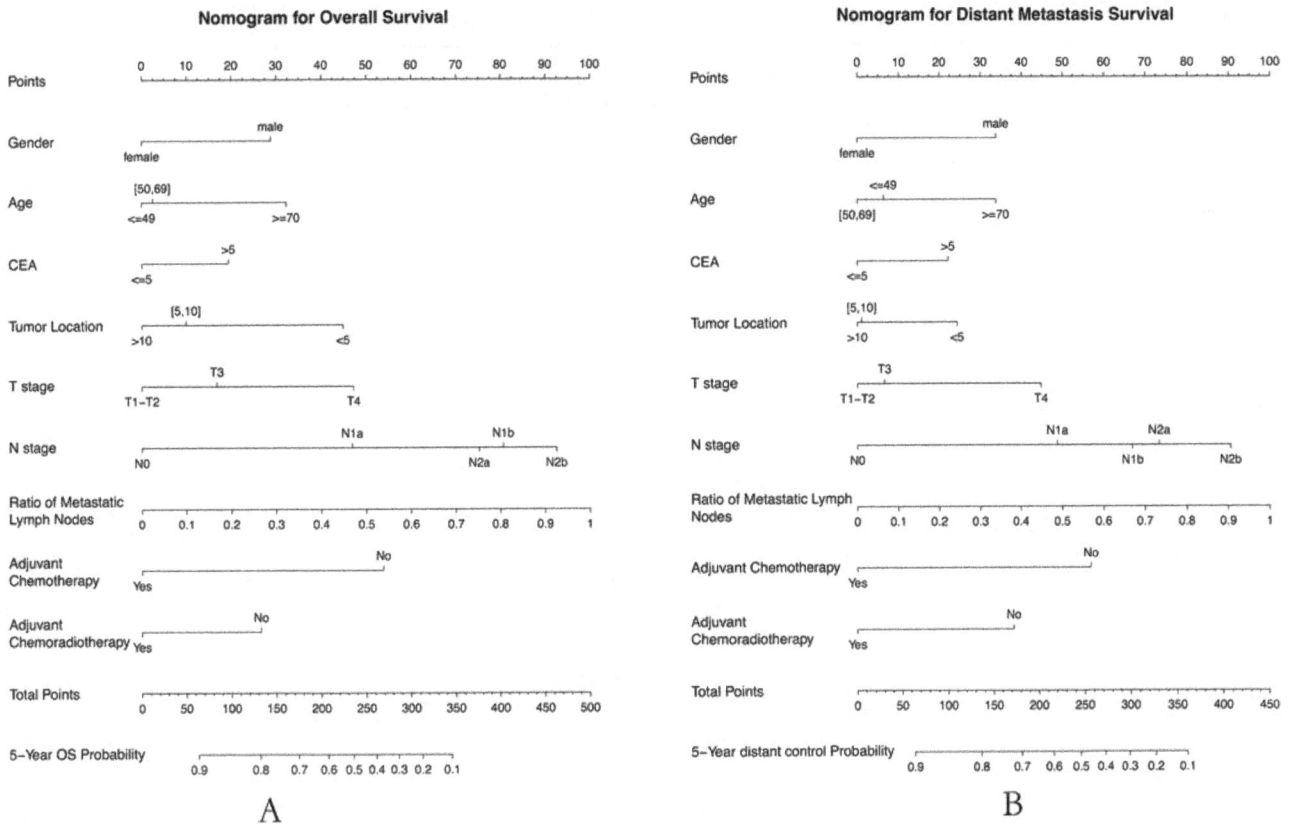

Figure 1. Nomograms developed for predicted 5-year overall survival (A) and distant control survival (B). Each variable value is assigned a score, and the sum of scores is converted to a probability of observed events in the lowest scale.

Predicted events within each AJCC stage classification

Within each AJCC stage (7th Edition), the 5-year OS rates were 82.2% (stage IIA), 70.2% (stage IIB–C), 70.1% (stage IIIA), 57.0% (stage IIIB) and 44.8% (stage IIIC); and the 5-year DM rates were 19.8% (stage IIA), 28.7% (stage IIB–C), 28.1% (stage IIIA), 34.9% (stage IIIB), and 52.0% (stage IIIC), respectively. The Kaplan-Meier survival probability curves by AJCC stage were plotted for OS and DM in Figure 2. The overall log-rank tests for testing whether the survival curves are the same among all AJCC stage groups are significant for both OS and DM (p<0.001).

Based on our developed nomograms, the predicted probability of 5-year overall survival and distant control for each patient was computed, and the corresponding histograms were produced by AJCC stage classification from stage IIA to stage IIIC, respectively (Figure 3). The histograms showed that even within the same AJCC stage category, there are still a substantive amount of variability in terms of the predicted 5-year OS and DM-free probabilities, while in average the later stage patients have a smaller probabilities compared to earlier stage patients for both survival outcomes. Greater variations were observed for later stage patients (stage IIIB and IIIC) than earlier stage patients (stage IIA to IIIC) in terms of both 5-year OS and DM-free predicted probabilities.

Discussion

In current study, for AJCC stage II–III (7th edition) rectal cancers without neoadjuvant treatment, we have developed prognostic nomograms with independent validation samples for predicting OS and DM, based on demographic, clinicopatholog-

ical and adjuvant treatment information. Our models were developed using a 20-year period institutional database; during that time, neoadjuvant RT or CRT was not well applied in China. Our predictive models are helpful to support decision-making in clinical practice and follow-up protocols, especially in patients with rectal cancer who are preoperatively under-staged and undergo surgical resection first.

The purpose of treatment in rectal cancer is to potentially improve symptoms through local control, increase chance of cure, or prolong survival. Although the German Rectal Cancer Study Group established the significant improvements in local control and toxicity for patients with locally advanced rectal cancer treated with preoperative CRT [4], long-term follow-up and other clinical trials didn't show benefit in overall survival and distant control for patients undergoing preoperative CRT[18–21]. A variety of factors ultimately influence a patient's decision to receive preoperative CRT, such as proximal tumor location, suboptimal preoperative staging methods, inaccessible facilities for optimal radiotherapy, patient preference, and/or financial considerations. The potential benefits of receiving preoperative CRT must be carefully evaluated with the potential risks. Currently, there is no nationwide or international report about the accurate proportion of preoperative CRT in locally advanced rectal cancer. The US National Cancer Database (NCDB) reported that in 2008, 41% of patients with stage I–II rectal cancer received proctocolectomy with chemotherapy or radiotherapy, in which 80% of chemotherapy, which is mainly accompanied by radiotherapy, was delivered preoperatively. However, the percentage of preoperative CRT in stage II–III rectal cancer was not reported [2]. In Canada, only an average of 45% of stage II–III rectal cancers treated in 2007–2008

Table 2. Multivariate analyses of 5-year outcomes: the final predictors for developing the nomograms.

Variable	Cox PH Regression			Nomogram	
	HR	95% CI	*p*-value	C-index	95% CI
Distant Metastases					
Gender					
Male vs Female	1.42	[1.07,1.88]	0.014		
Age (years)					
50–69 vs <=49	0.94	[0.69,1.27]	0.672		
>=70 vs <=49	1.33	[0.92,1.93]	0.134		
Tumor location					
Mid ([5 cm, 10 cm]) vs Low (<5 cm)	0.79	[0.58,1.07]	0.122		
High (>10 cm) vs Low (<5 cm)	0.78	[0.46,1.31]	0.344		
Adjuvant chemotherapy					
Yes vs No	0.55	[0.41,0.74]	<0.0001		
Adjuvant chemoradiotherapy					
Yes vs No	0.67	[0.50,0.90]	0.008	Training Data: 0.68	[0.64,0.72]
pT classification				Validation Data:0.73	[0.63,0.83]
T3 vs T1–T2	1.07	[0.66,1.72]	0.781	Ten-fold Cross	
'T4' vs 'T1–T2'	1.59	[1.03,2.47]	0.038	Validation	
pN classification				(Training Data): 0.65	
'N1a' vs 'N0'	1.66	[1.05,2.62]	0.031		
'N1b' vs 'N0'	2.00	[1.23,3.27]	0.005		
'N2a' vs 'N0'	2.14	[1.21,3.80]	0.009		
'N2b' vs 'N0'	2.56	[1.23,5.32]	0.012		
CEA					
>5 vs <=5	1.26	[0.96,1.64]	0.093		
LNR					
Continuous*	1.11	[1.02,1.20]	0.013		
Overall Survival					
Gender					
Male vs Female	1.37	[1.06, 1.78]	0.017		
Age (years)					
50–69 vs <=49	1.03	[0.77,1.36]	0.854		
>=70 vs <=49	1.42	[1.00,2.02]	0.049		
Tumor location					
Mid ([5 cm, 10 cm]) vs Low (<5cm)	0.68	[0.52, 0.90]	0.007		
High (>10 cm) vs Low (<5 cm)	0.61	[0.37, 1.01]	0.053		
Adjuvant chemotherapy					
Yes vs No	0.56	[0.42, 0.73]	<0.0001		
Adjuvant chemoradiotherapy					
Yes vs No	0.75	[0.57, 0.98]	0.033	Training data: 0.70	[0.66, 0.73]
pT stage				Validation data: 0.76	[0.67, 0.86]
'T3' vs 'T1–T2'	1.20	[0.77, 1.87]	0.414	Ten-fold Cross	
'T4' vs 'T1–T2'	1.68	[1.11,2.52]	0.013	Validation	
pN stage				(Training Data): 0.67	
'N1a' vs 'N0'	1.67	[1.08, 2.59]	0.021		
'N1b' vs 'N0'	2.42	[1.54, 3.79]	0.00012		
'N2a' vs 'N0'	2.28	[1.33, 3.91]	0.0028		
'N2b' vs 'N0'	2.75	[1.40, 5.44]	0.0035		
CEA					
>5 vs <=5	1.24	[0.96, 1.59]	0.097		

Table 2. Cont.

Variable	Cox PH Regression			Nomogram	
	HR	95% CI	*p*-value	C-index	95% CI
LNR					
Continuous*	1.12	[1.03, 1.20]	0.0046		

Note: The concordance index (c-index) for the training and external validation are given for the nomogram as a performance measure; Tumor location was determined the distance from anal verge by preoperative colonoscopy or digital examination.
*LNR was analyzed as a continuous variable.
Abbreviations: HR, hazard ratio; PH, proportional hazards; c-index, concordance index; CEA, carcinoembryonic antigen; LNR, metastatic lymph nodes ratio.

were reported to undergo preoperative RT or CRT in a Canadian nationwide cancer performance report [1,22]. In Asian countries, much lower percentage of stage II–III rectal cancers undergo preoperative RT or CRT, as most surgeons in Asia do not usually recommend preoperative CRT for clinical T2 or T3 rectal cancers [3]. The wide variation in indications and clinical applications of neoadjuvant RT or CRT reflect the complexity of the disease, which should alert international rectal cancer expert organizations as well as health-care administrators. Therefore, in current clinical circumstance, there are still a great number of patients with locally advanced rectal cancer receiving curative surgical treatment prior to RT or CRT. Our study will help rectal cancer patients and physicians to pursue more individualized postoperative treatment according to their risks of disease control and survival expectations.

With the wide utilization of neoadjuvant CRT in clinical practice and randomized clinical trials, several studies focused on the outcome prediction in patients with combined modality treatment. Recently, a prediction nomogram was developed to predict local recurrence, distant metastases, and survival for patients with locally advanced rectal cancer treated with long-course chemoradiotherapy (CRT) followed by surgery in five

European phase III clinical trials [16]. Postoperative ypT stage and ypN stage were most relevant to overall survival. However, as downstaged by preoperative CRT, the two most important prognostic factors (ypT and ypN classfications) could not be well applied to patients treated with curative surgery prior to adjuvant treatment. Otherwise, the decision of neoadjuvant CRT mainly relies on preoperative staging of the primary tumor. The accuracy of T and N stage by preoperative MRI or endorectal ultrasound varies, especially in N stage. A number of patients with locally advanced rectal cancer will be under-staged preoperatively and undergo surgery first. The postoperative treatment and outcome prediction for this group of patients are currently lacking. Moreover, although perioperative CRT or CT has been proved to be effective in rectal cancer, in real clinical circumstance, there are still a part of patients with locally advanced rectal cancer undergoing surgery alone. According to a large-scale population-based study through the California Cancer Registry, there were still 33% and 18.6% of patients with stage II and stage III rectal cancer undergoing surgery alone from the year 1994 to 2008 [23]. Similarly, 57.4% and 13.0% of patients with stage II and stage III rectal cancer underwent surgery alone in our study. Currently, we are lacking of studies in defining characteristics of patients who

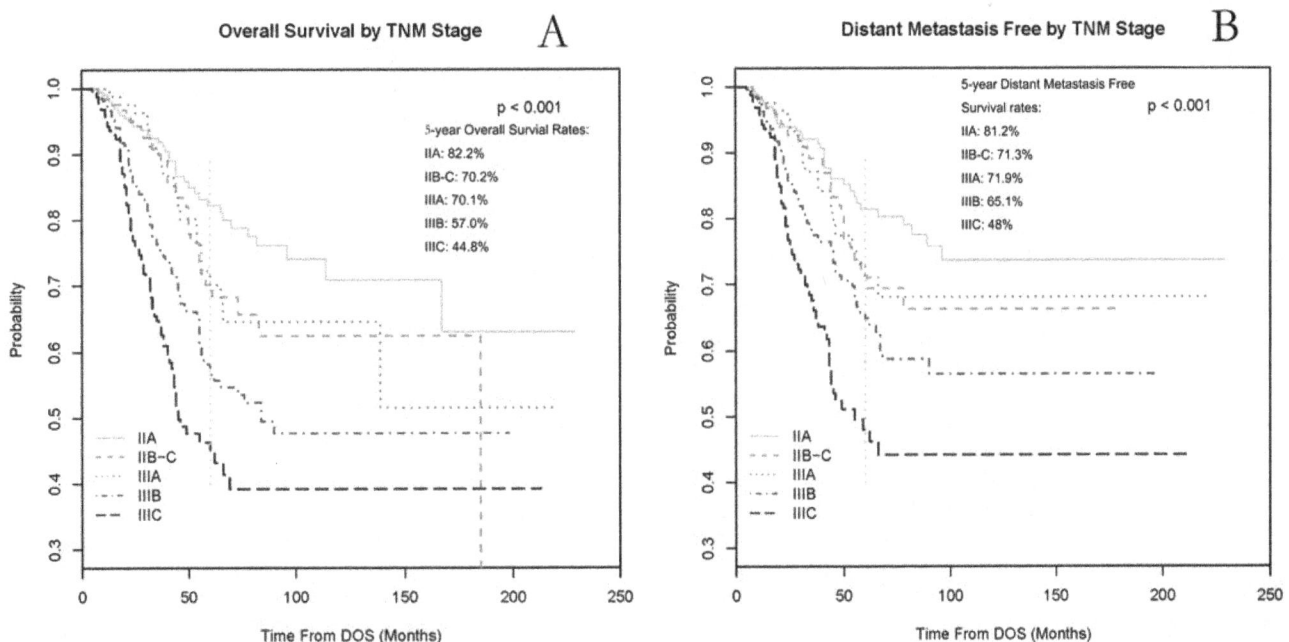

Figure 2. The overall survival (A) and distant metastases free (B) Kaplan-Meier probability curves within each stage (AJCC 7ᵗʰ Edition) classification in locally advanced rectal cancer.

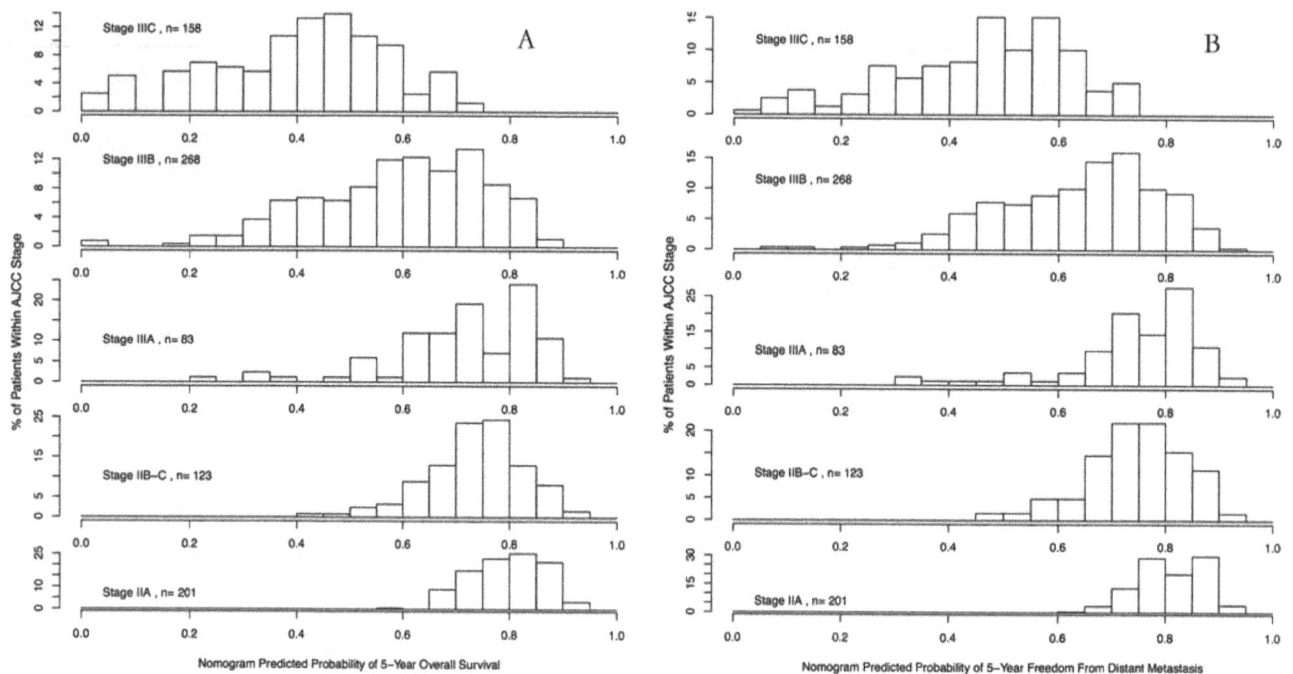

Figure 3. Histogram of nomogram-predicted 5-year overall survival rate (A) and distant control rate (B) within each subgroup of the 7th edition of American Joint Committee on Cancer (AJCC) stage.

have good outcomes without neoadjuvant therapy, particularly with surgery alone. Our nomogram provides a helpful tool for identifying patients with good outcomes if they were preoperatively under-staged and underwent surgery first. Meanwhile, as preoperative CRT contributed small improvements in overall survival and distant metastases, our study provided helpful tools and comparable dataset for predicting patients' distant control and overall survival in locally advanced rectal cancer with multiple treatment modalities.

The goal of our study is to develop monograms to predict overall survival and distant metastases for patients without preoperative treatment. To our knowledge, using the 7th edition of AJCC staging system was the first predicting model for OS and distant control in rectal cancer (Figure 2), especially in Asian patients who were less represented in the AJCC stage system. Similar survival differences among different AJCC stage categories were observed in our patient cohort, as compared with Surveillance, Epidemiology, and End Results (SEER) population-based data [24]. Postoperative T stage and N stage were still most significant factors to predict OS and DM rates. However, from the predicted outcomes based on our nomograms, heterogeneities in the risk of death and distant metastases still largely existed within each sub-category stage from stage IIA to stage IIIC. Specifically, from the histograms in Figure 3, the variability of predicted OS and DM rates was observed greater in patients in stage IIIB and IIIC than patients in stage IIA–IIIA. This suggests that the prediction value of OS and DM may be better in patients with stage IIIB and IIIC rectal cancer when adding these demographic and clinicopathological variables which were not included in TNM staging system; while for patients with stage IIA to IIIA, molecular markers (eg. microsatellite instability, loss of heterozygosity, etc.), rather than adding more clinicopathological variables, may be benefit to further improve the accuracy of outcome prediction. By integrating important demographic and clinico-pathological features, our nomogram helped further individualize

the outcome prediction based on current TNM staging system. More personalized postoperative treatment may be utilized for preoperatively under-staged patients with rectal cancer in the same AJCC stage.

In addition to the TN stage, metastatic lymph nodes ratio (LNR) was reported to be a reliable prognostic factor both in colon and rectal cancer[25–28]. However, utilization LNR in clinical practice is relatively difficult, as optimal cut-off of the continuous LNR value has not been established. We also found LNR was one of most important prognostic factors for predicting DM and OS, in addition to patients' N stage. LNR was treated as a continuous variable in our predicting nomograms, which contributed to improve the performance of our model in predicting patients' survival outcomes. Data from the five European trials found small but statistical significant improvement in distant control for patients with neoadjuvant CRT [16]. A recent meta-analysis of 21 randomized controlled trials from 1975 to 2011 concluded that adjuvant 5-Fu-based chemotherapy was beneficial for rectal cancer patients in improving overall survival and disease-free survival [29]. However, the benefit of adjuvant chemotherapy after combined treatment of rectal cancer is still not well defined in single randomized trials [4,19,21]. In our patient cohort, we only found improvements in local control in patients with any adjuvant treatment, compared with no adjuvant treatment. Further clinical trials are needed to explore the effect of adjuvant chemotherapy (single agent or combination) in improving distant control and overall survival.

Currently, there are emerged debates about adding adjuvant radiotherapy to node positive patients who receive surgical treatment first because of under-staged disease by preoperative imaging. Although randomized clinical trials proved the improvement of local control in node positive rectal cancer [30,31], the risks of treatment toxicities and decremented quality of life limited its clinical use [32,33]. A predicted nomogram for local recurrence including demographic and clincopathological variables may help physicians to choose patients who may benefit more from adjuvant radiotherapy. In our study, improved local control was observed in patients with any adjuvant treatment in univariate analysis, and the most optimal local control were observed in patients with adjuvant chemoradiotherapy followed by chemotherapy (Table 2). Unfortunately, our study was not able to develop a reliable nomogram for predicting local recurrence. Treatment variations in adjuvant setting, heterogeneous data, lacking of statistical power, less events in the validation group may be attributed to this. Further studies are needed to develop a reliable predictive model for local recurrence in preoperatively under-staged patients.

As a retrospective study, there are other limitations: detailed regimens of adjuvant chemotherapy could not be clearly provided for each patient; techniques of radiotherapy are changing over the 20 years; detailed information of recurrence may be unclear for part of patients, as well as loss of follow-up problems. However, our study still provides a valuable tool to help clinicians manage under-staged patients with rectal cancer who undergo surgery first.

Further study is needed to provide optimal postoperative treatment for these patients.

Conclusions

The prognostic nomograms integrated demographic and clinicopathological factors to account for tumor and patient heterogeneity, and thereby provided a more individualized outcome prognostication than that by the AJCC staging system alone. Our individualized prediction nomograms could help physicians counsel and advise patients about their personalized treatment strategies and follow-up protocols, especially in patients with preoperatively under-staged rectal cancer.

Author Contributions

Conceived and designed the experiments: JP SC. Performed the experiments: DS XL HW. Analyzed the data: LS YD ST SC. Contributed reagents/materials/analysis tools: XL HW. Wrote the paper: JP YD.

References

1. Rahal R, Forte T, Lockwood G, Klein-Geltink J, Bryant H (2012) Recently published indicators allow for comparison of radiation treatment rates relative to evidence-based guidelines for rectal cancer. Current oncology 19: 175–176.
2. Database NC American College of Surgeons Commission on Cancer, 2008 Data Submission.
3. Hyodo I, Suzuki H, Takahashi K, Saito Y, Tanaka S, et al. (2010) Present status and perspectives of colorectal cancer in Asia: Colorectal Cancer Working Group report in 30th Asia-Pacific Cancer Conference. Japanese journal of clinical oncology 40 Suppl 1: i38–43.
4. Sauer R, Becker H, Hohenberger W, Rodel C, Wittekind C, et al. (2004) Preoperative versus postoperative chemoradiotherapy for rectal cancer. The New England journal of medicine 351: 1731–1740.
5. Lai LL, Fuller CD, Kachnic LA, Thomas CR Jr (2006) Can pelvic radiotherapy be omitted in select patients with rectal cancer? Seminars in oncology 33: S70–74.
6. Peeters KC, van de Velde CJ, Leer JW, Martijn H, Junggeburt JM, et al. (2005) Late side effects of short-course preoperative radiotherapy combined with total mesorectal excision for rectal cancer: increased bowel dysfunction in irradiated patients–a Dutch colorectal cancer group study. Journal of clinical oncology : official journal of the American Society of Clinical Oncology 23: 6199–6206.
7. Tepper JE, O'Connell M, Niedzwiecki D, Hollis DR, Benson AB 3rd, et al. (2002) Adjuvant therapy in rectal cancer: analysis of stage, sex, and local control–final report of intergroup 0114. Journal of clinical oncology : official journal of the American Society of Clinical Oncology 20: 1744–1750.
8. Edge S, Byrd DR, Compton CC, Fritz AG, Greene FL, et al. (2010) AJCC Cancer Staging Manual (7th Edition). New York: Springer.
9. Green FL, Page DL, Fleming ID, Fritz A, Balch CM, et al. (2002) AJCC Cancer Staging Manual (6th edition). Chicago, IL, American Joint Committee on Cancer.
10. Capirci C, Valentini V, Cionini L, De Paoli A, Rodel C, et al. (2008) Prognostic value of pathologic complete response after neoadjuvant therapy in locally advanced rectal cancer: long-term analysis of 566 ypCR patients. International journal of radiation oncology, biology, physics 72: 99–107.
11. Quah HM, Chou JF, Gonen M, Shia J, Schrag D, et al. (2008) Pathologic stage is most prognostic of disease-free survival in locally advanced rectal cancer patients after preoperative chemoradiation. Cancer 113: 57–64.
12. Gronchi A, Miceli R, Shurell E, Eilber FC, Eilber FR, et al. (2013) Outcome Prediction in Primary Resected Retroperitoneal Soft Tissue Sarcoma: Histology-Specific Overall Survival and Disease-Free Survival Nomograms Built on Major Sarcoma Center Data Sets. Journal of clinical oncology : official journal of the American Society of Clinical Oncology.
13. Meretoja TJ, Strien L, Heikkila PS, Leidenius MH (2012) A simple nomogram to evaluate the risk of nonsentinel node metastases in breast cancer patients with minimal sentinel node involvement. Annals of surgical oncology 19: 567–576.
14. Wang Y, Li J, Xia Y, Gong R, Wang K, et al. (2013) Prognostic nomogram for intrahepatic cholangiocarcinoma after partial hepatectomy. Journal of clinical oncology : official journal of the American Society of Clinical Oncology 31: 1188–1195.
15. Giordano A, Egleston BL, Hajage D, Bland J, Hortobagyi GN, et al. (2013) Establishment and validation of circulating tumor cell-based prognostic nomograms in first-line metastatic breast cancer patients. Clinical cancer research : an official journal of the American Association for Cancer Research 19: 1596–1602.
16. Valentini V, van Stiphout RG, Lammering G, Gambacorta MA, Barba MC, et al. (2011) Nomograms for predicting local recurrence, distant metastases, and overall survival for patients with locally advanced rectal cancer on the basis of European randomized clinical trials. Journal of clinical oncology : official journal of the American Society of Clinical Oncology 29: 3163–3172.
17. Harrell FE Jr, Lee KL, Mark DB (1996) Multivariable prognostic models: issues in developing models, evaluating assumptions and adequacy, and measuring and reducing errors. Statistics in medicine 15: 361–387.
18. Gray R, Barnwell J, McConkey C, Hills RK, Williams NS, et al. (2007) Adjuvant chemotherapy versus observation in patients with colorectal cancer: a randomised study. Lancet 370: 2020–2029.
19. Bosset JF, Collette L, Calais G, Mineur L, Maingon P, et al. (2006) Chemotherapy with preoperative radiotherapy in rectal cancer. The New England journal of medicine 355: 1114–1123.
20. Sebag-Montefiore D, Stephens RJ, Steele R, Monson J, Grieve R, et al. (2009) Preoperative radiotherapy versus selective postoperative chemoradiotherapy in patients with rectal cancer (MRC CR07 and NCIC-CTG C016): a multicentre, randomised trial. Lancet 373: 811–820.
21. Sauer R, Liersch T, Merkel S, Fietkau R, Hohenberger W, et al. (2012) Preoperative versus postoperative chemoradiotherapy for locally advanced rectal cancer: results of the German CAO/ARO/AIO-94 randomized phase III trial after a median follow-up of 11 years. Journal of clinical oncology : official journal of the American Society of Clinical Oncology 30: 1926–1933.
22. Canadian Partnership Against Cancer (2011) The 2011 Cancer System Performance Report. Toronto, ON: CPAC.
23. Cho MM, Morgan JW, Knutsen R, Oda K, Shavlik D, et al. (2013) Outcomes of Multimodality Therapies for Patients With Stage II or III Rectal Cancer in California, 1994–2009. Diseases of the colon and rectum 56: 1357–1365.
24. Gunderson LL, Jessup JM, Sargent DJ, Greene FL, Stewart A (2010) Revised tumor and node categorization for rectal cancer based on surveillance, epidemiology, and end results and rectal pooled analysis outcomes. Journal of clinical oncology : official journal of the American Society of Clinical Oncology 28: 256–263.
25. Ferri M, Lorenzon L, Onelli MR, La Torre M, Mercantini P, et al. (2013) Lymph node ratio is a stronger prognostic factor than microsatellite instability in colorectal cancer patients: Results from a 7 years follow-up study. International journal of surgery.
26. Lu YJ, Lin PC, Lin CC, Wang HS, Yang SH, et al. (2013) The Impact of the Lymph Node Ratio is Greater than Traditional Lymph Node Status in Stage III Colorectal Cancer Patients. World journal of surgery 37: 1927–1933.
27. Greenberg R, Itah R, Ghinea R, Sacham-Shmueli E, Inbar R, et al. (2011) Metastatic lymph node ratio (LNR) as a prognostic variable in colorectal cancer patients undergoing laparoscopic resection. Techniques in coloproctology 15: 273–279.
28. Peng J, Xu Y, Guan Z, Zhu J, Wang M, et al. (2008) Prognostic significance of the metastatic lymph node ratio in node-positive rectal cancer. Annals of surgical oncology 15: 3118–3123.
29. Petersen SH, Harling H, Kirkeby LT, Wille-Jorgensen P, Mocellin S (2012) Postoperative adjuvant chemotherapy in rectal cancer operated for cure. The Cochrane database of systematic reviews 3: CD004078.
30. Tveit KM, Guldvog I, Hagen S, Trondsen E, Harbitz T, et al. (1997) Randomized controlled trial of postoperative radiotherapy and short-term time-scheduled 5-fluorouracil against surgery alone in the treatment of Dukes B and C rectal cancer. Norwegian Adjuvant Rectal Cancer Project Group. The British journal of surgery 84: 1130–1135.
31. Fisher B, Wolmark N, Rockette H, Redmond C, Deutsch M, et al. (1988) Postoperative adjuvant chemotherapy or radiation therapy for rectal cancer: results from NSABP protocol R-01. Journal of the National Cancer Institute 80: 21–29.

21

Whole Brain Radiotherapy Plus Concurrent Chemotherapy in Non-Small Cell Lung Cancer Patients with Brain Metastases: A Meta-Analysis

Hong Qin, Feng Pan, Jianjun Li, Xiaoli Zhang, Houjie Liang*, Zhihua Ruan*

Department of Oncology, Southwest Hospital, the Third Military Medical University, Chongqing, PR China

Abstract

Objective: The aim of the present meta-analysis is to evaluate the response rate, median survival time (MST) and toxicity in patients with brain metastases (BM) originating from non-small cell lung cancer (NSCLC) and who were treated using either whole brain radiotherapy (WBRT) plus concurrent chemotherapy or WBRT alone.

Methods: PubMed, EMBASE, Web of Science, The Cochrane Library, clinical trials and current controlled trials were searched to identify any relevant publications. After screening the literature and undertaking quality assessment and data extraction, the meta-analysis was performed using Stata11.0 software.

Results: In total, six randomized controlled trials (RCT) involving 910 participants were included in the meta-analysis. The results of the analysis indicate that WBRT plus concurrent chemotherapy was more effective at improving response rate (RR = 2.06, 95% CI [1.13, 3.77]; P = 0.019) than WBRT alone. However, WBRT plus concurrent chemotherapy did not improve median survival time (MST) (HR = 1.09, 95%CI [0.94, 1.26]; P = 0.233) or time of neurological progression (CNS-TTP) (HR = 0.93, 95%CI [0.75, 1.16]; P = 0.543), and increased adverse events (Grade≥3) (RR = 2.59, 95% CI [1.88, 3.58]; P = 0.000). There were no significant differences in Grade 3–5 neurological or hematological toxicity between two patient groups (RR = 1.08, 95%CI [0.23, 5.1]; P = 0.92).

Conclusion: The combination of chemotherapy plus WBRT in patients with BM originating from NSCLC may increase treatment response rates of brain metastases with limited toxicity. Although the therapy schedule did not prolong MST or CNS-TTP, further assessment is warranted.

Editor: Matthew B. Schabath, H. Lee Moffitt Cancer Center, United States of America

Funding: These authors have no support or funding to report.

Competing Interests: The authors have declared that no competing interests exist.

* Email: zhihuaruan@gmail.com (ZR); lianghoujie@sina.com (HL)

Introduction

Approximately 20% to 40% of patients with cancer develop brain metastases (BM) during their disease course. Patients with solid tumors, such as lung and, breast cancer or melanoma, are at high risk for BM. In particular, it has been estimated that approximately 50% of primary lung cancers develop into BM [1]. Furthermore, non-small cell lung cancer (NSCLC) accounts a large percentage of lung cancer cases. It has also been estimated that 25% to 30% of newly diagnosed NSCLC patients also suffer from brain metastases [2]. NSCLC patients who develop BM often have poor prognoses, severe neurological symptoms, poor quality of life and dismal survival rates. The overall survival time (OS) for NSCLC patients with BM is less than 3–6 months when left untreated [3]; effective treatment options for NSCLC patients with BM are needed urgently.

Whole brain radiotherapy (WBRT) has been the standard therapy for most patients with multiple BM.WBRT can palliate neurological symptoms and control the local disease. However, it has been difficult to eradicate the tumors due to the limitations of radiation therapy. One study reported that one-third of included patients had uncontrollable localized tumors following WBRT treatment and that 50% of patients died of intracranial tumor progression [4]. Systemic chemotherapy has also been used to reduce tumor burden in patients with BM originating from NSCLC. However, the treatment's effectiveness is limited due to the brain-blood barrier (BBB). Clinical doctors, therefore, faced a dilemma when treating NSLCL patients with BM. Some researchers have suggested that chemical drugs can infiltrate the brain tissue when radiation destroys the BBB, and several clinical trials have indicated that WBRT combined with chemotherapy is not only more effective than WBRT alone, but also improves the response rate and prolongs survival [5–7]. Other studies have failed to confirm the efficacy of chemotherapy and suggest that chemotherapy concurrent with WBRT increases the incidence of adverse events and does not benefit NSCLC patients with BM [8–10]. The role of chemotherapy concurrent with WBRT for the treatment of patients with BM originating from NSCLC is controversial. We have therefore conducted a meta-analysis assessing the efficacy and safety of chemotherapy combined with WBRT versus treatment with WBRT alone.

Materials and Methods

Search strategy

PubMed, EMBASE, the Cochrane Library, Web of Science, clinical trials and current controlled trials were searched to identify relevant studies in the published literature. The search was performed on September 25, 2013, using both Mesh and free text words. The following basic search terms were used: lung neoplasms, lung tumor, lung cancer, brain metastasis, brain neoplasms, radiotherapy and chemotherapy. The search was performed without any language limitations.

Inclusion criteria

All articles which met the following criteria were eligible: (1) randomized controlled trials (RCT) with voluntarily enrolled patients; (2) patients had histologically or cytologically confirmed NSCLC and had been diagnosed with multiple brain metastases using CT or MRI; (3) the trials compared WBRT plus chemotherapy with WBRT alone; (4) trials did not include patients with chemotherapy contraindications or serious vital organ dysfunction and Karnofsky performance status (KPS) scores ≥ 70; (5) the analyses included response rate, median survival time (MST), the time to neurological progression (CNS-TTP), adverse events (Grade≥ 3) or hematological toxicity (Grade≥ 3); (6) response rate was determined using the Response Evaluation Criteria in Solid Tumors (RECIST) or WHO evaluation criteria on solid tumors. complete remission (CR) was defined as tumor completely disappearing for at least four weeks without any new lesions, partial response (PR) was defined as more than 50% tumor regression for at least for four weeks without new lesions, Progressive disease (PD) was defined as an increase in the sum of the longest diameters (LD) of the target lesions by 25% or higher, using as reference the smallest sum LD recorded since treatment started or the appearance of one or more new lesions. Stabilized disease (SD) was defined as a $\leq 50\%$ tumor regression or an increase $\leq 25\%$. (7) Toxicity was evaluated according to the National Cancer Institute Common Terminology Criteria for Adverse Events.

Study selection

The eligibility assessment was first performed by screening titles and abstracts and subsequently reviewing the full text of articles. The selection of all studies was performed independently, according to the inclusion criteria, by two reviewers. Disagreement on whether an article should be included was resolved using a third reviewer.

Data extraction

Two authors independently extracted data from all the eligible studies. When the extracted data were not uniform, consultation was needed to make a final determination. All of the studies included in the analysis contain the following data: first author's name, published year, type of study, trial phase, country of origin study, percentage of men, performance status, number of patients, average ages, interventions and outcomes.

Quality assessment

All of the selected studies were evaluated by two reviewers according to the Cochrane Handbook for RCT, based on the following criteria: (1) randomized method; (2) allocation concealment; (3) blinding of participants, personnel and outcome assessment; and (4) intention-to-treat analysis if the trials lost participants to follow-up or if participants quit. Each trial for bias based on the criteria listed above was marked as 'low risk', 'high risk' or 'unclear risk'. Trials judged as low risk of bias (i.e. A rating) when all criteria are assessed as low risk; Trials judged as moderate risk of bias (i.e. B rating) when one or more criteria are assessed as unclear risk; Trials judged as high risk of bias (i.e. C rating) when one or more criteria are assessed as high risk.

Statistical analysis

Statistical analyses were performed using Stata software11.0. Chi-square and I-square tests were used to test the heterogeneity of different studies [11]; no heterogeneity was considered to exist when $P > 0.1$ and $I^2 < 50\%$. A fixed-effect model was applied to pool the study results. Significant heterogeneity was found if $P < 0.1$ and $I^2 > 50\%$, and a random-effects statistical model was used [12]. Response rate, severe hematological toxicity and advent events were analyzed using dichotomous variables. MST and CNS-TTP were calculated using effect variables.

Results

Selection of studies

In total, we identified 2104 studies that met our selection criteria after searching the relevant databases; 236 of these studies were excluded due to duplication. By verifying related terms in the titles and abstracts, we excluded 1847 irrelevant articles, and another 15 articles were excluded after the full text was read. Finally, six RCTs [10,13–17] were selected for the present meta-analysis. A flowchart depicting the study selection is shown in figure 1.

General characteristics of included studies

There were 910 patients with BM originating from NSCLC in the six selected RCT trials, with 478 patients having received WBRT concurrent with chemotherapy and 432 patients having received only WBRT; these results are summarized in table 1. Of the six RCTs, three were phase III clinical trials [10,14,16], two were phase II studies [15,17], and one was a study [13] that did not mention a trial phase. The analyzed interventions were WBRT plus chemotherapy and WBRT alone, except in the case

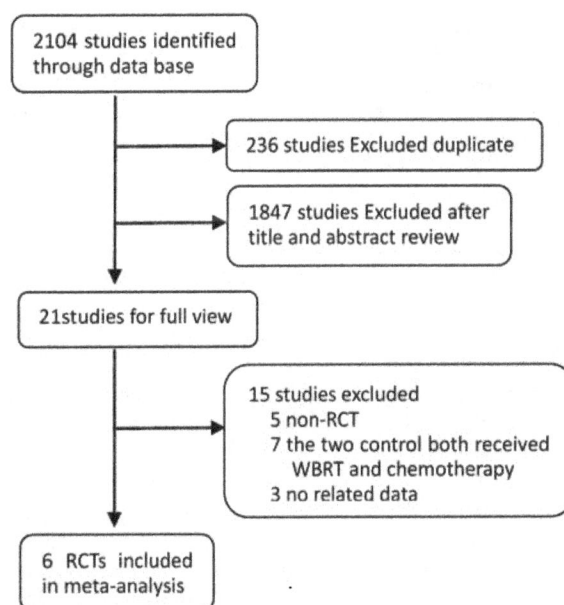

Figure 1. A flow chart on selection included of trials in the Meta-analysis.

of Sperduto, P. W.2013, which compared the combination treatment WBRT, stereotactic radiotherapy (SRS) and chemotherapy with WBRT+SRS treatment. Among all of the included studies, chemotherapy drugs included temozolomide (TMZ), carboplatin, motexafin gadolinium (MGD), chloroethylnitrosoureas and tegafur. TMZ was used in three of the trials. Outcomes included response rate, adverse events, hematological toxicity, median survival time (MST) and time to central nervous system progression (CNS-TTP).

Methodological quality

In accordance with the recommendations of the Cochrane Handbook for Systematic Reviews, two authors evaluated the eligible studies using the four aspects mentioned above. Four studies [10,15–17] mentioned the use of random allocation, but only two articles discussed the methods [13,14]. None of the studies performed or reported their allocation concealment and blinding methods. The Hassler, M.R.2013 [15] trial reported follow-up information, but the other studies did not. All of the articles applied the intent-to-treat analysis. The six eligible studies all received B quality scores, as shown in table 1.

Response rate

Three of the included studies [13,15,16] reported the efficacy of treatment using WBRT plus concurrent chemotherapy and WBRT alone. Ushio, Y.1991 [13] reported tumor response rates in the WBRT and WBRT plus chemotherapy groups were 36% and 71%, respectively. Hassler, M.R.2013 [15] reported two cases of PR in the WBRT arm, and two CR and three PR cases in the WBRT plus chemotherapy arm. Guerrieri, M.2004 [16] reported response rates were 10% and 29% in the WBRT and WBRT plus carboplatin arms, respectively. There was no heterogeneity ($P = 0.801$, $I^2 = 0.0\%$) among the three studies, and as a result, the fixed effect model was used for the meta-analysis. The results indicate that WBRT plus concurrent chemotherapy resulted in superior response rates when compared with WBRT alone ($RR = 2.06$, 95%CI [1.13, 3.77]; $P = 0.019$) (figure 2).

Adverse events

Three studies [10,15,17] reported the occurrence of drug-related hematological toxicity (Grade≥3). A random effects model was used for the meta-analysis of these studies based on the heterogeneity values ($P = 0.041$, $I^2 = 68.8\%$). The results indicate no significant difference in hematological toxicity between WBRT plus chemotherapy and WBRT alone ($RR = 1.08$, 95% CI [0.23, 5.1]; $P = 0.92$) (figure 3). However, another four studies [10,14,15,17] described adverse events (Grade≥3) and included both hematological and non-hematological toxicity. A fixed effect model was used for the meta-analysis of these studies because heterogeneity did not exist ($P = 0.500$, $I^2 = 0.0\%$). The results indicate that the incidence of severe adverse events was higher in the group treated using WBRT concurrent with chemotherapy ($RR = 2.59$, 95% CI [1.88, 3.58]; $P = 0.000$) (figure 4).

Survival

Five of the studies [10,14–17] reported MST for both patient groups; the studies were not heterogeneous ($P = 0.425$, $I^2 = 0.0\%$). Analysis using a fixed effect model suggests that in NSCLC patients diagnosed with BM, there was no significant MST difference between those who were treated with chemotherapy and those who were not ($HR = 1.09$, 95% CI [0.94, 1.26]; $P = 0.233$) (figure 5). The most meaningful outcome was the time to neurological progression (CNS-TTP). Three studies [10,14,17]

Table 1. Characteristics of trials included in the Meta-analysis.

Studies	Country	Trial phase	N (T/C)	Male (T/C,%)	Ages (T/C, years)	ECOG	Interventions T	Interventions C	Outcomes	Study quality
Ushio, Y.1991	Japan	NM	69/31	80/87	57/63	NM	WBRT+methyl-CCNU/ACNU/tegafur	WBRT	Response rate	B
Sperduto, P.W.2013	American	3	40/44	NM	63/64	0–1	WBRT+SRS+TMZ	WBRT+SRS	MST, OS, CNS-TTP, toxicity	B
Mehta, M.P.2009	France	3	279/275	59/55	59/59	0–2	WBRT+MGD	WBRT	MST, CNS-TTP, Adverse event	B
Hassler, M.R.2013	Austria	2	22/13	59/62	69/64	0–2	WBRT+TMZ	WBRT	Response rate, MST, Toxicity, Adverse events	B
Guerrieri, M.2004	Australia	3	21/21	71/71	60/63	0–2	WBRT+ carboplatin	WBRT	MST, Response rate	B
Chua, D.2010	China	2	47/48	64/67	59/62	0–2	WBRT+TMZ	WBRT	MST, CNS-TTP, Toxicity, Adverse event	B

T: treatment group (chemotherapy plus WBRT group); C: control group (WBRT group); NM: not mentioned; ECOG: ECOG/WHO performance status WBRT: Whole brain radiotherapy; TMZ: temozolomide; MST: median survival time; OS: overall survival; CNS: central nervous system; MGD: motexafin gadolinium; TTP: time to progression.

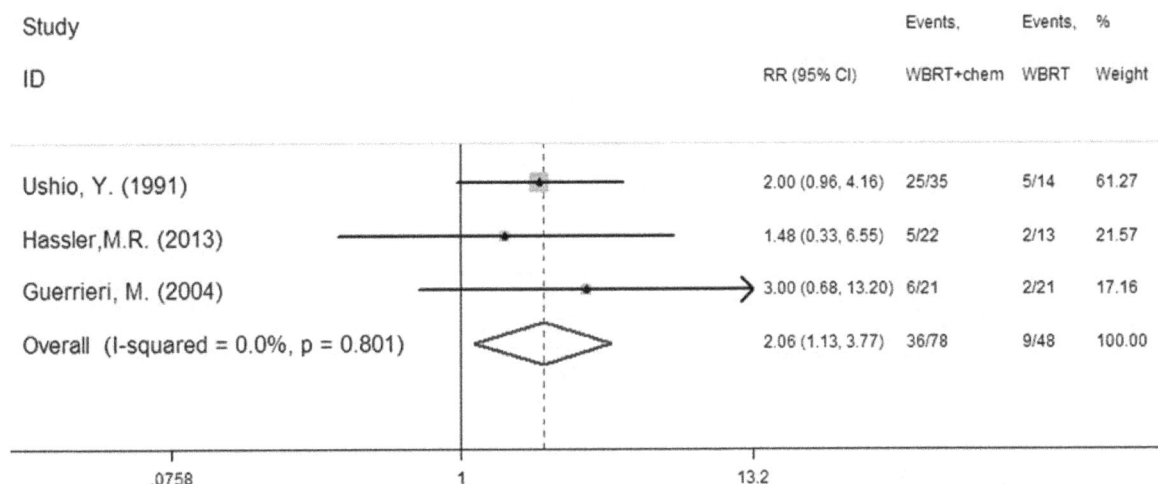

Figure 2. Response rate (P = 0.019).

reported CNS-TTP, and there was no significant heterogeneity between them (P = 0.186, I^2 = 40.5%); accordingly, a fixed effect model was used for the meta-analysis of CNS-TTP. The results suggest that combining chemotherapy with WBRT could prolong the time of neurological progression (HR = 0.93, 95% CI [0.75, 1.16]; P = 0.543) (figure 6). In conclusion, this meta-analysis suggests that WBRT concurrent with chemoradiotherapy significantly increased response rate and potentially prolonged the time of neurologic progression for patients with BM originating from NSCLC. However, more hypotoxic chemotherapy drugs still need to be explored in future clinical research.

Discussion

Currently, WBRT is the standard therapy for NSCLC patients whose disease has metastasized to the brain. Several studies have verified that WBRT palliates the neurological symptom associated with BM. However, because radiotherapy doses are limited, the treatment has been unsuccessful at curing malignant lesions. Furthermore, the brain-blood barrier (BBB) prevents the transport of most anticancer agents to the central nervous system and restricts the delivery of drugs to infiltrating BM. These additional barriers restrict the use of chemotherapy for patients with BM.

Results of several trails have indicated that chemotherapy combined with WBRT benefits NSCLC patients with BM. Some clinicians found that WBRT could allow chemotherapy drugs to pass through the BBB. Additionally, chemotherapy had the potential to make brain tumor cells more sensitive to radiotherapy. Several studies have indicated that WBRT plus concurrent chemotherapy is playing an increasing role in the treatment of BM. Mehta, M. P. 2009 [14] reported that treatment using motexafin gadolinium (MGd) improved the neurologic progression interval when compared with WBRT alone (15 months vs.10 months). Verger, E. 2005 [18] reported results of patients who received the combination treatment of WBRT with TMZ, noting that they exhibited good tolerance and significantly better progression-free survival of BM at 90 days (54% vs. 72%; P = 0.03). Nonetheless, some studies have suggested that WBRT had a minor effect on promoting chemotherapy drugs across the BBB. Adding chemotherapy to WBRT treatment did not confer any benefits to the patients, but did increase the incidence of adverse events. For instance, Neuhaus, T.2009 [19] reported that concurrent radiochemotherapy (WBRT+topotecan) did not achieve significant curative effects in patients with lung cancer.

A total of six RCTs were included in present meta-analysis. The response rate was significantly improved in patients treated with

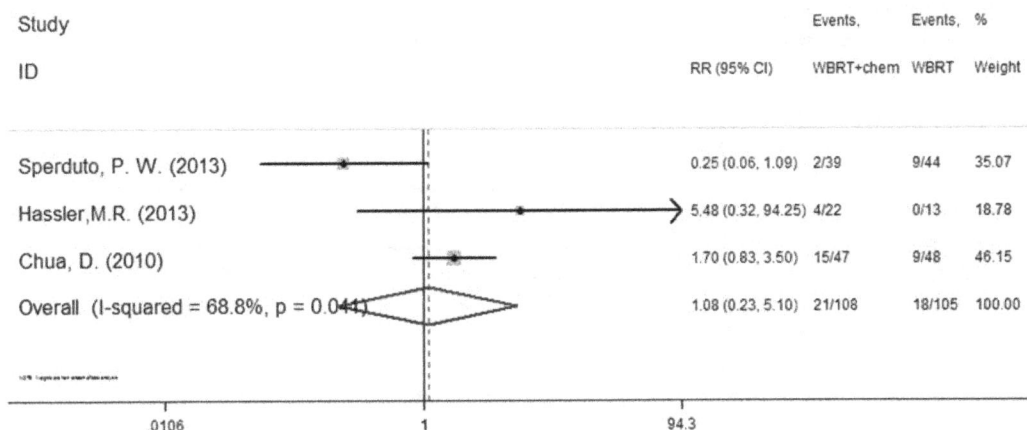

Figure 3. Severe haematological toxicity (P = 0.92).

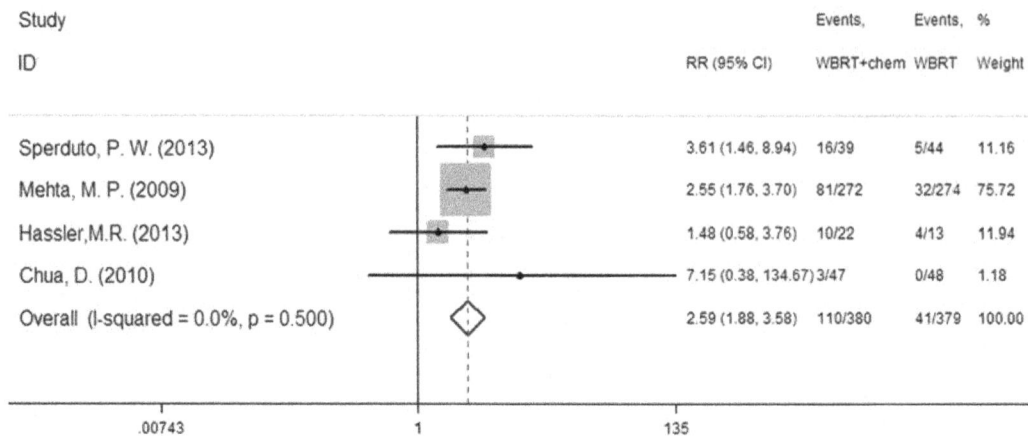

Figure 4. Severe adverse event (P = 0.000).

WBRT plus chemotherapy. However, WBRT plus chemotherapy did not improve MST and CNS-TTP for patients with malignant lesions. WBRT plus chemotherapy increased the incidence of adverse reactions, such as asthenia, fatigue, nausea, vomiting, infection, thrombocytopenia, anemia and neutropenia, but there were no significant differences in the rates of severe hematological toxicity. Each group of patients in the Sperduto, P. W.2013 study received SRS, which might have influenced the final outcomes of the meta-analysis; therefore, we extracted these data and re-analyzed MST and CNS-TTP. Although no significant statistical differences were found, treatment with both WBRT with concurrent chemotherapy tended to prolong MST and CNS-TTP (MST: HR = 1.06, 95% CI [0.91, 1.23], P = 0.462; CNS-TTP: HR = 0.84, 95% CI [0.65, 1.08], P = 0.183).

Researchers hold the opinion that the favorable therapeutic effects of combining chemotherapy with WBRT depend on the drugs crossing the BBB [20]. Temozolomide (TMZ) protocols have been recommended for the favorable distribution of the chemotherapy drug through the BBB and to achieve an effective concentration in the brain tissue [21]. A number of trials have shown that TMZ was well tolerated by patients with BM and achieved high release rates [22,23]. By contrast, some chemotherapy drugs, such as etoposide and cisplatin, had difficulty reaching the intracranial environment because of the BBB. Those agents did not improve response rates and only increased the incidence of neurological toxicity [8]. Due to a lack of response rates and CNS-TTP data, we did not analyze the differences between TMZ and non-TMZ treatments.

Our present systematic review suggests that the combination of chemotherapy and WBRT does not obviously improve MST and CNS-TTP. Moreover, we found a tendency toward prolonged CNS-TTP intervals in the concurrent chemoradiotherapy group.

Our results suggest that the combination of chemotherapy and WBRT significantly increased adverse events of Grade 3 or higher, although there was insufficient evidence to indicate that the treatment resulted in severe nervous-system toxicity. Sperduto, P. W.2013 [10] reported that rates of Grade 3–5 toxicity for WBRT/SRS and WBRT/SRS/TMZ were 11% and 41%, respectively. However, most of the adverse events were fatigue, dehydration and other aspecific symptoms. Chua, D.2010 [17] reported that three patients suffered adverse events (≥Grade 3), and none of these events were related to neurologic toxicity.

Meta-analysis is based on the results of published articles and several steps of integration; thus, certain biases are inevitable. Also, 6 studies included in the meta-analysis were published in the period 1991–2013. Although the dose of WBRT for the treatment of multiple brain metastases did not change during this 22-year period, more precisely delineated target regional and advanced equipment would affect the effectiveness of treatment as technology advances. In addition, as more and more researchers focused their attention on the investigation of targeted drug combine with WBRT in the treatment of multiple brain metastases, and many chemoradiotherapy-related studies were retrospective study and single-arm study, limited RCT were included in this study. Furthermore, the methods of randomization, allocation concealment, and blinding in most of the included studies are not clear. As

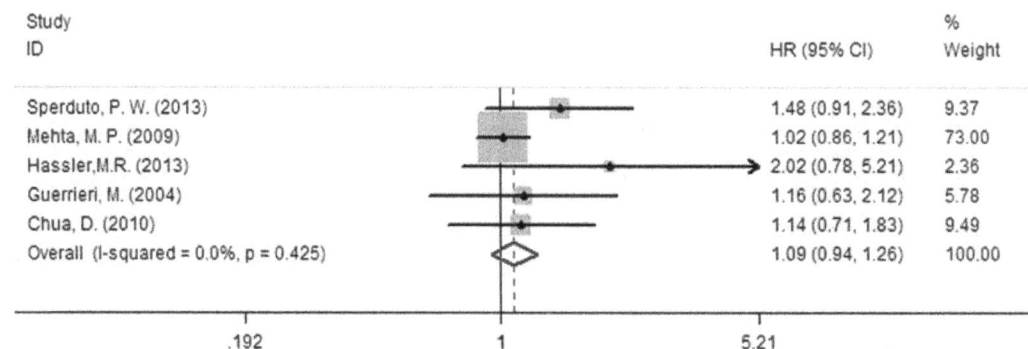

Figure 5. Median survival time (MST) (P = 0.233).

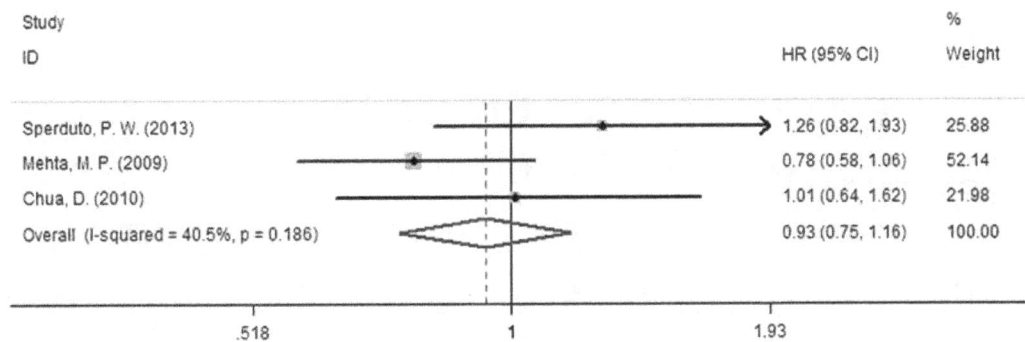

Figure 6. The time to CNS-progression (P = 0.543).

a result, the quality of the 6 RCTs was not high. The different strategies used to divide groups and the dose of WBRT and chemotherapy drugs were not clear; these procedures may have influenced the final outcomes. More high quality and large scale trials are necessary to confirm the efficacy and safety of WBRT plus concurrent chemotherapy for the treatment of patients with BM originating from NSCLC.

In conclusion, this meta-analysis reports that concurrent chemoradiotherapy significantly increased response rates and had the potential to prolong neurologic progression time NSCLC patients with BM. However, additional future clinical research is needed to explore the use of more hypotoxic chemotherapy drugs.

Acknowledgments

The authors thank all the participants in this study.

Author Contributions

Conceived and designed the experiments: HQ HL ZR. Performed the experiments: HQ FP JL XZ. Analyzed the data: HQ ZR. Wrote the paper: HQ FP.

References

1. Seoane J and De Mattos-Arruda L (2014) Brain metastasis: New opportunities to tackle therapeutic resistance. Mol Oncol 8: 1120–1131.
2. Berger LA, Riesenberg H, Bokemeyer C and Atanackovic D (2013) CNS metastases in non-small-cell lung cancer: Current role of EGFR-TKI therapy and future perspectives. Lung Cancer 80: 242–248.
3. Sperduto PW, Kased N, Roberge D, Xu Z, Shanley R, et al. (2012) Summary report on the graded prognostic assessment: an accurate and facile diagnosis-specific tool to estimate survival for patients with brain metastases. J Clin Oncol 30: 419–425.
4. Gijtenbeek JM, Ho VK, Heesters MA, Lagerwaard FJ, de Graeff A, et al. (2011) [Practice guideline Brain metastases' (revision)]. Ned Tijdschr Geneeskd 155: A4141.
5. Siu TL, Jeffree RL and Fuller JW (2011) Current strategies in the surgical management of cerebral metastases: an evidence-based review. J Clin Neurosci 18: 1429–1434.
6. Bailon O, Chouahnia K, Augier A, Bouillet T, Billot S, et al. (2012) Upfront association of carboplatin plus pemetrexed in patients with brain metastases of lung adenocarcinoma. Neuro-Oncology 14: 491–495.
7. Barlesi F, Gervais R, Lena H, Hureaux J, Berard H, et al. (2011) Pemetrexed and cisplatin as first-line chemotherapy for advanced non-small-cell lung cancer (NSCLC) with asymptomatic inoperable brain metastases: a multicenter phase II trial (GFPC 07-01). Ann Oncol 22: 2466–2470.
8. Kaba SE, Kyritsis AP, Hess K, Yung WK, Mercier R, et al. (1997) TPDC-FuHu chemotherapy for the treatment of recurrent metastatic brain tumors. J Clin Oncol 15: 1063–1070.
9. Nieder C (1999) Front-line chemotherapy with cisplatin and etoposide for patients with brain metastases from breast carcinoma, nonsmall cell lung carcinoma, or malignant melanoma. A prospective study. Cancer 86: 900–903.
10. Sperduto PW, Wang M, Robins HI, Schell MC, Werner-Wasik M, et al. (2013) A phase 3 trial of whole brain radiation therapy and stereotactic radiosurgery alone versus WBRT and SRS with temozolomide or erlotinib for non-small cell lung cancer and 1 to 3 brain metastases: Radiation Therapy Oncology Group 0320. Int J Radiat Oncol Biol Phys 85: 1312–1318.
11. Higgins JPT, Thompson SG, Deeks JJ and Altman DG (2003) Measuring inconsistency in meta-analyses. BMJ (Clinical research ed) 327: 557–560.
12. Ford AC, Forman D, Hunt RH, Yuan Y and Moayyedi P (2014) Helicobacter pylori eradication therapy to prevent gastric cancer in healthy asymptomatic infected individuals: systematic review and meta-analysis of randomised controlled trials. BMJ (Clinical research ed) 348: g3174.
13. Ushio Y, Arita N, Hayakawa T, Mogami H, Hasegawa H, et al. (1991) Chemotherapy of brain metastases from lung carcinoma: a controlled randomized study. Neurosurgery 28: 201–205.
14. Mehta MP, Shapiro WR, Phan SC, Gervais R, Carrie C, et al. (2009) Motexafin gadolinium combined with prompt whole brain radiotherapy prolongs time to neurologic progression in non-small-cell lung cancer patients with brain metastases: results of a phase III trial. Int J Radiat Oncol Biol Phys 73: 1069–1076.
15. Hassler MR, Pfeifer W, Knocke-Abulesz TH, Geissler K, Altorjai G, et al. (2013) Temozolomide added to whole brain radiotherapy in patients with multiple brain metastases of non-small-cell lung cancer: a multicentric Austrian phase II study. Wien Klin Wochenschr 125: 481–6.
16. Guerrieri M, Wong K, Ryan G, Millward M, Quong G, et al. (2004) A randomised phase III study of palliative radiation with concomitant carboplatin for brain metastases from non-small cell carcinoma of the lung. Lung Cancer 46: 107–111.
17. Chua D, Krzakowski M, Chouaid C, Pallotta MG, Martinez JI, et al. (2010) Whole-brain radiation therapy plus concomitant temozolomide for the treatment of brain metastases from non-small-cell lung cancer: a randomized, open-label phase II study. Clin Lung Cancer 11: 176–181.
18. Verger E, Gil M, Yaya R, Vinolas N, Villa S, et al. (2005) Temozolomide and concomitant whole brain radiotherapy in patients with brain metastases: a phase II randomized trial. Int J Radiat Oncol Biol Phys 61: 185–191.
19. Neuhaus T, Ko Y, Muller RP, Grabenbauer GG, Hedde JP, et al. (2009) A phase III trial of topotecan and whole brain radiation therapy for patients with CNS-metastases due to lung cancer. Br J Cancer 100: 291–297.
20. Biswas G, Bhagwat R, Khurana R, Menon H, Prasad N, et al. (2006) Brain metastasis-evidence based management. J Cancer Res Ther 2: 5–13.
21. Addeo R and Caraglia M (2011) Combining temozolomide with other antitumor drugs and target-based agents in the treatment of brain metastases: An unending quest or chasing a chimera? Expert Opin Investig Drugs 20: 881–895.
22. Adonizio CS, Babb JS, Maiale C, Huang C, Donahue J, et al. (2002) Temozolomide in non-small-cell lung cancer: preliminary results of a phase II trial in previously treated patients. Clin Lung Cancer 3: 254–258.
23. Addeo R, Caraglia M, Faiola V, Capasso E, Vincenzi B, et al. (2007) Concomitant treatment of brain metastasis with Whole Brain Radiotherapy WBRT and Temozolomide TMZ is active and improves Quality of Life. BMC cancer 7: doi: 10.1186/1471-2407-7-18.

22

Effectiveness and Safety of Chemotherapy Combined with Dendritic Cells Co-Cultured with Cytokine-Induced Killer Cells in the Treatment of Advanced Non-Small-Cell Lung Cancer: A Systematic Review and Meta-Analysis

Rui-xian Han[1,2&], Xu Liu[1&], Pan Pan[1,2], Ying-jie Jia[1]*, Jian-chun Yu[1]*

1 First Teaching Hospital of Tianjin University of Traditional Chinese Medicine, Tianjin, China, **2** Tianjin University of Traditional Chinese Medicine, Tianjin, China

Abstract

Background: Lung cancer, particularly non-small-cell lung cancer (NSCLC) is the leading cause of cancer mortality. Chemotherapy combined dendritic cells co-cultured with cytokine-induced killer cells (DC-CIK) immunotherapy has been applied in advanced NSCLC patients' treatment, but couldn't provide consistent beneficial results. Therefore, it is necessary to evaluate the efficiency and safety of combination therapy to promote the application.

Methods: A literature search for randomized controlled trials of NSCLC was conducted in PubMed database. Before meta-analysis was performed, studies were evaluated heterogeneity. Pooled risk ratios (RRs) were estimated and 95% confidence intervals (CIs) were calculated using a fixed-effect model. Sensitivity analysis was also performed.

Results: Six eligible trials were enrolled. Efficiency and safety of chemotherapy followed by DC-CIK immunotherapy (experimental group) and chemotherapy alone (control group) were compared. 1-year overall survival (OS) ($P = 0.02$) and progression free survival (PFS) ($P = 0.005$) in the experimental group were significantly increased compared with the control. Disease control rate (DCR) ($P = 0.006$) rose significantly in experimental group. However, no significant differences between the two groups were observed in 2-year OS ($P = 0.21$), 2-year PFS ($P = 0.10$), overall response rate (ORR) ($P = 0.76$) and partial response (PR) ($P = 0.22$). Temporary fever, anemia, leukopenia and nausea were the four major adverse events (AEs) treated by chemotherapy. The incidence of anemia, leukopenia and nausea in the experimental group was obviously lower than the control group. Temporary fever rate was higher in experimental group than that in the control, but could be alleviated by taking sufficient rest.

Conclusions: Chemotherapy combined with DC-CIK immunotherapy showed superiority in DCR, 1-year OS and PFS, and no more AEs appeared, however, there was no significant improvement in ORR, PR, 2-year OS and PFS. As a whole, the combination therapy is safer but modest in efficacy for advanced NSCLC patients.

Editor: Jian-Xin Gao, Shanghai Jiao Tong University School of Medicine, China

Funding: This work was supported by National Natural Science Foundation of China (No. 81273937), Key Project of Anti-Cancer of Tianjin (12ZCDZSY15800), Science and Technology Developing and Supporting Program from Tianjin (12CDZSY17000), Specialized Research Fund for the Doctoral Program of Higher Education (20121210110010). The funders had no role in study design, data collection and analysis, decision to publish, or preparation of the manuscript.

Competing Interests: The authors have declared that no competing interests exist.

* Email: yujianchun2000@hotmail.com (JCY); jiayingjie1616@sina.com (YJJ)

& These authors contributed equally to this work.

Introduction

Lung cancer has been considered as one of the most commonly diagnosed type of cancer affected by population aging and growth as well as change in lifestyle, such as smoking and physical inactivity [1]. Furthermore, lung cancer is a devastating disease, particularly non-small-cell lung cancer (NSCLC); NSCLC is among the leading causes of mortality worldwide and accounts for approximately 80% to 85% of all lung cancer cases [2].

Surgery, radiation and chemotherapy are the three most widely employed cancer treatments; however, these treatments elicit multiple side effects and often fail to completely remove the tumor

tissues, including small lesions and metastatic cells that may cause disease recurrence after treatment [3]. In chemotherapy, platinum-based regimens are considered as the most important form of treatment [4]. For example, a four-cycle regimen (i.e., cisplatin or carboplatin) is administrated, thereby improving the conditions of patients with NSCLC. However, five-year survival rate remains very poor, drug resistance and adverse effects appears subsequently, thus, the more effective and safer treatments are urgently require to prompt to improve the quality and duration of life. With progression in disease treatments, immunotherapy, particularly

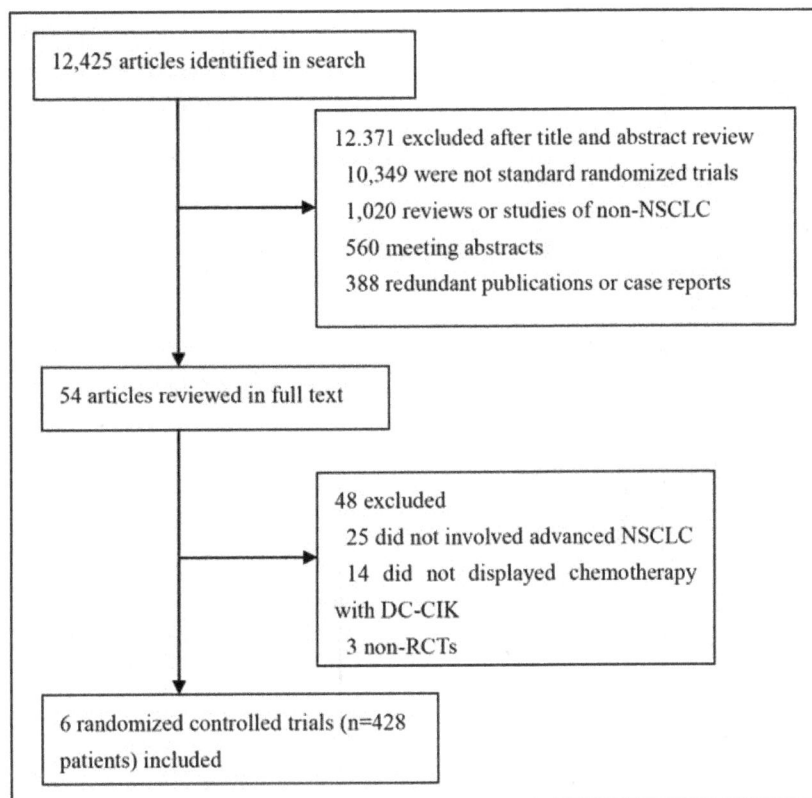

Figure 1. Flow diagram.

dendritic cells co-cultured with cytokine-induced killer cell (DC-CIK) therapy, has been applied as an important component of cancer treatment [5].

Ex vivo and *in vivo* experimental evidence has shown that CIK cells [6], which are cytotoxic lymphocytes generated from peripheral lymphocytes by a cytokine cocktail containing anti-CD3 monoclonal antibody, IFN-γand IL-2 and mainly consist of the $CD3^+CD56^+$ subset [7], can be used against solid tumors. These cells show a high level of cytotoxic activity and lyse a broad range of tumor cell lines, including multi-drug resistant and autologous tumor cells [8].

These biological features of CIK cells have been considered for adoptive immunotherapy and have yielded encouraging results in tumor therapy [9,10]. The anti-tumor activity of CIK cells can be improved after co-culturing with dendritic cells (DCs) [11].

DCs are the most potent antigen-presenting cells in the body and can promote the generation of helper and cytotoxic T cells, and are also stimulators of effective T cells that can present tumor antigens to T lymphocytes and induce anti-tumor immune responses [12–15]. Thus, the combination of DCs and CIKs can lead to a remarkable increase in cytotoxic activity; and show more effective than single treatment [16], which has gained encouraging clinical prospects and has been widely used to treat solid and hematological system carcinomas [17,18].

Meta-analysis based on data from pooled patient samples provides an avenue for evaluating the efficacy and side effects of chemotherapy combined with DC-CIK for advanced NSCLC patients. In this study, we used a meta-analysis to evaluate the efficacy and safety of the combination therapy on advanced NSCLC patients.

Materials and Methods

Literature Search Strategy

Electronic databases, including Cochrane Library, EMBASE, PubMed and Web of Science, were searched for studies that could be included in this meta-analysis from 2003 to 2014. Articles published in English and Chinese were enrolled. Search terms were "Dendritic Cells and Cytokine-Induced Killer Cells" or "DC-CIK immunotherapy", "non-small-cell lung cancer" or "NSCLC", and "Chemotherapy". Our search based on PRISMA guidelines [19].

Inclusion Criteria

Trials were eligible for inclusion in the present meta-analysis if they were randomized controlled trials (RCTs) of patients with advanced NSCLC. Patients in the control group received chemotherapy alone, whereas patients in the experimental group received chemotherapy combined with DC-CIK immunotherapy.

Study Selection

The following selection criteria were used: (1) studies were written in English and non-English languages and limited to human trials (2) studies that performed and completed randomize controlled trials (RCTs).

Quality Assessment

The quality of the included RCTs was assessed in accordance with the Cochrane Handbook [20] by recording seven items of bias risk: random sequence generation; allocation concealment;

Table 1. Clinical trials of the meta-analysis of advanced non-small-cell lung cancer (NSCLC).

Study	Patients (N=428)	Gender (F/M)		Median Age (Range)		Follow up (Years)	Stages	Treatment Design	
		Exp	Con	Exp	Con			Exp	Con
Wu 2008[25]	59	7/23	5/24	61.0(38–74)	60.0(41–78)	3	IIIa/IIIb/IV	TP+CIK	TP
Zhao 2009 [26]	75	13/23	13/26	50.2(44–72)	51.3(42–68)	2	IIIa/IIIb/IV	NP+CIK	NP
Zhong 2011 [27]	28	8/6	7/7	No	No	7	IIIa/IIIb/IV	NP+DC/CIK	NP
Shi 2012 [28]	60	13/17	12/18	60.5(40–77)	58.5(40–76)	3	IIIa/IIIb/IV	NP+DC/CIK	NP
Yang 2012 [29]	122	12/49	12/49	63.0(29–80)	63.5(28–82)	2	IIIb/IV	NP+DC/CIK	NP
Li 2009 [30]	84	14/28	14/28	61.0(44–78)	60.5(40–80)	2	I/II/III	NP+DC/CIK	NP

Note: A total of 428 patients were included in the meta-analysis; among these patients, 213 were assigned to the experimental group (Exp) treated with DC-CIK/CIK plus Chemotherapy and 215 were assigned to the control group (Con) treated with chemotherapy alone.
Abbreviations: F, Female; M, Male, CIK, cytokine-induced killer biotherapy; DC, dendritic cells; NP, vinorelbine-platinum chemotherapy; TP, tocetaxel-cisplatin chemotherapy.

Table 2. Adverse events in advanced non-small-cell lung cancer (NSCLC).

Adverse Events	Wu et al.		Li et al.		Yang et al.		Zhao et al.		Shi et al.		Zhong et al.	
Groups	N=59		N=84		N=122		N=75		N=60		N=28	
	Exp	Con	Exp	Con	Exp	Con	Exp	Con	Exp	Con	Exp	Con
Leukopenia	-	-	-	-	-	-	48.7%	83.3%	-	-	71.4%	92.8%
Nausea	-	-	-	-	-	nc	51.2%	86.1%	-	-	64.2%	92.8%
Anemia	-	-	nc	nc	nc	nc	17.8%	44.5%	-	-	28.5%	42.8%
Insomnia	-	-	-	-	-	-	7.7%	30.6%	-	-	-	-
Temporary Fever	nc	-	nc	-	nc	nc	-	-	13.3%	nc	71.4%	21.4%
Headache	nc	-	-	-	-	nc	-	-	-	-	-	-
Fatigue	-	-	-	-	-	-	-	-	10.0%	nc	7.1%	57.1%
Thrombocytopenia	-	-	-	-	-	-	20.5%	38.9%	-	-	-	-
Chest distress	-	-	-	-	-	-	-	-	3.3%	nc	-	-

Abbreviations: Exp: experimental group; Con: control group; Nc: not clear, that is, simply mentioned in the article but did not provide an exact number; -, no description.

Study or Subgroup	Experimental Events	Total	Control Events	Total	Weight	Risk Ratio M-H, Fixed, 95% CI	Risk Ratio M-H, Fixed, 95% CI
1.1 1-year OS							
Li 2009	41	42	40	42	13.6%	1.02 [0.94, 1.11]	
Shi 2012	30	30	28	30	9.7%	1.07 [0.96, 1.20]	
Wu 2008	29	29	26	30	8.8%	1.15 [0.99, 1.34]	
Yang 2012	60	61	58	61	19.7%	1.03 [0.97, 1.10]	
Zhong 2011	13	14	12	14	4.1%	1.08 [0.84, 1.40]	
Subtotal (95% CI)		176		177	55.8%	1.06 [1.01, 1.11]	
Total events	173		164				
Heterogeneity: Chi² = 2.34, df = 4 (P = 0.67); I² = 0%							
Test for overall effect: Z = 2.39 (P = 0.02)							
1.2 2-year OS							
Li 2009	40	42	38	42	12.9%	1.05 [0.93, 1.19]	
Wu 2008	58	61	56	61	19.0%	1.04 [0.94, 1.14]	
Yang 2012	11	14	9	14	3.0%	1.22 [0.76, 1.97]	
Zhong 2011	27	29	28	30	9.3%	1.00 [0.87, 1.14]	
Subtotal (95% CI)		146		147	44.2%	1.05 [0.97, 1.12]	
Total events	136		131				
Heterogeneity: Chi² = 0.91, df = 3 (P = 0.82); I² = 0%							
Test for overall effect: Z = 1.24 (P = 0.21)							
Total (95% CI)		322		324	100.0%	1.05 [1.01, 1.10]	
Total events	309		295				
Heterogeneity: Chi² = 3.23, df = 8 (P = 0.92); I² = 0%							
Test for overall effect: Z = 2.51 (P = 0.01)							
Test for subgroup differences: Chi² = 0.11, df = 1 (P = 0.75), I² = 0%							

0.01 0.1 1 10 100
Favours control   Favours experimental

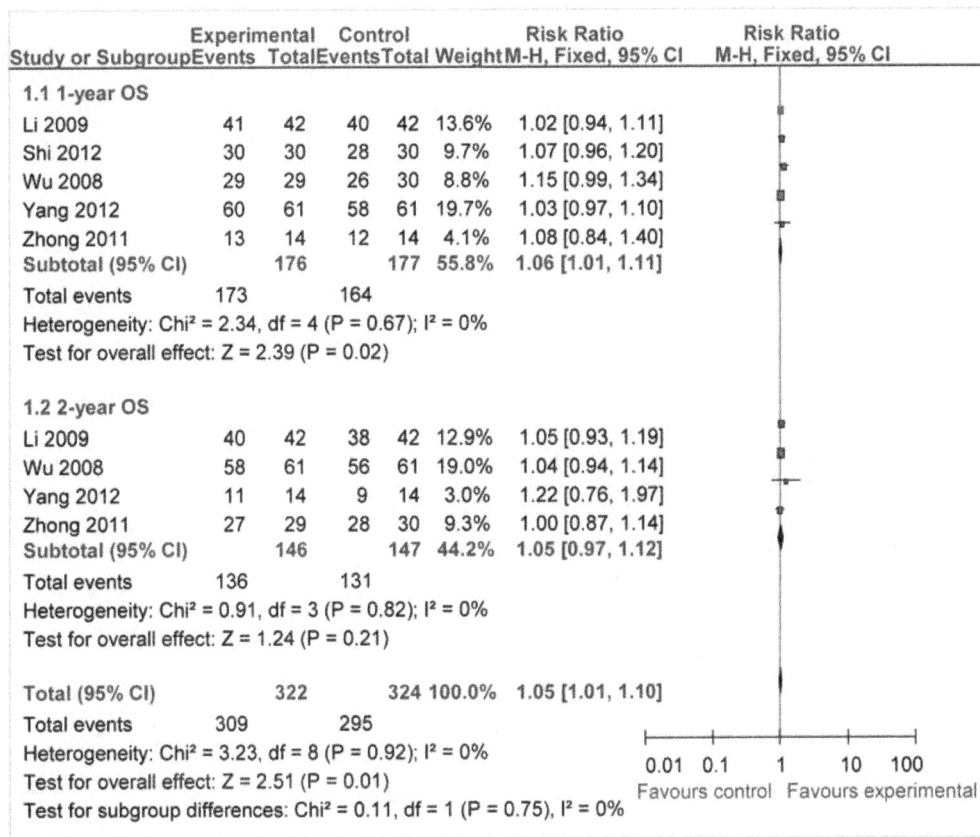

Figure 2. Forest plot of the comparison of overall survival (OS). *P* values are from P for the effect modification evaluation of heterogeneity within or across the groups of regimens. CI, confidence interval; RR, risk ratio; DC/CIK, DC-CIK immunotherapy; Chemo, chemotherapy; Con, control group; Exp, experimental group. A fixed-effect meta-analysis model (Mantel-Haenszel method) was used.

blinding of participants; blinding of outcome assessment; incomplete outcome data addressed; and free of selective reporting. Each of the seven items was scored as "low risk", "unclear risk" or "high risk".

Data Extraction

Two independent reviewers (RXH, PP) scanned titles and available abstracts to identify potentially relevant articles. Disagreements were discussed with a third investigator (XL). The following data were collected: the first author's last name; the year of publication; the country where the study was performed; study design; number of years of follow-up period or study period; age range; number of subjects; and NSCLC stages.

Curative Effects

Clinical responses were assessed in terms of the overall survival (OS) and progression free survival (PFS) to evaluate prognosis. Partial response (PR), overall response rate (ORR) and disease control rate (DCR) were considered to assess treatment efficacy. OS was defined as the time from the start of treatment to the time of death from any cause. PFS was defined as the length of time during and after treatment in which the patients lived with a disease that did not worsen. ORR was defined as the sum of partial and complete response rates, and the DCR was the sum of stable disease, partial response and complete response rates. These values were in accordance with the criteria provided by the World Health Organization.

Safety Assessment

Adverse events (AEs) during the follow-up periods of all of the included studies were determined. AEs [21,22] could be characterized as fatal, life threatening, required or prolonged existing hospitalization, or persistent or significant disability or indisposition and were graded in accordance with the criteria provided by the National Cancer Institute Common Toxicity [23].

Statistical Analysis

Statistical analysis was performed using Review Manager Version 5.0 provided by the Cochrane Collaboration. $P < 0.05$ was considered statistically significant. Heterogeneity [24] between trials was assessed to determine the most suitable model. Once heterogeneity was verified, a random-effect method was used; otherwise, a fixed-effect method was used. To evaluate whether or not the results of studies were homogenous, we performed Cochran's Q-test in which homogeneity was considered at $I^2 < 50\%$ or $P > 0.1$. Risk ratios (RR) were the principal measures of effect and presented with a 95% confidence interval (CI). Sensitivity analysis was conducted and two trials (Wu et al. [25], Zhao et al. [26]) were excluded because DC immunotherapy was not applied in experimental group.

Results

Search Results

A total of 12,479 articles were identified during the initial search. By scanning titles and abstracts, redundant publications,

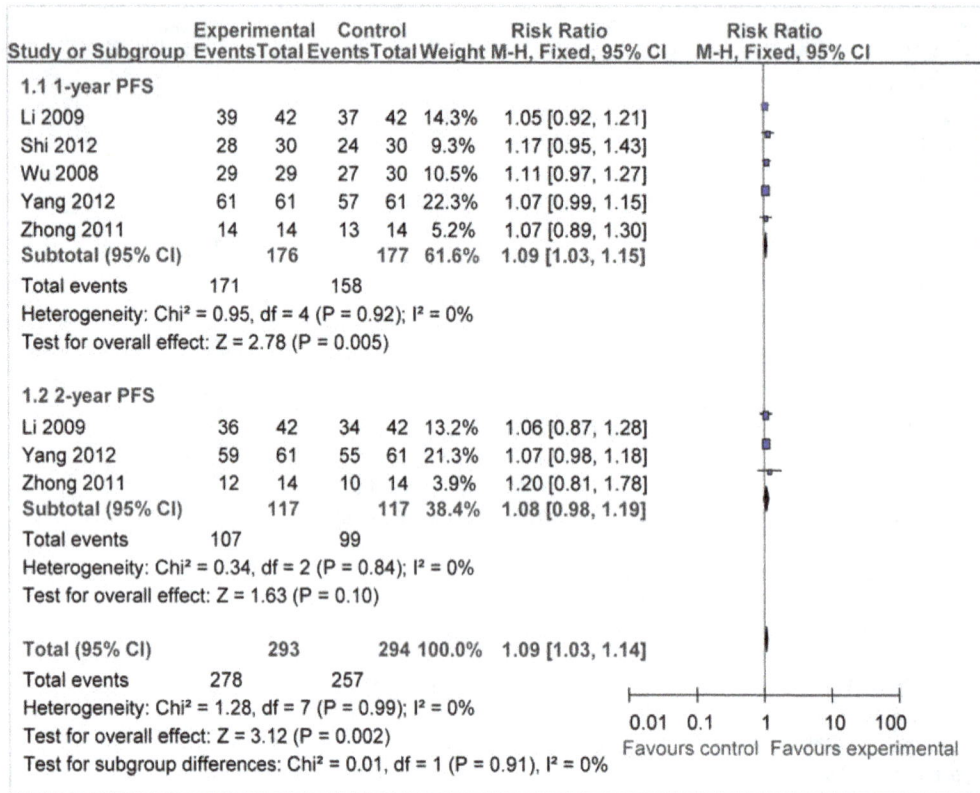

Figure 3. Forest plot of the comparison of progression free survival (PFS). *P* values are from P for the effect modification evaluation of heterogeneity within or across the groups of regimens. CI, confidence interval; RR, risk ratio; DC/CIK, DC-CIK immunotherapy; Chemo, chemotherapy; Con, control group; Exp, experimental group. A fixed-effect meta-analysis model (Mantel-Haenszel method) was used.

reviews, meeting abstracts, and case reports were excluded. After referring to full texts, we removed 12,473 articles that did not satisfy the selection criteria: (1) not involved advanced NSCLC; (2) not displayed chemotherapy with DC-CIK immunotherapy; and (3) non-RCTs. As a result, 6 trials that included a total of 428 patients were eligible in the present analysis. The exclusion reasons were illustrated in **Figure 1**.

Table 1 showed the characteristics of the six trials [25–30] included in the meta-analysis. All of the trials were conducted in mainland China. Among these trials, five provided the specific years of follow-up (two years to seven years). All of the six studies

were randomized, and items were ranked as "low risk" based on the Cochrane Handbook.

Meta-Analysis of Prognosis Evaluation

The prognosis included two parts, namely, OS and PFS.

Among the six trials, five reported 1-year OS rate and four reported 2-year OS rate (**Figure 2**). Considering that slightly significant heterogeneity was detected, we selected the fixed-effect model. Chemotherapy combined with DC-CIK immunotherapy showed significant increase in 1-year OS compared with that of chemotherapy alone (RR = 1.06, 95%CI = 1.01–1.11, *P* = 0.02)

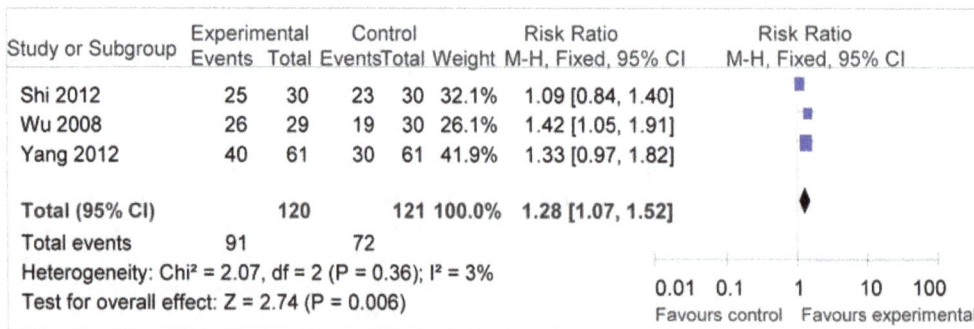

Figure 4. Forest plot of the comparison of disease control rate (DCR). *P* values are from P for the effect modification evaluation of heterogeneity within or across the groups of regimens. CI, confidence interval; RR, risk ratio; DC/CIK, DC-CIK immunotherapy; Chemo, chemotherapy; Con, control group; Exp, experimental group. A fixed-effect meta-analysis model (Mantel-Haenszel method) was used.

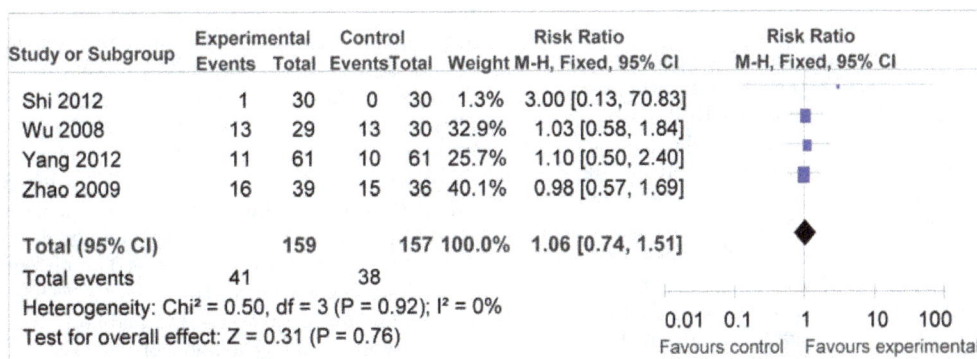

Figure 5. Forest plot of the comparison of overall response rate (ORR). *P* values are from P for the effect modification evaluation of heterogeneity within or across the groups of regimens. CI, confidence interval; RR, risk ratio; DC/CIK, DC-CIK immunotherapy; Chemo, chemotherapy; Con, control group; Exp, experimental group. A fixed-effect meta-analysis model (Mantel-Haenszel method) was used.

according to the test for overall effect, however, the 2-year OS in the experiment group was not significantly different from those in control group (RR = 1.05, 95%CI = 0.97–1.12, *P* = 0.21).

In terms of PFS, five studies presented relevant data of 1-year PFS and three reported 2-year PFS. In **Figure 3**, chemotherapy combined with immunotherapy significantly prolonged 1-year PFS (RR = 1.09, 95CI% = 1.03–1.15, P = 0.005) compared with chemotherapy alone. However, for 2-year PFS, the experimental group had no significant difference (RR = 1.08, 95CI% = 0.98–1.19, P = 0.10) compared with control group.

Meta-Analysis of Efficacy Assessment

Efficacy was assessed in terms of DCR, ORR and PR.

The analysis result of DCR was shown in **Figure 4**, revealing positive outcomes for the combination therapy (RR = 1.20, 95% CI = 1.07–1.52, P = 0.006). But the RR of ORR was 1.06 (95% CI = 0.74–1.51, *P* = 0.76), which showed in **Figure 5**, did not infer significantly difference between two groups.

Fix-effect models were chosen to analyze the PR rate because low heterogeneity was obtained. In **Figure 6**, RR was 1.23 (95% CI = 0.88–1.71, *P* = 0.22), suggesting no statistically significant improvement between two groups.

Sensitivity Analysis

Considering that not all of the **efficacy** parameters were presented in all of the reviewed studies, we performed sensitivity

analyses separately on each parameter in accordance with the alternative exclusion criteria of trials, such as the studies by Wu et al [25] and Zhao et al [26], which did not apply the DC method. The results of this analysis were similar to those obtained from the overall analysis of the pooled trials.

Assessment of AEs or Toxicity for advanced NSCLC

The current clinical trials with advanced NSCLC indicated considerable AEs or toxicity. The details of treatment-related AEs or toxicity were summarized in **Table 2**.

In **Table 2**, all of the six trials reported adverse effects. However, three of these trials [25,27,30] did not provide the exact numbers of AEs. In both groups, leukopenia, nausea, anemia, insomnia, temporary fever, headache, fatigue, thrombocytopenia, and chest distress were observed. Among them, temporary fever, anemia, leukopenia and nausea were the four main AEs.

The results indicated that chemotherapy combined with DC-CIK therapy could obviously alleviate leukopenia, nausea, anemia, insomnia, fatigue, and thrombocytopenia compared with chemotherapy alone. For temporary fever, the experimental group was a little more than the control group and could be relieved naturally in 24 hours without any medical treatment.

For chest distress, the effectiveness of chemotherapy combined with DC-CIK remained unclear because chemotherapy alone was not clearly described.

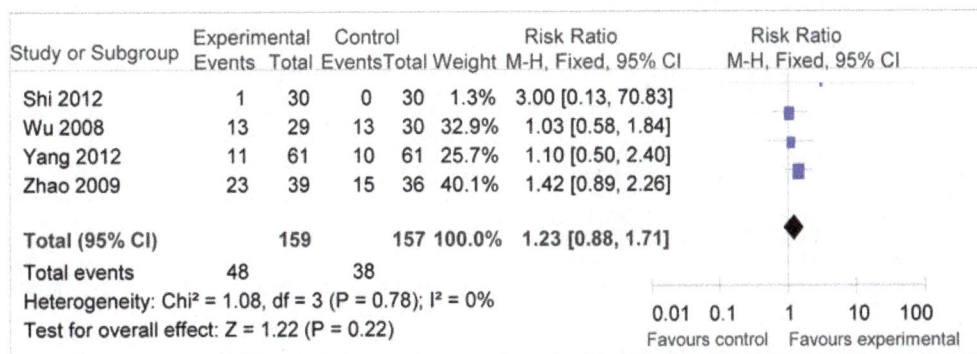

Figure 6. Forest plot of the comparison of partial response rate (PR). *P* values are from P for the effect modification evaluation of heterogeneity within or across the groups of regimens. CI, confidence interval; RR, risk ratio; DC/CIK, DC-CIK immunotherapy; Chemo, chemotherapy; Con, control group; Exp, experimental group. A fixed-effect meta-analysis model (Mantel-Haenszel method) was used.

Discussion

The 6 trials included in this meta-analysis adopted chemotherapy combined DC-CIK therapy for patients with advanced NSCLC. Hence, the number of published RCTs would affect the results of this study and the quality of the reported data influenced the power of our meta-analysis, and greater statistical reliability would be achieved if additional and more comprehensive trials including all of the efficacy parameters were enrolled. Nevertheless, sensitivity analysis supported the conclusions drawn from the overall unstratified analyses.

Other factors, such as individual difference of patients, different lengths of follow-up may confer limitations on this meta-analysis. In overall studies, no significant publication bias existed, in addition, as many RCTs as possible were included to improve the statistical reliability. Our literature search strategy guaranteed that there was less possibility of important published trials being overlooked. According to our meta-analysis, all patients with advanced NSCLC met quality-control specifications and protocol eligibility. Finally, risk ratios demonstrated that no statistical inconsistency existed between results from each of the original studies and those of overall efficacy suggested that the results were valid.

For clinical therapy, effectiveness and safety are the key factors [31]. At present, DC-CIK technology is widely used in clinic due to its higher security. Up to date, a large body of clinical evidence indicated that there was neither serious AEs nor death caused by DC-CIK therapy. The main side effects are temporary fever (usually below 39°C) and cold symptoms [32].

The present meta-analysis indicated that chemotherapy combined with DC-CIK had potential advantages in NSCLC treatment: firstly, its efficiency was observed in clinic. An outstanding characteristic was significant increase in 1-year OS ($P = 0.02$) and 1-year PFS ($P = 0.005$). Besides, DCR in the combined therapy was also improved significantly ($P = 0.006$), and patients obtained better quality of life, such as relieving pain, fatigue and insomnia; secondly, the AEs of chemotherapy combined with DC-CIK were alleviated obviously compared with

that of the chemotherapy alone, including leucopenia, nausea, anemia, insomnia, fatigue, and thrombocytopenia. Undoubtedly, these were the greatest benefits for patients.

However, the efficacy of chemotherapy combined with DC-CIK has been in argument, especially in long-term effectiveness. The analysis of 2-year OS ($P = 0.21$) and 2-year PFS ($P = 0.10$) showed no statistical significance between the two groups. For ORR ($P = 0.76$) and PR ($P = 0.22$), there appeared no statistical differences, too. These results suggested that the current DC-CIK immunotherapy is modest in efficacy. This may be related to large tumor burden in the advanced NSCLC as well as the shortages of the methods for generation of DC and CIK. It is possible that (a) current methods for generation of DCs are unable to generate sufficient number of immunogenic DCs; (b) these DCs are unable to efficiently process and present endogenous tumor antigens, and (c) CIKs are short on life if endogenous and exogenous DC could not provide sufficient help for their survival.

Taken together, although chemotherapy combined with DC-CIK is a recommendable method and applies successfully in clinic for patients with NSCLC [33,34], our meta analysis indicates that this type of therapy currently is modest for NSCLC. Especially, the quality of DC-CIK needs to be rigorously improved to enhance therapeutic efficacy and prolong the survival period of patients.

Acknowledgments

We thank Ling Li, Fanming Kong and Xuezhu Zhang for their professional suggestions and constructive comments on this manuscript.

Author Contributions

Performed the experiments: YJJ JCY. Analyzed the data: RXH PP. Contributed reagents/materials/analysis tools: RXH XL PP. Wrote the paper: RXH XL PP.

References

1. Jemal A, Bray F, Center M, Ferlay J, Ward E, et al. (2011) Global cancer statistics. Ca Cancer J Clin 61: 69–90.

2. Zheng Y, Li R, Zhang X, Ren X (2013) Current adoptive immunotherapy in non-small cell lung cancer and potential influence of therapy outcome. Cancer Invest 31: 197–205.

3. Thanendrarajan S, Nowak M, Abken H, Schmidt-Wolf IGH (2011) Combining cytokine-induced killer cells with vaccination in cancer immunotherapy: More than one plus one? Leukemia Research 35: 1136–1142.

4. DeVita V, Rosenberg S (2012) Two hundred years of cancer research. N Engl J Med 366: 2207–2013.

5. Kelly RJ, Gulley JL, Giaccone G (2010) Immunotherapy for non-small cell lung cancer. Clin Lung Cancer 11: 228–237.

6. Kakimi K, Nakajima J, Wada H (2009) Active specific immunotherapy and cell-transfer therapy for the treatment of non-small cell lung cancer. Lung Cancer 65: 1–8.

7. Jäkel CE, Schmidt-Wolf IG (2014) An update on new adoptive immunotherapy strategies for solid tumors with cytokine-induced killer cells. Expert Opin Biol Ther: Epub ahead of print.

8. Olioso P, Giancola R, Riti MD, Contento A, Accorsi P, et al. (2009) Immunotherapy with cytokine induced killer cells in solid and hematopoietic tumours: a pilot clinical trial. Hematol Oncol 27: 130–139.

9. Ma Y, Zhang Z, Tang L, Xu Y, Xie Z, et al. (2012) Cytokine-induced killer cells in the treatment of patients with solid carcinomas: a systematic review and pooled analysis. Cytotherapy 14: 483–493.

10. Tao L, Huang G, Shi S, Chen L (2014) Bevacizumab improves the antitumor efficacy of adoptive cytokine-induced killer cells therapy in non-small cell lung cancer models. Med Oncol 31: 777(771–778).

11. Wongkajornsilp A, Wamanuttajinda V, Kasetsinsombat K, Duangsa-ard S, Sangiamsuntorn K, et al. (2013) Sunitinib indirectly enhanced anti-tumor cytotoxicity of cytokine-induced killer cells and CD3+CD56+ subset through the co-culturing dendritic cells. PloS One 8: epub ahead of printing.

12. Wang X, Yu W, Li H, Yu J, Zhang X, et al. (2014) Can the dual-functional capability of CIK cells be used to improve antitumor effects? Cell Immunol 287: 18–22.

13. Wang QJ, Wang H, Pan K, Li YQ, Huang LX, et al. (2010) Comparative study on anti-tumor immune response of autologous cytokine-induced killer (CIK) cells, dendritic cells-CIK (DC-CIK), and semi-allogeneic DC-CIK. Chin J Cancer 29: 641–648.

14. Zhong R, Han B, Zhong H (2014) A prospective study of the efficacy of a combination of autologous dendritic cells, cytokine-induced killer cells, and chemotherapy in advanced non-small cell lung cancer patients. Tumour Biol 35: 987–994.

15. Holt GE, Podack ER, Raez LE (2011) Immunotherapy as a strategy for the treatment of non-small-cell lung cancer. Therapy 8: 43–54.

16. Huang X, Chen Y, Song H, Huang G, Chen L (2011) Cisplatin pretreatment enhances anti-tumor activity of cytokine-induced killer cells. World J Gastroenterol 17: 3002–3011.

17. Rao B, Han M, Wang L, Gao X, Huang J, et al. (2011) Clinical outcomes of active specific immunotherapy in advanced colorectal cancer and suspected minimal residual colorectal cancer: a meta-analysis and system review. J Transl Med 9: 17–27.

18. Liu L, Zhang W, Qi X, Li H, Yu J, et al. (2012) Randomized study of autologous cytokine-induced killer cell immunotherapy in metastatic renal carcinoma. Clin Cancer Res 18: 1751–1759.

19. Moher D, Liberati A, Tetzlaff J, Altman DG, The PG (2009) Preferred reporting items for systematic reviews and meta-analyses: the PRISMA statement. PLoS Med 6: e1000097.

20. Higgins J, Green S (2011) Cochrane Handbook for Systematic Reviews of Interventions Available: http://www.cochrane-handbook.org/. Accessed: 2012 Nov 13.

21. Chrischilles E, Pendergast J, Kahn K, Wallace R, Moga D, et al. (2010) Adverse events among the elderly receiving chemotherapy for advanced non-small-cell lung cancer. J Clin Oncol 28: 620–627.

22. Wu S, Keresztes RS (2011) Antiangiogenic agents for the treatment of nonsmall cell lung cancer: characterizing the molecular basis for serious adverse events. Cancer Invest 29: 460–471.

23. Kautio AL, Haanpaa M, Kautiainen H, Leminen A, Kalso E, et al. (2011) Oxaliplatin scale and National Cancer Institute-Common Toxicity Criteria in the assessment of chemotherapy-induced peripheral neuropathy. Anticancer Res 31: 3493–3496.

24. Jackson D, White I, Riley R (2012) Quantifying the impact of between-study heterogeneity in multivariate meta-analyses. Stat Med 31: 3805–3820.

25. Wu C, Jiang J, Shi L, Xu N (2008) Prospective study of chemotherapy in combination with CIK cells in patients suffering from advanced non-small cell lung cancer. Anticancer Res 28: 3997–4002.

26. Zhao G, Huang Y, Ye L, Duan L, Zhou Y, et al. (2009) Therapeutic efficacy of traditional vein chemotherapy and bronchial arterial infusion combining with CIKs on III stage non-small cell lung cancer. Chin J Lung Cancer 12: 1000–1004.

27. Zhong R, Teng J, Han B, Zhong H (2011) Dendritic cells combining with cytokine-induced killer cells synergize chemotherapy in patients with late-stage non-small cell lung cancer. Cancer Immunol Immunother 60: 1497–1502.

28. Shi S, Ma T, Li C, Tang X (2012) Effect of maintenance therapy with dendritic cells: cytokine-induced killer cells in patients with advanced non-small cell lung cancer. Tumori 98: 314–319.

29. Yang L, Ren B, Li H, Yu J, Cao S, et al. (2013) Enhanced antitumor effects of DC-activated CIKs to chemotherapy treatment in a single cohort of advanced non-small-cell lung cancer patients. Cancer Immunol Immunother 62: 65–73.

30. Li H, Wang CL, Yu JP, Cao S, Wei F, et al. (2009) Dendritic cell-activated cytokine-induced killer cells enhance the anti-tumor effect of chemotherapy on non-small cell lung cancer in patients after surgery. Cytotherapy 11: 1076–1083.

31. Tucker ZCG, Laguna BA, Moon E, Singhal S (2012) Adjuvant immunotherapy for non-small cell lung cancer. Cancer Treat Rev 38: 650–661.

32. Aerts J, Hegmans J (2013) Tumor-specific cytotoxic T cells arecrucial for efficacy of immunomodulatory antibodies in patients with lung cancer. Cancer Res 73: 2381–2388.

33. Hiret S, Senellart H, Bennouna J (2010) Molecular biology of lung cancer series. Rev Mal Respir 27: 954–958.

34. Wang J, Zou Z, Xia H, He J, Zhong N, et al. (2012) Strengths and weaknesses of immunotherapy for advanced non-small-cell lung cancer: a meta-analysis of 12 randomized controlled trials. PLoS One 7: 1–12.

23

The Glasgow Prognostic Score Predicts Poor Survival in Cisplatin-Based Treated Patients with Metastatic Nasopharyngeal Carcinoma

Cui Chen[1,9], Peng Sun[2,3,9], Qiang-sheng Dai[1,9], Hui-wen Weng[1], He-ping Li[1], Sheng Ye[1]*

1 Department of Oncology, The First Affiliated Hospital, Sun Yat-Sen University, Guangzhou, China, 2 Department of Medical Oncology, Sun Yat-sen University Cancer Center, Guangzhou, China, 3 Collaborative Innovation Center for Cancer Medicine, State Key Laboratory of Oncology in South China, Guangzhou, China

Abstract

Background: Several inflammation-based prognostic scoring systems, including Glasgow Prognostic Score (GPS), neutrophil to lymphocyte ratio (NLR) and platelet to lymphocyte ratio (PLR) have been reported to predict survival in many malignancies, whereas their role in metastatic nasopharyngeal carcinoma (NPC) remains unclear. The aim of this study is to evaluate the clinical value of these prognostic scoring systems in a cohort of cisplatin-based treated patients with metastatic NPC.

Methods: Two hundred and eleven patients with histologically proven metastatic NPC treated with first-line cisplatin-based chemotherapy were retrospectively evaluated. Demographics, disease-related characteristics and relevant laboratory data before treatment were recorded. GPS, NLR and PLR were calculated as described previously. Response to first-line therapy and survival data were also collected. Survival was analyzed in Cox regressions and stability of the models was examined by bootstrap resampling. The area under the receiver operating characteristics curve (AUC) was calculated to compare the discriminatory ability of each scoring system.

Results: Among the above three inflammation-based prognostic scoring systems, GPS ($P<0.001$) and NLR ($P=0.019$) were independently associated with overall survival, which showed to be stable in a bootstrap resampling study. The GPS consistently showed a higher AUC value at 6-month (0.805), 12-month (0.705), and 24-month (0.705) in comparison with NLR and PLR. Further analysis of the association of GPS with progression-free survival showed GPS was also associated independently with progression-free survival ($P<0.001$).

Conclusions: Our study demonstrated that the GPS may be of prognostic value in metastatic NPC patients treated with cisplatin-based palliative chemotherapy and facilitate individualized treatment. However a prospective study to validate this prognostic model is still needed.

Editor: Konradin Metze, University of Campinas, Brazil

Funding: The authors received no specific funding for this work.

Competing Interests: The authors have declared that no competing interests exist.

* Email: yes20111212@163.com

⑨ These authors contributed equally to this work.

Introduction

Nasopharyngeal carcinoma (NPC) is a distinct disease with unique ethnic and geographic characteristics, whose incidence varies from 0.5–3/100 000/year in North Africa to 20–30 in some areas of southern China. [1,2] Although the cure rate has been significantly improved owing to advances in diagnostic imaging, radiotherapeutic techniques and chemotherapy regimens recently, distant metastases remain the main reason for failure of treatment. [3] In these cases, palliative systemic therapy remains the primary therapeutic option and cisplatin-based combination chemotherapy is considered the standard front-line regimen for decades, offering response rates in the range of 50–80% and a significant prolongation of overall survival (OS). [4] However, there are still wide individual differences in clinical response and outcomes. Some reports indicate that overall survival may exceed ten years for specific subgroups of patients. It is therefore of paramount interest to find an easily available model to help evaluate individual prognosis which will greatly improve the ability of clinical decision-making.

Currently, clinical characteristics are dominating indexes for judging prognosis of metastatic NPC patients, such as performance status and disease-free interval. [5] The prognostic value of circulating Epstein–Barr virus (EBV) DNA load has also been well established in various reports. [6,7] Besides aforementioned prognostic factors representing tumor status and clinical characteristics, it is now recognized that the host inflammatory response, in particular the systemic inflammatory response, plays an important role in disease development and progression by inhibition of apoptosis, promotion of angiogenesis, and damage of DNA. [8,9,10] Several inflammation-based prognostic scoring systems have been devised and found to be strongly correlated with prognosis in patients with a variety of neoplasms. These include a combination of neutrophil and lymphocyte counts as the neutrophil to lymphocyte ratio (NLR) and a combination of platelet and lymphocyte counts as the platelet to lymphocyte ratio (PLR), both of which reflect full blood count derangements induced by the acute phase reaction, while the Glasgow Prognostic Score (GPS) incorporates raised circulating C-reactive protein (CRP) and hypoalbuminemia. [11,12,13,14,15] Recently some researches have also shown that markers of systemic inflammatory response represent reliable prognostic factors in patients with early nasopharyngeal carcinoma. [16] However, to the best of our knowledge, there is no data regarding the prognostic impact of systemic inflammation-based scoring systems in metastatic NPC. In the present study, we therefore evaluated the clinical value of several inflammation-based prognostic scoring systems including GPS, NLR and PLR in a cohort of cisplatin-based treated patients with metastatic NPC.

Patients and Methods

Patient selection

From October 2005 to October 2011, 211 patients with histologically proven metastatic NPC treated with first-line cisplatin-based chemotherapy were included in the study at Sun Yat-Sen University Cancer Center. Entry criteria consisted of: (1) radiologically measurable disease; (2) treated with at least two cycles of first-line cisplatin-based palliative chemotherapy; (3) Karnofsky Performance Scores (KPS) ≥60; (4) normal hepatic and renal function. Exclusion criteria included: (1) patients with other types of malignancy; (2) patients with brain metastases; (3) patients with clinical evidence of infection or other inflammatory conditions. This study was approved by the institutional review board and ethics committee of Sun Yat-Sen University Cancer Center. All patients provided written informed consent to

participate in this study. Parental written consent was obtained for minors in current study.

Treatment

All eligible patients received 1 of the following cisplatin-based chemotherapy regimens as the first-line treatment: (1) cisplatin (25 mg/m^2 intravenously [IV] on Days 1–3 of a 21-day cycle) plus 5-fluorouracil (500 mg/m^2 IV on Days 1–5 of a 21-day cycle), (2) paclitaxel (175 mg/m^2 IV over 3 hours with standard premedication on Day 1 of a 21-day cycle) plus cisplatin (25 mg/m^2 IV on Days 1–3 of a 21-day cycle), (3) paclitaxel (135 mg/m^2 IV over 3 hours with standard premedication on Day 1 of a 21-day cycle) plus cisplatin (25 mg/m^2 IV on Days 1–3 of a 21-day cycle) plus 5-fluorouracil (800 mg/m^2, continuous IV infusion for 24 hours, on Days 1–5 of a 21-day cycle). Of the 211 eligible patients, 78 (37.0%) patients were given the PF regimen, 24 (11.4%) patients were given the TP regimen, and 109 (51.6%) patients received the TPF regimen.

Relevant Evaluation

Basic demographics, baseline characteristics, detailed medical history as well as relevant laboratory data before treatment (C-reactive protein (CRP), Serum lactate dehydrogenase (LDH), albumin, neutrophil, lymphocyte, platelet (Plt) count and plasma EBV DNA level) were recorded. The GPS, NLR and PLR were constructed as described previously. In GPS, patients with both an elevated CRP level (>1.0 mg/dl) and hypoalbuminemia (<3.5 g/dl) were allocated a score of 2, patients with only one of these biochemical abnormalities were allocated a score of 1, and patients with neither of these abnormalities were allocated a score of 0. NLR was divided into two groups (<5 and ≥5) while PLR was categorized into three groups (<150, 150–300 and >300).

Progression-free survival (PFS) and overall survival (OS) were defined as the time from the first diagnosis of metastasis to the date of documented progression and to the date of death, respectively. Tumor response was evaluated according to the Response Evaluation Criteria in Solid Tumors (RECISTs) 1.0.

Table 1. Demographic and Baseline Characteristics of Patients.

Patient characteristics	Number (%)
Total evaluated	211 (100)
Age, years (median/range)	46/14–72
Gender (male/female)	181/30 (85.8/14.2)
KPS (median/range)	90/60–100
Number of involved sites (median/range)	2/1–6
Synchronous metastasis (yes/no)	53/158 (25.1/74.9)
Liver metastasis (yes/no)	73/138 (34.6/65.4)
Lung metastasis (yes/no)	97/114 (45.9/54.1)
Bone metastasis (yes/no)	88/123 (41.7/58.3)
Disease-free interval, months (median/range)	6/0–65
Chemotherapy regimen (PF/TP/TPF)	78/24/109 (37.0/11.4/51.6)
Serum LDH, U/L (median/range)	247/81–632
Pre-treatment EBV DNA, copies/mL (median/range)	4.93×10^4/0–9.73×10^7
GPS (0/1/2)	125/66/20 (59.2/31.3/9.5)
NLR (median/range)	3.12/0.81–11.03
PLR (median/range)	71.2/31.3–422.5

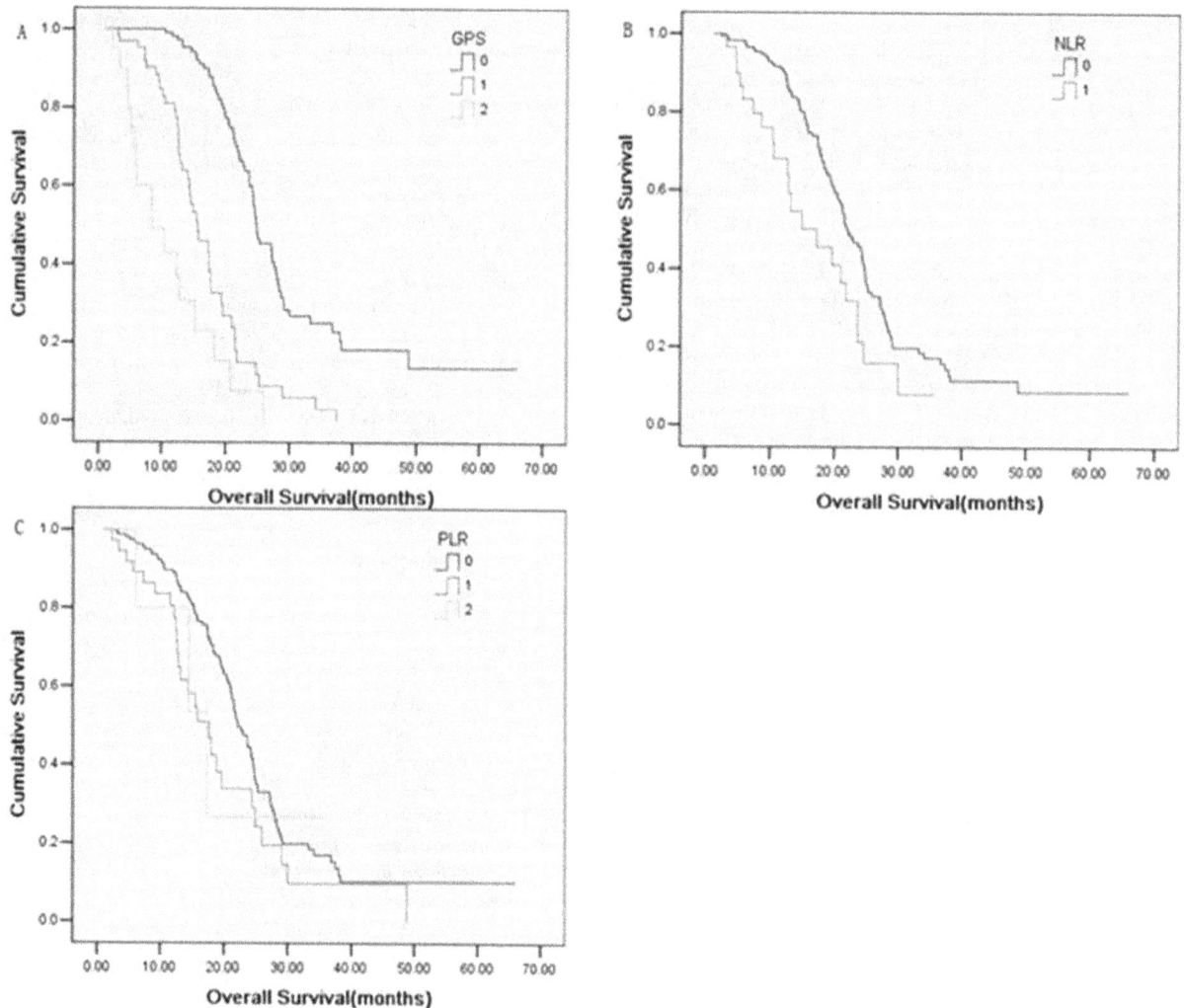

Figure 1. Comparison of overall survival according to scoring systems, GPS (A), NLR (B) and PLR (C).

Follow up

Patients were regularly followed up after chemotherapy until death or their last follow-up appointment. Physical examination and imaging studies of the relevant region(s) were performed every 3 months after the completion of the chemotherapy or when clinical indications dictated for follow-up. The start date of follow-up period was the date of initial metastatic NPC diagnosis. The time of last follow-up was 31st December 2013 or death.

Statistical analysis

All statistical analysis was performed using SPSS version 13.0 software or WinStat software. PFS and OS were obtained by using the Kaplan–Meier method and differences between the groups were compared by the log-rank test. A univariate analysis was performed for the potential prognostic factors. Age, karnofsky performance score before treatment, number of involved sites, disease-free interval, serum LDH, pre-treatment EBV DNA entered the calculations in a continuous way. NLR and PLR were also tested at first as continuous variables in order to avoid the bias induced by binarization of continuous data. And we tested the GPS and the other variables entering the analysis as categorical variables. Multivariable analysis including variables that proved to be significant in the univariate analysis was

performed subsequently using the Cox model to analyse factors related to prognosis (P<0.05 was used as the cut-off value of statistical significance). The stability of the COX model was tested by bootstrap resampling. New data sets of equal size were created by random sampling of the original data with replacement. In each new bootstrap data set, a patient may be represented once, multiple times or not at all. Cox regressions with the same conditions as in the original data set were then calculated for the new data sets in order to obtain the bootstrap parameter estimates. Descriptive statistics for the patient groups are reported as mean, median, and range. Categorical variables were presented numbers and percentages. Non-parametric test was applied for comparison of data among groups. A receiver operating characteristics (ROC) curve was also generated and the area under the curve (AUC) was calculated to evaluate the discriminatory ability of each scoring systems. A two-tailed P value less than 0.05 was considered to be statistically significant.

Results

Patient characteristics and Outcomes

A total of 211 patients with metastatic NPC were included in the present study. All of the patients were from epidemic areas in

Table 2. Univariate and Multivariate Analysis of Prognostic Factors of Overall Survival.

| Variable | Univariate analysis | | Multivariate analysis | |
	P	HR (95% CI)	*P*	HR (95% CI)
Age	0.444	1.006 (0.990–1.023)		
Gender (male/female)	0.631	1.147 (0.655–2.008)		
KPS	0.934	1.020 (0.637–1.633)		
Liver metastasis (yes/no)	0.989	1.003 (0.694–1.449)		
Lung metastasis (yes/no)	0.848	1.035 (0.726–1.476)		
Number of involved sites	0.020	1.282 (1.040–1.580)	0.560	1.064 (0.864–1.310)
Synchronous metastasis (yes/no)	0.696	0.920 (0.604–1.400)		
Disease-free interval	0.278	1.218 (0.853–1.739)		
Chemotherapy regimen (PF/TP/TPF)	0.358	0.767 (0.435–1.351)		
Serum LDH	0.014	1.210 (1.040–1.409)	0.911	1.011 (0.835–1.225)
Pre-treatment EBVDNA	0.024	1.234 (1.028–1.481)	0.037	1.239 (1.013–1.515)
GPS (0/1/2)	<0.001	3.078 (2.393–3.959)	<0.001	2.520 (1.977–3.212)
NLR	0.025	1.732 (1.071–2.800)	0.019	1.800 (1.103–2.940)
PLR	0.125	1.311 (0.928–1.853)		

China, with a male predominance (85.8%). The mean age of diagnosis of metastatic NPC was 46 (range 14–72) years. About half of the patients had more than one metastatic site with lung being the most common site (45.9%). The pretreatment plasma EBV DNA ranged from 0 to 9.73×10^7 copies/mL, with a median of 4.93×10^4 copies/mL. One hundred and fifty (71.1%) patients showed an elevated pretreatment EBV DNA level ($>1 \times 10^3$ copies/mL). One hundred and twenty-five (59.2%) patients were allocated to GPS 0, 66 (31.3%) patients were allocated to GPS 1, and 20 (9.5%) patients were allocated to GPS 2, respectively. The median NLR level was 3.12 (range 0.81~11.03). Thirty patients (14.2%) had an NLR≥5 and the rest had an NLR<5. The PLR ranged from 31.3 to 422.5, with a median of 71.2. A PLR greater than 300 was seen in 5 patients (2.4%), 168 patients (79.6%) had PLR<150, and the rest had a PLR in between. Other patient characteristics are summarized in Table 1.

At the time of analysis, 124 (58.8%) patients had died, and the median PFS and OS were 7.9 and 21.6 months, respectively. The overall clinical response rate was 70.1% for all 211 patients.

Prognostic factor analysis for overall survival

Various potential prognostic factors including age, gender, karnofsky performance score before treatment, metastasis sites (liver and lung), number of involved sites, synchronous metastasis, disease-free interval, chemotherapy regimen, serum LDH, pre-treatment EBV DNA, GPS status, NLR and PLR were analyzed. Univariate analysis revealed that a larger number of involved sites ($P = 0.020$), higher baseline serum LDH level ($P = 0.014$), higher pretreatment EBV DNA level ($P = 0.024$), higher score of GPS ($P<0.001$) and higher value of NLR ($P = 0.025$) were considered adverse factors for overall survival (Table 2, Fig. 1). Age, gender, PLR and the other variables in the analysis had no prognostic relevance. In multivariate analysis, pre-treatment EBV DNA ($P = 0.037$), GPS ($P<0.001$) and NLR ($P = 0.019$) were independent prognostic factors (Table 2). The stability of this model was confirmed in a bootstrap resampling procedure. Among 1000 new

models, pre-treatment EBV DNA was present in 69%, GPS appeared in 89% and NLR in 71%.

Moreover, the two inflammation-based prognostic scoring systems constructed by categorizing the continuous variables of NLR and PLR as described before were compared with the GPS. Receiver operating characteristic curves were constructed for survival status at 6-month, 12-month, and 24-month of follow-up, and the area under the ROC curve (AUC) was compared (Fig. 2) to assess the discrimination ability of each scoring system. The GPS consistently show a higher AUC value at 6-month (0.805), 12-month (0.705), and 24-month (0.705) in comparison with other inflammation-based prognostic scores.

Association of GPS with clinicopathologic characteristics

Baseline patient and disease-related characteristics for each GPS group and comparisons between groups are depicted in Table 3. Although the difference was not statistically significant, a trend towards an association of GPS with BMI was observed. Of note, an elevated GPS was significantly associated with higher serum LDH and higher pretreatment EBV DNA.

Association of GPS with progression-free survival

GPS was further associated with PFS. Kaplan–Meier curves for PFS for the total cohort according to GPS was shown in Fig. 3. Median PFS (95% CI) was 8.73 (7.64–9.82), 5.27 (4.51–6.02) and 3.40 (1.21–5.59) months for patients with GPS 0, 1 and 2, respectively. As shown in Table 4, multivariate analysis including the aforementioned parameters and GPS revealed that GPS was also the independent predictor for PFS ($P<0.001$). The stability of this model was also confirmed in a bootstrap resampling procedure. In the bootstrap resampling, GPS entered in 100% and pre-treatment EBV DNA appeared in 25%.

Discussion

Markers of systemic inflammatory response represent reliable prognostic factors in patients with advanced cancer.

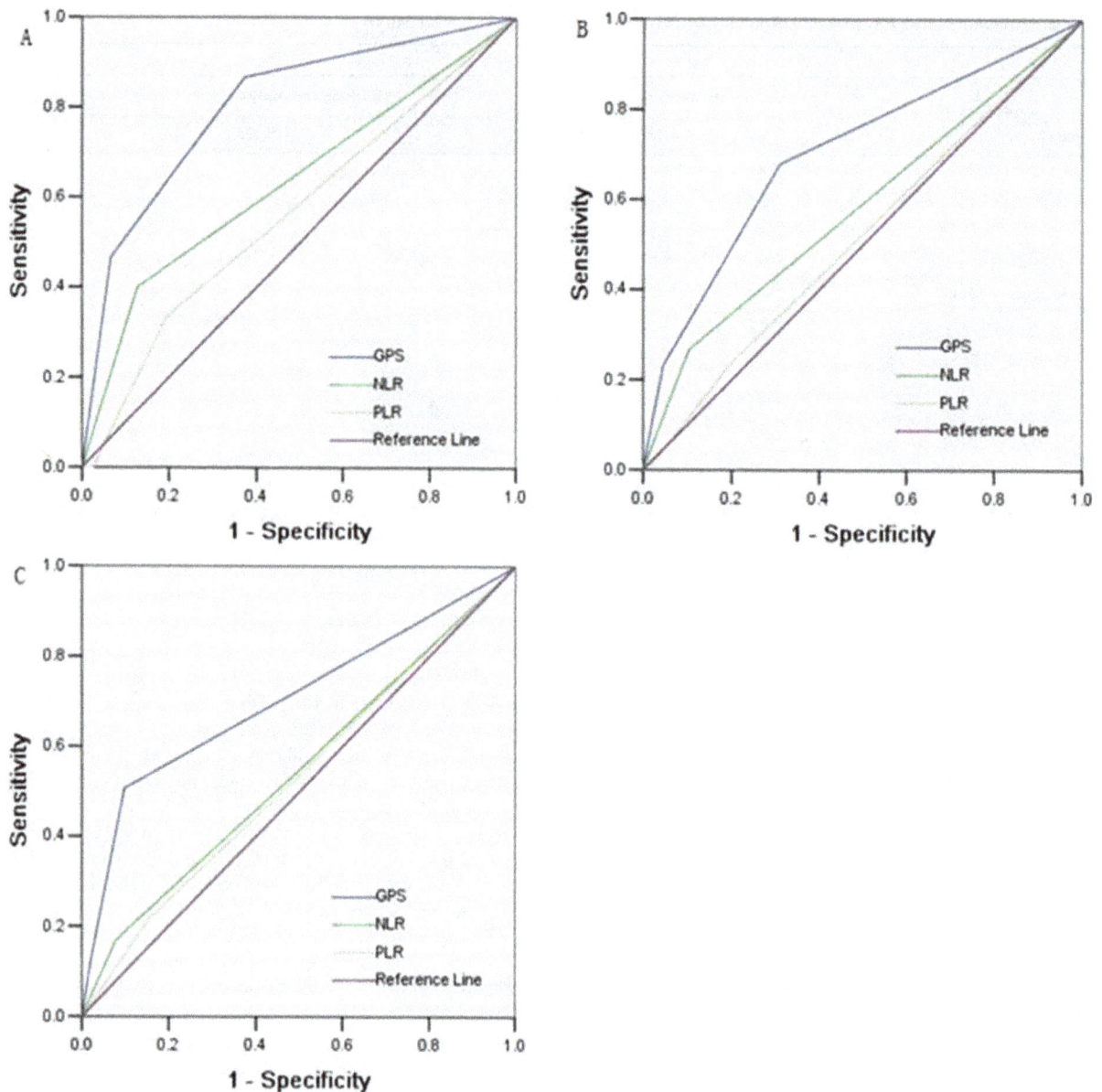

Figure 2. Comparisons of the area under the receiver operating curve for survival status between scoring systems at 6 month (A), 12 month (B) and 24 month (C).

[8,11,12,13,14,16] To the best of our knowledge, this study has firstly demonstrated that the GPS, an inflammation-based prognostic score, is an independent marker of poor prognosis in patients with metastatic NPC and is superior to the NLR in terms of prognostic ability. Furthermore, our data demonstrated a significant, independent association between GPS and PFS.

Accumulating evidence indicates the prognostic importance of GPS in various solid cancers, such as colorectal cancer, [17,18] esophageal cancer, [19] lung cancer, [13] pancreatic cancer, [12] and gastric cancer. [14] A similar result was achieved in our study. The biological basis for the correlation between the GPS and survival are not completely understood. Below are some supposed mechanisms. First, cachexia, which often manifests as nutritional depletion (weight loss, elevated resting energy expenditure and loss of lean tissue) and functional decline, is common in patients with advanced cancer and has been recognized to be associated with

poorer outcome. [20,21,22] CRP has been reported to be associated with the nutrition status and development of cachexia while albumin represents a negative acute phase protein and also represents a marker of nutritional status. [8] As we know, lower serum albumin correlates to nutritional depletion closely. Our study also shows a trend towards an association of GPS with BMI. Based on these reports, GPS, incorporating CRP and serum albumin levels, may reflect both presence of the nutritional depletion and functional decline, resulting in poor survival outcome. Second, a strong association was found between EBV infection and NPC in previous studies. [23] Plasma EBV DNA has been identified to be prognostic in metastatic NPC patients. [6,7] EBV infection stimulated the release of pro-inflammatory cytokine including IL-1, IL-6, and TNF-α from the tumor microenvironment, which results in the induction of CRP synthesis from the liver and the reduction of albumin by hepatocytes. [24,25] In

Table 3. Association of GPS with characteristics of patients.

characteristics	GPS = 0	GPS = 1	GPS = 2	P
Age (≤45/>45)	65/60	30/36	12/8	0.472
Gender (male/female)	103/22	60/6	18/2	0.236
KPS (≤80/>80)	24/101	12/54	4/16	0.978
BMI (≤18.5/>18.5)	21/104	20/46	6/14	0.070
Number of involved sites (1/≥2)	61/64	36/30	8/12	0.493
Synchronous metastasis (yes/no)	26/99	22/44	5/15	0.165
Liver metastasis (yes/no)	43/82	21/45	9/11	0.553
Lung metastasis (yes/no)	53/72	35/31	9/11	0.373
Bone metastasis (yes/no)	50/75	28/38	10/10	0.694
Serum LDH, U/L (<245/≥245)	83/42	27/39	8/12	0.001
Pre-treatment EBV DNA, copies/mL (<median/≥median)	99/26	5/61	2/18	0.0001

other words, GPS level may be a marker of inflammation from EBV infection and may indicate the magnitude of inflammation and the prognosis of patients as EBV DNA load. Previous studies have also indicated that inflammation in the tumor microenvironment play an important role in promoting tumor growth, invasion, and metastasis. [9,10] Our data shows that an elevated GPS is significantly associated with higher EBV-DNA level, which will, to certain extent, add further support to the proposal. In addition to these explanations, because our data find an elevated GPS is also significantly associated with elevated LDH, which has been reported to be an indicator of high tumor burden, an

elevated GPS score may indirectly reflect a high tumor burden. [26] In general, these explanations suggest that it is reasonable that GPS is a significant and independent predictor of survival outcome.

Recently a study by Wei-xiong Xia et al also showed that elevated CRP and CRP kinetics correlated with poor prognosis in patients with metastatic NPC. This study had similar aims and results compared with our study. However there are still some differences between the two studies. Firstly, the GPS incorporates CRP and hypoalbuminemia and may be more suitable to reflect systemic inflammatory response than CRP alone. Secondly, the

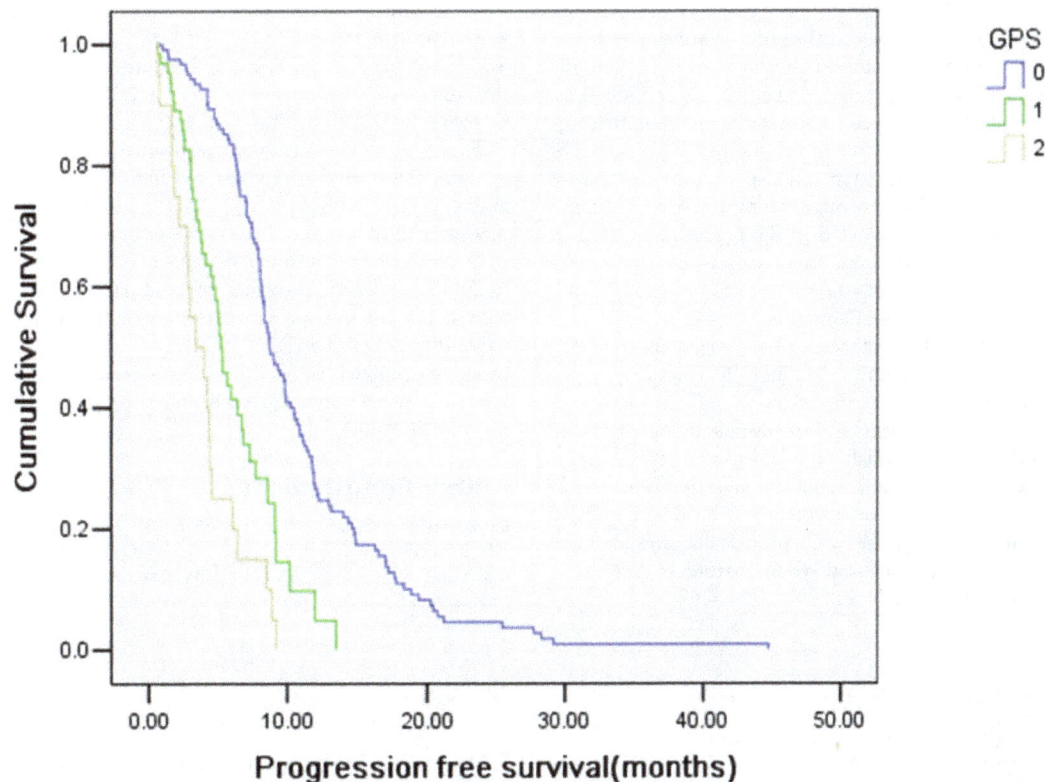

Figure 3. Kaplan–Meier estimates for progression-free survival according to GPS.

Table 4. Univariate and Multivariate Analysis of Prognostic Factors of Progression-free Survival.

Variable	Univariate analysis		Multivariate analysis	
	P	HR (95% CI)	P	HR (95% CI)
Age	0.613	0.996 (0.981–1.011)		
Gender (male/female)	0.489	1.162 (0.760–1.776)		
KPS	0.372	0.998 (0.994–1.002)		
Liver metastasis (yes/no)	0.477	0.893 (0.655–1.219)		
Lung metastasis (yes/no)	0.127	1.261 (0.936–1.698)		
Number of involved sites	0.043	1.201 (1.0066–1.435)	0.493	1.063 (0.893–1.266)
Synchronous metastasis (yes/no)	0.933	1.015 (0.719–1.434)		
Disease-free interval	0.238	1.198 (0.887–1.617)		
Chemotherapy regimen (PF/TP/TPF)	0.609	0.884 (0.552–1.417)		
Serum LDH	0.340	1.072 (0.93–1.235)		
Pre-treatment EBVDNA	<0.001	1.426 (1.170–1.739)	0.133	1.206 (0.945–1.539)
GPS (0/1/2)	<0.001	2.417 (1.916–3.050)	<0.001	2.248 (1.753–2.833)
NLR	0.054	1.400 (0.995–1.971)		
PLR	0.611	1.061 (0.844–1.334)		

eligibility criteria are different. All patients enrolled in current study received first-line cisplatin-based regimens. Thus, it is helpful to exclude the potential confounding effect of different regimens.

The GPS test is simple and based on standardized, wildly available protein assays. Therefore assessment of the GPS can be routinely in most clinical centers. Based on the present results, the significant value of GPS test is that it can identify patients at high risk of disease progression and death as a clinically convenient and useful biomarker. Thus it not only provides guidance of follow-up care at clinic but also has the potential to be a stratification factor or a selection criterion in randomized clinical trials for metastatic NPC. Moreover, in our study, most of the patients evaluated as disease progression at the end of second cycle of chemotherapy were allocated a score of 2. Patients in the good GPS group (GPS 0) had a more prolonged progression-free survival. As a consequence we believe that the presence of a systemic inflammatory response should be evaluated in the pretreatment period and might become the promising new targets of anti-tumor therapy. Nowadays there was an amount of ongoing research into the effect of non-steroidal anti-inflammatory drugs on anti-tumor treatment, including colon cancer, [27] lung cancer, [28] esophagus cancer [29] and so on. Accordingly, it is also interesting and significant to study the modification of the systemic inflammatory response in patients with metastatic nasopharyngeal carcinoma. And the GPS which is inexpensive, reliable, and widely available may have a certain guiding significance for selecting patients who might be candidates for modulation of systemic inflammatory response and provide a well defined therapeutic target for future clinical trials. Further evaluation is required to confirm this hypothesis.

In addition, the NLR and PLR have been reported to be important prognostic models in patients with a variety of solid cancers, such as colorectal cancer, esophageal cancer, gastric cancer, pancreatic cancer, and lung cancer. Several studies have also shown that an elevated NLR is associated with poor prognosis in patients with NPC. [12,14,30,31] In accord with the study of Jian-rong He et al. who tested the prognostic value of NLR in 1410 patients with various stages of NPC [32] and the study of Xin An et al. who tested the prognostic value of NLR in 363 patients with non-disseminated NPC, [16] we also found a significant association between NLR and OS. However, the COX model and the AUC analysis have shown that the GPS was superior to NLR in terms of discriminating ability and prognostic accuracy. For PLR, it was not independently associated with overall survival. In general, this study is the first to show the superior prognostic ability of the GPS over the NLR and PLR in patients with metastatic NPC.

In conclusion, our study demonstrated that the GPS may be useful to predict the prognosis of metastatic NPC patients treated with cisplatin-based palliative chemotherapy and facilitate individualized treatment. A prospective study to validate this prognostic model is needed. The mechanisms underlying the relationship between high GPS and poor prognosis in NPC still need further study.

Author Contributions

Conceived and designed the experiments: SY. Performed the experiments: CC PS HPL. Analyzed the data: CC PS QSD. Contributed reagents/materials/analysis tools: PS SY HWW. Contributed to the writing of the manuscript: CC PS.

References

1. Yu MC, Yuan JM (2002) Epidemiology of nasopharyngeal carcinoma. Semin Cancer Biol 12: 421–429.
2. Chang ET, Adami HO (2006) The enigmatic epidemiology of nasopharyngeal carcinoma. Cancer Epidemiol Biomarkers Prev 15: 1765–1777.
3. Chiesa F, De Paoli F (2001) Distant metastases from nasopharyngeal cancer. ORL J Otorhinolaryngol Relat Spec 63: 214–216.
4. Bensouda Y, Kaikani W, Ahbeddou N, Rahhali R, Jabri M, et al. (2011) Treatment for metastatic nasopharyngeal carcinoma. Eur Ann Otorhinolaryngol Head Neck Dis 128: 79–85.
5. Liu MT, Hsieh CY, Chang TH, Lin JP, Huang CC, et al. (2003) Prognostic factors affecting the outcome of nasopharyngeal carcinoma. Jpn J Clin Oncol 33: 501–508.

6. Twu CW, Wang WY, Liang WM, Jan JS, Jiang RS, et al. (2007) Comparison of the prognostic impact of serum anti-EBV antibody and plasma EBV DNA assays in nasopharyngeal carcinoma. Int J Radiat Oncol Biol Phys 67: 130–137.

7. An X, Wang FH, Ding PR, Deng L, Jiang WQ, et al. (2011) Plasma Epstein-Barr virus DNA level strongly predicts survival in metastatic/recurrent nasopharyngeal carcinoma treated with palliative chemotherapy. Cancer 117: 3750–3757.

8. McMillan DC (2009) Systemic inflammation, nutritional status and survival in patients with cancer. Curr Opin Clin Nutr Metab Care 12: 223–226.

9. Grivennikov SI, Greten FR, Karin M (2010) Immunity, inflammation, and cancer. Cell 140: 883–899.

10. Chiang AC, Massague J (2008) Molecular basis of metastasis. N Engl J Med 359: 2814–2823.

11. Kinoshita A, Onoda H, Imai N, Iwaku A, Oishi M, et al. (2013) The Glasgow Prognostic Score, an inflammation based prognostic score, predicts survival in patients with hepatocellular carcinoma. BMC Cancer 13: 52.

12. Wang DS, Luo HY, Qiu MZ, Wang ZQ (2012) Comparison of the prognostic values of various inflammation based factors in patients with pancreatic cancer. Med Oncol 29: 3092–3100.

13. Gioulbasanis I, Pallis A, Vlachostergios PJ, Xyrafas A, Giannousi Z, et al. (2012) The Glasgow Prognostic Score (GPS) predicts toxicity and efficacy in platinum-based treated patients with metastatic lung cancer. Lung Cancer 77: 383–388.

14. Wang DS, Ren C, Qiu MZ, Luo HY, Wang ZQ, et al. (2012) Comparison of the prognostic value of various preoperative inflammation-based factors in patients with stage III gastric cancer. Tumour Biol 33: 749–756.

15. McMillan DC (2013) The systemic inflammation-based Glasgow Prognostic Score: a decade of experience in patients with cancer. Cancer Treat Rev 39: 534–540.

16. An X, Ding PR, Wang FH, Jiang WQ, Li YH (2011) Elevated neutrophil to lymphocyte ratio predicts poor prognosis in nasopharyngeal carcinoma. Tumour Biol 32: 317–324.

17. Maeda K, Shibutani M, Otani H, Nagahara H, Sugano K, et al. (2013) Prognostic value of preoperative inflammation-based prognostic scores in patients with stage IV colorectal cancer who undergo palliative resection of asymptomatic primary tumors. Anticancer Res 33: 5567–5573.

18. Ishizuka M, Nagata H, Takagi K, Iwasaki Y, Kubota K (2013) Inflammation-based prognostic system predicts survival after surgery for stage IV colorectal cancer. Am J Surg 205: 22–28.

19. Vashist YK, Loos J, Dedow J, Tachezy M, Uzunoglu G, et al. (2011) Glasgow Prognostic Score is a predictor of perioperative and long-term outcome in patients with only surgically treated esophageal cancer. Ann Surg Oncol 18: 1130–1138.

20. Laviano A, Meguid MM, Inui A, Muscaritoli M, Rossi-Fanelli F (2005) Therapy insight: Cancer anorexia-cachexia syndrome–when all you can eat is yourself. Nat Clin Pract Oncol 2: 158–165.

21. Donohoe CL, Ryan AM, Reynolds JV (2011) Cancer cachexia: mechanisms and clinical implications. Gastroenterol Res Pract 2011: 601434.

22. Fearon KC, Voss AC, Hustead DS (2006) Definition of cancer cachexia: effect of weight loss, reduced food intake, and systemic inflammation on functional status and prognosis. Am J Clin Nutr 83: 1345–1350.

23. Senba M, Zhong XY, Senba MI, Itakura H (1994) EBV and nasopharyngeal carcinoma. Lancet 343: 1104.

24. Eliopoulos AG, Stack M, Dawson CW, Kaye KM, Hodgkin L, et al. (1997) Epstein-Barr virus-encoded LMP1 and CD40 mediate IL-6 production in epithelial cells via an NF-kappaB pathway involving TNF receptor-associated factors. Oncogene 14: 2899–2916.

25. Pepys MB, Hirschfield GM (2003) C-reactive protein: a critical update. J Clin Invest 111: 1805–1812.

26. Liaw CC, Wang CH, Huang JS, Kiu MC, Chen JS, et al. (1997) Serum lactate dehydrogenase level in patients with nasopharyngeal carcinoma. Acta Oncol 36: 159–164.

27. Fuchs CS, Ogino S (2013) Aspirin therapy for colorectal cancer with PIK3CA mutation: simply complex!. J Clin Oncol 31: 4358–4361.

28. Gridelli C, Gallo C, Ceribelli A, Gebbia V, Gamucci T, et al. (2007) Factorial phase III randomised trial of rofecoxib and prolonged constant infusion of gemcitabine in advanced non-small-cell lung cancer: the GEmcitabine-COxib in NSCLC (GECO) study. Lancet Oncol 8: 500–512.

29. Szumilo J, Burdan F, Szumilo M, Lewkowicz D, Kedzierawska-Kurylcio A (2009) Cyclooxygenase inhibitors in chemoprevention and treatment of esophageal squamous cell carcinoma. Pol Merkur Lekarski 27: 408–412.

30. Kwon HC, Kim SH, Oh SY, Lee S, Lee JH, et al. (2012) Clinical significance of preoperative neutrophil-lymphocyte versus platelet-lymphocyte ratio in patients with operable colorectal cancer. Biomarkers 17: 216–222.

31. Feng JF, Huang Y, Chen QX (2014) Preoperative platelet lymphocyte ratio (PLR) is superior to neutrophil lymphocyte ratio (NLR) as a predictive factor in patients with esophageal squamous cell carcinoma. World J Surg Oncol 12: 58.

32. He JR, Shen GP, Ren ZF, Qin H, Cui C, et al. (2012) Pretreatment levels of peripheral neutrophils and lymphocytes as independent prognostic factors in patients with nasopharyngeal carcinoma. Head Neck 34: 1769–1776.

24

Chemobrain Experienced by Breast Cancer Survivors: A Meta-Ethnography Study Investigating Research and Care Implications

Maryam Hafsah Selamat[1], Siew Yim Loh[2,3]*, Lynette Mackenzie[3], Janette Vardy[4,5]

1 Department of Postgraduate Studies, University of Malaya, Kuala Lumpur, Malaysia, 2 Department of Rehabilitation Medicine, Faculty of Medicine, University of Malaya, Kuala Lumpur, Malaysia, 3 Discipline of Occupational Therapy, Faculty of Health Sciences, University of Sydney, Sydney, Australia, 4 Concord Cancer Centre, Concord Repatriation and General Hospital, Concord, Sydney, Australia, 5 Sydney Medical School, The University of Sydney, Sydney, Australia

Abstract

Background: Cognitive impairment, colloquially termed "chemobrain", occurs in 10–40% of all cancer patients, and is an emerging target of cancer survivorship research.

Aim: This study reviews published qualitative studies to explore cognitive impairments or chemobrain among breast cancer survivors, with particular attention given to the impact on quality of life.

Method: Using keywords, we searched ten electronic databases (CINAHL, EMBASE, Proquest, OVID SP, MEDLINE, Oxford Journal, Science Direct, PubMED).

Findings: Of 457 papers, seven relevant papers were included. Data was extracted and concepts were analysed using a meta ethnography approach. Four second order intepretations were identified, on the basis of which, four third order intrepretations were constructed. Linked together in a line of argument, was a consistent account on their struggles to self-manage the chemobrain impairments that impact their daily lives. Five concepts emerged from the analysis of the primary findings: i) real experiences of cognitive changes, ii) calls for help, iii) impact of cognitive impairments, iv) coping and v) survivorship and meaning. Further synthesis resulted in four new order intepretations: i) The chemobrain struggle, ii) The substantial impact of chemobrain on life domains, iii) The struggle to readjust and to self manage, and iv) 'thankful yet fearful' representation.

Discussion: Awareness of cognitive changes were context-dependent on healthcare settings and cultural contexts as strong determinants. Subjects verified the existence of chemobrain but healthcare providers mis-recognised, under-recognised, and sometimes negated it perhaps due to its unknown aetiology. Asian breast cancer survivors appear less vocal than their western counterparts.

Conclusion: The current literature on the lived experiences of how women experienced chemobrain provides a consistent report that chemobrain is real, persistent and with detrimental impacts on quality of life - manifested as a constant struggles. A greater awareness of the effects of chemobrain with improved functional assessment and interventions is warranted.

Editor: Gayle E. Woloschak, Northwestern University Feinberg School of Medicine, United States of America

Funding: This study is funded by the University Malaya Research Grant (UMRG 477/12htm). The funders had no role in study design, data collection and analysis, decision to publish, or preparation of the manuscript.

Competing Interests: The authors have declared that no competing interests exist.

* Email: syloh@um.edu.my

Introduction

Cancer survivorship is an emerging field of study and development. Today, there is a steep rise in numbers of cancer survivors internationally, due to earlier detection, better chemo-therapeutic regimens and multidisciplinary collaborative care approaches [1,2]. In the United State alone, the 5-year relative survival rate for female breast cancer has improved significantly from 63% in the early 1960s to 90% in 2011 [3]. With the rise in survivors, attention is turning to studying the longer-term adverse effects of treatment and the impact they can have on daily activities of living, participation and functioning by occupational therapists. The phenomena of cognitive impairment after cancer, is gaining increasing attention as one of the key foci of cancer survivorship research by health professionals.

Cognitive impairment is being acknowledged as an after-effect of cancer treatment, and is also commonly known as 'chemofog' or 'chemobrain' [4–9]. Matsuda et al. [7] reported that chemotherapy-induced cognitive deficits occurred in 10–40% of all cancer patients, with up to 23% in women with breast cancer [6]. Overall, the estimated prevalance of chemobrain varies in the literature from 15% to 70% [10]. The aetiology of chemobrain remains unknown. However, there are indications that it may be due to toxicity from chemotherapy agents, especially high dose treatments [11]. Hypotheses of the mechanisms involved include vascular injuries and oxidative damage, inflammation, direct injuries to neurons, autoimmune responses, chemotherapy-induced anaemia and the presence of the apolipoprotein Eε4 (APOE ε4) allele [12]. Studies also suggest cognitive changes may be due to a combination of psychological and medical factors associated with adjuvant systemic therapy (e.g. low oestrogen and progesterone from chemotherapy) as well as anticancer hormonal treatments (e.g. tamoxifen or aromatase inhibitors) [10,13,14]. Cognitive impairments have also been shown to occur prior to chemotherapy, making it difficult to determine what is actually due to the chemotherapy [6,14,15]. Cognitive performance can also be influenced by common problems faced by cancer survivors that may include pain, insomnia, depression and fatigue [16].

Many survivors of breast cancer complain of increased difficulties with multi-tasking and slower mental processing time, which become more noticeable once they try to resume their normal activities. This is especially evident when they return to work and particularly for those in intellectually demanding occupations [17]. In a study by Wagner et al. [18] 63% of cancer survivors reported problems with concentration and attention, 50% problems with memory, and 38% problems with abstract reasoning. The review by Matsuda et al. [7] identified cognitive impairments related to memory loss and inattention [15]; and problems with concentration, visuo-spatial skills, and motor function [6]. This had detrimental consequences on work performance (75%) that required patients to utilize compensatory strategies (58%), with accompanying patient frustration (50%) as well as adverse impacts on family relationships (33%) [18]. Overall these studies highlighted that cancer survivors commonly reported greater difficulties in work related activity with either a decrease in functional ability or maintenance of functional ability levels that required increased mental effort [19].

However, none of these studies captured the lived experiences or the levels of severity of chemobrain symptoms experienced by cancer survivors. It is therefore important for several reasons to undertake an in-depth exploration of this issue, to understand the cognitive changes experienced by breast cancer survivors. Firstly: i) due to high survival rates, breast cancer patients are likely to live with these problems for a considerable time – making it highly pertinent to explore the impact of these cognitive impairments on their quality of life. Secondly, there is no published meta-review of qualitative studies addressing the chemobrain experience. A qualitative review is a relevant approach to evaluate the meaning that breast cancer survivors ascribe to cognitive changes, and it represents an area of concern that would not be feasible to be examined using quantitative approaches. Qualitative approach variables are flexible and better able to explore specific relationships while taking into account the complexity of individual contexts [20–22]. Therefore, the aim of this study was to review qualitative studies that explored the lived experience of chemobrain among breast cancer survivors, with particular attention given to the impact of chemobrain on daily living and quality of life.

Methods

This study is the first part of a larger study involving focus group on survivors. The ethic to conduct the study was approved by University Malaya Ethical Committee Boards. Using a meta-ethnography method, the interpretation of results from a range of original studies were compared and translated to acquire a greater understanding of the cognitive changes experienced by breast cancer survivors [22–25]. We used the 7–step process of meta-ethnography by Noblit and Hare [25] -: 1. Developing a specific research question; 2. Deciding what is relevant to the research question; 3. Reviewing each study to identify key concepts and recording them; 4. Determining how the studies are related, and comparing study approaches to the key concepts; 5. Translating the studies into one another; 6. Synthesising the translation outcomes, and 7. Expressing the synthesis.

Step 5 above involved the researchers interpreting and translating the key concepts via:- i) reciprocal translation (i.e. studies with similar findings were directly compared and synthesised), ii) refutational translation (i.e. studies rebutting each other with conflicts of findings), and iii) Lines of Argument (i.e. translation of the studies to build a final interpretation using both differences and similarities among studies) [23].

Based on these steps, the researchers (MHS &SYL) independently appraised the selected papers and undertook the steps to extract the information and synthesize the findings. Further discussions took place between the reviewers when any discrepancies arose. Next, second order intepretations were identified, on the basis of which, third order intrepretations (based on key concepts and second-order interpretations) were constructed. These were all linked together in a line of argument [(i.e. the final interpretation using both differences and similarities among studies) to present the intrepetation of cognitive impairments experienced by women. The synthesis can be expressed as text as well as in summary tables, diagrams or models, which can produce significant new insights into the topic [23]. Finally a table synthesis of concepts and order interpretation was built to connect each of the papers.

Search strategy

We undertook a systematic search of the literature for all published English language articles from 2002–2013 that used qualitative methods to investigate post-chemotherapy cognitive impairments for women with breast cancer. The following databases were searched: CINAHL, Web of Knowledge, EMBASE, Proquest, OVID SP, MEDLINE, Oxford Journal, Science Direct, PubMED, and Wiley.

Researchers performed free text searches by using keywords of chemobrain OR (chemotherapy AND mild cognitive impairment) OR post-chemotherapy cognitive changes. Next, we add in, the term " breast cancer survivors" AND qualitative. The search filters were used at this stage to address the inclusion criteria for the study.

The inclusion criteria were: 1) breast cancer and chemobrain. The terms used were chemofog, cognitive dysfunction, cognitive changes. Chemobrain was referred to as any domain of cognition decline or dysfunction experienced by survivors who had chemotherapy; 2) qualitative study. Terms used included lived experience and qualitative experience; 3) studies published from 2002 to 2014. All papers published within the last 10 years; 4) English language text and; 5) full text publication. The exclusion criteria included: 1) study design other than a qualitative design methodology; 2) studies with patients with cancers other than breast cancer; and 3) non English papers.

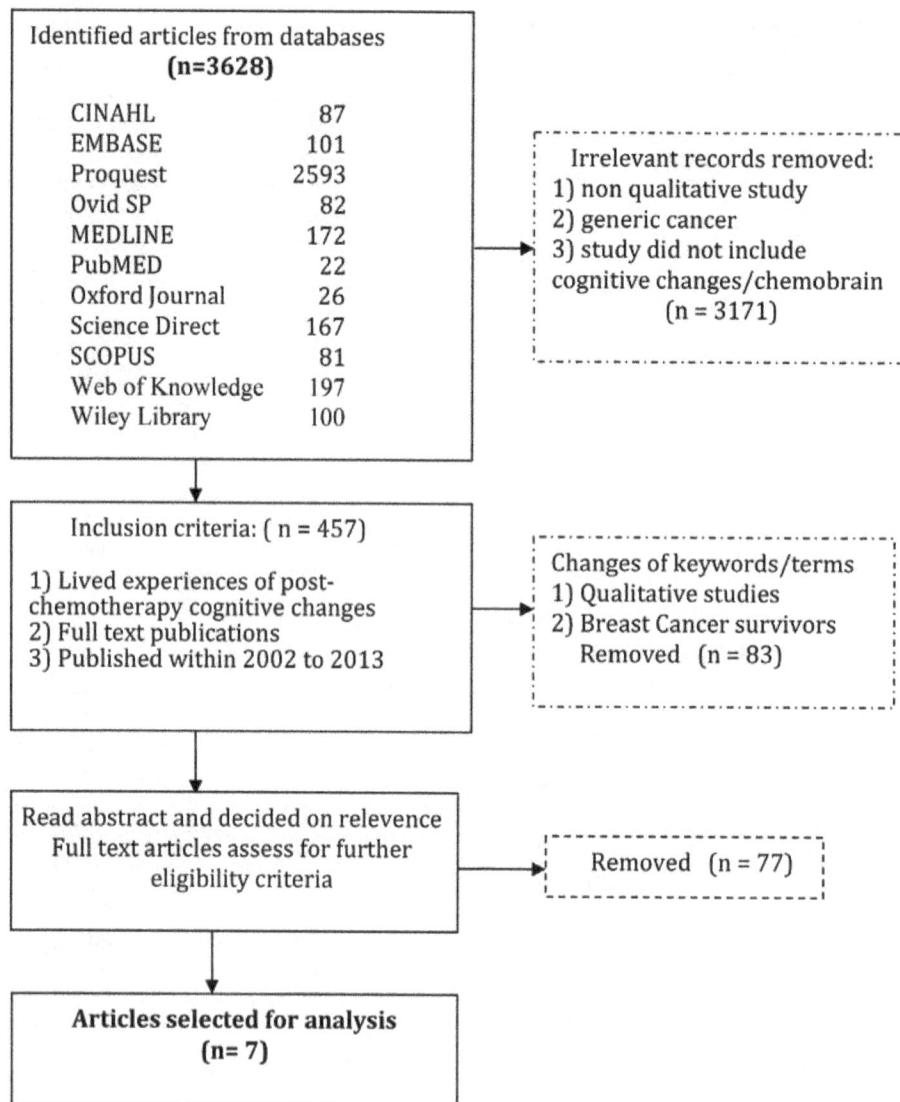

Figure 1. This is the Figure 1 Search strategy.

The second step of the Noblit and Hare process [23] involved deciding what studies were relevant to our research question and aims. In particular, the research team were interested to understand women's lived experience of chemobrain. The process of the search strategy is detailed in Figure 1.

Quality Appraisal

Quality appraisal instruments are available to apply to qualitative research reviews in a consistent manner, to ensure credibility or trustworthiness of the findings [26]. We adopted the 'Critical Appraisal Skills Program', or CASP [27] format to appraise each article in order to apply a valid, reliable and objective method prior to synthesis. The CASP checklist is a 10-item tool to appraise qualitative papers without using a numerical score. This is to remind researchers of the importance of every criterion in a qualitative paper in order to reduce bias. Bias in qualitative research is usually related to the influence of researchers and a lack of transparency in data collection and analysis, whereas in positivist quantitative studies, bias is related to representativeness and generalizability. Therefore, qualitative

studies are usually evaluated using agreed criteria about data collection and analysis processes that need to be fulfilled in order to contribute to a review of findings. The first two questions act as the core criteria in selecting the qualitative reports [28]. Nevertheless, the process itself is useful as it may contribute to the richness and the focus of discussion [23]. Appraisal of the selected studies contributed to the synthesis of the findings of the review, as any critique of the studies could be identified [29] and incorporated into the review. Table 1 outlines the CASP criteria used to evaluate quality. The first two questions are screening questions. If the answer to both is "yes", it is worth proceeding with the remaining questions.

Interpretation with an analytic lens

This study used a seven-step process of meta-ethnography as outlined by Noblit and Hare [25]. Two of the authors (MHS & SYL) independently reviewed the identified studies from the search and appraised the selected papers and undertook the seven steps [22] to extract information and synthesize the findings. Next, discussions took place between the reviewers and other authors

Table 1. Critical Appraisal Skill Program (CASP Quality appraisal criteria).

1. Was there a clear statement of the aims of the research?
2. Is a qualitative methodology appropriate?
3. Was the research design appropriate to address the aims of the research?
4. Was the recruitment strategy appropriate to the aims of the research?
5. Were the data collected in a way that addressed the research issue?
6. Has the relationship between researcher and survivors been adequately considered?
7. Have ethical issues been taken into consideration?
8. Was the data analysis sufficiently rigorous?
9. Is there a clear statement of findings?
10. How valuable is the research?

The first two questions are screening questions. If the answer to both is "yes", it is worth proceeding with the remaining questions. Record a "yes", "no" or "cannot tell" to most of the questions.

where discrepancies arose from collecting and categorising data of each selected study to form the primary dataset. Table 2 outlines the idea of the first process, or gathering of all concepts across the studies, based on subjects' experiences, as reported by each of the study authors and suggested by Schultz [30]. During this early stage, interpretation was avoided to maintain the original outcomes of each article.

During steps three to five (Noblit and Hare 1988) the research team identified key concepts through reciprocal translation (similar findings) and refutational translation (conflicting findings) and the interpretation of findings were taken together. These processes of explicitly relating the papers occurs on three levels [30]. We systematically followed Schultz's process to interpret and explain the results via analysis of key metaphors, and were careful not to reduce the qualitative accents but to retain the sense of the account of the women as reported in the papers. Schultz's concepts of first-order refer to the daily perceptions of the common people; the second-order construct refers to the constructs of findings from the scientific view in the papers, and the third order constructs are final synthesis derived from the key concepts and second order contructs based on the interpetations of the review authors [24].

Theoretical framework for the review: The Illness Representation Theory

To guide the synthesis for this review, the Model of Illness Representation by Laventhal et al. [31] was adopted. This allowed researchers to capture individual perceptions of illness related to cognitive impairments experienced. This model consists of seven components of illness representation: 1) *Identity*, or the name or label of a threat; 2) *Timeline*, or the belief about the time trajectory for the illness; 3) *Consequences*, or the perceived consequence of a threat from the illness; 4) *Cause*, or the perceived causal mechanism of any threats; 5) *Control/Cure*, or whether something can be done to control the threat; 6) *Illness Coherence*, or whether a person thinks about the threat in a coherent way, and 7) *Emotional representation*, or the emotions associated with the illness experience. This framework is particularly relevant to the review topic and enabled the researchers to interpret and capture the reasoning and self management issues for women experiencing chemobrain.

Researcher positionality

Inevitably the interpretations of the study data from the review will be influenced in some way by the interests and experiences of the researchers, as researchers were the instruments of both the data collection and the data analysis for the review. Therefore, it was important that the researchers reflected on their own biases in order to overcome them in the data analysis process. MH

contributed the theoretical perspectives for the review, SYL is experienced in self management of women following breast cancer, JV contributed medical and clinical encounters with women being treated for breast cancer and LM brought the perspective of an expert-patient with personal experience of breast cancer.

Results

Qualitative studies identified for review

A total of 3628 papers were identified electronically following the search using the keywords "chemobrain" and "chemotherapy" and "mild cognitive impairment". These papers were further scanned for their relevance and this process reduced the number to 457 articles. Next, the criteria for inclusion were applied to the abstracts and this resulted in 83 articles. Further examination of the full versions of these papers, according to the boundaries set by the focused research aim for this study resulted in seven papers that met the inclusion criteria for the review. Some of the qualitative papers did not include the study design in the titles of the publications, so it was necessary for the researchers to read and screen the methodology sections to ensure that a qualitative design was used. The full text for each of these seven papers was obtained and each study was appraised. Figure 1 outlines the search results for the review.

Results of the quality appraisal process

Based on the CASP checklist (Table 1) as outlined in the methodology section, five of the seven papers were considered to have met all the quality criteria as judged by the reviewers. Table 2 below showed the result of the critical appraisal skill program (CASP)'s quality appraisal for the seven selected papers. The researchers record a "yes", "no" or "cannot tell" to each questions and then discuss to reach a consensus. Two studies did not meet one quality criterion, which concerned the adequacy of consideration of the relationship between researchers and survivors. These two studies were still included in the review since the unmet criterion was judged to be a minor issue and did not adversely affect the relevance of the studies to the objectives of this review.

Results of the qualitative review of data extracted

Table 3 outlines the summary of each of the selected papers for review and identifies the themes from each individual study. Based on the synthesis-of-order [25,26,29,30] process, this table summarises the first order constructs that reflect the understandings of the participants from each study and are usually summarised in the results section of each article. Four themes emerged from the

Table 2. Critical Appraisal Skill Program (CASP)'s Quality appraisal for selected papers.

CASP Criteria from Table 1	[1]	[2]	[3]	[4]	[5]	[6]	[7]	[8]	[9]	[10]
Mulrooney Tamsin 2007 [32]	Y	Y	Y	Y	Y	Y	Y	Y	Y	Y
Von Ah et al. 2013 [33]	Y	Y	Y	Y	Y	N	N	Y	Y	Y
Cheung et al. 2012 [34]	Y	Y	Y	Y	Y	Y	Y	Y	Y	Y
Munir et al. [35]	Y	Y	Y	Y	Y	Y	Y	Y	Y	Y
Myers 2012 [36]	Y	Y	Y	Y	Y	Y	Y	Y	Y	Y
Boykoff et al. 2009 [37]	Y	Y	N	Y	Y	N	N	Y	Y	Y
Thielen 2008 [38]	Y	Y	Y	Y	Y	N	N	Y	Y	Y

Index N = No, Y = Yes, C = Cannot tell.

analysis of the seven selected papers-: i) The chemobrain struggles, ii) The substantial impact from chemobrain, iii) The struggle to adjust and self manage and iv) The 'thankful yet fearful' attitudinal representation. Four second order intepretations were identified, on the basis of which four third order intrepretations (based on key concepts and second-order interpretations) were constructed. These were all linked together in a line of argument that accounts for survivors struggles to self-manage the chemobrain impairment that impacted their activities of daily living.

Table 4 outlines the meta-ethnography process that utilises the Schultz [30] notions of first, second, and third order constructs as the follow-up analysis.

i) The chemobrain struggle. Chemobrain or chemotherapy-associated cognitive impairment was reported consistently as a real experience. The signs and symptoms were noticed by women with breast cancer, who described them in various ways. The term *chemobrain* offers a quick reference to a concept that may easily encapsulate a range of experiences and enable women to attribute their experiences to a concrete term. However, chemobrain was experienced as a *struggle* as the manifestation of the signs and symptoms triggered the survivors to continually question its existence, and to question if their experience was 'real or not'. There was a need to seek confirmation via various means, yet the situation remained unresolved as there was no clear answer to their question, leading to a persistent struggle within themselves and with significant others.

Most women felt that chemobrain was an outcome of cancer and its treatment, and perceived themselves to be "chemobrain victims" [32]. Studies used indirect probes to gain descriptions of the experience of chemobrain. and these validated the cognitive changes by providing descriptions such as not being 'as-sharp or quick' as before, or feeling 'foggy' or 'spacey' after treatment [33]. In a study involving Asian women, participants were only able to identify the term chemobrain or describe the symptoms when they were being indirectly probed about their experiences [34]. Survivors noticed cognitive changes during and after chemotherapy treatment [35]. Most of the breast cancer survivors reported changes in the cognitive domains of short and long term memory, processing speed, attention, concentration, language, verbal memory and executive functioning [32,33,35,36].

Although other confounding factors (e.g. cancer related fatigue, mood changes, lack of mental and physical activity, the cancer condition, ageing, hormonal therapy, lack of social support and menopausal status [33,34], have been found to induce or worsen sustained cognitive issues, many survivors disagreed with this. They justified that they had problems with attention and concentration, although they agreed that they may be more easily distracted when they were tired [33,34]. Multi-tasking in particular seemed to cause concern and often resulted in feelings of anxiety and frustration [32,35]. Survivors often described chemobrain as "frustrating", "upsetting" and some were frightened by problems in processing new information. This phenomenon was perceived to affect their emotions as they struggled to understand the changes occurring.

Timing of onset of Chemobrain

The onset of chemobrain has been reported at different times across the illness trajectory. Survivors had difficulty giving an exact time of onset of the chemobrain symptoms; however they seemed to lessen over time but not fully resolve [32,36]. Some survivors reported they experienced changes in cognitive functioning after diagnosis, during chemotherapy or after one to two months of treatment [33,34,36], with most reporting that they continued to experience it after the completion of chemotherapy [33,34]. A

Table 3. Characteristics of the selected studies.

	Aim	Sample & method	Findings	Conclusion	Limitation
Von Ah et al. (2013) USA. [31]	To obtain a better understanding of breast cancer survivors' experiences of perceived cognitive impairment, its trajectory, and its impact on relationship, daily functioning, work and overall life satisfaction after breast cancer diagnosis and treatment.	**n = 22** breast cancer survivors who reported cognitive impairment at least 1 year postchemotherapy treatment. **Interview** and content analysis approach.	Expressed concern in 6 major domains of cognition: short term memory, long term memory, speed of processing, attention and concentration, language and executive functioning. Chemobrain is frustrating, affects self-confidence and social relationships. Difficulties in work and adapt using compensatory strategies. Validation of perceived cognitive impairment is important for adjustment.	Perceived cognitive deficits have broad implications for wellbeing. Study provides direction for theory development, measurement selection and additional targets. Greater understanding leads to development of effective treatment of these symptoms.	Limited by sample characteristics (geographic area and homogenous). Self report might be influenced by previous participation in cognitive behavioral trial.
Myers, (2012) USA. [34]	To provide an in depth description of the experience of chemotherapy-related cognitive impairment for women with breast cancer and identify related information that women would find useful prior to chemotherapy and cognitive changes	**n = 18** breast cancer survivors who reported cognitive changes within 6–12months postchemotherapy. **Focus group discussion**, semi structured interview and content analysis approach.	Survivors describe difficulty of cognitive changes and the impact in daily living. Survivors shares their coping skills strategies. Survivors want to get information prior to intiating chemotherapy and psychosocial education.	It provides a framework for better understanding regarding the changes that can be used as a guide for patient and family education and generates questions for additional research.	Coding was performed by single investigator and as such may be biased. Interpretation by only one individual poses bias.
Cheung et al. (2012) Singapore. [32]	To gather descriptions from multiethnic breast cancer survivors on their experiences and impact of chemotherapy- associated cognitive changes on daily lives and the coping strategies.	**n = 43** breast cancer patient receiving chemotherapy- **Focus group discussion** and thematic analysis.	Survivors were unfamiliar with the term 'chemobrain' and viewed it as a result of physical and psychosocial adverse effects. Encoutered memory loss, difficulty in decision making, speech problems. Married women claimed frustrations that limited their role as homemaker. Self-identification of coping strategies.	This phenomenon is unfamiliar to most Asians yet it impacted their daily lives. Results suggested that a culturally relevant approach should be adopted to evaluate and manage cognitive changes in these patients.	Selection bias due to nonrandomized sample recruitment and response rate was low. No baseline assessment was conducted. Heterogenous group. Priming effects and preexisting knowledge of chemobrain.
Munir et al. (2009) UK. [33]	To investigate women's awareness of chemotherapy-induced cognitive changes, their perception of cognitive limitations in carrying out daily tasks and subsequent return to work decision and perception of work ability.	**n = 13 breast cancer** survivors who completed chemotherapy between 12 months to 10 years ago who have returned to work. **Semi structured interview** with two focus groups. Using template analysis.	Survivors noticed decline lasting about a year or longer in concentration, confusion and lack of clear thinking. Chemobrain negatively affects self confidence in cognitive ability and return to work, but support from collegues and employers increased confident in cognitive skills. Impact related to work ability: poor memory, concentration, difficulties in thinking quickly, organising information and decision making. Insufficient information regarding cognitive side effects from oncology team or support groups.	Chemotherapy-induced cognitive impairment affected returning to work and subsequent work ability. Return to work and ability to manage work were influenced by three interrelated factors: 1) actual cognitive ability following chemotherapy, (2) awareness of cognitive failures by the women and their families, & 3) subsequent impact on their confidence in carrying out daily tasks including work tasks.	This study does not explore issues in sufficient depth.
Boykoff et al. (2009) USA. [35]	To document in-depth the effects that cognitive impairment has on women's personal and professional lives.	**n = 74 white and African American breast cancer** survivors who experienced side effects at least 1 year beyond completion. Focus group/in-depth interviews and content analysis approach	Cognitive impairment can be problematic for survivors. Survivors reported it diminished quality of life and daily functioning. Survivors suggested a range of coping strategies to manage social and profesional lives.	Chemobrain impacts survivors' economically, emotionally and interpersonally. More research needed on psychosocials aspect of post treatment symptoms to inform the efforts of medical and mental health communities.	This study was non randomised and participants self nominated for the study.

Table 3. Cont.

	Aim	Sample & method	Findings	Conclusion	Limitation
Thielen (2008) USA. [36]	To explore the lived experiences of the neurological changes women describe while undergoing chemotherapy for breast cancer	n = **13 breast cancer** patients undergoing or completed adjuvant chemotherapy within 12 months. **Interviews.** A Descriptive phenomenological method guided analysis	Validated the existence of chemobrain phenomenon Women described it affects daily living. These findings may be useful for designing questionaires, educational products and interventional strategies.	A decrease in cognitive function is multifactorial in origin. The womens' feelings, meaning and perceptions contribute to the fundamental of the lived phenomenon.	Small sample size: Participants were not of mixed ethnicity: sample were from caucasian women. Inexperienced researcher.
Mulrooney Tamsin (2007) USA. [30]	To describe lived experiences of self reported cognitive impairment in a sample of women who were treated with chemotherapy for breast cancer.	n = 10 women with breast cancer – treated with chemotherapy within last 15–52 months. **Interviews.** A descriptive and interpretative Gadamerian phenomenological theory	Survivors described problems with memory, learning, concentration, language and multitasking. Incidents of chemobrain could occur at anytime and affected the ability to perform usual activities at home and work. Relationship changed among friends and family Chemobrain caused by necessary treatment of breast cancer. Survival was paramount.	The experiences of chemobrain can impact all aspects of life including work. Despite the belief of chemotherapy as a cause, other factors should be acknowledged.	Small numbers, homogenous participants with similar demographic background, educational levels.

1st order construct - Constructs that reflect participants' understandings, as reported in the included studies and usually found in the results section of an article.

rationale offered was that during chemotherapy, many other acute physical symptoms (such as nausea, vomiting, fatigue) could not be ignored, and so survivors did not focus on the subtler cognitive symptoms. Women tend to be overwhelmed by having to suddenly adjust to the reality of a cancer diagnosis, starting chemotherapy and having a potentially life-threatening illness, so that they initially disregarded changes in memory or attention [33,37]. The present information suggests that cognitive changes can remain a long-term problem for breast cancer survivors.

Dealing with the symptoms or side effects of cancer treatment is a challenge that requires support from others. Family and friends were regarded as good social support systems who encouraged survivors to engage in activities and return to their role in the community. Healthcare providers were also seen as a potential source of support since they work closely with survivors. It has been reported that many healthcare providers are more nonchalant about the phenomena of chemobrain. Survivors reported that their healthcare providers did not discuss any issues relating to chemobrain [33,36,37] and some were insensitive when survivors made complaints about their experiences of cognitive deficits. It seemed that the survivors were dissatisfied as they wanted professional validation of their experience of chemobrain symptoms but they were largely ignored.

Healthcare providers often assumed that reported cognitive changes were due to other variables such as, stress or the natural ageing process, and were quick to label chemobrain as a misnomer

Table 4. Synthesis of concepts, with second and third order interpretations.

Concepts	Second order interpretations	Third order interpretations
Experiences of cognitive changes: Trajectory of cognitive changes, types of cognitive changes, cognitive domains affected, experiences of cognitive changes, awareness of cognitive changes. **Call for help and support:** Healthcare providers to inform of possible cognitive changes, respond to medical community, how to teach me, Looking for answers in all the wrong places, underwhelming information for an overwhelming experience	(a) Patients want validation that it is real and to be prepared for cognitive changes; want health staff to be proactive in addressing the issue; a strategy viewed as able to reduce tension and frustration of family members also	(b) The chemobrain struggle
Impact of chemobrain: Self and social relationship – how I changed, daily functioning, working life, psychosocial, financial, overall life satisfaction, change in all aspects of functioning	(c) Significant impact of chemobrain phenomena on self, family, social circle, daily living and work performances.	(d) The substantial impact of chemobrain across life domains
Coping: Trying my best to fit in, coping strategies, adjusting to fit in, prior needs of information on cognitive side effects	(e) Ways of coping derived by survivors with multiple strategies to help themselves to overcome the phenomena.	(f) Struggling to self manage (without support from health professionals)
Reflect on survivorship: Thankfulness - I am still alive, Apprehension - what the future holds.	(g) Reflection on survivorship to attain normality and regain function	(h) Thankful for life, yet fearful of the future

2nd order construct interpretations of participants' understandings made by authors of these studies (and usually found in the discussion and conclusion section of an article). 3rd order construct the synthesis of both first and second order constructs into a new model or theory about a phenomenon.

[37,38]. Conversely, some women reported that they did receive general information about the possibility of cognitive side-effects from chemotherapy from the oncologists or oncology nurses [38], although conversations were usually initiated by the survivors as they sought explanations [32]. Women felt that early warnings and validation of these changes from healthcare providers with patient-information could help them cope proactively with these changes [33,36,38]. Support groups may help survivors to identify or recognise cognitive changes and to be better prepared [36].

ii) A substantial impact of chemobrain across life domains. Women described the impact of chemobrain on themselves, their social relationships, working life and daily living [33]. Survivors reported that family and friends ranged from being supportive to being unconcerned about their chemobrain experiences. Some women reported that the cognitive changes had affected their psychological well-being and they lost selfconfidence and self-esteem in the company of family members and friends. Survivors were often confused by their cognitive changes and then felt misunderstood or embarrassed. Survivors who were home-makers described memory difficulties adversely affecting their roles in the family, and that some family members had a lack of awareness about these changes. Some suggested their difficulties maintaining their homemaker roles were related to their own expectations about what they should be able to achieve [33,34,37,38]. Some families provided considerable support as they understood the issues and were aware of the cognitive changes and this was related to positive cultural values. For instance, Cheung et al. [34] reported that the Asian value for living in communities and having a kindred spirit meant that members of the community became a source of support.

Cognitive changes often impacted on working life and school related activities. Survivors indicated that cognitive impairment affected their confidence in returning to work because returning to work would highlight their problems further and be too challenging [35]. Survivors who had returned to work reported that they were struggling to perform and complete tasks. Their job performance had decreased due to an inability to maintain attention or focus at work, to maintain their thoughts during conversations and inability to comprehend a text without reading it more than once. As a result, work tasks required more time and they were less productive. For some, this difficulty contributed to loss of employment and difficulties finding work [33,36,37]. Professional women in jobs that required a high level of cognitive functioning were more negatively affected by chemobrain [32]. They reported that they needed more effort to perform tasks than previously, and that as their jobs required several skill sets that incorporated multiple cognitive domains, this created additional challenges. Survivors found they required more attention to complete work tasks to a sufficient standard [32,33,38]. Munir et al. [35] found that survivors sometimes hid cognitive difficulties from their employer. However the findings suggest that good support from employers and colleagues, helped survivors to regain confidence in returning to work.

iii) Struggling to adjust and to self manage. While struggling to overcome cognitive changes, often without real support or acknowledgement from health professionals, most survivors developed their own strategies to overcome the effects of chemobrain, to prevent further complications and to help them cope with daily living and work functioning These are listed in Table 5. Two studies out of the seven reviewed [33,35] did not discuss any coping strategies.

The majority of the survivors used non pharmacological strategies such as mental activities, psychosocial management and practical reminders, while some survivors trained themselves

in memory strategies to remember things more easily. In the Asian study by Cheung et al. [34] the use of complementary or alternative medicine was more popular than pharmacological intervention as participants perceived these remedies would enhance energy and improve blood circulation to the brain. Coping strategies for some survivors meant avoiding situations that required them to remember names and engage in social conversation. Many survivors decided not to focus on their disabilities and adapted their enviroment to cope with chemobrain by telling people about their cognitive changes [37]. Other survivors relied on their family members and co-workers to remind them about important things [36,37].

iv) Thankful for life, yet fearful of the future. In spite of the challenges of daily living activities, the psychosocial impact, and the lack of support from many health providers during the chemobrain experience, these factors did not cause women with breast cancer to withdraw from chemotherapy treatment. Survivors appreciated receiving chemotherapy as it reduced their risk of mortality. Most were grateful that they had survived and some took their diagnosis as a turning point in their life. They worked towards personal goals for self-satisfaction and some women placed a higher priority on developing relationships with family and friends and contributing to wider society [33,34].

"Life isn't guaranteed, and I try not to be real pessimistic, but it is sort of a wakeup call. You are not guaranteed that tomorrow will come" [32], p. 122.

However, Thielen [38] reported that survivors were still living in doubt about their cancer prognosis and the likely duration of their chemobrain symptoms. They were apprehensive about the situation as they had received little information about chemobrain. This created additional stress for survivors who were attempting to self-manage what they saw as obvious impairments, which were not acknowledged by their health providers. This also led them to adopt the belief that they should be grateful (to be alive), and 'downplay' cognitive impairment as a lesser issue to self manage their return to their normal state.

Application of the experience of chemobrain to the Leventhal [31] framework

The line-of argument synthesis [24] using the Laventhal model enabled us to frame the significance of the burden of cognitive impairment in cancer survivors. In Table 6 we attempted to present each dimension of Illness Representation Theory [31] in the context of the experiences of chemobrain from the reviewed studies. The cognitive and emotional processes experienced by women were captured and may influence their mental image of potential threats attributable to chemobrain. The interpretation that chemobrain is a relatively small issue (in comparison with death for example), may underestimate the threat of the debilitating effect chemobrain can have on everyday functioning and quality of life. The burden of cognitive impairment in cancer survivors appeared grossly underestimated. This warrants it to be addressed promptly as studies have shown that illness perceptions have associations with a number of negative outcomes in the experience of chronic illness including self-management behaviours and quality of life [39], and this can be anticipated within the breast cancer population.

Table 5. Coping strategies adopted by survivors.

COPING STRATEGIES	32	34	36	37	38
Pharmacological					
Nutritional products		X			
Complementary and alternative medicine		X			
Non Pharmacological					
Healthy lifestyle practices		X	X		
Physical activities		X	X		
Mental activities	x	x	X		
Practical reminders					
Written	X	X	X	X	x
Use of technology	x	x			

Discussion

Implications of the experience of chemobrain

The meta-ethnography method facilitated the synthesis of seven qualitative research studies, and the creation of a preliminary notion to highlight the perceptions women with breast cancer have about their experience of chemobrain. The application of the Illness Representation Theory to the findings allowed further interpretation of the meanings attributed to the chemobrain experience. Although our analytical approach was inductive in nature, it was helpful to consider a theoretical framework that addressed meaning such as the construct of illness representation. The Illness Representation Theory informed the analysis about the 'vague but real' cognitive symptoms experienced by breast cancer survivors, portrayed as broader health problems involving identity, timeline, consequences, cause, control, illness coherence,

and emotional representations [31]. The idea of illness perceptions is derived from self-regulation theory [31,40]. This theory proposes that individuals form common-sense beliefs about their symptoms to cope with any potential health threats. Our review suggests that the breast cancer survivors were actively trying to find some meaning to their chemobrain symptoms which became more confronting when they resumed their daily activities.

Illness Representation Theory dictates that illness representations are mediated by influencing factors that have not been adequately explained by the biomedical model of illness. A strong thread of 'struggling' with the 'why', 'how' and 'when' of chemobrain is manisfested cognitively and in survivors' self management behaviour. There is thus, a real gap in survivorship care, as chemobrain becomes a consistently reported phenomena associated with the rise in breast cancer survival rates. Coupled with the unusual terminology of 'chemobrain', survivors have

Table 6. Interpretation based on Illness Representation Theory – the struggle of Chemobrain.

Dimension	Potential Manifestations (per illness representation theory)
1. Identity	Matching or nonmatching of cognitive symptoms to the chemobrain experience (e.g., matching symptoms like feeling foggy, not as sharp, not as quick refering to the chemobrain syndrome; or rationalizing it as 'deficits are unimportant compared to getting through treatment, surviving from cancer)
2. Timeline	Beliefs about the expected onset/duration of it (e.g., acute vs chronic or cyclical). Increasing reports of survivors belief that chemobrain starts after they resume work, but most are unsure of exact timing. Some belief it is transient but others fear its persistent impact. There will be some degree of struggle- transient to persistent
3. Consequences	The perceived and anticipated impact of chemobrain (e.g., reversible vs static vs progressive or permanent). Subjects highlighted that chemobrain affected their daily functioning, economic status, and their social relationships. Some believed these impacts may get better whilst others feared that the cognitive deficits may be permanent loses. The underlying finding is that they will have to struggle with it.
4. Causes	They perceived the contextual factors or antecedent causes (e.g., aging, stress of having cancer and treatment, rather than from treatment since there is no evidence on the mechanism and since their health providers did not validate chemobrain) leading to a constant struggle.
5. Controllability	An expectation that chemobrain symptoms can be somewhat controlled via coping strategies, but may not be cured and may even be permanent damage. Survivors were struggling to adjust. A belief that they should just self-manage since "it does not seems to be a significant according to the health providers'.
6. Illness coherence	The subjects' perceived understanding of the chemobrain phenomena – (ie vague, subtle, foggy, spacey) but the health team did not validate it, suggesting a period of uncertain struggle.
7. Emotional representa-tions	Panic and frustrated in response to chemobrain experience Sense of dissatisfaction and anger that they were not forewarned Neutral or matter-of-fact emotional state (for some) Again mansifesting a constant struggle within themselves and with significant others

Based on the Leventhal's Common Sense Model of Illness Representation [31,40].

expressed that their health providers are negating its presence, and are therefore not validating its existence. Common sense reasoning is then left to fill the gap, so that cognitive issues are attributed to stress or aging or other potential contextual factors. This leads the survivors to arrive at a state of problem-solving where they struggle to self manage an 'unknown' but real issue. The idea that women should just manage as well as they can suggests a constant struggle to cope. The final dimension of illness representation is a cognitive representation of the issue, and this amounts to chemobrain being considered insignificant compared to surviving cancer, despite dissatisfaction with the situation and having to live with the consequences.

Implications for health services across health settings

Chemobrain or mild cognitive impairment associated with chemotherapy treatment is consistently reported by breast cancer survivors. There is a growing body of research, but the incidence and causes remain uncertain due to inconsistent methods of objective assessment of cognitive changes and subjective reports from survivors [41,42]. Although many studies suggest that chemobrain is related to cancer treatment such as chemotherapy [43,44], it is essential to recognise the other confounding factors such as psychological factors and insomnia that could contribute to cognitive changes [45]. In order to enhance the quality of life of survivors, healthcare providers should be reliable sources of information about cognitive changes. A proactive inter-disciplinary team approach comprising the oncology medical staff and allied health professionals is essential to ensure a holistic partnership to provide better care, and to address the participation needs of cancer patients [46].

A consistent evaluation of potential causative factors by health professionals can help to explore the main causes and mechanisms of chemobrain and assist in developing interventions for survivors [46], however few studies have been completed to guide this development. It must be highlighted that some medical clinicians are reluctant to provide information on chemobrain, because of the belief that patients may reject chemotherapy if they believe there is a causal relationship between chemobrain and chemotherapy. Whilst the debate continues, women with breast cancer may face dilemmas about continuing treatment which may lead to worse adverse effects [8] Nevertheless, there are no data to suggest that fears about chemobrain are likely to lead to withdrawal from chemotherapy. In fact, the majority of participants indicated they were willing to undergo chemotherapy despite side effects [33,34,36]. However most of the participants stressed the importance of getting early information regarding potential cognitive changes. This needs to be a component of the informed consent process prior to treatment. Our review suggests that most survivors acknowledged their fears but were pragmatic and wanted to be informed early.

Addressing cognitive impairments

Despite the need for information about chemobrain for survivors, there are other needs to be considered. There is the potential for some psychological consequences of perceiving a threat from chemobrain which may be induced by the provision of information about it [47]. Health care professionals do acknowledge cognitive changes as an issue for the survivors, although there is a lack of scientific data regarding the aetiology [48] Health care professionals, particularly oncologists, tend to emphasise the management of physical side effects [49] or acute side effects which have been reported by patients, as these are more established in the literature.

Asian and western perspectives of women with breast cancer. Based on the qualitative papers available in the review, the researchers found emerging differences in approach to their chemobrain experience between the Asian and western subjects. Our review suggested that Asian women are less familiar with the chemobrain phenomena than their western counterparts, however this needs to be interpreted with caution as it was based on only one paper with a small sample size [34]. Asian cultures were emotionally less expressive in emotion [50]. It has been suggested that Asian women are more focused on completing their treatment rather than being concerned with survivorship issues [34,40]. Nevertheless, the uniqueness of the perceptions of Asian women should be taken into account in any discussion on the issue of chemobrain. These women clearly verified that chemobrain was not a myth, but a real daily experience for them, which became apparent when they resumed daily duties. Many expressed that they were thankful to be alive, and had adopted the belief that chemobrain was just one of the changes that they need to adapt to since survival was the ultimate outcome in overcoming breast cancer. This tolerance of chemobrain symptoms may be best explained by the medicalization of cancer treatment, and this has contributed to the lack of recognition of chemobrain from the medical fraternity.

For both Asian and western cancer survivors, medicalization of the cancer journey is focused on efforts to battle the disease and at the same time is a reminder to survivors that there is a risk of cancer recurrence.

'... undermining efforts at self-determination and self-care; and, keeping the patient's life suspended by continual reminders that death is just around the corner, and that all the time and energy left must be devoted to ferreting out and killing the disease' [40], p.53.

The refusal or reluctance by some medical practitioners to acknowledge the cognitive issues experienced by survivors may lead to a lack of referrals to allied health professionals to address issues like chemobrain. A lack of attention to chemobrain means that the measurement of chemobrain symptoms is neglected. This means that the extent of impairment cannot be defined, and may decrease the impetus to develop effective interventions as outcomes cannot be evaluated. This is a particular issue for the management of return to work for survivors.

Self-management of chemobrain symptoms

Our review identified a lack of self-awareness about when changes in cognitive functioning became obvious for survivors. It seemed to be most apparent when they struggled to get work done, engaged in their role as a home maker, socialised and tried to cope with being less productive at work. Chemobrain led to specific challenges in handling daily tasks. According to Vearncombe et al. [46] the greatest decline was experienced in verbal learning and memory for breast cancer survivors, with problems in concentration and memory functions, contributing to a decline in functional performance. Inability to perform functional tasks that required constant effort for survivors had resulted in emotional frustration, mood changes and higher anxiety.

Apart from the personal difficulties experienced, our review found that the impact of chemobrain extended to affecting survivors' social relationships. Survivors reported that they withdrew from social situations to avoid feelings of embarrassment about the effects of their chemobrain symptoms, and this caused changes in their social relationships among family members, friends and colleagues. If they had been prepared and had some self-management guidance, these social consequences may have been lessened or prevented.

In terms of self-managing chemobrain, cancer survivors struggled and tried many ways to cope with impairments. Most of the selected studies found that psychosocial interventions and practical reminders were good sources of coping strategies. There appeared to be some cultural differences in coping strategies for chemobrain. Asian women were more likely to use complementary and alternative medicine such as traditional Chinese medicine to improve their cognitive function [34]. Further studies are needed to explore how cultural beliefs and health setting models can influence early health intervention and the coping strategies of survivors. Research exploring how ethnicity or cultural background can affect how someone copes with chemobrain symptoms, and how they go about dealing with the situation, is a viable and timely topic to minimise the gap in this field of cancer survivorship studies.

Reflectivity of conducting the metaethnography study

We did encounter some challenges in developing a new synthesis of qualtitative research of a meta-ethnography study on 'chemobrain, in particular in synthesizing methods from different contexts and research traditions. Some issues we encountered were the need to appraise the papers to ensure they fit our research question, and the CASP quality.

Strengths and limitations of the study

The strength of this review is the direct insights obtained from reports by breast cancer survivors about the cognitive changes they experienced in real life. Synthesizing the data from various qualitative researchers helped identify the scope and depth of the key domains of cognitive impairments experienced across different cohorts, time periods, cultures and health settings using a variety of qualitative study methodologies. Using the meta-ethnography has allowed a body of qualitative research studies to be combined together in a systematic way, where we have attempted to inductively analyse them through extracting concepts, metaphors and themes arising from the seven different studies. Meta ethnography has been proven useful where reflection on such interpretative approaches are needed and it has been used widely in health studies [22,23,51,52]. In short, the strength of this approach lies in the way it was constructed to preserve the meaning of the primary data and the help it gives us to look into a theoretical underpinning to understand the chemobrain phenomenon in a new intepretation of synthesis [53,54]. However, whilst the method followed a systematic process, it remained fundamentally inductive as it re-interpreted qualitative data presented across several qualitative studies. Therefore, we conclude that these findings can inform the development of recommendations for health care professionals, including clinical practice guidelines on patient education, assessment and interventions for breast cancer survivors to address chemobrain symptoms.

Several limitations have been acknowledged in this review study. We recognised the importance of maximum variation sampling, however the number of studies included and the sample size within each study was small. The inclusion criterion of published sources with full text availability may have omitted the inclusion of other potential sources such as unpublished theses or published book chapters, and this may have reduced the richness of the data. Five out of seven of the studies were from the United States, one was from the United Kingdom and one was from the Asian region. There is clearly a gap in studies from many other geographical locations. Future studies should explore the differences between less developed countries and developed countries, where the healthcare systems are uniquely different. Despite the limitations, meta-ethnography is a useful method for synthesising qualitative research conducted on a specific issue, and for developing models that interpret findings across multiple studies [28].

Conclusion

Our review found clear verification and consistent reports that breast cancer survivors' experiences of cognitive impairments were real, with a reported disparity between health professional and survivor's viewpoints across different healthcare settings and cultures. Persistent chemobrain clearly has a detrimental impact on the economic, emotional and interpersonal status of breast cancer survivors. Subjective self-report were validated by the consistent findings across the studies, and it is likely that the severity of difficulties experienced (manifested as 'strugglings to self manage') was underestimated. Women may downplay the effect of these impacts because of the lack of recognition from health providers. The current literature on the lived experience of chemobrain symptoms by women with breast cancer provides (manifesting as a constant struggle on their daily living domains) evidence that chemobrain is real, persistent and has substantial, detrimental impacts on daily living and quality of life.

Recommendations

On the basis of the key findings discussed above, we recommend the development of an information resource to create awareness of potential cognitive changes associated with breast cancer treatment among patients, family caregivers and, perhaps most importantly, among healthcare providers. A more objective testing and monitoring of neurocognitive function in survivors complaining of cognitive changes is warranted. In addition, studies evaluating cognitive testing should be derived from reliable, functional and ecologically valid assessments which are culturally defined, rather than depending only on pen and paper assessments. Optimisation of some of the self-management strategies used by the some breast cancer survivors can be used to inform the development of educational information for survivors, and for enhancing awareness among healthcare providers. Further quantitative research is required to explore the causal mechanisms associated with chemobrain symptoms. Future research that includes systematic, longitudinal investigations of illness representation and its impact on health behaviours among survivors with cognitive impairment is needed. Greater awareness and culturally-specific therapy is critical to enhance functional return to daily tasks and quality of life during the cancer survivorship phase, especially related to return to work. Our study findings contribute to both theoretical and empirical implications for future research and the development of practice to address cognition in cancer survivorship.

Author Contributions

Conceived and designed the experiments: SYL MHS. Performed the experiments: MHS SYL. Analyzed the data: SYL MHS LM JV. Contributed reagents/materials/analysis tools: SYL. Contributed to the writing of the manuscript: MHS SYL LM JV.

References

1. Marin AP, Sanchez AR, Arranz EE, Aunon PZ, Baron MG (2009) Adjuvant Chemotherapy for Breast Cancer and Cognitive Impairment. Southern Medical Journal 102(9): 929–34.
2. Meade E, Dowling M (2012) Early breast cancer: diagnosis, treatment and survivorship. British Journal of Nursing 21(17): S4–7.
3. American Cancer Society (2012) Cancer Facts & Figures 2012. Atlanta: American Cancer Society. http://www.cancer.org/research/cancerfactsfigures/ cancerfactsfigures/cancer-facts-figures-2012#. Accessed 2012 November 28.
4. Argyriou A, Assimakopoulos K, Iconomou G, Fotini G, Haralabos K (2010) Either Called "Chemobrain" or "Chemofog," the Long-Term Chemotherapy-Induced Cognitive Decline in Cancer Survivors Is Real. Journal of pain and symptom management 41(1): 126–139.
5. Burstein H J. (2007) Cognitive side-effects of adjuvant treatments. The Breast 16(2): S166–8.
6. Jansen CE, Cooper BA, Dodd MJ, Miaskowski CA (2011) A prospective longitudinal study of chemotherapy-induced cognitive changes in breast cancer patients. Support Care Cancer 19(10): 1647–1656.
7. Matsuda T, Takayama T, Tashiro M, Nakamura Y, Ohashi Y, et al. (2005) Mild cognitive impairment after adjuvant chemotherapy in breast cancer patients–evaluation of appropriate research design and methodology to measure symptoms. Breast Cancer 12(4): 279–287.
8. Raffa RB, Duong PV, Finney J, Garber DA, Lam L, et al. (2006) Is " chemofog"/"chemo-brain " caused by cancer chemotherapy? Journal of Clinical Pharmacy and Therapeutics 31: 129–138.
9. Weiss B (2008) Chemobrain: a translational challenge for neurotoxicology. Neurotoxicology 29 (5): 891–8.
10. Sherwood G (October 2011). Survivorship in cancer. Torch: IWMF Newsletter. http://www.iwmf.com/docs/Torch%20October%202011.pdf. Accessed 2013 February 20.
11. Christie LA, Acharya MM, Parihar VK, Nguyen A, Martirosian V, et al. (2012) Impaired cognitive function and hippocampal neurogenesis following cancer chemotherapy. Clin Cancer Res 18(7): 1954–1965.
12. Nelson CJ, Nandy N, Roth AJ (2007) Chemotherapy and cognitive deficits: Mechanisms, findings, and potential interventions. Palliative & Supportive Care 2007 5(3): 273–280.
13. Ahles AT, Saykin JA (2007) Candidate mechanism for chemotherapy-induced cognitive changes. Nature Reviews Cancer 7: 195–201.
14. Schilder CM, Seynaeve C, Linn SC, Boogerd W, Beex LV, et al. (2010) Cognitive functioning of postmenopausal breast cancer patients before adjuvant systemic therapy, and its association with medical and psychological factors. Crit Rev Oncol Hematol 76(2): 133–141.
15. Biglia N, Bounous VE, Malabaila A, Palmisano D, Torta DME, et al. (2012) Objective and self-reported cognitive dysfunction in breast cancer women treated with chemotherapy: a prospective study. Eur J Cancer Care 21(4): 485–492.
16. Asher A. (2011) Cognitive dysfunction among cancer survivors. Am J Phys Med Rehabil 90: 16–26.
17. Vardy J. (2009) Cognitive function in breast cancer survivors. Cancer Treat Res 151: 387–419.
18. Wagner LI, Sweet J, Lai JS, Cella D. (2009) Measuring patient self-reported cognitive function: development of the functional assessment of cancer therapy-cognitive function instrument. J Support Oncol 7(6): W32–W39.
19. Wefel JS, Witgert ME, Meyers CA. (2008) Neuropsychological Sequelae of Non-Central Nervous System Cancer and Cancer Therapy. Neuropsychology Review 18(2): 121–131.
20. Creswell JW. (2007) Qualitative inquiry & research design: choosing among five approaches. Thousand Oaks: Sage Publication. 395 p.
21. Henwood KL. (1996) Qualitative inquiry: Perspectives, methods, and psychology. In Richardson JTE (Ed.), Handbook of qualitative research methods for psychology and the social sciences. Leicester, UK: BPS Books. pp. 25–42.
22. Britten N, Campbell R, Pope C, Donovan J, Morgan M, et.al. (2002) Using meta ethnography to synthesise qualitative research: a worked example. Journal of Health Services Research & Policy 7(4): 209–215.
23. Campbell R, Pound P, Morgan M, Daker-White G, Britten N, et al. (2011) Evaluating meta-ethnography: systematic analysis and synthesis of qualitative research. Health Technol Assess 15(43): 1–164.
24. Dixon-woods M, Cavers D, Agarwal S, Annandale E, Arthur A, et al. (2006) Conducting a critical interpretive synthesis of the literature on access to healthcare by vulnerable groups. BMC Medical Research Methodology 6(1): 35.
25. Noblit GW, Hare RD. (1988) Meta-ethnography: Synthesizing qualitative studies. Newbury Park, CA:Sage.
26. Toye F, Seers K, Allcock N, Briggs M, Carr E, et al. (2013) "Trying to pin down jelly" - exploring intuitive processes in quality assessment for meta-ethnography. BMC medical research methodology. doi: 10.1186/1471-2288-13-46.
27. Critical Appraisal Skill Programme.(2013) 10 questions to help you make sense of qualitative research. Available at http://www.casp-uk.net/wp-content/ uploads/2011/11/CASP-Qualitative-Research-Checklist-31.05.13.pdf. Accessed 2013 March 15.
28. Campbell R, Pound P, Pope C, Britten N, Pill R, et al. (2003) Evaluating meta-ethnography: a synthesis of qualitative research on lay experiences of diabetis and diabetes care. Social Science & Medicine 56: 671–684.
29. Atkins S, Lewin S, Smith H, Engel M, Fretheim A, et al. (2008) Conducting a meta-ethnography of qualitative literature: Lessons learnt. BMC Medical Research Methodology 8(1): 21.
30. Schutz A. (1962) Collected papers, Vol. 1. The Hague: Nijhoff.
31. Leventhal H, Benyamini Y, Brownlee S et al. (1997) Illness representations: Theoretical foundations. In K. J. Petrie & J. Weinman (Eds.), Perceptions of health and illness. Amsterdam: Harwood Academic Press. 19–46 p.
32. Mulrooney Tamsin. (2007) The experience of neurocognitive changes in women undergoing chemotherapy for breast cancer. Proquest Dissertation and Theses. http://search.proquest.com/docview/304627599?accountid=28930. Accessed 2013 January 20.
33. Von Ah D, Habermann B, Carpenter JS, Schneider BL (2013) Impact of Perceived cognitive impairment in breast cancer survivors. European Journal of Oncology Nursing 17: 236–241.
34. Cheung YT, Shwe M, Tan YP, Fan G, Ng R, Chan A. (2012) A Cognitive changes in multiethnic Asian breast cancer patient: a focus group study. Annals of Oncology 23: 2547–2552.
35. Munir F, Burrows J, Yarker J, Kalawsky K, Bains M. (2010) Women's perceptions of chemotherapy-induced cognitive side affects on work ability: a focus group study. Journal of clinical nursing 19(9–10): 1362–70.
36. Myers JS. (2012) Chemotherapy-related cognitive impairment: the breast cancer experience. Oncology Nursing Forum 39(1):E31–40.
37. Thielen JZ. (2008) The lived experience of cognitive imapairment in women treated with chemotherapy for breast cancer. Proquest Dissertation and Theses. http://search.proquest.com/docview/304804657?accountid=28930. Accessed 20 January 2013.
38. Boykoff N, Moieni M, Subramaniam SK. (2009) Confronting chemobrain: an in depth look at survivors' reports of impact on work, social network, and health care reponse. Journal cancer survivor 3(4): 223–232.
39. Petrie KJ, Jago LA, Devcich DA. (2007) The role of illness perceptions in patients with medical conditions. Current opinion in psychiatry 20(2): 163–7.
40. Leventhal H, Nerenz DR, Steele DJ. (1984) Illness representation and coping with health threats. In A. Baum, S. E. Taylor, & J. E. Singer (Eds.), Handbook of psychology. Hillsdale, NJ: Erlbaum: 219–252 p.
41. Shilling V, Jenkins V, Morris R, Deutsch G, Bloomfield D. (2005) The effects of adjuvant chemotherapy on cognition in women with breast cancer–preliminary results of an observational longitudinal study. The Breast 14(2): 142–50.
42. Castellon S, Ganz PA. (2009) Neuropsychological studies in breast cancer: in search of chemobrain. Breast cancer research and treatment 116(1): 125–7.
43. Breitbart WS, Alici Y. (2009) Psycho Oncology. Harvard Review of Psychiatry 17(6): 361–376
44. Baumgartner K. (2004) Neurocognitive changes in cancer patient. Seminars in Oncology Nursing 20(4): 284–290.
45. Hall B. (2003) An essay on an authentic meaning of medicalization. Adv Nurs Sci 26(1): 53–62.
46. Vearncombe KJ, Rolfe M, Wright M, Panchana NA, Andrew B, et al. (2009) Predictors of cognitive decline after chemotherapy in breast cancer patients. J Int Neuropsychol Soc 15(6): 951–962.
47. Schagen SB, Das E, Vermeulen L. (2012) Information about chemotherapy-associated cognitive problems contributes to cognitive problems in cancer patients. Psychooncology 21(10): 1132–5.
48. Cheung YT, Shue M, Tan EHJ, Chai WK, Ng R, et al. (2013). Acknowledging the relevance of cognitive changes in cancer patients: perspectives of oncology practitioners in Asia. J. Cancer Surviv 7(1): 146–54.
49. Pirl WF, Muriel A, Hwang V, Kornblith A, Greer J, et al. (2007) Screening for psycosocial distress: a national survey of oncologists. J Support Oncol 5(10): 499–504
50. Hirokawa K, Nagata C, Takatsuka N, Shimizu H. (2004) The relationship of a rationality/antiemotionality personality scale to mortalities of cancer and cardiovascular disease in a community population in Japan. J Psychosom Res 56(1): 103–11.
51. Furuta M, Sandall J, Bick D. (2014) Women's perception and experiences of severe maternal morbidity: A synthesis of qualitative studies using a meta-ethnographic approach. Midwifery 30: 158–169.
52. Banning M. (2011) Employment and breast cancer: a meta ethnography. European Journal of Cancer Care 20: 708–719
53. Campbell R, Pound P, Pope C, Britten N, Pill R, et al. (2003) Evaluating meta-ethnography: a synthesis of qualitative research on lay experiences of diabetis and diabetes care. Social Science & Medicine 56: 671–684.
54. Dixon-Woods M, Agarwal S, Jones D, Young B, Sutton A. (2005) Synthesising qualitative and quantitative evidence: a review of possible methods. Journal of Health Services & Policy 10: 45–53.

25

A miRNA Signature of Chemoresistant Mesenchymal Phenotype Identifies Novel Molecular Targets Associated with Advanced Pancreatic Cancer

Alakesh Bera[1], Kolaparthi VenkataSubbaRao[1], Muthu Saravanan Manoharan[3], Ping Hill[1], James W. Freeman[1,2,3]*

1 Department of Medicine, Division of Hematology and Oncology, University of Texas Health Science Center at San Antonio, San Antonio, Texas, United States of America, **2** Cancer Therapy and Research Center, Experimental and Developmental Therapeutics Program, San Antonio, Texas, United States of America, **3** Research and Development, Audie Murphy Veterans Administration Hospital, San Antonio, Texas, United States of America

Abstract

In this study a microRNA (miRNA) signature was identified in a gemcitabine resistant pancreatic ductal adenocarcinoma (PDAC) cell line model (BxPC3-GZR) and this signature was further examined in advanced PDAC tumor specimens from The Cancer Genome Atlas (TCGA) database. BxPC3-GZR showed a mesenchymal phenotype, expressed high levels of CD44 and showed a highly significant deregulation of 17 miRNAs. Based on relevance to cancer, a seven-miRNA signature (miR-100, miR-125b, miR-155, miR-21, miR-205, miR-27b and miR-455-3p) was selected for further studies. A strong correlation was observed for six of the seven miRNAs in 43 advanced tumor specimens compared to normal pancreas tissue. To assess the functional relevance we initially focused on miRNA-125b, which is over-expressed in both the BxPC3-GZR model and advanced PDAC tumor specimens. Knockdown of miRNA-125b in BxPC3-GZR and Panc-1 cells caused a partial reversal of the mesenchymal phenotype and enhanced response to gemcitabine. Moreover, RNA-seq data from each of 40 advanced PDAC tumor specimens from the TCGA data base indicate a negative correlation between expression of miRNA-125b and five of six potential target genes (*BAP1*, *BBC3*, *NEU1*, *BCL2*, *STARD13*). Thus far, two of these target genes, *BBC3* and *NEU1*, that are tumor suppressor genes but not yet studied in PDAC, appear to be functional targets of miR-125b since knockdown of miR125b caused their up regulation. These miRNAs and their molecular targets may serve as targets to enhance sensitivity to chemotherapy and reduce metastatic spread.

Editor: Shrikant Anant, University of Kansas School of Medicine, United States of America

Funding: Funding provided by National Institutes of Health-RO1CA069122 to JWF, Veterans Affairs Merit Award 1I01BX000927 to JWF and William and Eula Owens Medical Research Foundation to JWF. The funders had no role in study design, data collection and analysis, decision to publish, or preparation of the manuscript.

Competing Interests: The authors have declared that no competing interests exist.

* Email: freemanjw@uthscsa.edu

Introduction

PDAC continues to have the worst prognosis of any solid tumor. In 2013, it is estimated that more than 45,000 new cases will be diagnosed in the United States with mortality to incidence ratio almost equal to one [1]. Gemcitabine is the most commonly used chemotherapy for pancreatic cancer but is significantly metabolized in plasma and therefore requires high doses leading to toxicity [2]. Many PDAC are initially resistant to gemcitabine and responsive ones generally develop resistance during the course of treatment [3].

It remains to be determined whether the chemoresistant phenotype is induced as a result of therapy or whether there is a subpopulation of cancer cells within the tumor that are innately more resistant to therapy. Recent evidence indicates that most solid tumors, including PDAC possess a distinct subpopulation of cancer stem cells (CSCs). Evidence also suggests that CSCs are inherently more resistant to chemotherapy and utilize their self-renewal potential to regenerate new tumor growth [4]. A previous study links CSCs with epithelial to mesenchymal transition (EMT) [5].

EMT represents a trans-differentiation program that is required for tissue morphogenesis during different cellular developmental progression [6]. The EMT process can be regulated by a diverse array of cytokines and growth factors, such as TGF-β, whose activities are deregulated during tumor progression [7]. EMT induction in cancer cells results in the acquisition of invasive and metastatic properties. Studies also indicate that EMT also contributes to chemoresistance and that these cells possess CSC markers [8]. The development of chemoresistance in cancer cells to anticancer drugs including gemcitabine may be regulated or contributed to by micro-RNAs (miRNAs). miRNAs are small non-coding RNA molecules (22 nucleotides), which play crucial roles in transcriptional regulation of gene expression. The development of chemoresistance through an increase in the number of CSCs has been attributed to alterations at the level of miRNAs in pancreatic and other solid tumors [9].

Recent findings indicate an interrelationship between miRNAs, EMT phenotype, CSCs and chemoresistance [10,11]. Studies also suggest that miRNAs play a role in regulating the EMT process [3,11]. For instance, miRNAs have been shown to drive EMT by regulating cadherin 1 and additional EMT related molecules [12]. MiR-200a, miR-200b and miR-200c were down regulated in gemcitabine-resistant pancreatic cancer cells [13]. Studies also indicate that re-expression of the miR-200 family of miRNAs up regulated cadherin 1 and down regulated ZEB1 and vimentin [14]. Additionally, cancer cells with an EMT phenotype and that were resistant to gemcitabine showed down regulation of let-7 members [5,15,16]. In vitro studies of PDAC indicate a linkage among EMT, invasiveness and resistance to chemotherapy and other studies support the notion that miRNAs play a role in these processes by regulating gene expression [3,11].

In this study we sought to identify a miRNA signature for PDAC cells that possess chemoresistant and a mesenchymal phenotype (CRMP). Because patients with advanced PDAC tend to show minimal response to chemotherapy we further determined whether this miRNA signature might be reflected in their tumor tissues. These studies show that gemcitabine treatment induces a population of cells with CRMP in vitro and that a miRNA signature selected for this CRMP is shared with tumors specimens from advanced PDAC. Moreover, this study was able to initially establish a functional relevance of one over expressed miRNA (miR-125b) from this signature and potential tumor suppressor target genes. This study provides the basis for further dissecting the roles of miRNAs in CRMP. These miRNAs and their molecular targets may provide novel therapeutic strategies to eliminate a tumor cell population that is generally resistant to gemcitabine and possibly other chemotherapy.

Materials and Methods

Materials

Gemcitabine purchased from LKT Laboratories, Inc (St. Paul, MN) was dissolved in sterile PBS solution. Reverse transcription reagents and TaqMan real-time PCR master-mix were purchased from Applied Biosystems/Life Technologies (Foster city, CA). All other chemicals were obtained from Sigma–Aldrich (St. Louis, MO).

Cell lines

The human pancreatic adenocarcinoma cell line BxPC3, Capan-2, AsPC-1 and Panc-1 were purchased from ATCC and cultured them in DMEM media (except BxPC3) with 1% penicillin/streptomycin and 10% fetal bovine serum (FBS) in a humidified incubator containing 5% CO_2 at 37°C. BxPC3 was cultured in RPMI media with 1% penicillin/streptomycin and 10% FBS. This PDAC cell line BxPC3 was transiently exposed for four hours every seven days with increasing concentrations (50 ng to 1.5 μg/ml) of gemcitabine over a six-week period. The resulting gemcitabine resistant cell line referred to as BxPC3-GZR. For maintenance, BxPC3-GZR cells were expanded in culture medium and frozen in aliquots. For experiments BxPC3-GZR cells were thawed and allowed to expand in culture for two days and then treated with gemcitabine (1.5 μg/ml) for four hours. Gemcitabine was removed and BxPC3-GZR cells were harvested the following day for experiments including quality control Westerns blots to show that the acquired EMT phenotype was maintained.

Western blots analyses and immunofluorescence staining

Western blot analysis was performed as described previously [17]. Primary antibodies used were as follows: E-cadherin and Neu1 from Santa Cruz Biotechnology, Inc. (Santa Cruz, CA); CD44, beta-actin and PUMA (BBC3) were purchased from Cell Signaling Technology (Beverly, MA), vimentin from Life Technologies (Carlsbad, CA). Horseradish peroxidase-conjugated secondary antibodies were purchased from Amersham Biosciences (Piscataway, NJ). For immunofluorescence (IF) staining, cells grown on round cover slips in a 24-well plate. Fixing and immunostaining followed by capturing images were performed as described previously [18].

Matrigel Cell Invasion Assays

The invasive behavior of cells was analyzed by Matrigel invasion assays as described previously [17,18].

The expression profiling of miRNAs

Total RNA including small non-coding miRNA was isolated from BxPC3 and BxPC3-GZR using mirNeasy kit (Qiagen) per manufacturer procedures. Expression analysis of miRNA in both control BxPC3 and BxPC3-GZR cells were performed by LC Sciences (Houston, TX) using a proprietary μParaflo microfluidic biochip technology. Significant changes in miRNA expression were analyzed by t-test as provided by LC Sciences (Houston, TX). Only the most highly significant changes of both over and under expressed miRNAs were considered for further analysis (Table 1).

Reverse transcription and TaqMan quantitative PCR

TaqMan gene-expression assays (Life Technologies, Carlsbad, CA) were used to quantify the expression levels of both mRNA and mature miRNA. Total RNA extracted by mirVana (Life Technologies, Carlsbad, CA) RNA isolation kit and followed by reverse transcribed in a reaction mixture containing random hexamer primers (for mRNA RT-PCR) and miR-specific stem-loop RT primers (for miRNA RT-PCR). Quantitative PCR was performed in triplicate with reactions containing amplified cDNA and TaqMan primers in Universal Master Mix without AmpErase UNG (Applied Biosystems, Carlsbad, CA) by following manufacturer's protocol. All mRNA data and miRNA data are expressed relative to 18S and U6 respectively by TaqMan PCR performed on the same samples, unless otherwise specified. Fold expression was calculated from the triplicate of C_T values following the $2^{-\Delta\Delta C}{}_T$ method.

Stable cell line generation for miR-125b knockdown

Gemcitabine resistant BxPC3-GZR and Panc-1 cells were used in the miR-125b knock down study. System Bioscience's (SBI, Mountain View, CA) miRZipTM anti-sense miRNAs are stably expressed RNAi hairpins that inhibit miRNA activity. The miRZip shRNAs produce short, single-stranded anti-miRNAs that competitively bind their endogenous miRNA target and inhibit its function. The miRZip short hairpin RNAs are cloned into SBI's pGreenPuroTM shRNA expression vector, an improved third generation HIV-based expression lenti-vector. The lentiviral vector contains the genetic elements responsible for packaging, transduction, and stable integration of the viral construct into genomic DNA, inducing expression of the anti-miRNA effector sequence. For production of a high titer of viral particles, we used the ViraPowerTM Lentiviral Support Kit (Invitrogen, Carlsbad, CA) employing LipofectamineTM 2000

Table 1. The list of miRNAs that are highly significant in terms of expression in the gemcitabine resistant BxPC3-GZR cells compared to control BxPC3 cells.

miRNA ID	p Value	Log2 (R/Wt)
Positively correlated miRNAs (Bx-GZR> BxPC3)		
hsa-miR-125b	0.004	1.78
hsa-miR-155	0.00427	1.48
hsa-miR-100	0.00482	1.55
†hsa-miR-4324	0.00676	2.93
hsa-miR-21	0.00237	0.8
hsa-miR-15b	0.00388	1.19
hsa-miR-25	0.00516	0.53
†hsa-miR-424*	0.00756	0.57
has-miR-99b	0.00379	1.19
Negatively correlated miRNAs (Bx-GZR< BxPC3)		
hsa-miR-1246	0.00007	−4.03
hsa-miR-205	0.00445	−2.14
hsa-miR-4443	0.00504	−1.27
hsa-miR-30d	0.00185	−0.83
hsa-miR-27b	0.00877	−0.61
hsa-miR-4485	0.00456	−0.81
†hsa-miR-378*	0.00649	−0.96
hsa-miR-455-3p*	0.00485	−0.9

†These transcripts are statistically significant but very low signal.

(Invitrogen) for transfecting the miRzip vectors into HEK-293T cells. Because infected cells stably express GFP and puromycin, as well as the anti-miRNA cloned into the miRZipTM vector, we used puromycin to select for the infected cells harboring the miRzip. After screening we isolated BxPC3-GZRΔmiR-125b or Panc-1ΔmiR-125b cells. In the similar way we also generated Zip control of both cell-lines with miRZipTM vector. For determining drug sensitivity, cells were treated with indicated concentrations of gemcitabine for 96 h and MTT assays were performed as previously described [19].

MiRNA and transcriptome profiling of tumor data from The Cancer Genome Atlas (TCGA)

miRNA: Level 3.1.1.0 miRNA sequence data from TCGA data portal was downloaded for 43 tumor samples with one normal tissue. A data matrix was prepared by combining the raw read counts of 1046 miRNAs from 44 [43 tumor and 1 normal] samples. Based on the assumption that miRNA sequence data follow a negative binomial distribution [20], [21] the read counts were size-factor normalized using DESeq version 1.10.1 [22] package in R version 2.15.3. Normalized read count data was used to compute log2 fold change between tumor and normal samples.

Transcriptome: Level 3.1.1.0 RNA sequence data from TCGA data portal was downloaded for 40 tumor samples with one normal tissue as control. We used RSEM software for determining quantity of transcripts from RNA-Seq data. RSEM upper quartile normalized read counts data from 41 (40 tumors and 1 normal) tissue samples were used to compute log2 fold change between tumor and normal samples.

Statistical analysis

The Student's unpaired t-test was used to compare individual group means. A p-value of <0.05 was considered as statistically significant. All values in the figures and text were expressed as the mean ± S.D.

Results

Generation of a pancreatic cancer CRMP cell line model

The PDAC cell line BxPC3 was transiently exposed to increasing concentrations of gemcitabine over a six-week period. The resulting gemcitabine resistant BxPC3-GZR cells were compared with the parental BxPC3 cells for differences in morphology, response to gemcitabine, expression of mesenchymal, epithelial markers and CD44. Comparisons for morphology show that the parental BxPC3 cells grew in tightly packed areas and showed a flat and rounded appearance, characteristic of an epithelial like morphology; whereas, BxPC3-GZR cells grew as loosely-associated cells with a spindle-like morphology characteristic of a mesenchymal phenotype (Fig. 1A). The sensitivity to treatment with gemcitabine was compared between BxPC3-GZR and parental BxPC3 cells. BxPC3-GZR cells showed greater than a twofold decrease in response to gemcitabine compared to its parental cells BxPC3 (Fig. 1C). To determine whether BxPC3-GZR cells are also cross resistant to another chemotherapeutic compound, cells were treated with paclitaxel and MTT assays were performed. While BxPC3-GZR cells showed more than a twofold decrease in sensitivity to gemcitabine, these cells showed only a modest decrease in sensitivity to paclitaxel (Fig. S1). These observations suggest that different signaling pathways may be responsible for resistance against different drugs. A recent study with side population of PDAC cells with properties of cancer stem cells and that were selected for resistance to gemcitabine were not resistant to 5-FU [23]. Western blot analysis of cells collected at each week over the six weeks of increasing gemcitabine treatment revealed that the level of epithelial marker E-cadherin gradually decreased with concomitant increase in the levels of mesenchymal marker vimentin and the stem cell marker CD44 (Fig. 1B).

More importantly, we have also monitored and compared the expression levels of same proteins of BxPC3 and BxPC3-GZR cells that where expanded and passed for successive generations in culture. The stability of the BxPC3-GZR phenotype was confirmed in short term cultures with BxPC3-GZR cells showing a lower level of E-cadherin, up regulation of vimentin expression and elevated expression of stem cell markers CD44 (Fig. 1D). In agreement with the Western blot data, immunofluorescence analysis indicated a much stronger staining of both CD44 and vimentin in BxPC3-GZR cells compared to the parental BxPC3 counterpart (Fig. 1E, F).

Identification of a miRNA signature associated with CRMP in PDAC

Studies indicate that various miRNAs such as miR-100, miR-21, let-7, miR- 34a and miR - 200c play critical role in regulating tumorigenesis and chemoresistance in different cancers including pancreatic cancer [24–26]. Studies also showed a role for miRNAs in development of drug resistance in a variety of malignancies

[11]. The expression level of miRNA was compared in BxPC3 and BxPC3-GZR cells by µParaflo microfluidic chip miRNA profiling. After calculation and eliminating non-significant miRNAs (in terms of expression), a highly significant miRNA profile was established that distinguished BxPC3-GZR cells from parental BxPC3 cells (Fig. 2, *Table 1*). This profile showed most significant nine miRNAs that were up regulated in BxPC3-GZR cells compared to BxPC3 (miR-125b, miR-155, miR-100, miR-4324, miR-21, miR-15b, miR-25, miR-424*, miR-99b) and eight that were down regulated (miR-1246, miR-205, miR-4443, miR-30d, miR-27b, miR-4485, miR-378*, miR-455-3p).

Based on relevance to cancer and chemoresistance, seven of these miRNAs were selected for further study. Real Time–PCR using TaqMan assays were done to validate over or under-expressed miRNAs identified by miRNA arrays (Fig. 2B). Finally we identified four of the over-expressed miRNAs (miR-125b, miR-155, miR-100, miR-21) and three under expressed miRNAs (miR-27b, mir-205, and miR-455-3p) by miRNA microarrays were validated by Real-Time PCR (Fig. 2B).

The miRNA signature from the CRMP cell line model is also detected in clinical specimens from patients with advanced PDAC

To establish the potential relevance of the validated CRMP miRNA signature with miRNAs found in advanced PDAC, whole

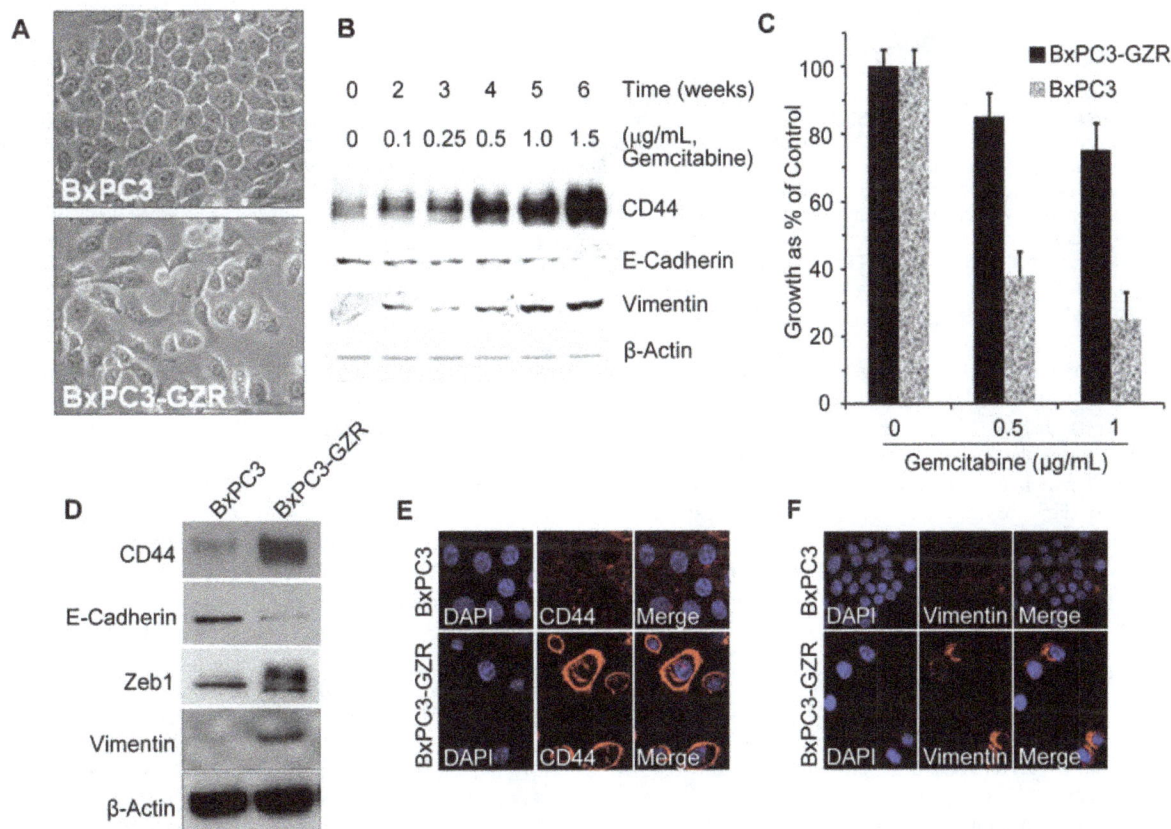

Figure 1. Characterization of BxPC3-GZR, a cell line model for CRMP. A. Morphological differences between parental BxPC3 and chemoresistance mesenchymal BxPC3-GZR cells. **B.** Western blot showing that BxPC3-GZR cells possess an EMT phenotype, which is demonstrated by increased expression of vimentin and a decrease of E-cadherin and express the stem cell marker CD44. **C.** MTT assay comparing the growth of the parental BxPC3 and BxPC3-GZR at 96 hrs after treatment with different concentrations of gemcitabine. **D.** Western blot comparing the expression of CD44, E-cadherin, Zeb-1 and vimentin after four passages of BxPC3 and BxPC3-GZR. **E** and **F.** Immunofluorescence confocal microscopy images show the differential expression of CD44 and vimentin in BxPC3 and BxPC3-GZR cells.

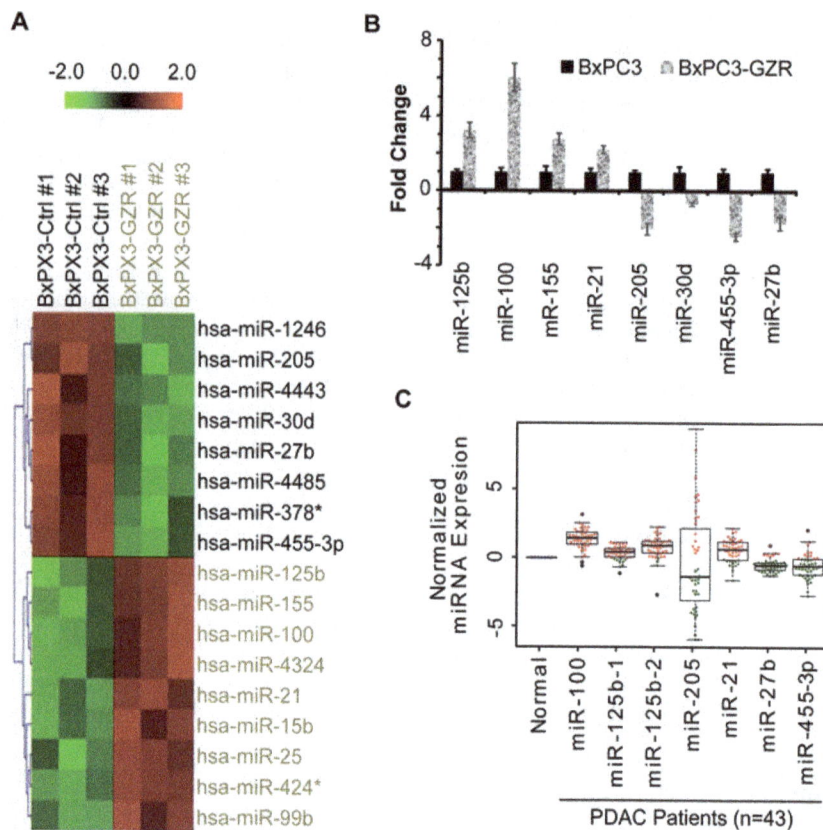

Figure 2. miRNA signature of BxPC3-GZR cells. A. Heat map data analysis of the miRNA microarray assays comparing BxPC3 parental cells and drug resistant BxPC3-GZR cells. Only miRNAs were chosen which had significantly over or under expressed as compared to parental cells (high fold changes based on log2 values and very low p-values) were taken for further validation. The statistical values are represented in the *Table 1*. **B.** Validation of miRNA microarray data was done for eight differentially expressed miRNAs using TaqMan qPCR assay. In each cell line, the expression level of indicated miRNA was compared between parental BxPC3 cells and BxPC3-GZR cells. RNU43 or U6 was used as an internal miRNA control. **C.** TCGA data analysis showing that 6 of the 7 miRNAs validated for being deregulated in BxPC3-GZR cells also showed differential expression in tumor specimens from patients with advanced PDAC. Tumor specimens from 43 patients with advanced PDAC were analyzed for miRNA expression compared to normal pancreas tissue.

transcriptome analyses (miRNA and mRNA-seq, expression levels) were performed with the PDAC patient specimen data from the TCGA data sets. In the TCGA database there are a total 43 PDAC patients samples containing expression level of miRNAs with a normal pancreas tissue. Forty of these patients' tumor specimens had data for both mRNA and miRNA expression levels. A comparison of the over and under expressed miRNAs in the TCGA with those in our miRNA array is presented in *Table 2*. As shown in *table 2*, of the seventeen miRNAs comprising the miRNAs aberrantly deregulated in BxPC3-GZR (9 over expressed and 8 under expressed) miRNA data for 14 of these were available in the TCGA analyses and for all seven of the validated miRNAs. A further comparison was done on the six-miRNA signature validated from the array data and for which there were matching data for advanced PDAC specimens. An analysis of this data is shown in Figure 2C. Interestingly there was a significant correlation with common expression levels of miRNAs in advanced PDAC tumor specimens with the validated CRMP miRNA signature for five of the six miRNAs (Fig. 2C, *Table 2*). It is important to note that the miR-125b data for the tumor specimens is given as both miR-125b-1 and miR-125b-2 isoforms, whereas in cell lines we only determined miR-125b-1 isoform (designated as miR-125b). Interestingly, the precursors of miR-125b-1 and miR-125b-2 isoforms were known to originate

independently from different chromosomal loci although their mature sequences and targets are same [27]. The most notable miRNAs over expressed in both BxPC3-GZR and clinical specimens were miR-100, miR-21, miR-125b-1, miR-125b-2 whereas miR-205, miR-27b and miR455 were under-expressed.

miR-125b plays a role in regulating the CRMP in PDAC

Initial studies were undertaken to determine whether the miRNAs identified in BxPC3-GZR cells and that were common to clinical specimens played a role in the CRMP. The miR-125b that was commonly over expressed in both advanced PDAC clinical specimens and in BxPC3-GZR cells (Fig. 2) was chosen for these analyses. For further studies, three PDAC cell lines (AsPC-1, Capan-2, Panc-1) in addition to BxPC3 were screened for expression levels of EMT markers along with miR-125b and miR-30d (Fig. 3 A, B). MiR-30d was used for comparison of differential expression of miRNA since it showed equal expression level in both parental (BxPC3) and resistant cells by qPCR analysis. In these cell lines the epithelial marker E-cadherin is inversely related to the expression of miR-125b; whereas, the mesenchymal marker vimentin and the stem cell marker CD44 were proportionally related to the expression of miR-125b (Fig. 3A, B). These data further suggests that the EMT phenotype may be regulated in part by the constitutive expression

Table 2. Comparison and validation of in vitro data with the patient samples.

Name of miRNA	Expression in patient samples relative to normal	
	(n = 43 TCGA Samples)	
	# of *Over* expressed	# of *Under* expressed
Over expressed in BxPC3-GZR		
hsa-miR-125b-1	34	9
hsa-miR-125b-2	39	4
hsa-miR-155	16	27
hsa-miR-100	41	2
hsa-miR-4324	ND*	ND
hsa-miR-21	31	12
hsa-miR-25	32	11
hsa-miR-99b	27	16
Under expressed in BxPC3-GZR		
hsa-miR-1246	ND	ND
hsa-miR-205	18	25
hsa-miR-4443	NA	NA
hsa-miR-30d	41	2
hsa-miR-27b	7	36
hsa-miR-4485	NA	NA
hsa-miR-378	10	33
hsa-miR-455	11	32

TCGA data was analyzed to determine the differential expression of different miRNAs indentified in BxPC3-GZR cells.
*ND = Not detected (very low copy number). NA = these micro-RNA data are not available in the database.

of miR-125b in Capan-2 and BxPC3 cells show an epithelial like phenotype and express low levels of miR-125b; however, AsPC-1 and Panc-1 cells are mesenchymal like and show higher levels of miR-125b (Fig. 3 A, B). Besides we have also monitored the expression of miR-125b in BxPC3 cells upon treatment with gemcitabine. Data indicates that 72 hours treatment with gemcitabine induced the expression of miR-125b in BxPC3 cells in a dose dependent manner (Fig. 3C). Therefore, these findings indicate that both chemoresistance and mesenchymal phenotypes are regulated by the differential expression of miR-125b.

In order to determine whether miR-125b expression is directly related to CRMP, we knocked down the expression of miR-125b by using Zip technology and stable cell lines generated and assayed for expression of miR-125b in both BxPC-GZR-Zip-Ctrl and in BxPC3-GZR-ΔmiR-125b cells (Fig. 4A). The morphology of miR-125b knockdown cells was also assessed and knockdown of miR-125b restored the epithelial like morphology (Fig. 4A). TaqMan qPCR assay indicated an approximate 80% knockdown of miR-125b in BxPC3-GZR cells (Fig. 4B). Knockdown of anti-miR125b reversed EMT markers as shown by the increased expression of the epithelial marker E-cadherin and the decreased expression of the mesenchymal marker vimentin and also decreased CD44 expression (Fig. 4C). Knockdown of miR-125b decreased cell migration (Fig. 4D, E) and partially reversed the gemcitabine resistance of BxPC3-GZR cells (Fig. 4F).

In order to confirm that this effect of miR-125b knockdown was not unique to BxPC3-GZR cells, miR-125b was also knocked down in Panc-1 cells. Similar to that seen in miRNA-125b knockdowns for BxPC3-GZR cells, Western blot and MTT assay data indicated that knockdown of miR-125b expression in Panc-1

cell partially reversed the mesenchymal phenotype (Fig. 4G,H) and enhanced response to gemcitabine (Fig. 4I).

Gene targets of miR-125b

Since miRNAs act by either repressing or cleaving their target mRNAs, we carried out gene expression analysis of several known downstream targets of miR-125b. Several studies indicated that mRNA targets of miR-125b are *BBC3* (PUMA), *ITCH*, *BAK1*, *BCL2*, *NEU1*, *PPP1CA*, *PPP2CA* [28] [29]; *STARD13* (DLC2) [30]; *AP1M1*, *STK11IP*, *PSMD8*, *TBC1D1*, *TDG*, *MKNK2*, *DGAT1*, BAP1, *GAB2*, *SGPL1* [28]. We analyzed the clinical tumor data for these above mRNA expression levels (Fig. 5). RNA-seq from TCGA showed that the expressions of some of these genes (*BAP1*, *BBC3* or PUMA, *BCL2*, *NEU1*, *STARD13*) are negatively correlated with the expression of miR-125b. We analyzed both the general expression trend of the targeted genes in the PDAC specimens from the TCGA database (Fig. 5A), as well as the expression level of targeted gene in relation to the expression of miRNA-125b within the same tumor specimens (Fig. 5B). Next, we have monitored the expression level of p53 up-regulated modulator of apoptosis (PUMA). PUMA also known as Bcl-2-binding component 3 (BBC3) is a pro-apoptotic protein and member of the Bcl-2 protein family [31,32]. PUMA is involved in both p53-dependent and -independent apoptosis pathway induced by a variety of signals [33]. Recent studies also indicate that *NEU1* product Neu1 salidase is important in regulation of integrin β4-mediated signaling, leading to suppression of cancer metastasis [34]. However, a separate study indicates that Neu1 salidase enhances EGFR signaling and thus could be tumor promoting [35]. The present findings along with the web-based miRNA target scan data suggest that miR-125b directly targets the

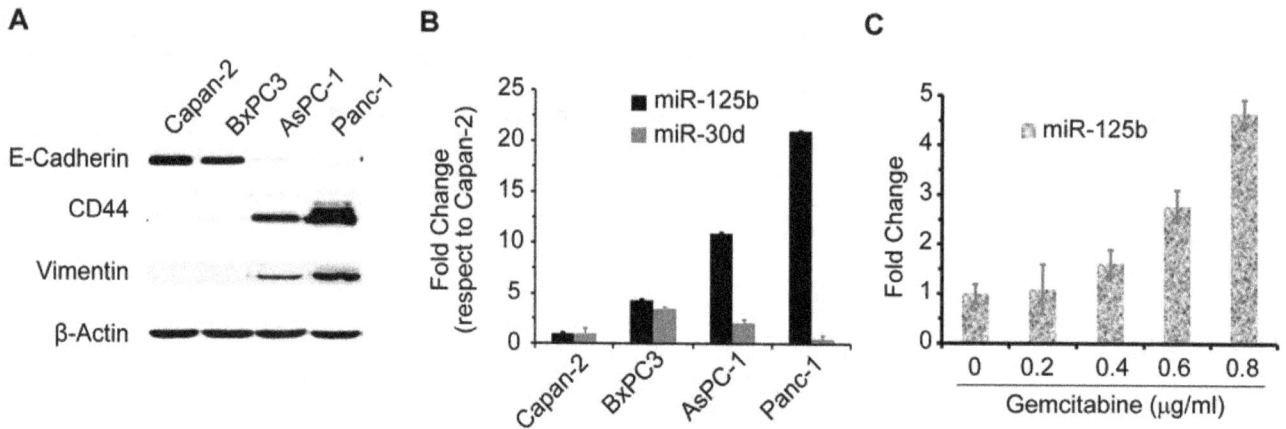

Figure 3. Micro-RNA-125b partially regulates CRMP. A. Western blot analyses showing the expression levels of EMT markers in PDAC cells in which miR-125b expression was determined. **B.** TaqMan qPCR analysis showing the relative expression of miRNAs (miR-125b and miR-30d) in different PDAC cells. MiR-30d is used as a control. **C.** Induction of miR-125b expression in BxPC3 upon treatment of gemcitabine. Quantitative PCR (TaqMan) were performed after 72 hrs of incubation with the drug in order to monitor the expression level of miR-125b in BxPC3 cells. Data indicates that expression of miR-125b is increased by the treatment of gemcitabine in a dose dependent manner.

3'UTRs of PUMA (BBC3) and Neu1 (Fig. 6. F,G). In support of this, the mRNA expressions for *BBC3* (PUMA) and *NEU1* were inversely correlated with the expression of miR-125b (Fig. 6A) in BxPC3-GzR cells.

Next, we compared the expression of three different potential miR-125b target genes PUMA (*BBC3*) (most under-expressed gene in patient samples), *NEU1* and *BAK1* (up-regulated gene) mRNAs between BxPC3 parental and BxPC3-GZR cells (Fig. 6B). In a similar manner, we also compared the expression of these genes between BxPC3-GZR cells and the BxPC3-GZR cells expressing anti-miR-125b (Fig. 6B). The data indicated that the expression of PUMA and Neu1 are negatively regulated by miR-125b expression. Cellular and clinical data indicated that expression of PUMA is most negatively regulated by the expression of miR-125b. It is also important to note that *BAK1* (another potential miR-125b target) expressions remain unchanged with respect to expression of miR-125b. The expression of PUMA and Neu-1 in BxPC3-GZR cells and the BxPC3-GZR-ΔmiR-125b cells was also determined by Western blot analysis (Fig. 6C). The data indicates that the expression of PUMA is negatively regulated by the expression of miR-125b (Fig. 6C). Similar analyses of PUMA, Neu1 and *BAK1* expression were performed for the Panc-1 and Panc-1ΔmiR-125b cells. These data suggests that the PUMA and Neu1 are functional targets of miR-125b and based on their known functions likely play a role in regulating CRMP (Fig. 6D, E).

Discussion

Recent evidence indicates a link between chemoresistance and metastatic potential of cancer cells that possess an EMT phenotype and express stem cell markers [36]. Other studies indicate that expression pattern of specific miRNAs regulate expression of genes involved in chemoresistance and metastatic potential [10,37,38]. To further investigate the role of miRNAs in regulating the chemoresistant and mesenchymal phenotype (CRMP), we developed a PDAC cell line model (BxPC3-GZR) of CRMP and compared its miRNA expression profile with that of an isogenically matched parental cell line (BxPC3) that possesses an epithelial phenotype. Based on q-RT-PCR validation and potential relevance to cancer we selected a molecular signature

of six miRNAs that were differentially expressed in BxPC3-GZR (four with increased expression and two with decreased expression). Finally, we compared this miRNA signature with miRNA expression and gene expression of 43 advanced PDAC clinical specimens and normal pancreas tissue from the TCGA database.

To develop a chemoresistant cell line model, BxPC3 cells were transiently exposed to increasing doses of gemcitabine over a six weeks time period. In agreement with a previous study [15], the selection of a more chemoresistant cancer cell population (BxPC3-GZR) was associated with EMT and stem cell-like properties (Fig. 1). To our knowledge this is the first study to identify a miRNA signature associated with a gemcitabine induced CRMP in PDAC. Our original eight miRNA signature validated by qPCR showed that miR-125b, miR-155, miR-100, miR-21 were up regulated and miR-1246, miR-205, miR-27b, miR455-3p were down regulated. In another study miRNA profiles were compared between a PDAC cell line that is drug resistant with a cell line that is more sensitive. In that study miR-21 was shown to be up regulated and miR-200b, miR-200c, let-7b, let-7c, let-7d, and let-7e were dramatically down regulated in gemcitabine resistant cells [39]. In agreement with this previous study we showed that miR-21 is significantly up regulated in BxPC3-GZR, our CRMP model. Further, miRNAs of the miR-200 family (miR-200a, b, c, miR-141 and miR-429) and miR-205 have been identified as key negative regulators of both EMT and the metastatic potential of cancer cells. The miR-200 family targets the key regulators of EMT including Zeb1 and Sip1 (also known as Zeb2), leading to increased E-cadherin expression levels [40,41].

MiR-125b that is over-expressed in BxPC3-GZR model was recently reported to play a role in chemoresistance in breast cancer and as a biomarker for screening non-small-cell lung cancer as well as a diagnostic or prognostic biomarker for advanced NSCLC patients receiving cisplatin-based chemotherapy [42–44]. This latter finding prompted us to further assess the role of miR-125b in regulating the CRMP in BxPC3-GZR model.

We sought to establish whether this miRNA signature associated with the CRMP could differentiate distinct subpopulations of cells in clinical specimens by assessing the miRNA expression profile from 43 clinical pancreatic cancer specimens from the TGCA database. Five of the six miRNAs (four up regulated and two down regulated) showed similar levels of

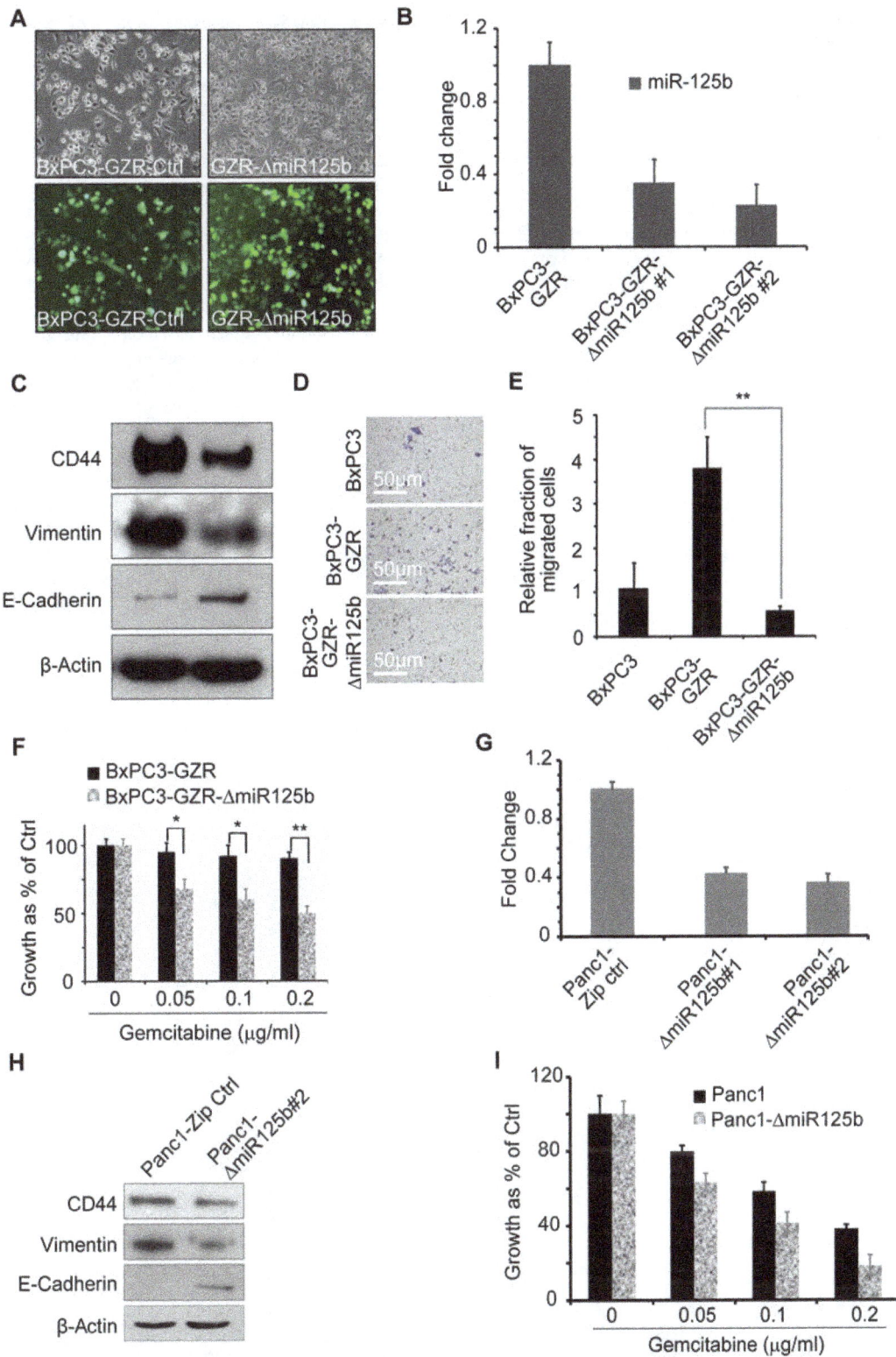

Figure 4. Knockdown of micro-RNA-125 reverses the mesenchymal phenotype and increases the drug sensitivity in BxPC3-GZR cells. A. Establish the Lenti-viral based stable cells expressing anti-miR-125b in BxPC3-GZR (Zip-control and miR-125b knock-down). **B.** TaqMan qPCR assays showing the knockdown of miR-125b in BxPC3-GZR-Zip ctrl cells compared to BxPC3-GZRΔmiR-125b cells. **C.** Expression of anti-miR-125b (Zip technology, SBI) decreases the expression of EMT and stemness marker monitored by Western bolt assays. Panels **D** and **E** show the attenuation of cell migration by knocking down miR-125b expression. Images were taken after crystal violet staining of migrated cells and the data was plotted as a graph (Bar = 50 μm). **F.** Knockdown of miR-125b increases response to gemcitabine. BxPC3-GZR-ZiP-Ctrl and BxPC3-GZRΔmiR-125b cells were treated with gemcitabine at different concentrations and the MTT assays were performed after 96 hours of treatment. **G.** Knockdown of miR-125b in Panc-1 cells. Lenti-viral based stable cells were generated to inhibit miR-125b expression (Zip technology,). TaqMan qPCR assays were performed to measure the expression of miR-125b in Zip-control Panc-1 cells and knock down cells (Panc-1 ΔmiR-125b). **H.** Inhibiting miR-125b decreases CD44 and

vimentin expression while up regulating the expression of E-cadherin. **I.** Knockdown of miR-125b increases the response of Panc-1 to gemcitabine. MTT assays were done after 96 hours of gemcitabine treatment. Statistical significance values *p<0.05 and **p<0.01 were calculated using student's T-tests.

deregulation in the advanced PDAC tumor specimens compared to normal pancreas tissues (Fig. 2). Only miR-155 that was up regulated in the BxPC3-GZR model showed a more equal distribution of being either up or down regulated in the tumor specimens. Out of the 43-pancreatic cancer specimens, miR-100, miR-125b (isoform 1 and 2), and miR-21 was over expressed in 41, 39 and 31 tumor specimens, respectively. Of the two miRNAs down regulated in BxPC3-GZR, analyses of the clinical specimens showed that miR-27b and miR-455 were down regulated in 36 and 32 specimens, respectively (*Table 2*). The results clearly suggest a commonality in the deregulation of five of the six miRNAs found in the BxPC3-GZR model with advanced human PDAC specimens. Future studies will be needed to determine whether this five-miRNA profile is related to patient survival or response to therapy. Moreover, these five miRNAs or their target genes may have potential as novel therapeutic targets.

Because of the broad range of possible roles of miR-125b in oncogenesis and since there are limited studies of this miRNA in PDAC, we chose to further determine its functional significance in relation to CRMP. Interestingly, screening of additional PDAC cell lines showed that miR-125b correlated directly with an EMT

phenotype (Fig. 3 and 4). Inhibiting the expression of miR-125b partially reversed the EMT phenotype, reduced the invasiveness and partially restored response to gemcitabine suggesting a direct role for miR-125b in maintenance of the CRMP. This result is consistent with the recent finding that miR-125b plays a role in chemoresistance of breast cancer [45,46]. However, other studies suggest a role for miR-125b as tumor suppressor in cancers of the ovary, bladder and breast, as well as in hepatocellular carcinoma, melanoma, squamous cell carcinoma and osteosarcoma [31], [47,48]. In contrast to the tumor-suppressive properties mentioned above, the members of miR-125 family, especially miR-125b, also act as oncogene in several cancers including prostate cancer [31,49].

Targeting miR-125b has potential to reverse the CRMP. As mentioned above, miR-125b is deregulated in many differentiated cancer cells. For example, among 328 known and 152 novel human microRNAs, miR-125b was one of the most down-regulated microRNAs in prostate cancer [13]. Our present data demonstrated that in PDAC cells miR-125b is up regulated in both EMT and chemoresistance phenomena by attenuating expression of PUMA and Neu-1.

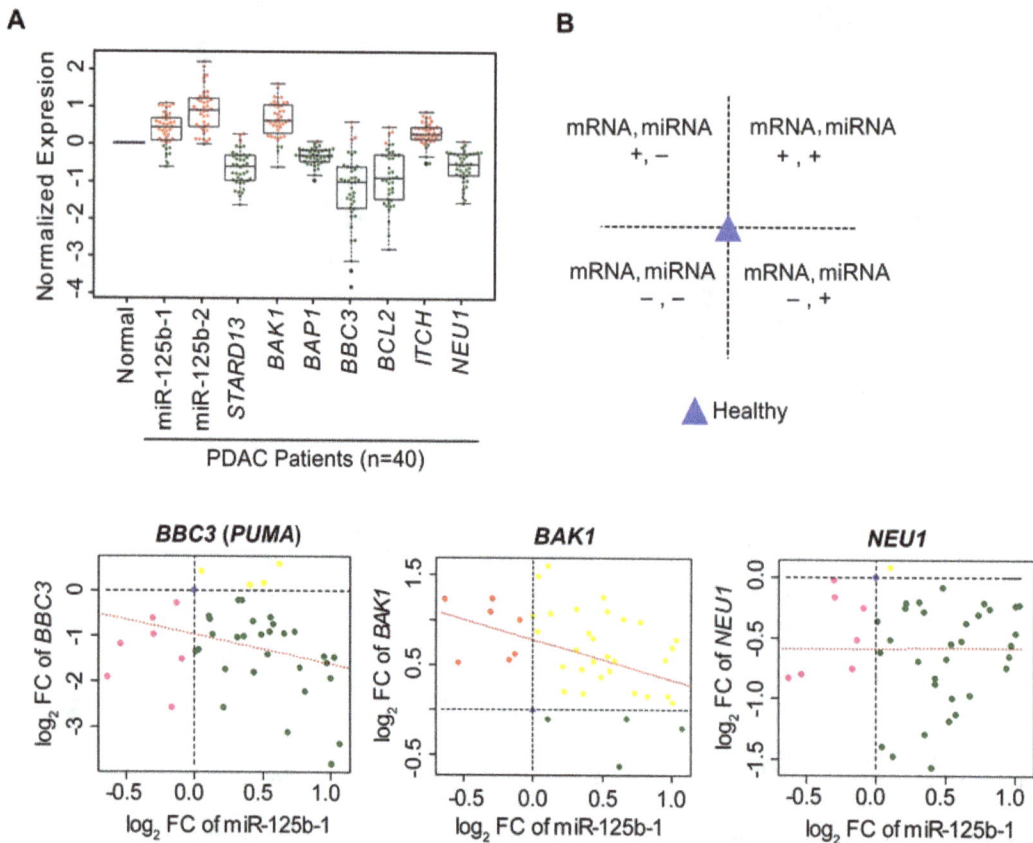

Figure 5. Gene targets of miR-125b. TCGA data analyses were performed with the clinical pancreatic tumor specimens (n = 40) for miRNA expression with the corresponding target mRNAs. A. Target mRNA expression profile analyses for miR-125b. Determined the expression of known miR-125b targets (*BBC3* (PUMA), *BCL2, STARD13, BAK1, BAP1, ITCH* and *NEU1*). **B.** A direct co-relation of the target mRNA and miR-125b expression level were measured in the same tumor from pancreatic adenocarcinoma [PDAC] patient's sample. First panel explains the different quadrants which includes up-regulation (+ Ve sign) or down regulation (- Ve sign) of mRNA and miRNA expression levels. Other panels are representing expression level of different mRNA (*BBC3, Neu1 and BAK1*) compared with the expression of miR-125b in the same tumor.

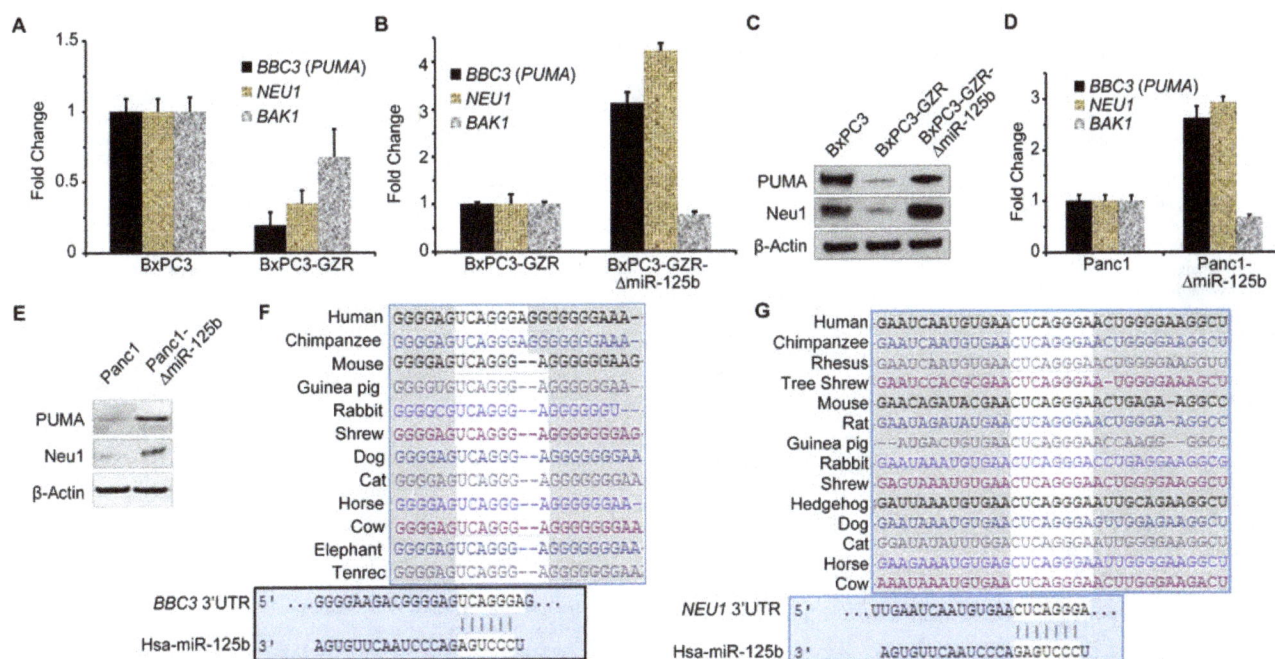

Figure 6. Validation of miR-125b target genes by qPCR and Western blot assays. A. PUMA (*BBC3*) and Neu1 are most prominent mRNA targets of miR-125b. The TaqMan qPCR analyses were performed to validate clinical data. The qPCR results indicating the expression level of different mRNA (*BBC3, Neu1 and BAK1*) which are direct target of miR-125b compared between BxPC3 parental cells and resistant GZR cells. **B.** Comparison of mRNA expression level of *BBC3, Neu1 and BAK1* in BxPC3-GZR cells and stable BxPC3-GZR cells expressing anti-miR-125b. **C.** Western blots analysis to monitor the expression level of PUMA and Neu1 in BxPC3, BxPC3-GZR, and miR-125b knockdown cells. **D** and **E**. Inhibiting miR-125b restores BBC3 and Neu-1 expression in Panc-1 cells, qPCR (D) and Western blot (E). **F, G**. Species conservation and matching of the seed sequence in 3'UTR of *BBC3* and *NEU1* mRNAs with miR-125b sequence were monitored by using Targetscan free web-based software.

PUMA is known to be important in chemotherapy induced apoptosis suggesting that down regulation of PUMA promotes chemoresistance [50]. Luciferase assay including rescue experiments with mutated seed sequence of 3'UTR of PUMA was used to establish the direct involvement of miR-125b to target mRNA of PUMA and represses its expression [28,49]. Neu1 plays an important role in regulating invasion and metastasis in different cancer types including human colon cancer and is reported to be a direct target of miR-125b [49]. A negative correlation was observed in invasion with the over-expression of Neu1 [34]. Our present data indicate that knockdown of miR-125b expression induced the up-regulation of Neu1 expression. A study in colon cancer indicates that it is a tumor suppressor gene and plays role in reducing invasive phenotype [34]. However, a separate study indicates that Neu1 facilitates EGFR signaling in pancreatic cancer and thus could have a tumor promoting effect [35]. Thus further studies are needed to weigh the effects of Neu1 effects on inhibiting invasion versus its role in EGFR signaling.

In summary we identified a set of six miRNAs that are deregulated in a PDAC model of CRMP. Analyses of 43 clinical specimens of PDAC from the TCGA data set revealed that five of the six miRNAs were commonly also deregulated in PDAC. One of the miRNAs, miR-125b, was further studied on the bases of its potential role in chemoresistance and inhibiting the expression of miR-125b partially reversed the EMT phenotype and enhanced response to chemotherapy. In addition, we found that several miR-125b target genes were down regulated and two of these *BBC3* (PUMA) and Neu1 are known tumor suppressors. We further found that knockdown of miR-125b restored the expression of PUMA and Neu1 and partially reversed CRMP. The present study identified a set of five miRNAs that are deregulated in PDAC cells showing a CRMP and in advanced PDAC tumor specimens. These miRNAs or their molecular targets may serve as the basis of new therapeutic strategies for overcoming gemcitabine resistance.

Supporting Information

Figure S1 Response of BxPC3 and BxPC3-GZR cells to paclitaxel were compared by MTT assays. Cells were treated with indicated concentrations of paclitaxel and MTT assays were performed after 96 hours. A graph of the data shows only a modest reduction of sensitivity of BxPC3-GZR cells to paclitaxel as compared to control BxPC3 cells. Bars represent mean +/−SE.

Author Contributions

Conceived and designed the experiments: JWF AB MSM KV. Performed the experiments: AB KV MSM PH. Analyzed the data: JWF AB MSM KV. Contributed reagents/materials/analysis tools: JWF MSM. Contributed to the writing of the manuscript: AB JWF KV.

References

1. Siegel R, Naishadham D, Jemal A (2013) Cancer statistics, 2013. CA Cancer J Clin 63: 11–30.

2. Beumer JH, Eiseman JL, Parise RA, Joseph E, Covey JM, et al. (2008) Modulation of gemcitabine (2′,2′-difluoro-2′-deoxycytidine) pharmacokinetics,

metabolism, and bioavailability in mice by 3,4,5,6-tetrahydrouridine. Clin Cancer Res 14: 3529–3535.

3. Wang Z, Li Y, Ahmad A, Banerjee S, Azmi AS, et al. (2011) Pancreatic cancer: understanding and overcoming chemoresistance. Nat Rev Gastroenterol Hepatol 8: 27–33.

4. Ricci-Vitiani L, Lombardi DG, Pilozzi E, Biffoni M, Todaro M, et al. (2007) Identification and expansion of human colon-cancer-initiating cells. Nature 445: 111–115.

5. Van den Broeck A, Gremeaux L, Topal B, Vankelecom H (2012) Human pancreatic adenocarcinoma contains a side population resistant to gemcitabine. BMC Cancer 12: 354.

6. Thiery JP (2003) Epithelial-mesenchymal transitions in development and pathologies. Curr Opin Cell Biol 15: 740–746.

7. Derynck R, Akhurst RJ, Balmain A (2001) TGF-beta signaling in tumor suppression and cancer progression. Nat Genet 29: 117–129.

8. Singh A, Settleman J (2010) EMT, cancer stem cells and drug resistance: an emerging axis of evil in the war on cancer. Oncogene 29: 4741–4751.

9. Liu C, Kelnar K, Vlassov AV, Brown D, Wang J, et al. (2012) Distinct microRNA expression profiles in prostate cancer stem/progenitor cells and tumor-suppressive functions of let-7. Cancer Res 72: 3393–3404.

10. Singh S, Chitkara D, Mehrazin R, Behrman SW, Wake RW, et al. (2012) Chemoresistance in prostate cancer cells is regulated by miRNAs and Hedgehog pathway. PLoS One 7: e40021.

11. Danquah M, Singh S, Behrman SW, Mahato RI (2012) Role of miRNA and cancer stem cells in chemoresistance and pancreatic cancer treatment. Expert Opin Drug Deliv 9: 1443–1447.

12. Korpal M, Lee ES, Hu G, Kang Y (2008) The miR-200 family inhibits epithelial-mesenchymal transition and cancer cell migration by direct targeting of E-cadherin transcriptional repressors ZEB1 and ZEB2. J Biol Chem 283: 14910–14914.

13. Ozen M, Creighton CJ, Ozdemir M, Ittmann M (2008) Widespread deregulation of microRNA expression in human prostate cancer. Oncogene 27: 1788–1793.

14. Park SM, Gaur AB, Lengyel E, Peter ME (2008) The miR-200 family determines the epithelial phenotype of cancer cells by targeting the E-cadherin repressors ZEB1 and ZEB2. Genes Dev 22: 894–907.

15. Wang Z, Li Y, Kong D, Banerjee S, Ahmad A, et al. (2009) Acquisition of epithelial-mesenchymal transition phenotype of gemcitabine-resistant pancreatic cancer cells is linked with activation of the notch signaling pathway. Cancer Res 69: 2400–2407.

16. Singh S, Chitkara D, Kumar V, Behrman SW, Mahato RI (2013) miRNA profiling in pancreatic cancer and restoration of chemosensitivity. Cancer Lett 334: 211–220.

17. Zhao S, Ammanamanchi S, Brattain M, Cao L, Thangasamy A, et al. (2008) Smad4-dependent TGF-beta signaling suppresses RON receptor tyrosine kinase-dependent motility and invasion of pancreatic cancer cells. J Biol Chem 283: 11293–11301.

18. Bera A, Zhao S, Cao L, Chiao PJ, Freeman JW (2013) Oncogenic K-Ras and loss of Smad4 mediate invasion by activating an EGFR/NF-kappaB Axis that induces expression of MMP9 and uPA in human pancreas progenitor cells. PLoS One 8: e82282.

19. Venkatasubbarao K, Choudary A, Freeman JW (2005) Farnesyl transferase inhibitor (R115777)-induced inhibition of STAT3(Tyr705) phosphorylation in human pancreatic cancer cell lines require extracellular signal-regulated kinases. Cancer Res 65: 2861–2871.

20. Hu HY, Guo S, Xi J, Yan Z, Fu N, et al. (2011) MicroRNA expression and regulation in human, chimpanzee, and macaque brains. PLoS Genet 7: e1002327.

21. Hamfjord J, Stangeland AM, Hughes T, Skrede ML, Tveit KM, et al. (2012) Differential expression of miRNAs in colorectal cancer: comparison of paired tumor tissue and adjacent normal mucosa using high-throughput sequencing. PLoS One 7: e34150.

22. Anders S, Huber W (2010) Differential expression analysis for sequence count data. Genome Biol 11: R106.

23. Niess H, Camaj P, Renner A, Ischenko I, Zhao Y, et al. (2014) Side population cells of pancreatic cancer show characteristics of cancer stem cells responsible for resistance and metastasis. Target Oncol. DOI 10.1007/s11523-014-0323-z

24. Dong J, Zhao YP, Zhou L, Zhang TP, Chen G (2011) Bcl-2 upregulation induced by miR-21 via a direct interaction is associated with apoptosis and chemoresistance in MIA PaCa-2 pancreatic cancer cells. Arch Med Res 42: 8–14.

25. Kent OA, Mendell JT (2006) A small piece in the cancer puzzle: microRNAs as tumor suppressors and oncogenes. Oncogene 25: 6188–6196.

26. Cochrane DR, Spoelstra NS, Howe EN, Nordeen SK, Richer JK (2009) MicroRNA-200c mitigates invasiveness and restores sensitivity to microtubule-targeting chemotherapeutic agents. Mol Cancer Ther 8: 1055–1066.

27. Nakanishi H, Taccioli C, Palatini J, Fernandez-Cymering C, Cui R, et al. (2014) Loss of miR-125b-1 contributes to head and neck cancer development by dysregulating TACSTD2 and MAPK pathway. Oncogene 33: 702–712.

28. Le MT, Shyh-Chang N, Khaw SL, Chin L, Teh C, et al. (2011) Conserved regulation of p53 network dosage by microRNA-125b occurs through evolving miRNA-target gene pairs. PLoS Genet 7: e1002242.

29. Le MT, Xie H, Zhou B, Chia PH, Rizk P, et al. (2009) MicroRNA-125b promotes neuronal differentiation in human cells by repressing multiple targets. Mol Cell Biol 29: 5290–5305.

30. Tang F, Zhang R, He Y, Zou M, Guo L, et al. (2012) MicroRNA-125b induces metastasis by targeting STARD13 in MCF-7 and MDA-MB-231 breast cancer cells. PLoS One 7: e35435.

31. Yang S, Sun W, Zhang F, Li Z (2013) Phylogenetically diverse denitrifying and ammonia-oxidizing bacteria in corals Alcyonium gracillimum and Tubastraea coccinea. Mar Biotechnol (NY) 15: 540–551.

32. Nakano K, Vousden KH (2001) PUMA, a novel proapoptotic gene, is induced by p53. Mol Cell 7: 683–694.

33. Yu J, Zhang L (2008) PUMA, a potent killer with or without p53. Oncogene 27 Suppl 1: S71–83.

34. Uemura T, Shiozaki K, Yamaguchi K, Miyazaki S, Satomi S, et al. (2009) Contribution of sialidase NEU1 to suppression of metastasis of human colon cancer cells through desialylation of integrin beta4. Oncogene 28: 1218–1229.

35. O'Shea LK, Abdulkhalek S, Allison S, Neufeld RJ, Szewczuk MR (2014) Therapeutic targeting of Neu1 sialidase with oseltamivir phosphate (Tamiflu(R)) disables cancer cell survival in human pancreatic cancer with acquired chemoresistance. Onco Targets Ther 7: 117–134.

36. Collins AT, Maitland NJ (2006) Prostate cancer stem cells. Eur J Cancer 42: 1213–1218.

37. Song B, Wang Y, Xi Y, Kudo K, Bruheim S, et al. (2009) Mechanism of chemoresistance mediated by miR-140 in human osteosarcoma and colon cancer cells. Oncogene 28: 4065–4074.

38. Vecchione A, Belletti B, Lovat F, Volinia S, Chiappetta G, et al. (2013) A microRNA signature defines chemoresistance in ovarian cancer through modulation of angiogenesis. Proc Natl Acad Sci U S A 110: 9845–9850.

39. Li Y, VandenBoom TG, 2nd, Kong D, Wang Z, Ali S, et al. (2009) Up-regulation of miR-200 and let-7 by natural agents leads to the reversal of epithelial-to-mesenchymal transition in gemcitabine-resistant pancreatic cancer cells. Cancer Res 69: 6704–6712.

40. Ebert MS, Neilson JR, Sharp PA (2007) MicroRNA sponges: competitive inhibitors of small RNAs in mammalian cells. Nat Methods 4: 721–726.

41. Peter ME (2009) Let-7 and miR-200 microRNAs: guardians against pluripotency and cancer progression. Cell Cycle 8: 843–852.

42. Cui EH, Li HJ, Hua F, Wang B, Mao W, et al. (2013) Serum microRNA 125b as a diagnostic or prognostic biomarker for advanced NSCLC patients receiving cisplatin-based chemotherapy. Acta Pharmacol Sin 34: 309–313.

43. Wang H, Tan G, Dong L, Cheng L, Li K, et al. (2012) Circulating MiR-125b as a marker predicting chemoresistance in breast cancer. PLoS One 7: e34210.

44. Yuxia M, Zhennan T, Wei Z (2012) Circulating miR-125b is a novel biomarker for screening non-small-cell lung cancer and predicts poor prognosis. J Cancer Res Clin Oncol 138: 2045–2050.

45. Wang L, Zhang D, Zhang C, Zhang S, Wang Z, et al. (2012) A microRNA expression signature characterizing the properties of tumor-initiating cells for breast cancer. Oncol Lett 3: 119–124.

46. Akhavantabasi S, Sapmaz A, Tuna S, Erson-Bensan AE (2012) miR-125b targets ARID3B in breast cancer cells. Cell Struct Funct 37: 27–38.

47. Scott GK, Goga A, Bhaumik D, Berger CE, Sullivan CS, et al. (2007) Coordinate suppression of ERBB2 and ERBB3 by enforced expression of micro-RNA miR-125a or miR-125b. J Biol Chem 282: 1479–1486.

48. Huang L, Luo J, Cai Q, Pan Q, Zeng H, et al. (2011) MicroRNA-125b suppresses the development of bladder cancer by targeting E2F3. Int J Cancer 128: 1758–1769.

49. Shi XB, Xue L, Ma AH, Tepper CG, Kung HJ, et al. (2011) miR-125b promotes growth of prostate cancer xenograft tumor through targeting pro-apoptotic genes. Prostate 71: 538–549.

50. Chen Y, Qian H, Wang H, Zhang X, Fu M, et al. (2007) Ad-PUMA sensitizes drug-resistant choriocarcinoma cells to chemotherapeutic agents. Gynecol Oncol 107: 505–512.

26

Comparison of Immunity in Mice Cured of Primary/Metastatic Growth of EMT6 or 4THM Breast Cancer by Chemotherapy or Immunotherapy

Reginald M. Gorczynski[1,2]*, Zhiqi Chen[1], Nuray Erin[3], Ismat Khatri[1], Anna Podnos[1]

1 University Health Network, Toronto General Hospital, Toronto, Canada, 2 Department of Immunology, Faculty of Medicine, University of Toronto, and Institute of Medical Science, University of Toronto, Toronto, Ontario, Canada, 3 Department of Medical Pharmacology, Akdeniz University, School of Medicine, Antalya, Turkey

Abstract

Purpose: We have compared cure from local/metastatic tumor growth in BALB/c mice receiving EMT6 or the poorly immunogenic, highly metastatic 4THM, breast cancer cells following manipulation of immunosuppressive CD200:CD200R interactions or conventional chemotherapy.

Methods: We reported previously that EMT6 tumors are cured in CD200R1KO mice following surgical resection and immunization with irradiated EMT6 cells and CpG oligodeoxynucleotide (CpG), while wild-type (WT) animals developed pulmonary and liver metastases within 30 days of surgery. We report growth and metastasis of both EMT6 and a highly metastatic 4THM tumor in WT mice receiving iv infusions of Fab anti-CD200R1 along with CpG/tumor cell immunization. Metastasis was followed both macroscopically (lung/liver nodules) and microscopically by cloning tumor cells at limiting dilution in vitro from draining lymph nodes (DLN) harvested at surgery. We compared these results with local/metastatic tumor growth in mice receiving 4 courses of combination treatment with anti-VEGF and paclitaxel.

Results: In WT mice receiving Fab anti-CD200R, no tumor cells are detectable following immunotherapy, and CD4+ cells produced increased TNFα/IL-2/IFNγ on stimulation with EMT6 in vitro. No long-term cure was seen following surgery/immunotherapy of 4THM, with both microscopic (tumors in DLN at limiting dilution) and macroscopic metastases present within 14 d of surgery. Chemotherapy attenuated growth/metastases in 4THM tumor-bearers and produced a decline in lung/liver metastases, with no detectable DLN metastases in EMT6 tumor-bearing mice-these latter mice nevertheless showed no significantly increased cytokine production after restimulation with EMT6 in vitro. EMT6 mice receiving immunotherapy were resistant to subsequent re-challenge with EMT6 tumor cells, but not those receiving curative chemotherapy. Anti-CD4 treatment caused tumor recurrence after immunotherapy, but produced no apparent effect in either EMT6 or 4THM tumor bearers after chemotherapy treatment.

Conclusion: Immunotherapy, but not chemotherapy, enhances CD4+ immunity and affords long-term control of breast cancer growth and resistance to new tumor foci.

Editor: Fabrizio Mattei, Istituto Superiore di Sanità, Italy

Funding: Supported by a grant (RG-11) to RMG from the Canadian Cancer Society (www.cancer.ca). The funders had no role in study design, data collection and analysis, decision to publish, or preparation of the manuscript.

Competing Interests: The authors have declared that no competing interests exist.

* Email: rgorczynski@uhnres.utoronto.ca

Introduction

The immunoregulatory molecule CD200 has been reported to regulate growth of human solid tumors [1,2] and hematological tumors [3–5]. Using a transplantable EMT6 mouse breast cancer line CD200 expression, by tumor cells or host, increased local tumor growth and metastasis to DLN [6,7], which was abolished by neutralizing antibody to CD200, or following growth in mice lacking the primary inhibitory receptor for CD200 (CD200R1KO mice). In contrast to these observations, growth of the highly metastatic 4THM breast tumor (derived from a 4T1 parent line) was increased in CD200R1KO mice, with somewhat diminished growth in CD200[tg] animals [8]. Surgical resection in CD200R1KO EMT6 tumor-bearing mice, followed by immunization with CpG as adjuvant, cured CD200R1KO mice of breast cancer recurrence in the absence of lung/liver metastases, and of micro metastases (defined by limiting dilution cloning in vitro) in DLN [9].

Multiple factors both intrinsic to tumor cells themselves and host associated elements are implicated in tumor metastasis [10–14]. Many such factors are associated with altering trafficking of either host inflammatory-type cells to the local tumor environment where they can facilitate metastasis through a variety of mechanisms [15–17], including regulation of host resistance mechanisms [18–21]. Metastatic tumor cells are known to undergo changes in gene expression profile leading to increased cancer stem cell- like properties and the ability to survive, establish and grow in a foreign environment [22–24]. Like CD200, an inhibitory member of the B7 family of T cell co stimulation, expression of another such molecule, B7× (B7-H4) has been reported to influence metastasis using 4T1 tumor cells and B7KO mice [25]. B7KO mice with 4T1 tumors, like CD200R1KO with EMT6, showed enhanced survival and a memory response to tumor re-challenge, which was correlated with decreased infiltration of immunosuppressive cells, including tumor-associated neutrophils, macrophages, and regulatory T cells, into tumor-bearing metastatic lung tissue [25]. CD200R1KO mice showed increased growth of 4THM tumors [24].

The studies below compared protection seen in surgically treated/immunized EMT6 or 4THM tumor injected WT mice with/without manipulation of CD200:CD200R interactions using Fab anti-CD200R, with attenuation of disease after surgical resection followed by chemotherapy.

Materials and Methods [9]

Ethics approval and animal use guidelines

This study was carried out in strict accordance with the recommendations of the Canadian council for Animal Care (CCAC). The protocol was approved by the Committee on the Ethical use of Animals for experimentation at the University Health Network (Permit Number:AUP.1.5). All surgery was performed under sodium pentobarbital anesthesia, and all efforts were made to minimize suffering.

Mice

CD200KO and CD200R1 knockout mice are described elsewhere [9]. WT BALB/c mice were from Jax Labs. All mice were housed 5/cage in an accredited facility at UHN. Female mice were used at 8 wk of age.

Monoclonal antibodies, and CpG deoxyoligonucleotide for adjuvant use, are described elsewhere [6,9,26]

Rabbit Fab anti-CD200R1 antibody was prepared using a commercial kit (Pierce Protein Products, Rockford, IL, USA) and rabbit IgG isolated by Cedarlane Labs (Hornby, Ontario, Canada), following immunization of rabbits with 500 μg mouse CD200R1 emulsified in Freund's Adjuvant. In independent studies (not shown) this antibody (1:1000 dilution) inhibited binding (FACS analysis) of FITC-labeled mouse CD200 to Hek cells transduced to over-express murine CD200R1.

EMT6 breast tumor cells, induction of tumor growth in BALB/c mice, and limiting dilution cultures to establish frequency of metastasis to draining lymph nodes (DLN) were as described earlier [9,26]

4THM tumors, a highly metastatic variant of 4T1, were derived by Erin et al as reported elsewhere [24].

Surgical resection and immunotherapy/chemotherapy of tumor-bearing mice [9]

Mice receiving 5×10^5 EMT6 or 1×10^5 4THM tumor cells injected into the mammary fat pad in 100 μl PBS underwent surgical resection 14–16 d later. For immunotherapy, mice received intraperitoneal immunization with 3×10^6 EMT6 (or 4THM) tumor cells (irradiated with 2500Rads) mixed with 100 ug CpG ODN (see above) in 100 μl PBS, emulsified with an equal

volume of Incomplete Freund's adjuvant, 2 days after surgery. Mice treated with chemotherapy post surgical resection, received 4 injections of paclitaxil intraperitoneally in 0.15 ml PBS (Taxol: 10 mg/Kg), beginning on the day of surgery, and at 21 day intervals thereafter. In addition, beginning on the day following surgery, and at 14 day intervals for a total of 6 injections, the same mice also received anti-VEGF (30 mg/Kg) iv in 0.3 ml PBS.

All animals were monitored ×3/week for weight loss and general health and sacrificed at the times indicated in individual experiments (>10% weight loss), with visible tumor colonies in the lung/liver enumerated. DLN cell suspensions were prepared from individual mice and cloned under limiting dilution in 96-well flat-bottomed microtitre plates to assess tumor colony formation [7]. Important variables measured were time post treatment to sacrifice, and tumor growth-note that aggressive uncontrolled tumor growth in some groups in individual experiments led to certain groups being sacrificed before others (see text).

Preparation of cells and cytotoxicity, proliferation and cytokine assays: see [9,26]

In brief, 5×10^6 splenocytes from mice treated as described in the text were stimulated in vitro in triplicate with 2×10^5 irradiated (2500Rads) tumor cells in 2 ml αMEM with 10% fetal calf serum. 100 μl aliquots of supernatants were assayed at 48 hr for various cytokines using commercial kits (BioLegend, San Diego, USA). Cells were harvested from cultures at 6 d, washed ×2, and incubated for 18 hr with 1×10^3 ^{3}HTdR-labelled tumor target cells at varying effector:target ratios to determine direct anti-tumor cytotoxicity.

Statistics

Cloneable tumor cell frequency was determined as before [6]. Within experiments, comparison between groups used ANOVA, with subsequent paired Student's t-tests as indicated.

Results

Surgical resection followed by immunization along with Fab anti-CD200R, or chemotherapy alone, prevents metastasis of EMT6, but not 4THM, in BALB/c mice

Surgical resection of a primary tumor in CD200R1KO mice followed by immunization prevented macroscopic lung/liver metastases enumerated at 90 d post tumor inoculation, compared with surgery alone [9]. As shown in Figure 1 (data pooled from 2 independent studies) no protection was seen in wild type (WT) mice Figure 1, panel a), but WT mice were cured if given Fab anti-CD200R following surgery/immunization (panel b). Note that aggressive tumor growth led to WT control mice having to be sacrificed within 18 d or 21 d of surgery (panels a/b), unlike immunotherapy-treated mice receiving anti-CD200R (panel b) where mice were able to be followed for ≥90 d post surgery. When mice in this latter group were sacrificed earlier (18–21 d post surgery) again no lung/liver colonies were observed (not shown, but note no colonies at 90 d). Both CD200R1KO and WT mice showed no evidence of macroscopic metastases following chemotherapy instead of immunotherapy post surgery (Figure 1, panels c/d respectively). Again note that addition of chemotherapy treatment allowed mice to be monitored for tumor metastases (90 d post surgery) much longer than non-chemotherapy controls (21 and 18 d in panels c, d respectively-however, in studies where chemotherapy mice were deliberately sacrificed early, no metastases were observed on days 18/21 (not shown-but note data for 90 d). In mice receiving 4THM tumors, attenuation of lung/liver metastasis was achieved using surgery+chemotherapy, but not by surgery followed by immunotherapy (see Figure 1, panels e and f respectively). Failure of immunotherapy to protect from 4THM tumors again led to these mice (panel e) being sacrificed much earlier (10 d post surgery) than with EMT6 mice (panels a–d) or 4THM mice receiving chemotherapy (panel f). Once again, in studies where chemotherapy-treated 4THM injected mice were sacrificed at 10 d post surgery, no metastases were seen (not

shown-but seen marked attenuation of metastases even at 90 d in panel f).

DLN cell suspensions of mice sacrificed at the times shown in Figure 1 were cultured under limiting dilution conditions with cultures monitored over a 21-day period for colony growth, to enumerate the frequency of tumor cells in the initial DLN samples (Figure 2: panel a shows data for EMT6 tumors, panel b for 4THM) [7]. Data to the far left in each panel show the frequency of tumor cells cloned from DLN of mice sacrificed on the day of

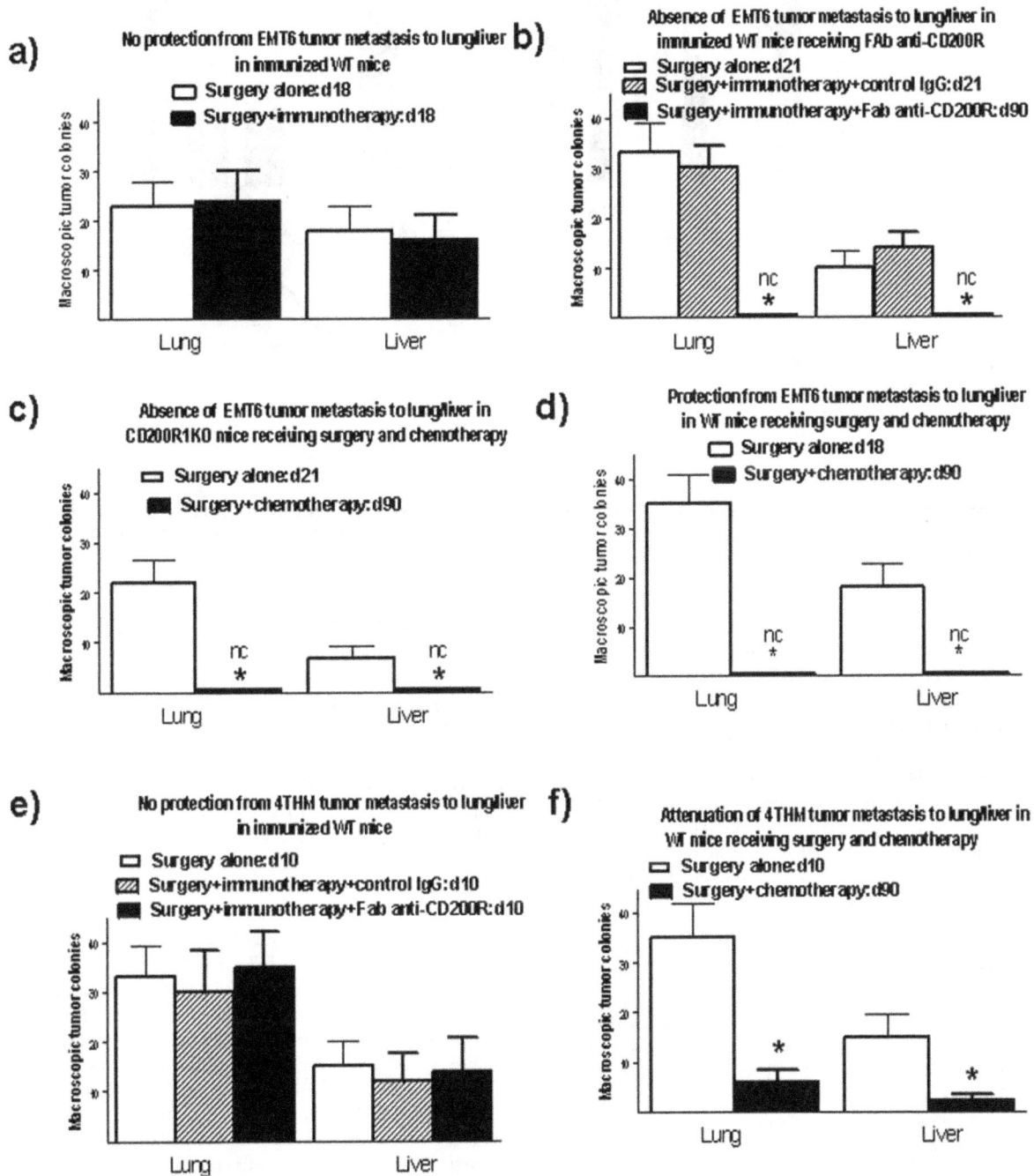

Figure 1. Comparison of lung and liver metastases of tumor cells in WT BALB/c mice receiving EMT6 or 4THM tumor cells and subsequently treated with surgical resection and chemotherapy/immunotherapy (see)Methods. 4 mice were used per group, with mice sacrificed at the times show post surgery (number above histogram bars) to measure macroscopic tumor metastases in the lung/liver. All data represent arithmetic means (±SD) for each group. nc indicates no metastatic colonies detected; *, p<0.05 relative to similar group receiving either immunotherapy or chemotherapy.

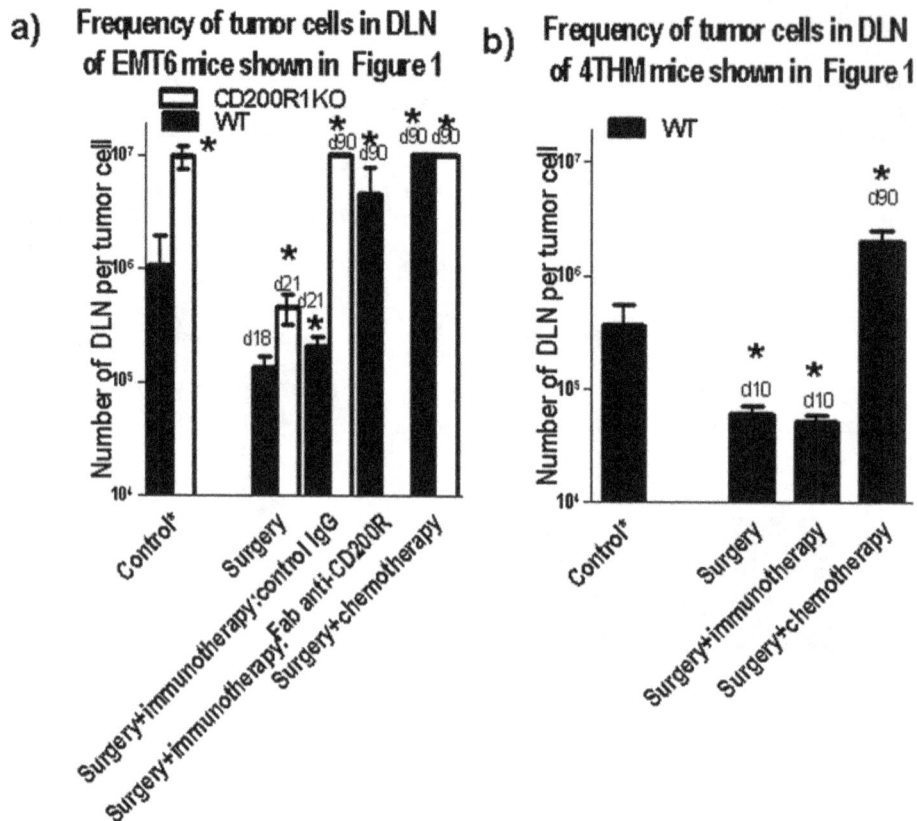

Figure 2. Attenuation of outgrowth of tumor from DLN of mice shown in Figure 1 as assessed by limiting dilution frequency (see Methods). DLN cells from separate mice were also cloned alone at the time of surgery (data to far left of each panel-control*). All frequencies were calculated based on the input numbers of cells from DLN of control mice only. *, p<0.05 compared with control* mice

tumor resection. Cells in all clones were stained (~100% positive) with anti-BTAK (anti-tumor) antibody (data not shown-see [7]).

The frequency of tumor cells cloned from DLN of both WT and CD200R1KO EMT6-injected mice treated only by surgical resection increased over 18–21 d post resection, relative to the frequency seen in DLN at the time of surgical resection (panel a). Surgical resection followed by immunotherapy and control IgG led to little decrease in the DLN tumor frequency in WT mice sacrificed at 21 d post surgery. Fab anti-CD200R along with surgery/immunization resulted in a marked decrease (>7x) in tumor cells cloned from DLN of WT mice (d90). In similarly treated CD200R1KO mice no tumor cells were detected (detection limits in assay ~1 in 1×10^7) at 90 d post surgery. No detectable tumor cells could be cloned from DLN of either WT or CD200R1KO mice 90 d post surgery if animals received chemotherapy following surgical resection (data to far right in Figure 2a). In 4THM tumor-bearers (panel b), sacrifice of mice 10 d after surgery with either no additional treatment, or immunotherapy (CpG+ irradiated 4THM), indicated an increase (~8x) in frequency of cloned tumor cells in DLN compared with the numbers present at the time of surgery. Surgery followed by chemotherapy decreased the number of cloned tumor cells at d90 (far right in Figure 2b).

In separate studies (not shown), no WT or CD200R1KO mice survived following treatment with surgery and anti-VEGF alone, and survival with paclitaxil as the sole chemotherapeutic agent was ≤50% of that seen using the combination shown, in both CD200R1KO and WT mice with each tumor used. Combined surgery and chemotherapy "cured" WT mice of EMT6 tumor

growth, as defined by an absence of macroscopic metastases at 300 d post surgery, and undetectable tumor cells cloned from DLN of mice at this time (limits of detection ~1 in 2×10^7 DLN cells)-see also [9]. All 4THM mice treated in this fashion died before110days post surgery (data not shown).

Absence of cells attenuating ability to clone tumor from DLN of mice receiving chemotherapy

Figure S1 investigated whether DLN of either immunotherapy- or chemotherapy-treated WT mice contained populations of cells which non-specifically attenuated growth of tumor cells, leading to inaccurate estimation of tumor cell frequency in limiting dilution [9]. Groups of 5WT mice were treated as in Figure 1 with EMT6 or 4THM tumor cells, followed by surgical resection and combined chemotherapy with anti-VEGF and paclitaxil. Mice were sacrificed 90 days post surgery. DLN cells from WT mice receiving either EMT6 or 4THM tumor cells 14d earlier (WT* in Figure S1) were cultured under limiting dilution conditions (from 2×10^3 to 1×10^5 cells/well) alone, or with a five-fold excess of DLN cells from the 90d chemotherapy-treated mice (from 1×10^4 to 5×10^5). Cells from these WT or CD200R1KO mice were also cloned alone. All tumor cells frequencies were subsequently calculated based on the input numbers of control cells only. Data shown in this Figure are pooled from 3 separate studies.

The frequency of detected tumor cells in the mice at 90 d post combined surgery/chemotherapy was below the limits of detection in this assay (see data to far right in each of the EMT6/4THM groups of Figure S1). Addition of a 5-fold excess of cells from the

DLN of these populations **did not** alter the measured frequency of cloneable tumor cells from DLN of WT* mice sacrificed at 14 d post tumor injection.

CD4+ cells in immunotherapy-treated, but not in chemotherapy-treated mice, are responsible for decreased metastasis

Protection (in CD200KO or CD200R1KO mice) was not related to a direct immune response from recipient mice to CD200 expressed on tumor cells themselves [9,25]. CD200/CD200R is not expressed on 4THM tumors, and thus an immune response to such tumor-bearing epitopes could not explain the differences observed above. Immunotherapy of EMT6 tumor growth was abolished by infusion of anti-CD4 mAb [9]. To investigate whether an active CD4-dependent immune process was implicated in protection afforded by (surgery + chemotherapy) we performed the following study.

Groups of 30 WT mice received EMT6 or 4THM cells into the mammary fat pad, followed by surgical resection. 5 mice/group received no further treatment. Two subgroups of 15 mice each then received either combination chemotherapy, or immunotherapy with irradiated tumor cells, CpG and Fab anti-CD00R. 10 d after immunotherapy/chemotherapy was initiated 5mice/group began a course of anti-CD4mAb or control IgG injections (3 injections of 75 µg in 300 µlPBS at 72 hr intervals iv). Mice were monitored for overall health, with sacrifice of all mice when there was evidence of respiratory distress and/or weight loss (10%) in any individual. Note that in the case of 4THM mice not receiving chemotherapy, this necessitated sacrifice at 10 d post surgery, while for EMT6 control mice, or EMT6 mice receiving immunotherapy and anti-CD4 treatment, this necessitated sacrifice at18, 26 d post surgery respectively (see also text to Figure 1 above). All surviving mice were terminated at 90 d post surgery, and macroscopic liver/lung metastases determined, along with frequency of tumor cells in DLN (see Figure 2). In addition (see Figure S2), splenocytes from individual mice were stimulated in vitro with irradiated tumor cells for 6 d, with cytokine production measured (48 hr) and CTL assayed at 6 days, as described in the Methods. Data for 1 of 3 such studies are shown in Figure 3.

Macroscopically visible metastases in lung/liver (Figure 3a), along with increased frequency of tumor cells cloned from DLN (Figure 3b), was seen in EMT6 tumor injected mice receiving immunotherapy and anti-CD4 relative to mice receiving control Ig (see also [9])-as noted in Figure 1, where other immunotherapy-treated (but no anti-CD4) EMT6 groups were sacrificed at d18/26 (not 90 d as shown) there were, as expected, no metastases seen. Also as noted in Figure 1, immunotherapy afforded no protection from 4THM growth, regardless of subsequent anti-CD4 treatment, and these mice had to be sacrificed early in the study (10 d post surgery, by comparison to chemotherapy-treated mice, sacrificed at 90 d post surgery). In contrast to these data, following both EMT6 and 4THM tumor injection, the protection from macroscopic (lung/liver) and microscopic (DLN) metastases afforded by chemotherapy was apparently resistant to anti-CD4mAb therapy (Figure 3a/b). In separate studies (not shown) no affect was seen after infusion of anti-CD8 mAb into chemotherapy treated mice either. These in vivo studies need to be seen in the context of data from Figure S2, showing elevated cytotoxicity (CD4+-dependent) only using splenocytes from immunotherapy-treated EMT6 tumor-injected mice (panel b), while in turn CD4+ cells from these same mice produced increased cytokines (TNFα, IL-2 and IFNγ) relative to mice receiving surgery alone. Note that in the cytotoxicity assay used in Figure

S2b, killing itself was a function of CD8+ cells in all groups (data not shown).

Resistance to implantation of fresh EMT6, but not 4THM, tumor in immunotherapy-treated EMT6-injected mice, but not in chemotherapy-treated EMT6/4THM-injected mice

The data in Figure 3 show that cure of both EMT6- and 4THM-injected mice of macroscopic and microscopic (DLN) tumor metastases following surgical resection and chemotherapy is resistant to anti-CD4 treatment, unlike mice cured of EMT6 tumor following surgery and immunotherapy. We next investigated resistance to fresh tumor implants of the same or different tumor in mice cured following immunotherapy/chemotherapy.

Groups of mice receiving EMT6/4THM tumors underwent surgical resection, followed by either chemotherapy (for all of 15 4THM- and 15 EMT6-injected mice) or immunotherapy (15 EMT6- injected mice). 90 d post surgical resection, with all animals free of obvious tumor growth and gaining weight, 5 mice/group, and 5 fresh mice, received either 5×10^5 EMT6 or 1×10^5 4THM tumors in the contralateral mammary fat pad to that used previously. Primary tumor growth was followed daily for all mice, and animals sacrificed 20 d later, with DLN harvested to assess tumor cells by limiting dilution. Data in Figure 4 show results (1 of 2 studies) for this experiment. None of the mice not receiving further tumor inoculation developed overt tumor recurrence in this time-data not shown to retain clarity.

Figure 4a shows that mice which undergo surgical eradication of EMT6, followed by immunotherapy, are refractory to re-challenge with EMT6 as monitored over 20 d by either visible tumor (panel a) or microscopic DLN metastases (panel b). There was no such protection seen if re-challenge was with 4THM tumor cells. Growth of either EMT6 or 4THM in mice receiving EMT6 followed by surgery/chemotherapy was equivalent to that seen in naive mice. Mice receiving primary injections with 4THM, and subsequently treated with chemotherapy, showed no resistance to re-challenge with either EMT6 or 4THM (Figure 4b). These data were mirrored by analysis of tumor cells frequencies in DLN of treated/re-challenged mice (Figure 4c). Only EMT6 tumor bearers cured by immunotherapy showed decreased DLN micro-metastasis after re-challenge with EMT6, but not 4THM, tumors. Note however, that in these mice (and mice cured of 4THM and re-challenged with EMT6) we cannot discern whether tumor cells measured were of EMT6 or 4THM origin.

Further evidence suggesting that immunotherapy, but not chemotherapy, treatment of EMT6-injected mice resulted in protective immunity to re-challenge with the same tumor came from studies using splenocytes pooled from 4mice/group 90 d post either surgical resection of primary tumors followed by either chemotherapy or immunotherapy. 50×10^6 of these cells were infused iv into fresh mice initially receiving 5×10^5 EMT6, or 1×10^5 4THM, tumor cells (Figure 5) 15 d earlier, and surgically removed 1 d before spleen cell transfer. Lung tumor colonies were enumerated in all groups at 15 days after surgery (14 d after spleen cell transfer), and DLN used to estimate tumor cell frequency by limiting dilution. Data for 1 of 2 studies are shown in Figure 5.

In this independent assay, protection from metastatic tumor colony growth, either macroscopic (to lung) or microscopic (DLN metastases assayed by limiting dilution), was afforded only by transfer of splenocytes from mice cured of EMT6 by surgical resection and immunotherapy, and not from mice cured by chemotherapy. Furthermore, no protection from growth of 4THM tumors was observed.

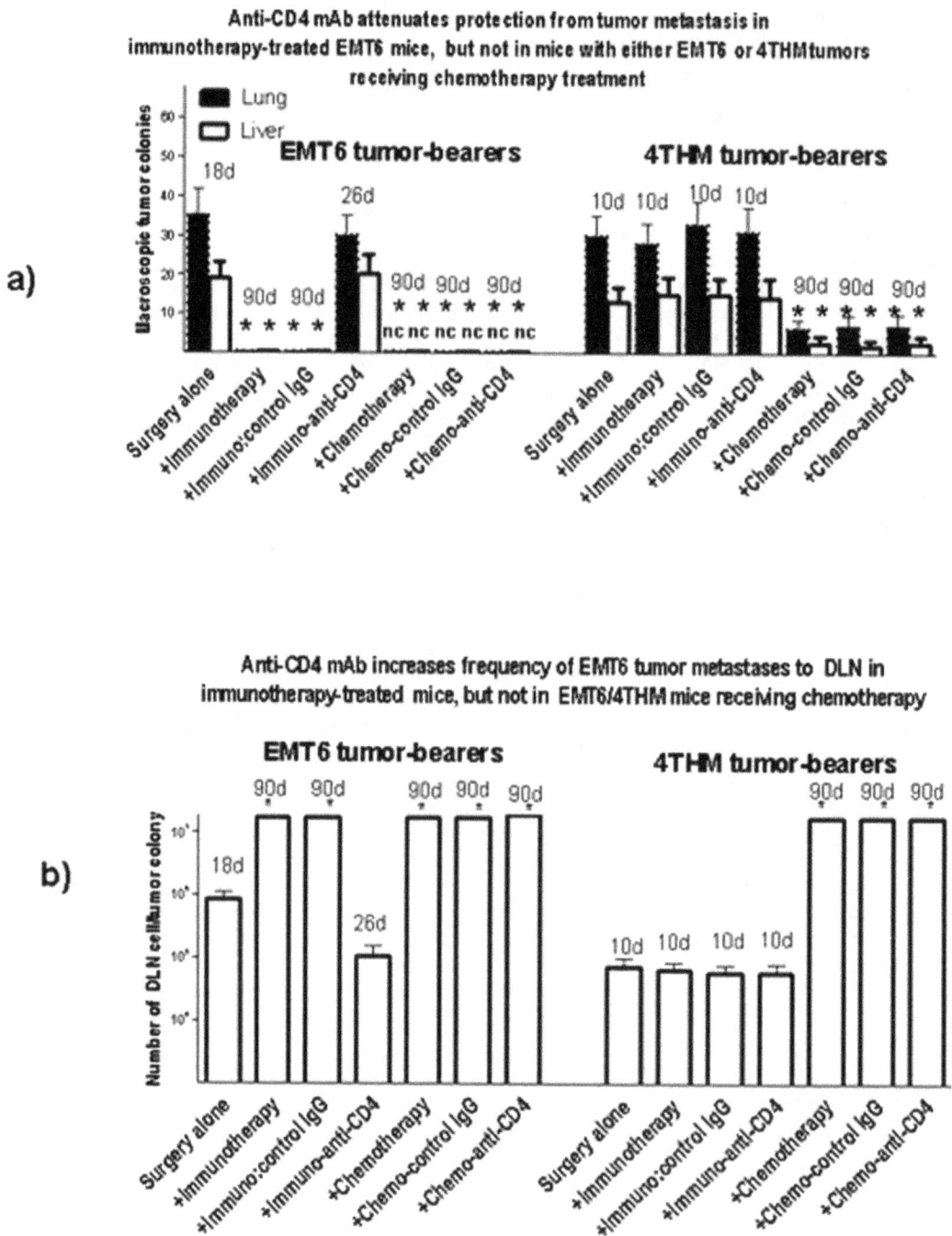

Figure 3. Effect of anti-CD4 mAb on lung/liver (panel a) or DLN (panel b) metastases in mice receiving EMT6 or 4THM tumor cells and treatment as in Figure 1. 5 mice were used per group for sacrifice at the time post surgery points shown (numbers above histogram bars). Data show means for macroscopic tumor colonies/group; nc = no visible tumor colonies. * indicates p<0.05, compared with control treated with surgery alone;

Discussion

Breast cancer cells are thought to be continuously monitored by host resistance mechanisms (immunosurveillance [27]), as evidenced by linkage of MHC expression (Class I) with breast cancer growth [28–30], as well as analysis of the role of other immune parameters on disease incidence/progression [31–34]. Included amongst such studies are several reporting on the possible importance of regulation of inflammation by T lymphocytes

[35–37]. Consistent with these concepts, lymphocyte infiltration into breast tumors is correlated with improved overall survival [38], and peripheral blood of breast cancer patients show evidence at both the cellular and humoral level of immunity to antigens (MUC-1 and Her-2/neu) associated with human breast cancer [39,40]. This in turn is reflected in the moderate success seen using Her-2/neu peptides, and other antigenic moieties, as a cancer vaccine [41,42]. While there remains controversy concerning whether development of CD4 or CD8 immunity will best predict

Specific host resistance to fresh EMT6 reinjection in mice cured of EMT6, but not 4THM, tumors by immuno- but not chemo-therapy

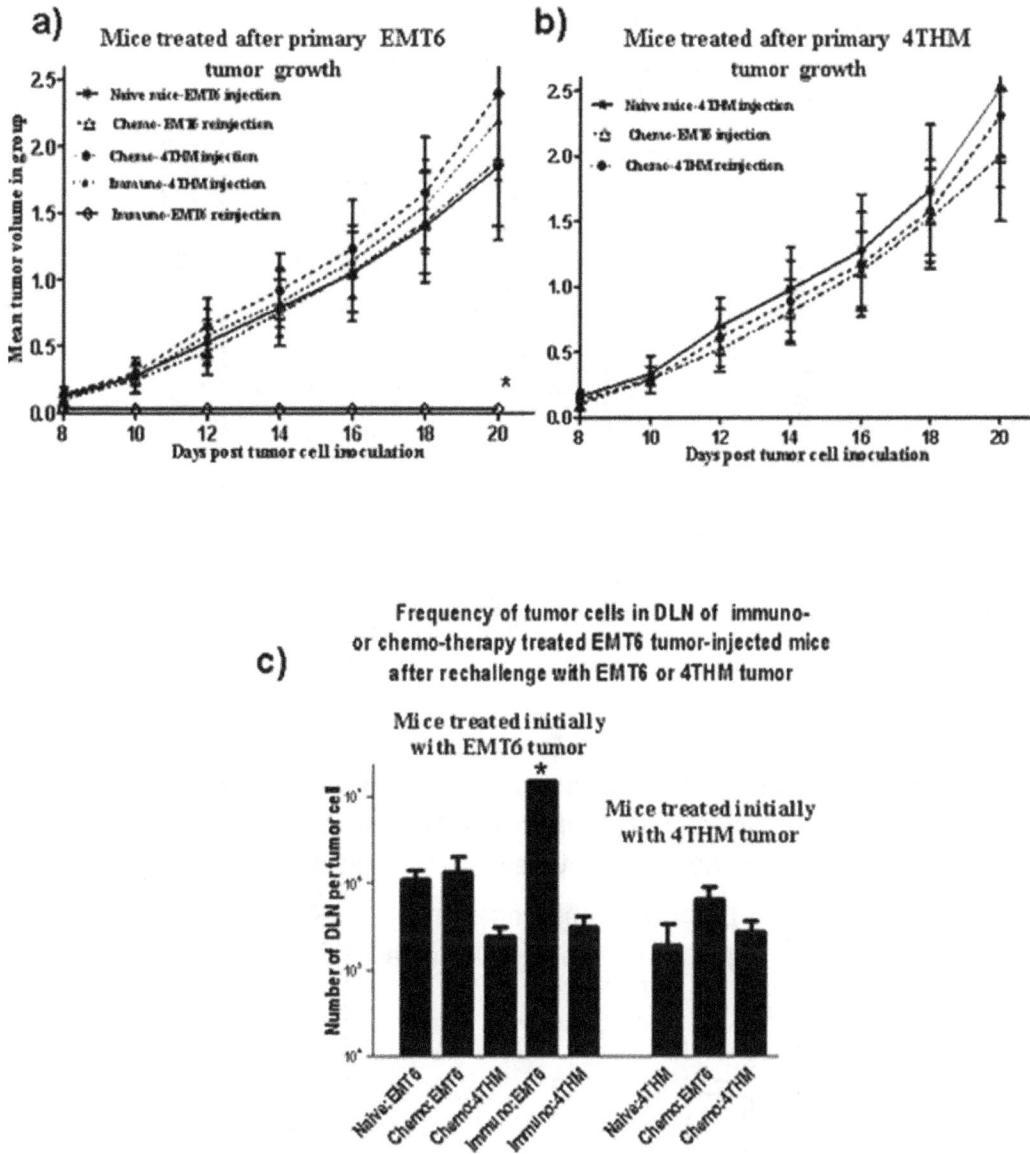

Figure 4. Specific protection from re-challenge with EMT6, but not 4THM, assaying either local tumor growth (panel a) or DLN metastases (panel c) in mice treated 90 d earlier by surgical tumor resection and immunotherapy. Naïve mice had had no previous EMT6 or 4THM tumor implants. All mice were sacrificed at 20 d post re-challenge. Data represent means for group. No protection was seen in mice initially treated with 4THM tumors before treatment/re-challenge (panel b). *, p<0.05 compared with equivalent fresh control mice.

host-resistance [43,44], there is also concern that vaccination may augment induction of Tregs to block effective tumor immunity [45,46]. Compounding the complexity of understanding the role of immunotherapy in breast cancer treatment is the potential effect of concomitant chemotherapy on the immune system of the tumor host. Conventional cyclophosphamide-methotrexate-5-fluoroura-cil (CMF) chemotherapy decreases both NK cell activity [47]. In contrast, in studies of taxane-based chemotherapy in 30 women with advanced breast cancer, increased NK and LAK cell activity and increased IL-6, GM-CSF, and IFNγ levels with decreased IL-1 and TNFα levels were reported in cancer patients following chemotherapy, and correlated with clinical responses [48].

Similarly, cyclophosphamide which is known to suppress T reg cells, has been incorporated into some vaccine *HER2/neu* vaccine trials [39].

Anti-CD200 mAb protects mice from micro-metastasis of EMT6 to DLN, while EMT6 over-expressing a CD200 transgene, or growing in CD200[tg] hosts, grew more aggressively and metastasized at higher frequency [7]. CD200RKO mice were more resistant both to primary and metastatic growth of tumor [25]. In CD200R1KO mice cured (tumor-free for >300 d) by surgical tumor resection and immunotherapy, CD4[+] cells, rather than effector CD8[+] cells, were critical for protection [9]. Growth and metastasis of a highly aggressive metastatic variant (4THM) of

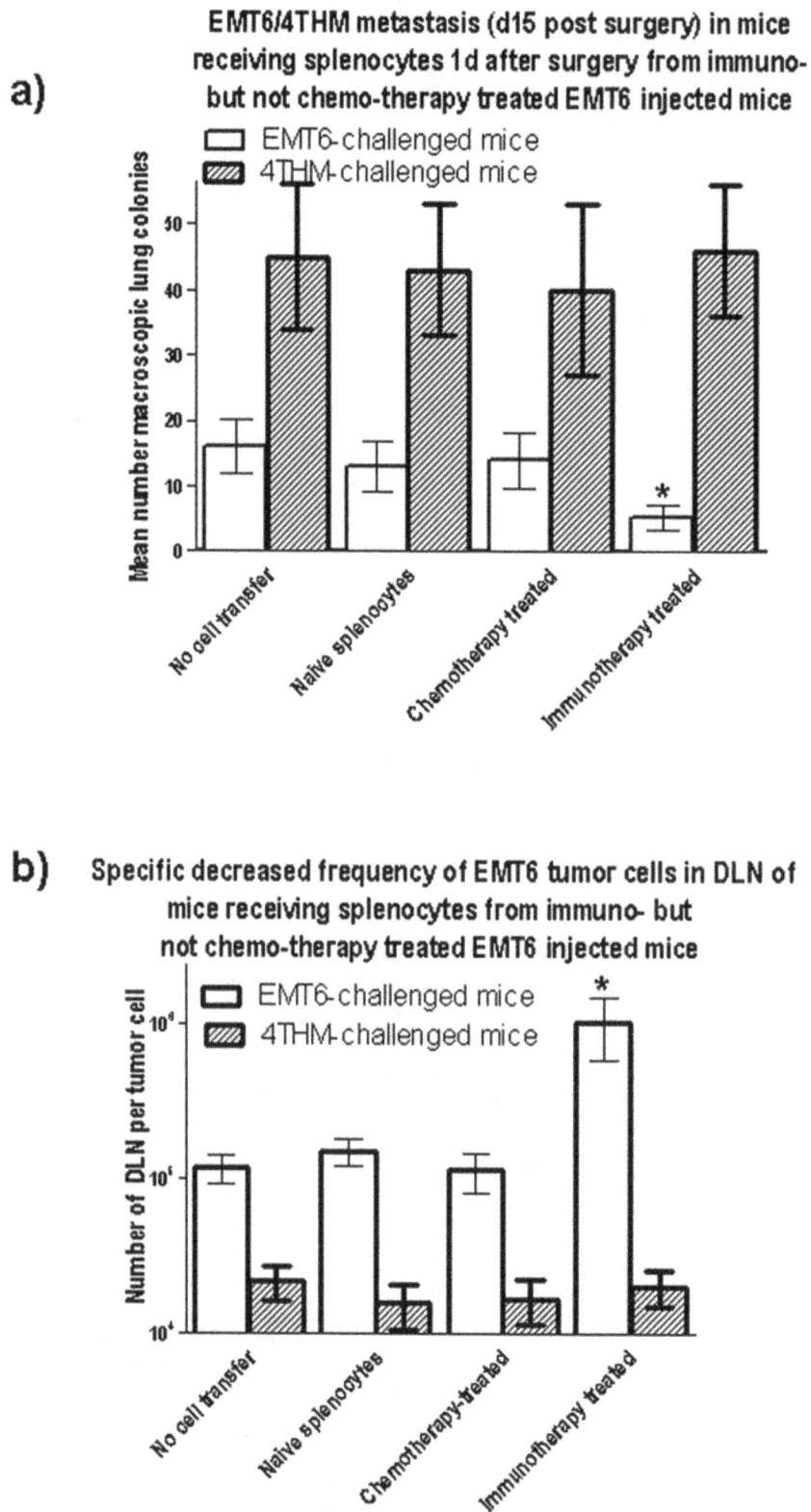

Figure 5. Adoptive transfer of splenocytes from immune- but not chemo-therapy treated mice receiving EMT6 tumors can decrease lung (panel a) and DLN (panel b) metastases in mice which had previously received EMT6 but not 4THM tumors. The tumors in the latter mice were surgically removed 1 d before spleen transfer, and all mice sacrificed 14 d after spleen cell transfer. Data show means (±SD). *, p< 0.01 relative to control (no cell transfer).

the breast tumor 4T1 was reported to be refractory to attenuation of CD200:CD200R interactions in CD200R1KO mice [8].

The current studies have extended our understanding of host resistance to EMT6 tumors using WT mice as tumor recipients, and, following surgical resection of tumor, by augmenting immunization with tumor cells (with CpG as adjuvant) with infusion of Fab anti-CD200R to block CD200:CD200R interactions. We compared this treatment with a more conventional approach using surgery followed by chemotherapy with anti-VEGF and paclitaxel, and compared results with EMT6 and the less immunogenic tumor, 4THM. 4THM mice were not effectively treated with immunotherapy, as was evident from the different times at which mice were sacrificed to measure tumor metastases endpoints in Figures 1–3. In contrast, chemotherapy was effective for both EMT6 and 4THM tumors, allowing us to study mice up to 90 d post surgery (Figures 1–3). Data in Figures 3–5, show that: (i) cure following chemotherapy in both tumor models is not abolished by anti-CD4 treatment, unlike cure of EMT6 tumors by immunotherapy (Figure 3-see also [9]). Immunotherapy in the EMT6 tumor model led to increased induction of direct killing (by CD8$^+$ effector cells) using splenocytes from treated mice, along with increased cytokine production in vitro-both effects were attenuated in mice receiving anti-CD4 treatment in vivo (Figure S2). (ii) following chemotherapy, mice initially cured of either 4THM or EMT6 tumors were not resistant to re-challenge with the same tumor, though immunotherapy of EMT6 tumors afforded resistance to re-challenge with the same tumor, but not with 4THM (Figure 4); and finally, (iii) only splenocytes from immuno- but not chemo-therapy treated EMT6 mice, could adoptively transfer protection from macroscopic/microscopic metastases to surgically treated WT mice (Figure 5) previously injected with the same tumor. Again no protection was afforded against 4THM tumors. Thus we were able to induce a tumor-protective immune response in WT mice with EMT6 tumors, but not mice with the more aggressive 4THM tumors. Additional features differentiating host inflammatory responses to EMT6 and 4THM have been described elsewhere by Erin et al (8). Given that the sensitivity of detection of metastases from DLN in our limiting dilution assay is $\sim 1{:}10^7$ cells, and that anti-CD4 treatment of immunotherapy-treated EMT6 tumor injected mice reveals increased metastases in mice otherwise "cured" of disease, we speculate that such mice may harbor quiescent tumor cells, whose growth is held in check by mechanisms which are CD4-dependent.

The nature of the resistant mechanism(s) in mice undergoing chemotherapy in the regimen prescribed is not yet clear. Preliminary data show a difference in intra-tumoral cytokine profiles in such animals, and a difference in phenotype of cells infiltrating the re-challenged EMT6 tumor in WT mice compared with those infiltrating a primary tumor challenge, with increased CD4$^+$ cells. This in itself is of interest given the data of Figure S2a, showing a CD4$^+$-dependent augmented cytokine production

(TNFα, IL-2 and IFNγ) in mice receiving immunotherapy, but not chemotherapy. Infusion of exogenous soluble CD200 into mice undergoing chemotherapy treatment did not attenuate cure or increase metastasis (RMG-unpublished), confirming the independence of this protection from an effect mediated by CD200:CD200R interactions, which is clearly implicated in the immunotherapy described. Our data suggest that optimal treatment of breast cancer should take into consideration the importance in "trade-off" between cancer cell sterilization by immunosuppressive drug treatment and the potential benefit of enhancing immune resistance by manipulation of co-inhibitory (CD200) pathways.

Supporting Information

Figure S1   DLN cell from (surgery+chemotherapy) treated WT mice do not antagonize outgrowth of tumor clones from DLN of WT mice sacrificed 14d post EMT6/4THM tumor cell injection. DLN cells from 5/group WT mice were harvested at 90 d post tumor resection and chemotherapy treatment (see Figures 1 and 2), and from separate groups of WT mice 14 d post EMT6/4THM injection-WT* in Figure). Cells from the latter were cultured under limiting dilution conditions (from 2×10^3 to 1×10^5 cells/well) alone, or with a 5-fold excess of cells from the 90 d treated mice. DLN cells from the latter were also cloned alone (data to far left in each subgroup in the Figure). All tumor cell frequencies cloned were calculated based on the input numbers of cells from DLN of WT* only.

Figure S2   Cytokine production (panel a) and CD8$^+$-dependent antigen specific lyses of ^{3}HTdR tumor target cells (panel b), using splenocytes from mice described in Figure 3. Control mice in each panel received no tumor cells-in this case only data are pooled for groups stimulated with either EMT6 or 4THM cells. Other mice shown were injected with EMT6 (left side of each panel) or 4THM tumor (right side of each panel), and received surgery alone, or followed by chemotherapy/immunotherapy. For all these studies splenocytes were harvested at 90 d post surgery, or earlier as necessary for groups where tumor growth was not controlled (see Figure 3), and re-stimulated in vitro with the same tumor cells (EMT6 or 4THM). Data show mean ($\pm$SD) for triplicate cultures, with a minimum of 4 individual spleen cells assayed/group. * p<0.05 compared with a surgery-only control group.

Author Contributions

Conceived and designed the experiments: RMG. Performed the experiments: RMG ZC IK AP. Analyzed the data: RMG NE IK. Contributed reagents/materials/analysis tools: RMG IK. Wrote the paper: RMG.

References

1. Petermann KB, Rozenberg GI, Zedek D (2007) CD200 is induced by ERK and is a potential therapeutic target in melanoma. J Clin Invest 117: 3922–3929.
2. Siva A, Xin H, Qin F, Oltean D, Bowdish KS, et al. (2008) Immune modulation by melanoma and ovarian tumor cells through expression of the immunosuppressive molecule CD200 Cancer Immunol Immunotherapy 57: 987–996.
3. Moreaux J, Veyrune JL, Reme T, DeVos J, Klein B (2008) CD200: A putative therapeutic target in cancer. Biochem Biophys Res Commun 366: 117–122.
4. McWhirter JR, KretzRommel A, Saven A (2006) Antibodies selected from combinatorial libraries block a tumor antigen that plays a key role in immunomodulation. Proc Nat Acad Sci Usa 103: 1041–1046.
5. Tonks A (2007) CD200 as a prognostic factor in acute myeloid leukemia. Leukemia 21: 566–571

6. Gorczynski RM, Chen Z, Diao J (2010) Breast cancer cell CD200 expression regulates immune response to EMT6 tumor cells in mice. Breast Cancer Res Treat 123: 405–415.
7. Gorczynski RM, Clark DA, Erin N, Khatri I (2011) Role of CD200 in regulation of metastasis of EMT6 tumor cells in mice. Breast Cancer Res Treatment 130: 49–60.
8. Erin N, Podnos A, Tanriover G, Duymus O, Cote E, Khatri I, et al. (2014) Bidirectional effect of CD200 on breast cancer development and metastasis, with ultimate outcome determined by tumor aggressiveness and a cancer-induced inflammatory response Oncogene: in press

9. Gorczynski RM, Chen Z, Khatri I, Podnos A, Yu K (2013) Cure of metastatic growth of EMT6 tumor cells in mice following manipulation of CD200:CD200R signaling. Breast Cancer Res Treatment 142: 271–282.

10. Pandit TS, Kennette W, MacKenzie L (2009) Lymphatic metastasis of breast cancer cells is associated with differential gene expression profiles that predict cancer stem cell- like properties and the ability to survive, establish and grow in a foreign environment. Int J Oncol 35: 297–308.

11. Pfeffer U, Romeo F, Noonan DM, Albini A (2009) Prediction of breast cancer metastasis by genomic profiling: where do we stand? Clin Exp Metastas 26: 547–558.

12. Pollard JW (2008) Macrophages define the invasive microenvironment in breast cancer. J Leukocyte Biol 84: 623–630.

13. Olkhanud PB, Baatar D, Bodogai M (2009) Breast Cancer Lung Metastasis Requires Expression of Chemokine Receptor CCR4 and Regulatory T Cells. Cancer Res 69: 5996–6004.

14. Lu X, Kang YB (2009) Chemokine (C-C Motif) Ligand 2 Engages CCR2(+) Stromal Cells of Monocytic Origin to Promote Breast Cancer Metastasis to Lung and Bone. J Biol Chem 284: 29087–29096.

15. Liang ZX, Yoon YH, Votaw J, Goodman MM, Williams L, et al. (2005) Silencing of CXCR4 blocks breast cancer metastasis. Cancer Res 65: 967–971.

16. Takahashi M, Miyazaki H, Furihata M (2009) Chemokine CCL2/MCP-1 negatively regulates metastasis in a highly bone marrow-metastatic mouse breast cancer model. Clin Exp Metastas 26: 817–828.

17. Ma XR, Norsworthy K, Kundu N (2009) CXCR3 expression is associated with poor survival in breast cancer and promotes metastasis in a murine model. Mol Cancer Ther 8: 490–498.

18. Huang B, Pan PY, Li QS (2006) Gr-1(+)CD115(+) immature myeloid suppressor cells mediate the development of tumor-induced T regulatory cells and T-cell anergy in tumor-bearing host. Cancer Res 66: 1123–1131.

19. Yang L, Debusk LM, Fukuda K (2004) Expansion of myeloid immune suppressor GR1+CD11b+ cells in tumor-bearing host directly promotes tumor angiogenesis. Cancer Cell 6: 409–421.

20. Qin FXF (2009) Dynamic Behavior and Function of Foxp3(+) Regulatory T Cells in Tumor Bearing Host. Cell Mol Immunol 6: 3–13.

21. Yang L, Huang JH, Ren XB (2008) Abrogation of TGF beta signaling in mammary carcinomas recruits Gr- 1+CD11b+ myeloid cells that promote metastasis. Cancer Cell 13: 23–35.

22. Pandit TS, Kennette W, MacKenzie L, Zhang GH, AlKatib W, et al. (2009) Lymphatic metastasis of breast cancer cells is associated with differential gene expression profiles that predict cancer stem cell- like properties and the ability to survive, establish and grow in a foreign environment. Int J Oncol. 35: 297–308.

23. Pakala SB, Rayala SK, Wang R, Ohshiro K, Mudvari P, et al. (2013) MTA1 Promotes STAT3 Transcription and Pulmonary Metastasis in Breast Cancer. Cancer Res. 73: 3761–3770

24. Erin N, Zhao W, Bylander J, Chase G, Clawson G (2006) Capsaicin-induced inactivation of sensory neurons promotes a more aggressive gene expression phenotype in breast cancer cells. Breast Cancer Res Treat 99: 351–364.

25. Abadi YM, Jeon H, Ohaegbulam KC, Scandiuzzi L, Ghosh K, et al. (2013) Host B7× Promotes Pulmonary Metastasis of Breast Cancer. J Immunol 190: 3806–3814

26. Podnos A, Clark DA, Erin N, Yu K, Gorczynski RM (2012) Further evidence for a role of tumor CD200 expression in breast cancer metastasis: decreased metastasis in CD200R1KO mice or using CD200-silenced EMT6. Breast Cancer Res Treatment 136: 117–127.

27. Standish LJ, Sweet ESND, Novack J, Wenner CA, Bridge C, et al. (2008) Breast Cancer and the Immune System. J Soc Integr Oncol. 6: 158–168.

28. Chaudhuri S, Cariappa A, Tang M (2000) Genetic susceptibility to breast cancer: HLA DQB*03032 and HLA DRB1*11 may represent protective alleles. Proc Natl Acad Sci USA 97: 11451–11454.

29. Marincola FM, Jaffee EM, Hicklin DJ (2000) Escape of human solid tumors from T-cell recognition: molecular mechanisms and functional significance. Adv Immunol 74: 181–273.

30. Camploi M, Changg CC, OLdford SA (2004) HLA antigen changes in malignant tumors of mammary epithelial origin: molecular mechanisms and clinical implications. Breast Dis 2004: 105–125.

31. Hamilton G, Reiner A, Teleky B (1988) Natural killer cell activities of patients with breast cancer against different target cells. J Cancer Res Clin Oncol. 114: 191–196.

32. Jarnicki AG, Lysaght J, Todryk S, Mills KH (2006) Suppression of antitumor immunity by IL-10 and TGF-beta-producing T cells infiltrating the growing tumor: influence of tumor environment on the induction of CD4+ and CD8+ regulatory T cells. J Immunol. 177: 896–904.

33. Ramsey-Goldman R, Mattai SA, Schilling E (1998) Increased risk of malignancy in patients with systemic lupus erythematosus. J Investig Med. 46: 217–222.

34. Calogero RA, Cordero F, Forni G, Cavallo F (2007) Inflammation and breast cancer. Inflammatory component of mammary carcino-genesis in ErbB2 transgenic mice. Breast Cancer Res. 9: 211–212.

35. Denardo DG, Coussens LM (2007) Inflammation and breast cancer. Balancing immune response: crosstalk between adaptive and innate immune cells during breast cancer progression. Breast Cancer Res. 9: 212–213.

36. Tan TT, Coussens LM (2007) Humoral immunity, inflammation and cancer. Curr Opin Immunol. 19: 209–216.

37. Einav U, Tabach Y, Getz G (2005) Gene expression analysis reveals a strong signature of an interferon-induced pathway in childhood lymphoblastic leukemia as well as in breast and ovarian cancer. Oncogene. 24: 6367–6375.

38. Menard S, Tomasic G, Casalini P (1997) Lymphoid infiltration as a prognostic variable for early onset breast carcinomas. Clin Cancer Res 3: 817–819.

39. Disis ML, Calenoff E, McLaughlin G (1994) Existent T cell and antibody immunity to Her-2/neu protein in patients with breast cancer. Cancer Res 54: 16–20.

40. Jerome KR, Domenech N, Finn OJ (1993) Tumor-specific cytotoxic T cell clones from patients with breast and pancreatic adenocarcinoma recognize EBV-immortalized B cells transfected with polymorphic epithelial mucin complementary DNA. J Immunol 151: 1654–1662.

41. Baxevanis CN, Sotiriadou NN, Gritzapis AD (2006) Immunogenic HER-2/neu peptides as tumor vaccines. Cancer Immunol Immunother 55: 85–95.

42. Anderson KS (2009) Tumor vaccines for Breast Cancer. Cancer Invest 27: 361–368.

43. Assudani DP, Horton RBV, Mathieu MG, McArdle SEB, Rees RC (2007) The role of CD4(+) T cell help in cancer immunity and the formulation of novel cancer vaccines. Cancer Immunol Immunother 56: 70–80.

44. Beyer M, Karbach J, Mallmann MR (2009) Cancer Vaccine Enhanced, Non-Tumor-Reactive CD8(+) T Cells Exhibit a Distinct Molecular Program Associated with "Division Arrest Anergy". Cancer Res 69: 4346–4354.

45. Zhou G, Drake CG, Levitsky HI (2006) Amplification of tumor-specific regulatory T cells following therapeutic cancer vaccines. Blood 107: 628–636.

46. Duraiswamy J, Kaluza KM, Freeman GJ, Coukos G (2013) Dual Blockade of PD-1 and CTLA-4 Combined with Tumor Vaccine Effectively Restores T-Cell Rejection Function in Tumors. Cancer Research 73: 3591–3603.

47. Tichatschek E, Zielinski CC, Muller C (1988) Long-term influence of adjuvant therapy on natural killer cell activity in breast cancer. Cancer Immunol Immunother. 27: 278–282.

48. Tsavaris N, Kosmas C, Vadiaka M (2002) Immune changes in patients with advanced breast cancer undergoing chemotherapy with taxanes. Br J Cancer. 87: 21–27.

27

Retrospective Analysis of 234 Nasopharyngeal Carcinoma Patients with Distant Metastasis at Initial Diagnosis: Therapeutic Approaches and Prognostic Factors

Lei Zeng[1,2,3&]**, Yun-Ming Tian**[1,2&]**, Ying Huang**[1]**, Xue-Ming Sun**[1]**, Feng-Hua Wang**[2]**, Xiao-Wu Deng**[1]**,
Fei Han[1]*****, Tai-Xiang Lu**[1]*****

1 Department of Radiation Oncology, Sun Yat-Sen University Cancer Center, State Key Laboratory of Oncology in South China, Collaborative Innovation Center of Cancer Medicine, Guangzhou, PR China, **2** Department of Medical Oncology, Sun Yat-Sen University Cancer Center, State Key Laboratory of Oncology in South China, Collaborative Innovation Center of Cancer Medicine, Guangzhou, PR China, **3** Department of Radiation Oncology, Jiangxi Cancer Hospital, Nanchang, PR China

Abstract

Purpose: The purpose of this retrospective study was to identify the independent prognostic factors and optimize the treatment for nasopharyngeal carcinoma (NPC) patients with distant metastasis at initial diagnosis.

Methods: A total of 234 patients referred between January 2001 and December 2010 were retrospectively analyzed. Among the 234 patients, 94 patients received chemotherapy alone (CT), and 140 patients received chemoradiotherapy (CRT). Clinical features, laboratory parameters and treatment modality were examined with univariate and multivariate analyses.

Results: The median overall survival (OS) time was 22 months (range, 2-125 months), and the 1-year, 2-year, 3-year overall survival rates were 82.2%, 51.3% and 34.1%. The overall response and disease control rates of metastatic lesions after chemotherapy were 56.0% and 89.8%. The factors associated with poor response were karnofsky performance score (KPS) < 80, liver metastasis, lactate dehydrogenase (LDH)>245 IU/L, and number of chemotherapy cycles <4. The 3-year OS of patients receiving CRT was higher than those receiving CT alone (48.2% vs. 12.4%, p<0.001). Subgroup analysis showed that significantly improved survival was also achieved by radiotherapy of the primary tumor in patients who achieved complete remission (CR)/partial remission (PR) or stable disease (SD) of metastatic lesions after chemotherapy. Significant independent prognostic factors of OS were KPS, liver metastasis, levels of LDH, and multiple metastases. Treatment modality, response to chemotherapy and chemotherapy cycles were also associated with OS.

Conclusion: A combination of radiotherapy and chemotherapy seems to have survival benefits for selected patients with distant metastases at initial diagnosis. Clinical and laboratory characteristics can help to guide treatment selection. Prospective randomized studies are needed to confirm the result.

Editor: Gayle E. Woloschak, Northwestern University Feinberg School of Medicine, United States of America

Funding: The authors have no support or funding to report.

Competing Interests: The authors have declared that no competing interests exist.

* Email: hanfei@sysucc.org.cn (FH); lutx@sysucc.org.cn (TXL)

& These authors contributed equally to this work.

Introduction

Nasopharyngeal carcinoma (NPC) is a common epithelial malignancy in southern China. The highest incidence has been reported in Guangdong province, where the rate is approximately 20 per 100,000 people per year [1,2]. Radiotherapy alone has become the standard treatment for early stage disease, and chemoradiotherapy for the advanced NPC [3]. Biologically different from other squamous cell cancers of the head and neck, approximately 95% of these cases were undifferentiated carcinomas with the highest incidence of distant metastases [4,5]. Once metastasis is diagnosed, the overall survival of patients is very poor after palliative chemotherapy. Furthermore, patients with distant

metastasis at initial diagnosis had been demonstrated with a significantly shorter survival when compared with those with subsequent metastases [6–10].

However, patients with distant metastasis at initial diagnosis do not behave in a uniform manner. It is hence not surprising to see significantly variable results between studies of similar therapeutic approaches in patients with metastatic NPC [11,12]. Although palliative chemotherapy has been demonstrated as the most effective way with high objective response rates, recurrence frequently occurs after chemotherapy ceases. However, the application of radiotherapy of the primary tumor remains controversial because of their short life expectancy and radiation-induced complications [11–13].

Therefore, determining the prognostic factors of survival outcomes in NPC patients with distant metastasis at initial diagnosis could help to select those patients who would most benefit from comprehensive treatment including radiotherapy of the primary tumor by retrospectively analyzing patients' clinical characteristics, treatment modalities and survival. These results might contribute to management of treatment and exploration of avenues of further research.

Materials and Methods

Patients and selection criteria

Between January 2001 and December 2010, 271 NPC patients presenting with distant metastases at initial diagnosis were referred to our cancer center. The selection criteria were as follows: (1) pathologically confirmed NPC in the nasopharynx, (2) diagnosis of distant metastasis based on physical examination and imaging, (3) receiving at least one anti-cancer treatment including the chemotherapy and the radiotherapy, (4) complete follow-up and clinical data, including laboratory and imaging data. Patients with other malignancies or unstable cardiac disease requiring treatment were excluded. Of the 271 NPC patients, 37 patients were excluded from the survival analysis, including 14 cases because of missing clinical data and 23 cases because of refusing any

treatment, leaving 234 patients for evaluation. The clinicopathological data of the 234 patients are presented in Tables 1, 2, 3.

Ethical Review Committee of Sun Yat-Sen University Cancer Center has approved the project. Written consent was given by the patients to be stored in the hospital database.

Pre-treatment evaluation

All patients had a pre-treatment evaluation including complete history, physical examination, hematology and biochemistry profiles, Epstein-Barr virus (EBV) serology, chest radiographs, sonography of abdomen, whole-body bone scan and magnetic resonance imaging (MRI) of head and neck regions. A titre of more than 1:20 was considered to be positive for the VCA-IgA antibodies as adopted in previous study on the marker [9]. Patients were evaluated according to the 2002 American Joint Committee on Cancer (AJCC) TNM stages.

Treatment

The treatment modalities were determined according to the experience of our center and the acceptance of the patients. Radiotherapy of the primary tumor was generally administrated to those patients who achieved disease control of the metastatic lesions after chemotherapy. It was also administered to reduce serious symptoms caused by the primary tumor that affected the

Table 1. Clinical characteristics.

Characteristics	N(%)
Gender	
Female	32(14)
Male	202(86)
Age (years)	
<48	116(50)
≥48	118(50)
Karnofsky performance score (KPS)	
<80	30(13)
≥80	204(87)
Histology	
WHO Type 2	8(3)
WHO Type 3	226(97)
Bony metastasis	
Present	157(67)
Absent	77(33)
Liver metastasis	
Present	75(32)
Absent	159(68)
Lung metastasis	
Present	36(15)
Absent	198(85)
Distant nodal metastasis	
Present	27(12)
Absent	207(88)
No. of metastatic sites	
Single	52(22)
Multiple	182(78)

Table 2. Laboratory characteristics.

Characteristics	N(%)
Haemoglobin (g/L)	
<120	29(12)
≥120	205(88)
Lactate dehydrogenase (LDH) (IU/L)	
≤245	154(66)
>245	80(34)
Alkaline phosphatase (ALP) (IU/L)	
≤110	182(78)
>110	52(22)
VCA-IgA	
Negative	13(5)
Positive	221(95)

quality of life. Among the 234 patients, 94 patients received chemotherapy alone (CT), and 140 patients received chemoradiotherapy (CRT).

All the patients were treated with cisplatinum-based chemotherapy. The median number of cycles of chemotherapy was 5 (range, 1–14).

Among of the patients who received RT, 116 (82.9%) were treated with conventional techniques, 20 (14.3%) underwent intensity-modulated radiotherapy (IMRT) and 4 underwent three-dimensional conformal radiotherapy (3D-CRT). Details regarding the RT techniques have been previously reported [14–15]. One hundred and seventeen patients received a radiation dose ≥66 Gy and 23 patients underwent a dose <66 Gy. The median dose was 70 Gy (range, 40–78 Gy).

Fifty-five patients received local therapy to metastases, including 39 patients received radiotherapy to bone lesion (30–66Gy/10-33f), 10 received radiofrequency ablation (RFA) and 3 received

interventional embolization of liver lesions, and 3 received surgery of lung lesions.

Treatment evaluations and follow up

Imaging of the metastasis was performed after every two courses of chemotherapy, and then every 3 months during follow-up. Objective response was measured according to the Response Evaluation Criteria in Solid Tumors (RECIST). The evaluation of bone metastasis was based on the imaging findings of recalcification shown in CT and the decreased concentration in the whole bone scanning and the clinical evidence of the pain relief.

Patients were followed up by direct telecommunication mean or by checking the clinic attendance records. The overall survival (OS) was defined as the duration from the date of diagnosis to the date of death from any cause or the censoring of the patient at the date of the last follow-up. The median follow-up for the whole was 22 months (range, 2-125).

Table 3. Treatment characteristics.

Characteristics	N(%)
Treatment modality	
Chemotherapy alone	94(40)
Chemoradiotherapy	140(60)
Chemotherapy regimen	
Cisplatin+fluorouracil	124(53)
Paclitaxel+cisplatin	110(47)
Chemotherapy response	
Progression of disease	24(10)
Stable disease*	79(34)
Complete remission+Partial remission†	131(56)
Chemotherapy cycles	
1–3 cycles	74(32)
≥4 cycles	160(68)

*52 patients received RT to primary lesions and 27 patients did not received RT;
†88 patients received RT to primary lesions and 43 patients did not received RT.

Statistical analysis

Statistical analysis was performed using SPSS 13.0 package. Overall survival (OS) was analyzed using the Kaplan-Meier method and was compared using the log-rank test. Univariate and multivariate analysis were performed using the Cox proportion hazards model. The multivariate analyses were undertaken with both forward and backward stepwise procedures for identifying variables correlated with overall survival. Covariates included patients' characteristics (Karnofsky performance score, gender and age), laboratory parameters (hemoglobin, lactate dehydrogenase, alkaline phosphatase and the EBV serology), metastatic features (extension and response to chemotherapy) and treatment approaches (number of chemotherapy cycles, radiotherapy of the primary tumor and local therapy of metastases). Furthermore, the relationship of response to chemotherapy and various factors was tested by logistic regression model. A two-tailed P-value <0.05 was considered statistically significant.

Results

Treatment response and overall survival

One hundred and fifty-four patients had been dead by the final evaluation date. The main cause of death was progression died of metastatic lesions, which occurred in 137/154 (89.0%) patients; 15/154 (9.7%) patients died of local failure and 2/154 (1.3%) die of cardiac disease. The median OS time was 22 months (range, 2-125 months), and the 1-year, 2-year, 3-year overall survival rates were 82.2%, 51.3% and 34.1%, respectively.

Of the 234 patients, 10/234 (4.3%) achieved complete response (CR) of metastatic lesions, 121/234 (51.7%) achieved partial response (PR), 79/234 (33.8%) had stable disease (SD) and 24/234 (10.2%) had progressive disease (PD). The overall response and disease control rates were 56.0% and 89.8%, respectively. Logistic regression analysis showed that the following factors were significantly associated with poor response to chemotherapy (PD+SD): KPS <80 (P=0.016); liver metastasis (P=0.001); LDH>245 IU/L (P=0.023); and number of chemotherapy cycles <4 (P<0.001).

Toxicities

Two of the patients died of treatment-related toxicity including one with severe infection caused by the grade IV leucopenia and one with the hepatic failure during chemotherapy exhibited. In total, 45.3% developed grade III–IV leucopenia or neutropenia and 16.7% exhibited grade II–III toxicity with vomiting and nausea. Among the patients receiving RT, the most significant toxicity was the grade 3/4 mucositis with a rate of 40.5%, and the skin reaction with a rate of 25.0%. All patients completed the full course of RT.

Univariate analysis and Multivariate analysis

The result of univariate analysis and multivariate analysis are summarized in Table 4 and Table 5. The negative prognostic factors in the univariate analysis for OS were as follows include KPS<80 (P<0.001), LDH>245 (P<0.001), ALP>110 (P<0.001), Liver metastasis (HR=2.204, P<0.001), and Multiple metastases (P<0.001). CT alone (P<0.001), Chemotherapy cycles<4 (P=0.001), Poor response to chemotherapy (P<0.001), and Without local therapy to metastatic lesions (P<0.001) were also associated with poor OS in the univariate analysis.

The multivariate analysis show that the significant prognostic factors for poor survival were KPS<80 (HR=4.077, P<0.001), LDH>245 (HR=1.748, P=0.004), Liver metastasis (HR=1.652, P=0.008), and Multiple metastases (HR=2.106, P=0.003). CT

alone (HR=2.066, P<0.001), Chemotherapy cycles<4 (HR=1.748, P<0.001), and Poor response to chemotherapy(PD group, HR=6.455, P<0.001; SD group, HR=2.251, P<0.001) were also associated with poor OS in the multivariate analysis. Patients with good performance status (KPS≥80) survived longer than those with poor performance status (3-year OS: 37.9% vs. 4.4%). Patients with normal LDH level had a better survival than those with high LDH level (3-year OS: 44.7% vs. 13.7%). The 3-year OS rate for patients with liver metastasis was poorer than those without liver metastasis (14% vs. 45.7%). Patients with single metastasis had a better survival than those with multiple metastases (the 3-year survival rates: 65.8% vs. 25.9%). Furthermore, the therapy related factors were also associated with OS. The 3-year OS rate for patients receiving chemotherapy cycles <4 was poorer than those receiving chemotherapy cycles ≥4 (23.2% vs. 39.1%). The 3-year survival of patients receiving CRT was 48.2%, better than those receiving CT alone with only 12.4%. Patient with response to chemotherapy of metastatic lesions also show better survival with 3-year OS rate of 38.0% for patients with PR or CR, and 14.2% for patients with SD, and none for patients with PD. These results are shown in Figure 1.

For patients who achieved CR or PR after chemotherapy of metastatic lesions, multivariate analysis showed that radiotherapy of the primary tumor was an independently significant favorable prognostic factor (HR=0.435, P=0.001). Significantly improved survival was achieved by radiotherapy of the primary tumor in these patients (3-year OS rate 59.6% vs. 20.3%, P<0.001, Figure 2a). For patients who achieved SD after chemotherapy of metastatic lesions, multivariate analysis also showed that radiotherapy of the primary tumor was an independently significant favorable prognostic factor (HR=0.363, P=0.001). Significantly improved survival was achieved by radiotherapy of the primary tumor in these patients (3-year OS 24.7% vs. 0%, P=0.003, Figure 2b).

Discussion

For patients presenting with distant metastases at initial diagnosis, the optimal treatment strategy remains a subject of debate [11–13]. The benefits of systemic chemotherapy have been demonstrated in some studies and considered as the only possibly curative option. Platinum-based combination regimen achieves high response rates and is the most widely used regimen [11,16,17]. For the number of cycles of chemotherapy was an independent factor associated with survival, it was important for patients receive a sufficient number of cycles. However, it was still uncertain regarding the optimal cycles of chemotherapy. In a retrospective study involving 20 long-term disease-free survivors with metastatic NPC reported by Fandi et al. [11], the results showed that approximately six cycles of chemotherapy were required. In the current study, the cut-off point of number of cycles was evaluated by the Receiver operating characteristic (ROC) and the patients with at least four cycles of chemotherapy had a significantly better survival than those with less than four cycles. The results indicated the importance of sufficient chemotherapy for patients with metastatic NPC. However, owing to the retrospective nature of this study, it was still hard to determine the optimal cycles of chemotherapy. Furthermore, the response of metastatic lesions to chemotherapy was demonstrated as a significant predictor of OS. The overall response rate (CR and PR) after chemotherapy was 56.0%, and poor response was associated with KPS <80, liver metastasis, LDH>245 IU/L and number of chemotherapy cycles <4, suggesting that these factors could be potential predictors of treatment response. The response

Table 4. Univariate analysis of variables correlated with overall survival.

Characteristic	Univariate Analysis	
	P	HR (95% CI)
Gender, men vs women	0.096	1.536(0.927–2.545)
Age, <48 vs ≥48	0.787	0.957(0.698–1.314)
KPS, <80 vs ≥80	<0.001[a]	4.712(3.018–7.358)
Liver metastasis, yes vs no	<0.001[a]	2.204(1.598–3.039)
Lung metastasis, yes vs no	0.377	0.819(0.525–1.276)
Bone metastasis, yes vs no	0.754	0.948(0.681–1.321)
Distant nodal metastasis, yes vs no	0.800	1.069(0.636–1.798)
Number of involved site,>1 vs 1	<0.001[a]	2.648(1.678–4.178)
Haemoglobin, <120 vs ≥120	0.933	1.021(0.624–1.672)
Serum LDH,>245 vs ≤245	<0.001[a]	2.554(1.843–3.538)
Serum ALP,>110 vs ≤110	<0.001[a]	2.124(1.497–3.014)
VCA-IgA, Positive vs Negative	0.370	0.734(0.374–1.443)
Local therapy to metastases, no vs yes	<0.001[a]	2.565(1.657–3.970)
Treatment modality, CT vs CRT	<0.001[a]	3.058(2.202–4.247)
Response to chemotherapy, PR+CR		Baseline
SD	<0.001[a]	2.251(1.583–3.202)
PD	<0.001[a]	6.455(3.876–10.735)
Chemotherapy cycles, <4 vs ≥4	0.001[a]	1.783(1.280–2.484)

HR: hazard ration; CI: confidence interval; CT: Chemotherapy CRT: Chemoradiotherapy; PD: Progression of disease; SD: Stable disease; PR: Partial remission; CR: Complete remission;
[a] Statistically significant.

of metastatic lesions to chemotherapy also plays a key part in the consideration of the treatment choice. The results indicated that patients with CR or PR were recommended for a more progressive treatment as this could significantly improve survival.

In the clinical practice, the most controversial issue for NPC patients initially with metastases was the application of radiotherapy to the primary tumor for the uncertain indications in the guideline of NCCN (National Comprehensive Cancer Network),

which posed great challenge for the oncologists [12,13]. It was often considered as inappropriate to give a prolonged course of radiotherapy to patients with stage IVC NPC because of their short life expectancy and serious late complications in the past era. However, due to the improvements in radiation techniques and increasing efficacy of platinum-based combination regimen, some studies show that the local control of primary tumor following the radiotherapy would improve the quality of life and contribute to

Table 5. Multivariate analysis of variables correlated with overall survival.

Variables	HR(95%CI)	P
Clinical and Laboratory Characteristic		
KPS, <80 vs ≥80	4.077(2.481–6.700)	<0.001[a]
Liver metastasis, yes vs. no	1.652(1.140–2.393)	0.008[a]
Number of involved site, >1 vs 1	2.106(1.288–3.444)	0.003[a]
Serum LDH, >245 vs ≤245	1.686(1.187–2.395)	0.004[a]
Treatment Characteristic		
Treatment modality, CT vs CRT	2.066(1.440–2.964)	<0.001[a]
Chemotherapy cycles, <4 vs ≥4	1.748(1.223–2.499)	<0.001[a]
Response to chemotherapy, PR+CR	Baseline	
SD	2.338(1.591–3.437)	<0.001[a]
PD	3.370(1.947–5.833)	<0.001[a]

HR: hazard ration; CI: confidence interval; CT: Chemotherapy CRT: Chemoradiotherapy; PD: Progression of disease; SD: Stable disease; PR: Partial remission; CR: Complete remission;
[a] Statistically significant.

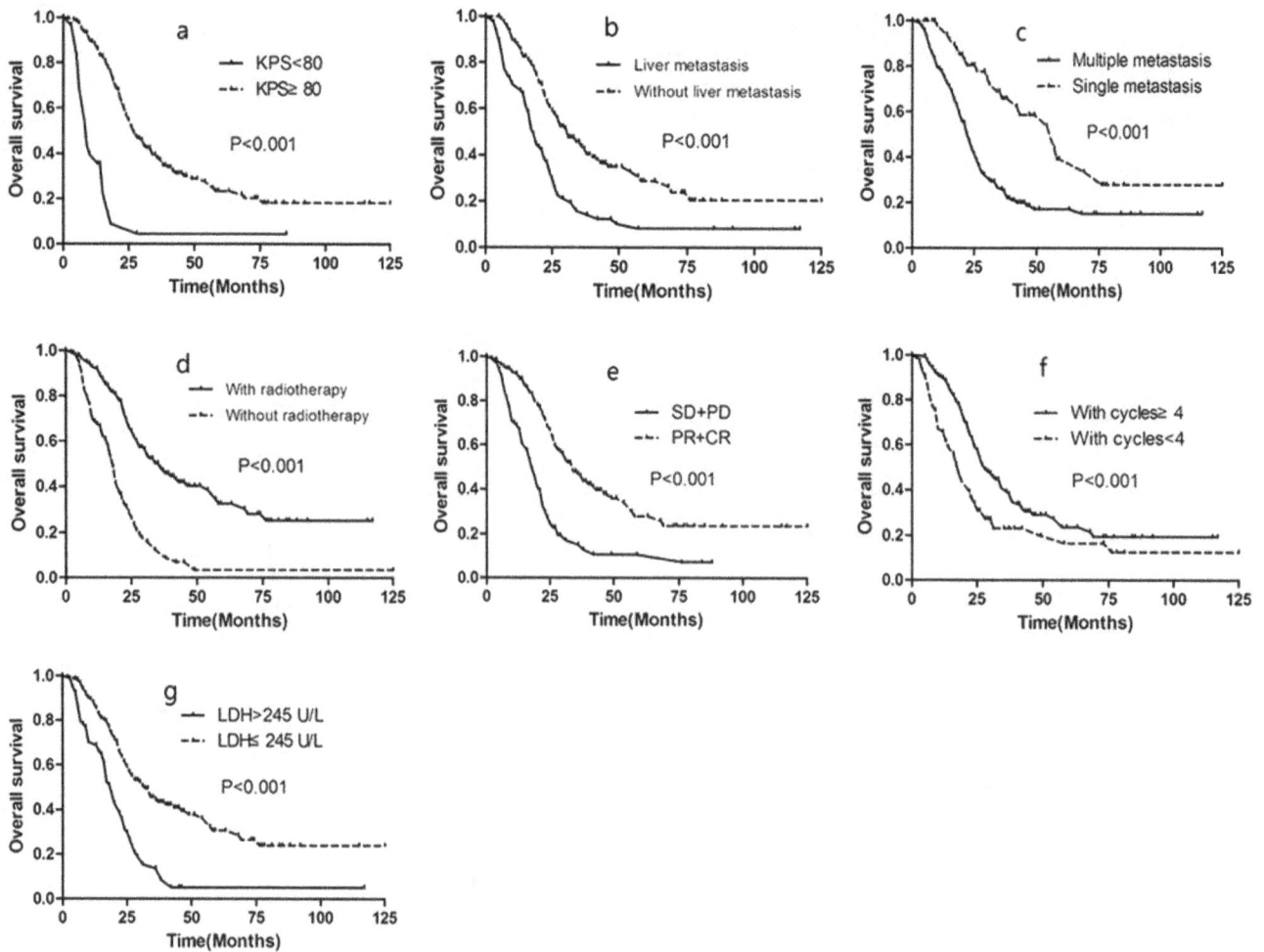

Figure 1. Overall survival rates according to KPS (a), liver metastasis (b), number of metastatic site (c), radiotherapy of primary tumor (d), response to chemotherapy (e), number of cycles of chemotherapy (f) and LDH (g).

prolonged survival. In a retrospective analysis of 125 NPC patients initially with metastases reported by Yeh et al. [13], the 2-year OS rate was 24.0% when they received radiotherapy alone when compared to 10% in those who received chemotherapy alone, and it also showed that the local control of the primary tumor improved the quality of life because of the reduced necrosis,

bleeding and severe headaches. In the current study, the application of radiotherapy after chemotherapy was a positive factor associated with survival. The 3-year OS of patients receiving radiotherapy after chemotherapy was up to 48.2%, significantly higher than those receiving chemotherapy alone with only 12.4%. However, the survival benefit may be also related to the selection

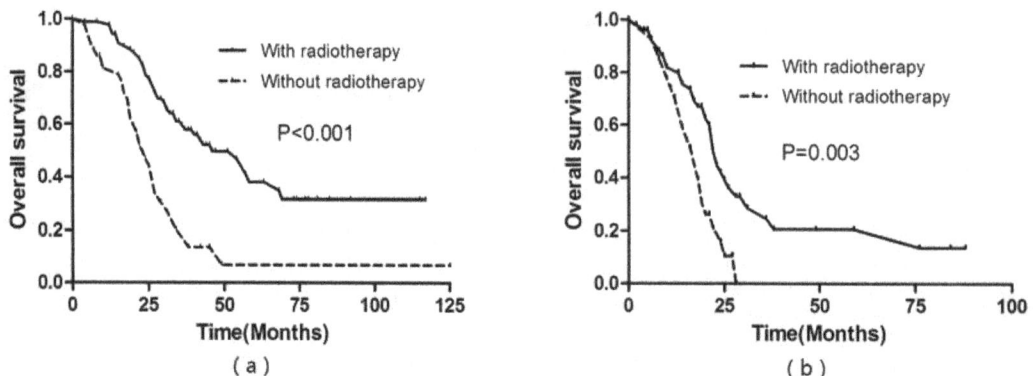

Figure 2. Overall survival rates for patients who achieved CR or PR after chemotherapy of metastatic lesions (a), for patients who achieved SD after chemotherapy of metastatic lesions (b).

for radiotherapy. Therefore, it was very important to select the patients who would most benefit from the radiotherapy. In the subgroup analysis, we found the radiotherapy could significantly improve the survival of patients who achieved the CR or PR of metastatic lesions after chemotherapy with a 3-year OS rate of 59.6%. Even though for patients who achieved SD after chemotherapy of metastatic lesions, significantly improved survival was achieved by radiotherapy of the primary tumor in (3-year OS 24.7% vs. 0%, P = 0.003).

These findings indicated that excellent local control may help reduce the tumor burden and the risks of death caused by progression of primary tumor, especially for the patients with CR/PR or SD of metastatic lesions after chemotherapy. Furthermore, the improvements of radiation technique such as the application of Intensity-modulated radiotherapy (IMRT) may further improve the treatment benefit.

Part of our results were consistent with those reported by Toe et al. [6], liver metastasis was associated with poor survival. In the current study, the 3-year OS rate of patients with liver metastasis was only about 14.0%, significantly poorer than those with other metastasis included the lung, bone or distant nodal metastasis with a 3-year OS rate of 43.7%. In the retrospective analysis of 379 NPC patients with subsequent metastases reported by Hui et al. [7], the lung metastasis alone was demonstrated as a positive factor of survival and long-term survival was possible for those patients. The reason for poor survival of liver metastasis may relate to the rich blood supply of liver and the low rate of the response to chemotherapy. Furthermore, the patients with single metastasis exhibited the excellent survival with 3-year OS rate of 65.8%, while only 25.9% for those patients with multiple metastases. It may be the sub-group of long-term survival after aggressive approach to treatment.

Elevated levels of LDH also demonstrated as a negative prognostic factor, which may be associated with large tumor burden, tumor extension and high risk of metastasis [18–20]. Serum LDH levels twice normal levels are rarely seen in loco-regional disease but are commonly observed in NPC patients with liver metastasis or multiple organ metastases. Studies have found that NPC patients with elevated baseline LDH levels were more likely to develop liver metastasis after treatment. In the study of Jin

et al. [20], elevated LDH levels were reported in over 55.0% of patients with metastatic NPC, the relative risk to die increased with LDH>245 IU/L by the factor 1.8. In our study, the 3-year OS rate of patients with normal level of LDH was about 47.7%, significantly higher those with elevated LDH levels with a 3-year OS rate of 13.7%. More than 60% of patients with liver metastasis had elevated levels of LDH. Furthermore, elevated LDH was also associated with poor response of metastatic lesions to chemotherapy. Pretreatment serum level of LDH may be a potential predictor.

This retrospective analysis has several weaknesses. First, the circulating EBV DNA load has been demonstrated as an independent prognostic factor in disseminated NPC [21]. However, only small part of patients' EBV DNA data was collected in our study, therefore we had excluded the factor to avoid the potential bias. Second, treatment modality has an impact on survival outcome in patients with disseminated NPC at initial diagnosis. Since the treatment modalities were selected according to the physician's policy of practice in our study, it is inevitable to cause selection bias when we identify prognostic factors for patients with distant metastases at initial diagnosis.

Conclusion

In this study we identified some negative prognostic factors for patients with distant metastases at initial diagnosis which included poor performance status, elevated levels of LDH, liver metastasis and multiple metastases. We also found that chemotherapy alone, chemotherapy cycles<4 and poor response to chemotherapy were associated with poor OS. It can help to select the appropriate patient for more progressive treatment of a combination of chemotherapy and radiotherapy. Long-term survival is possible for patients with less negative prognostic factors. Prospective randomized studies are needed to optimize treatment strategy.

Author Contributions

Conceived and designed the experiments: LZ TXL. Performed the experiments: LZ YMT FH. Analyzed the data: LZ YMT YH XMS FHW XWD. Contributed reagents/materials/analysis tools: YMT XMS. Wrote the paper: LZ.

References

1. Jemal A, Bray F, Center MM, Ferlay J, Ward E, et al. (2011) Global cancer statistics. CA Cancer J Clin 61: 69–90.
2. Parkin DM, Bray F, Ferlay J, Pisani P. (2005) Global cancer statistics, 2002. CA Cancer J Clin 55: 74–108.
3. Al-Sarraf M, LeBlanc M, Giri PG, Fu KK, Cooper J, et al. (1998) Chemoradiotherapy versus radiotherapy in patients with advanced nasopharyngeal cancer: phase III randomized Intergroup study 0099. J Clin Oncol 16: 1310–1317.
4. Lee AW, Ng WT, Chan YH, Sze H, Chan C, et al. (2012) The battle against nasopharyngeal cancer. Radiother Oncol 104: 272–278.
5. Wei WI, Sham JS. (2005) Nasopharyngeal carcinoma. Lancet 365: 2041–2054.
6. Teo PM, Kwan WH, Lee WY, Leung SF, Johnson PJ. (1996) Prognosticators determining survival subsequent to distant metastasis from nasopharyngeal carcinoma. Cancer 77: 2423–2431.
7. Hui EP, Leung SF, Au JS, Zee B, Tung S, et al. (2004) Lung metastasis alone in nasopharyngeal carcinoma: a relatively favorable prognostic group. A study by the Hong Kong nasopharyngeal carcinoma study group. Cancer 101: 300–306.
8. Ong YK, Heng DM, Chung B, Leong SS, Wee J, et al. (2003) Design of a prognostic index score for metastatic nasopharyngeal carcinoma. Eur J Cancer 39: 1535–1541.
9. Jin Y, Cai XY, Cai YC, Cao Y, Xia Q, et al. (2012) To build a prognostic score model containing indispensible tumor markers for metastatic nasopharyngeal carcinoma in an epidemic area. Eur J Cancer 48: 882–888.
10. Khanfir A, Frikha M, Ghorbel A, Drira MM, Daoud J, et al. (2007) Prognostic factors in metastatic nasopharyngeal carcinoma. Cancer Radiotherapy 11: 461–464.

11. Fandi A, Bachouchi M, Azli N, Taamma A, Boussen H, et al. (2000) Long-term disease-free survivors in metastatic undifferentiated carcinoma of nasopharyngeal type. J Clin Oncol 18: 1324–1330.
12. Setton J, Wolden S, Caria N, Lee N. (2012) Definitive treatment of metastatic nasopharyngeal carcinoma: Report of 5 cases with review of literature. Head Neck 34: 753–757.
13. Yeh SA, Tang Y, Lui CC, Huang EY. (2006) Treatment outcomes of patients with AJCC stage IVC nasopharyngeal carcinoma: benefits of primary radiotherapy. Jpn J Clin Oncol 36: 132–136.
14. Zhao C, Han F, Lu LX, Huang SM, Lin CG, et al. (2004) Intensity modulated radiotherapy for local-regional advanced nasopharyngeal carcinoma. Ai Zheng 23: 1532–1537.
15. Luo W, Deng XW, Lu TX. (2004) Dosimetric evaluation for three dimensional radiotherapy plans for patients with early nasopharyngeal carcinoma. Ai Zheng 23: 605–608.
16. Au E, Ang PT. (1994) A phase II trial of 5-fluorouracil and cisplatinum in recurrent or metastatic nasopharyngeal carcinoma. Ann Oncol 5: 87–89.
17. Foo KF, Tan EH, Leong SS, Wee JT, Tan T, et al. (2002) Gemcitabine in metastatic nasopharyngeal carcinoma of the undifferentiated type. Ann Oncol 13: 150–156.
18. Liaw CC, Wang CH, Huang JS, Kiu MC, Chen JS, et al. (1997) Serum lactate dehydrogenase level in patients with nasopharyngeal carcinoma. Acta Oncol 36: 159–164.
19. Zhou GQ, Tang LL, Mao YP, Chen L, Li WF, et al. (2012) Baseline serum lactate dehydrogenase levels for patients treated with intensity-modulated radiotherapy for nasopharyngeal carcinoma: a predictor of poor prognosis and subsequent liver metastasis. Int J Radiat Oncol Biol Phys 82: 359–365.

28

Ratio of Intratumoral Macrophage Phenotypes Is a Prognostic Factor in Epithelioid Malignant Pleural Mesothelioma

Robin Cornelissen[1⊙], **Lysanne A. Lievense**[1⊙], **Alexander P. Maat**[2], **Rudi W. Hendriks**[1], **Henk C. Hoogsteden**[1], **Ad J. Bogers**[2], **Joost P. Hegmans**[1], **Joachim G. Aerts**[1]*

1 Department of Pulmonary Medicine, Erasmus MC Cancer Institute, Rotterdam, The Netherlands, **2** Department of Cardio-Thoracic Surgery, Erasmus MC Cancer Institute, Rotterdam, The Netherlands

Abstract

Hypothesis: The tumor micro-environment and especially the different macrophage phenotypes appear to be of great influence on the behavior of multiple tumor types. M1 skewed macrophages possess anti-tumoral capacities, while the M2 polarized macrophages have pro-tumoral capacities. We analyzed if the macrophage count and the M2 to total macrophage ratio is a discriminative marker for outcome after surgery in malignant pleural mesothelioma (MPM) and studied the prognostic value of these immunological cells.

Methods: 8 MPM patients who received induction chemotherapy and surgical treatment were matched on age, sex, tumor histology, TNM stage and EORTC score with 8 patients who received chemotherapy only. CD8 positive T-cells and the total macrophage count, using the CD68 pan-macrophage marker, and CD163 positive M2 macrophage count were determined in tumor specimens prior to treatment.

Results: The number of CD68 and CD163 cells was comparable between the surgery and the non-surgery group, and was not related to overall survival (OS) in both the surgery and non-surgery group. However, the CD163/CD68 ratio did correlate with OS in both in the total patient group (Pearson r −0.72, p<0.05). No correlation between the number of CD8 cells and prognosis was found.

Conclusions: The total number of macrophages in tumor tissue did not correlate with OS in both groups, however, the CD163/CD68 ratio correlates with OS in the total patient group. Our data revealed that the CD163/CD68 ratio is a potential prognostic marker in epithelioid mesothelioma patients independent of treatment but cannot be used as a predictive marker for outcome after surgery.

Editor: Nupur Gangopadhyay, University of Pittsburgh, United States of America

Funding: Stichting Asbestkanker Rotterdam, Mesothelioma Applied Research Foundation (MARF) – Larry Davis Memorial Grant. The funders had no role in study design, data collection and analysis, decision to publish, or preparation of the manuscript.

Competing Interests: The authors have declared that no competing interests exist.

* Email: j.aerts@erasmusmc.nl

⊙ These authors contributed equally to this work.

Introduction

Malignant pleural mesothelioma is invariably a lethal tumor with a median survival of 9–12 months after the first signs of illness. It is one of the diseases caused by exposure to asbestos fibers. The incidence varies from two to 30 cases per 1 000 000 population worldwide. Most patients are older than 60 years, a reflection of the latency period of 30–50 years after asbestos fiber inhalation.

Chemotherapy is offered to patients as standard of care treatment, as it currently is the only treatment that improved survival in randomized controlled trials in mesothelioma patients [1,2]. The survival benefit of chemotherapeutic treatment is in general modest with 2–3 months but long-term survivors do exist.

For decades, clinicians have tried to improve survival by removal of the pleural-based lesions. In order to try to completely remove the disease, a pneumonectomy with the complete removal of the visceral and parietal pleura is considered necessary, a so-called extra-pleural pneumonectomy (EPP). EPP is mostly performed in a multi-modality setting with induction chemotherapy and adjuvant radiotherapy. Selection of patients appeared crucial in the case-series that were published [3]. A less invasive procedure, that does not include the removal of the affected lung but of the visceral and parietal pleura, if necessary pericardium and diaphragm, an extended pleurectomy/decortication (PD), is also performed in patients.

Whether surgery does lead to increased survival remains a matter of continuous debate, but it is evident that long-term survival after surgery occurs [4,5]. On the other hand, there are also patients in whom survival after surgery is extremely short. This points out the need for a biomarker to provide insight in which patients may benefit from surgery and which patients do not.

Gordon *et al.* described a four-gene expression ratio test that can predict good prognosis after surgery [6], however this test still has to be validated in a clinical setting. Suzuki *et al.* found in a patient group with predominantly surgical therapy that chronic inflammation in stroma is an independent predictor of survival [7], while other groups found a subset of immunological cell types to predict for better outcome in patients receiving surgical treatment with a special focus on CD8 tumor infiltrating lymphocytes [8,9]. The question remains whether these factors are prognostic or predictive for the effect of surgery.

The role of immune cells, like CD8 cells, within the tumor microenvironment has become a major area of interest in the last decade. It is now established in certain tumor types, that these infiltrating immune cells are capable of influencing tumor progression. One of the other involved immunological cell types are macrophages, which are known to have a dual role in cancer depending on their phenotype. Tumor associated macrophages (TAMs) can be divided in classically activated (M1) macrophages and alternatively activated macrophages (M2). M1 macrophages, following exposure to interferon-γ (IFN-γ), can secrete chemokines and promote T cell proliferation, thus activate type 1 T cell responses and have antitumor activity and tissue-destructive activity. However, M2 TAMs promote the development and metastatic capacity of tumors due to the production of multiple cytokines such as interleukin (IL)-1, IL-6 and IL-10, vascular endothelial growth factor (VEGF) and transforming growth factor beta (TGF-β) [10]. In mesothelioma, Burt *et al* showed that higher densities of tumor-infiltrating macrophages are associated with poor survival in patients after surgery, however, this was only in patients with non-epithelioid MPM [11].

A large proportion of M1 macrophages in the total macrophage count that can aid in tumoricidal activities could provide a better tumor control, since the overall balance in the tumor microenvironment shifts to an anti-tumor response. If the TAMs largely consist of M2 macrophages, this balance can shift to an overall pro-tumor micro-environment. The importance of the percentage of M2 macrophages of the total macrophage count (i.e. the CD163/CD68 ratio) and M1/M2 ratio has been found in other tumor types recently, such as melanoma, non-small cell lung carcinoma and angioimmunoblastic T-cell lymphoma [12–17]. In most of these studies, the ratio of M1/M2 macrophages predicts survival and metastatic ability of these cancers. Overall, a larger M2 component of the total macrophage count is inversely correlated with survival.

With CD8 T-cells and TAMS being the key immune cells in the tumor microenvironment [18,19], we analyzed if T cells and macrophage subtypes could be useful as a predictive marker to select mesothelioma patients for surgical treatment. Furthermore, the prognostic value of the different macrophage subtypes and CD8 positive tumor infiltrating lymphocytes (TILs) were tested.

Materials and Methods

Patients and specimens

The Erasmus Medical Center ethical commission gave approval for this study. Diagnostic paraffin-embedded tumor specimens were used from 8 MPM patients who underwent an extended PD during the course of a phase 1 clinical trial following induction chemotherapy in our institute between 2008 and 2010 (a local study which is identified as Erasmus MC Cancer Institute MEC

number 2008-405). The clinical trial randomized patients to P/D or best supportive care. Consent was obtained to use patient material for future research. Unfortunately, from the patients randomized to the best supportive care arm, adequate histology was not available in all cases. Therefore, we selected 8 MPM out of the total 89 patients that only were treated with chemotherapy during the course of the trial. The selection was matched to the surgical cases upon survival, EORTC prognostic score [20] and histology. Patient information was anonymized end de-identified prior to analysis. Histopathological diagnoses were established by pathologists from our institute and confirmed by the National Mesothelioma Pathology Board. Clinicopathological information was collected from patient charts. The TNM stage was based on the International Union Against Cancer (UICC) and the American Joint Committee on Cancer (AJCC) classification. Overall survival (OS) analysis of patients who underwent either chemotherapy or chemotherapy and PD was conducted. OS was defined as the time from the completion of chemotherapy to death. Three patients are still alive at the time of submitting this manuscript, since these are the 3 patients with the longest survival, last contact date was used instead of date of death.

Immunohistochemistry

The following primary antibodies were used: anti-human CD8 (clone C8/144B, Dako, Glostrup, Denmark), anti-human CD68 (clone KP-1, Dako), and anti-human CD163 (clone 10D6,Leica Biosystems Novocastra, Newcastle, UK). Paraffin-embedded tumor specimens were cut into sequential 5 µm thick sections and deparaffinized and stained using a fully automated Ventana BenchMark ULTRA Stainer (Ventana, Tucson Arizona, USA) according to manufacturers' instructions at the pathology department. Binding of peroxidase-coupled antibodies was detected using 3,3' - diaminobenzidine (DAB) as a substrate and the slides were counterstained with haematoxylin. The specificity of antibodies was checked using isotype-matched controls.

Evaluation of CD8, CD68 and CD163 stainings

The number of CD8-positive T-cells, CD68-positive total macrophages and CD163-positive M2-type macrophages were independently assessed by two investigators (R.C. and L.L.) who were not informed of the patients' clinicopathological data. To examine TILs and TAMs, the number of cells per microscopic field of $0,025$ cm^2 with immunoreactivity to CD8, CD68 and CD163 were counted in three independent tumor areas with the most abundant immunoreactive cells. For each antibody, the same area was used. Only cells with a visible nucleus were counted. We defined the average value of the three times the number of TILs and TAMs were counted for each case.

In vitro measurement of CD80, HLA-DR, IL-10, IL-12, VEGF, PD-L1, CD163, iNOS (NOS2) and Arginase-1 in macrophages by quantitative real time PCR

We investigated the influence of mesothelioma-derived factors on the phenotype and function of macrophages. Monocytes obtained from peripheral blood of an healthy control were cultured in the presence of 20 ng/ml recombinant M-CSF (R&D systems, Abingdon U.K.) in RPMI medium (Life Technologies, Bleiswijk, the Netherlands) containing 5% normal healthy AB serum (NHS) during 6 days at 37°C/5% CO$_2$. After six days of differentiation, macrophages were cultured in the presence of 30% mesothelioma cell line conditioned media (CM) during two days (n = 6). CM were obtained from mesothelioma cell lines at 80% confluency, centrifuged for 10 min at 400×g to remove cells and debris. These long-term tumor cell lines were established from the cellular fraction of 6 mesothelioma patient's pleural effusions as described earlier [21]. As a control we used standardized M1 (medium supplemented with 100 ng/ml LPS [Sigma-Aldrich, Zwijndrecht, the Netherlands] and 20 ng/ml IFN-gamma [R&D systems] and M2 cultures (medium supplemented with 40 ng/ml IL-10 [R&D systems]). Cells were harvested and mRNA was isolated by RNeasy micro kit according to manufacturer's instruction (Qiagen, Hilden, Germany). cDNA was prepared from 1 ug RNA sample using First Strand cDNA synthesis kit (Thermo Fisher, Pittsburgh, PA, USA). cDNA (5 µL) was amplified by RT-PCR reactions with 1× Maxima SYBR green/ROX qPCR mastermix (Thermo Fisher) in 96-well plates on an 7300 real time PCR system (Applied Biosystems), using the program: 10 min at 95°C, and then 40 cycles of 20 s at 95°C, 1 min at 58°C and 30 sec at 72°C. The primer sets used for different sets of genes are listed in Table 1. Specificity of the produced amplification product was confirmed by examination of dissociation curves. Expression levels were normalized to the internal control β-actin.

Statistical analysis

The numbers of CD8 TILs and CD163 and/or CD68 TAMs were expressed as mean ± SD. Statistical differences between the means were analyzed by the Mann–Whitney U test. Correlations were made calculating the Pearson r correlation. Statistical calculations were performed using IBM SPSS Statistics version 21.0.0.1. Statistical significance was established at the $p<0.05$ level, and all analyses were two-sided. Overall survival (OS) was calculated from the start date of treatment until patient death.

Results

Patient characteristics

The median age of all participating patients was 62 years (range 36-75 years). There were 12 men and 4 women. All histologies were of the epithelioid subtype. The patient characteristics of the surgery and the non-surgery group are listed in Table 2. Chemotherapeutic treatment was given in both groups and consisted of 4 cycles of pemetrexed combined with either cisplatin or carboplatin. In case of surgery, P/D was performed 8 to 10 weeks after induction chemotherapy in all cases.

CD8 tumor infiltrating lymphocytes in MPM

A representative image of immunohistochemical staining of CD8 TILs are shown in Figure 1. The mean CD8 numbers were comparable between the surgery and the non-surgery group ($p = 0.51$) and no correlation was found between CD8 cell count and OS in the surgery group ($p = 0.88$) and non-surgery group ($p = 0.96$) nor for the whole group ($p = 0.73$).

CD68 and CD163 TAMs in MPM

Representative images of immunohistochemical staining of TAMs are shown in Figure 2a and 2b. The total count of CD68 was comparable between surgery and the non-surgery group (mean 211.3, SD 80.2 vs. mean 213.9, SD 100.4, $p = 1.0$). Also, the total count of CD163 was comparable between surgery and the non-surgery group (mean 168.3, SD 80.2 vs. mean 164.1, SD 82.5, $p = 0.8$).

The CD68 count did not correlate with OS (Figure 3a, Pearson r -0.07, $p = 0.81$), the CD163 count showed an inverse trend with OS (Figure 3b, Pearson r -0.33, $p = 0.22$).

CD163/CD68 ratio correlating with overall survival

We calculated the CD163/CD68 ratio, i.e. the number of M2 macrophages within the total macrophage count. This ratio was significantly negatively correlated with OS in the total patient group (Figure 4, Pearson r -0.72, $p<0.05$). A correlation analysis for the individual groups in regards to the CD163/CD68 and OS showed a significant correlation in the non-surgery group (Pearson r -0.91 [$p = 0.001$]) and a trend for the surgery group (Pearson r -0.65 [$p = 0.08$]).

RT-PCR measurements for macrophage phenotype conditioned in mesothelioma environments

To investigate the influence of tumor-derived factors on macrophage phenotype, we cultured monocyte-derived macrophages in the presence of supernatant derived from six mesothelioma cell lines. Tumor cell supernatants (CM) induced macrophages towards a M2 prone phenotype with relatively high expression levels of the M2 cytokine IL-10 and low mRNA levels of the M1 markers IL-12, CD80 and HLA-DR. The standard M2 marker CD163 and the arginase1/iNOS ratio showed differential expressions dependent on the different CM. Furthermore, expression levels of the activation marker PD-L1 on macrophages cultured in CM were comparable to the M2 condition, in general these levels were lower than the M1 condition. Furthermore, results showed that CM have different abilities to influence macrophage phenotypes (Figure 5). Gene expression of IL-12 was only found when macrophages were cultured under M1 conditions

Table 1. Primer sequences of genes associated with macrophage phenotype used in RT-PCR.

Gene	Forward primer	Reverse primer
β-actin	CTGTGGCATCCACGAAACTA	AGTACTTGCGCTCAGGAGGA
CD80	AAACTCGCATCTACTGGCAAA	GGTTCTTGTACTCGGGCCATA
HLA-DR	AGTCCCTGTGCTAGGATTTTTCA	ACATAAACTCGCCTGATTGGTC
IL-10	TCAAACTCACTCATGGCTTTGT	GCTGTCATCGATTTCTTCCC
IL-12	GCGGAGCTGCTACACTCTC	CCATGACCTCAATGGGCAGAC
VEGF	CACACAGGATGGCTTGAAGA	AGGGCAGAATCATCACGAAG
PD-L1	TATGGTGGTGCCGACTACAA	TGCTTGTCCAGATGACTTCG
CD163	GCGGGAGAGTGGAAGTGAAAG	GTTACAAATCACAGAGACCGCT
iNOS	ATTCTGCTGCTTGCTGAGGT	TTCAAGACCAAATTCCACCAG
Arg1	GTTTCTCAAGCAGACCAGCC	GCTCAAGTGCAGCAAAGAGA

Table 2. Patient characteristics.

	Surgery	Non-surgery
Patients (n)	8	8
Mean age (SD)	60 (11,9)	55 (7)
Male (n)	6	6
EORTC (SD)	1,025 (0,6)	0,88 (0,5)
EORTC high (n)	2	1
EORTC low (n)	6	7
PR after chemotherapy (n)	1	2
TNM		
T1-2 (n)	6	5
T3-4 (n)	2	3
N0 (n)	5	5
N1-2 (n)	3	3
M0 (n)	8	7

and VEGF expression was low/absent in all conditions (data not shown). In conclusion, mesothelioma-derived factors influence macrophages towards a M2 phenotype to varying degrees.

Discussion

Macrophages in tumors are usually referred to as tumor-associated macrophages and their presence can be substantial (up to 60% of the tumor mass) [22]. A hallmark of macrophages is their plasticity, an ability to either aid or fight tumors depending on the tumor environment, which has given them the reputation of a double-edged sword in tumor biology [23]. At the extremes of this spectrum are the M1 and M2 macrophages. In an early phase of tumor development, the TAMs mainly consist of an M1-like phenotype and later in the tumorigenic process, when the tumor changes its local environment, there is a skewing toward the M2 phenotype [24–26]. Analysis of CD163/CD68 ratio in biopsy material before treatment showed a correlation with OS (combined groups: Pearson r -0.72 [p<0.05]; non-surgery group:

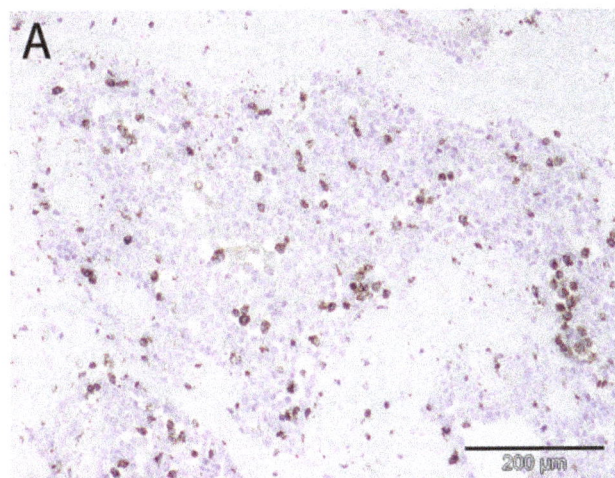

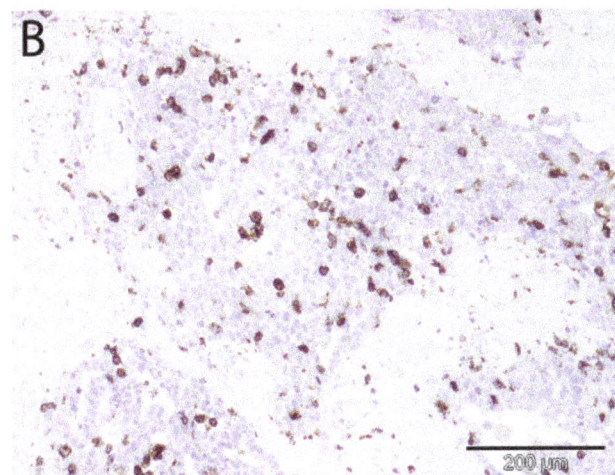

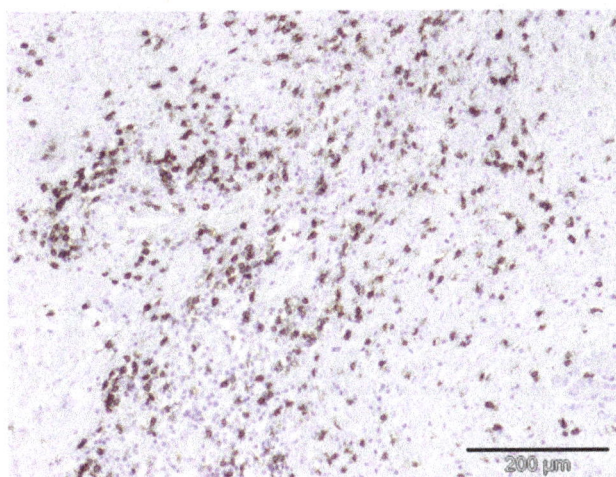

Figure 1. Representative image of CD8 staining in the tumor biopsy of one MPM patient.

Figure 2. Representative images of CD68 (a) and CD163 (b) staining in the tumor biopsy of one MPM patient.

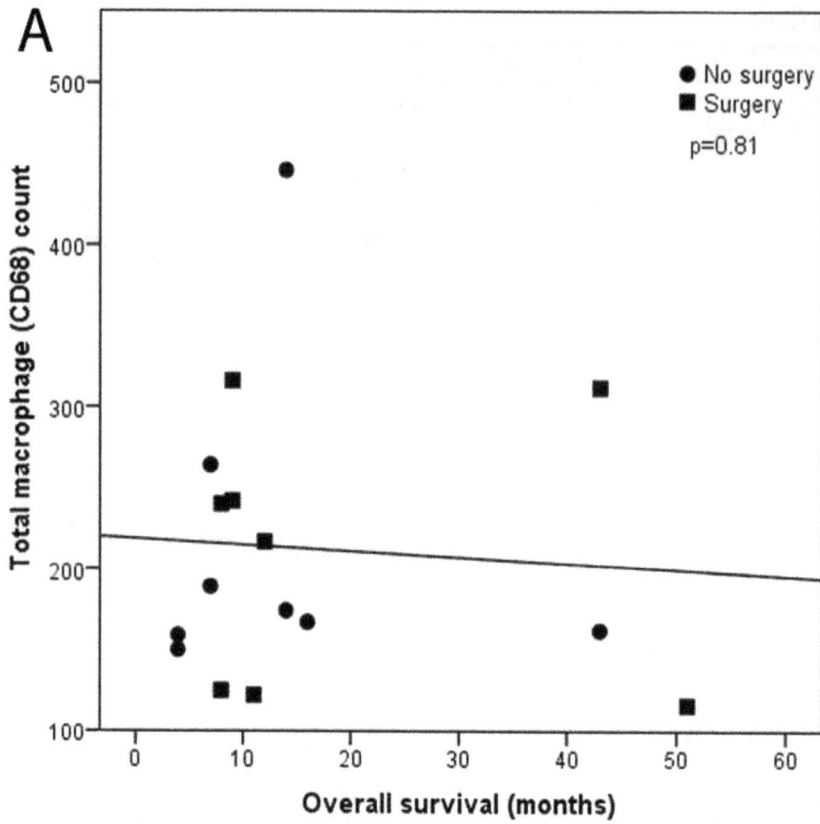

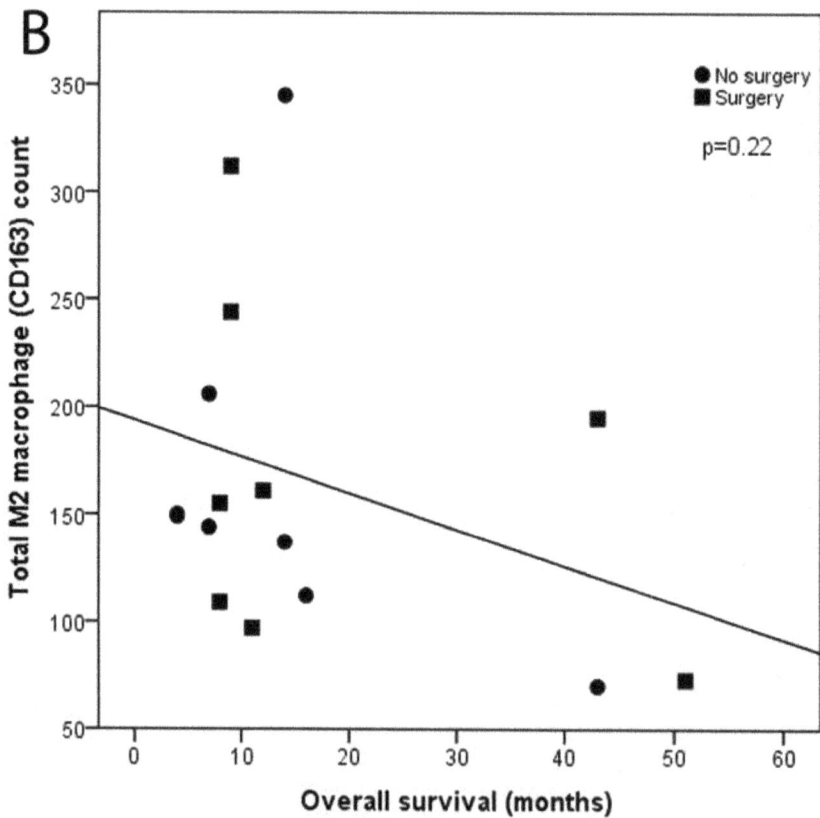

Figure 3. Correlation between CD68 (a) count or CD 163 (b) count and OS in both surgery and non-surgery groups. The CD68 count does not correlate with OS (Pearson r -0.07, p = 0.81), the CD163 count shows an inverse trend with OS (Pearson r -0.33, p = 0.22).

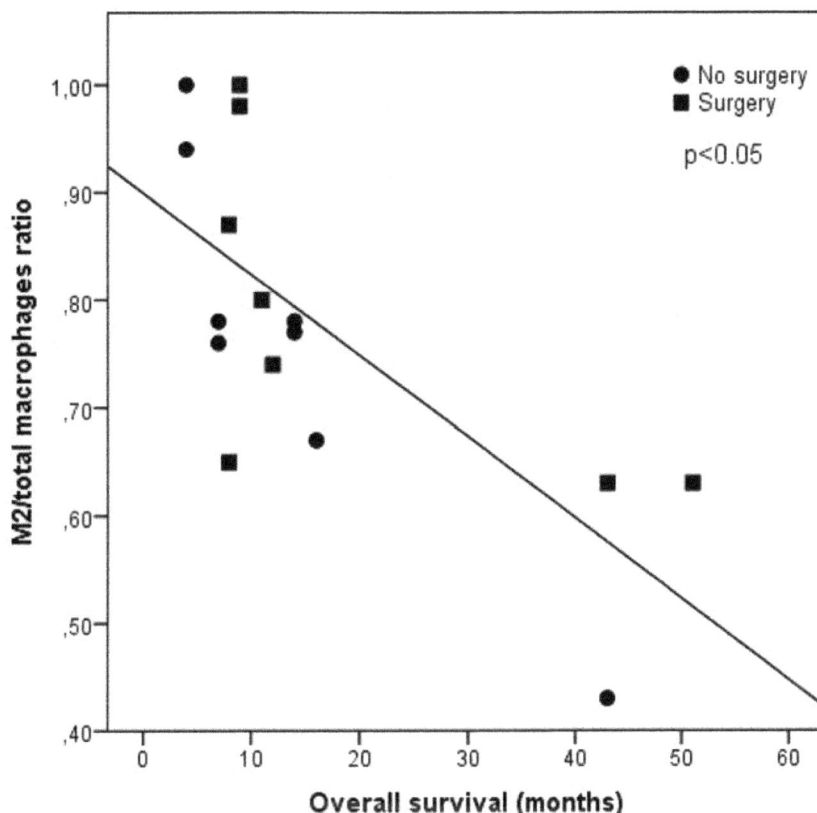

Figure 4. Correlation between CD163/CD68 ratio in tumor in both surgery and non-surgery patients and OS. This ratio is significantly negatively correlated with OS in the total patient group (Pearson r -0.72, p<0.05).

Pearson r -0.91 [p = 0.001]; surgery group: Pearson r -0.65 [p = 0.08]). The total number of macrophages did not correlate with OS, indicating that the absolute number of macrophages does not influence tumor progression. The percentage of M2 macrophages of the total macrophage count was comparable between the surgery and non-surgery group and therefore, the CD163/CD68 ratio does not discriminate in favor of surgery in mesothelioma patients.

Although the terms M1 and M2 macrophages are an oversimplification of reality, it can be used to explain the opposing effects of different macrophage subsets. Our findings indeed correspond with the negative prognostic capacities of the M2 macrophages; a large proportion of these CD163 positive macrophages in the total macrophage count correlates with a decreased survival. This emphasis that the balance between M1 and M2 macrophages seems to play a crucial role in the prognosis of MPM patient.

As mentioned before, the importance of the CD163/CD68 and M1/M2 ratio is found in several other tumor types [12–17]. In our study, a similar outcome is found regarding M1/M2 ratio based on CD163/68 ratio and the prediction of survival in patients with mesothelioma. This gives a clinical correlation to the hypothesis of the anti-tumor effect of M1 TAMs and the pro-tumor effect of the M2 TAMs. To our knowledge, this is the first publication showing the importance of the CD163/CD68 ratio in mesothelioma. Furthermore, this ratio proved to be significantly correlated with survival in epithelioid mesothelioma. Previously, it was only shown that the absolute number of macrophages was prognostic in non-epithelioid mesothelioma after EPP [11].

In previous studies looking at the number of CD8 TIL's a high number of CD8 TIL was associated with a better outcome in mesothelioma patients after surgery [8,9]. We could not reproduce these findings in our study. This could be due to the smaller numbers of surgical patients that were available for our study. Furthermore, the correlation between TIL count and survival was only found in patients that received chemotherapy and EPP, while in our study, P/D was performed.

The six mesothelioma cell lines showed evident heterogeneous effects on the macrophages in terms of macrophage polarization. Tumor-derived factors from cell lines induced M1 and M2 macrophage phenotypes in varying degrees, in concordance with the broad phenotype spectrum found in tumors. However, overall the tumor cell supernatants induced a more M2 prone phenotype with relatively high expression levels of IL-10 and low expression levels of M1 markers: IL-12, CD80 and HLA-DR. The standard M2 marker CD163 and the arginase1/iNOS ratio showed very differential results between the tumor cell lines. Furthermore, PD-L1 expression levels appeared to be relatively low. However, PD-L1 is known to be upregulated in a response to high IFN-γ levels as a negative feedback mechanism and therefore although PD-L1 is a co-inhibitory receptor, its presence can be indicative of an active T-cell response [27–29]. This was confirmed by the high PD-L1 level in the M1 condition. The *in vitro* experiments using tumor derived factors to influence macrophage phenotype complement the *in vivo* immunohistochemical findings by demonstrating that tumor-derived factors can directly modulate macrophage phenotype multiformity.

In addition to the impact of this finding on prognostic value of the OS of patients, macrophages may also reveal as a potential

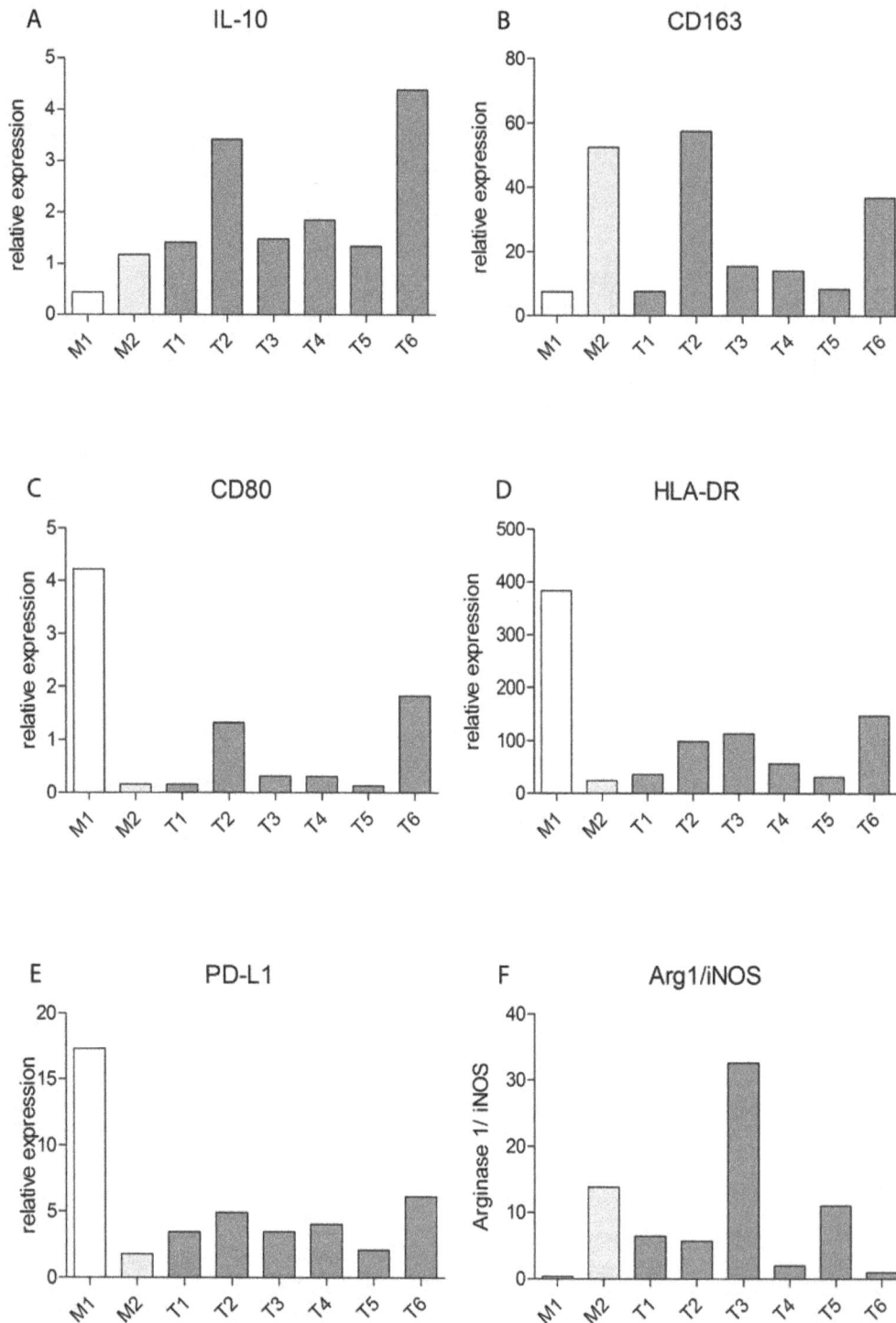

Figure 5. Tumor derived factors influence macrophages towards a M2 phenotype to varying degrees. Relative mRNA expression levels of IL-10 (a), CD163 (b), CD80 (c), HLA-DR (d), PD-L1 (e), and Arginase-1/iNOS (NOS2) ratio (f) in macrophages cultured in six mesothelioma cell line conditioned media (T1 - T6) compared to standard M1 and M2 conditions.

target for therapeutic intervention. Targeting the total macrophage population would not be the most optimal approach, since M1 macrophages would be decreased as well as the M2 macrophages. In an earlier trial we showed that this kind of intervention does not lead to increased survival in a murine model of mesothelioma [36]. There are several proposed strategies to counteract the M2 macrophages, including inhibiting M2 macrophage recruitment [37], M2 macrophage depletion [38] and blocking M2 tumor-promoting activity of TAMs [39]. However, since M2 macrophages remain the plasticity for polarization [40], re-polarization from M2 to M1-type could be the ideal method to tip the balance between M1 and M2 to a tumor-hostile situation. Recently, it has become clear that there is probably not one single compound that can achieve this goal [22]. A proposed strategy therefore is a combination of infusion of antibodies against CD40 in order to stimulate the secondary lymph node resident macrophages to migrate into the tumor tissue with IFN-γ to effectively reprogram tumor-induced M2-like macrophages into activated IL-12 producing M1 cells [41]. In addition, targeting the nuclear factor κB (NF-κB) signaling pathway, a crucial pathway in the activation of M2 TAMs, was shown to switch M2 TAMs to a M1 phenotype [42]. Furthermore, the combined use of Toll-like receptor 9 ligand CpG-ODN and anti-IL-10 blocking antibodies has been shown to induce the switch from M2 to M1 phenotype [43]. Also, several other therapeutic strategies are under investigation [44–47]. In mesothelioma, Fridlender et al. tested monocyte chemoattractant protein-1 (MCP-1/CCL2) blockade in a mouse model for mesothelioma and demonstrated an altered macrophage phenotype and improved survival. Currently there are no clinical compounds tested in mesothelioma patients which specifically aim at macrophage repolarization [48].

Our study has several limitations. First, the number of patients included is rather small. This is due to the fact that mesothelioma surgery in Europe is advised to be only performed in the setting of a clinical trial by the guidelines of the European Respiratory Society and the European Society of Thoracic Surgeons for the management of malignant pleural mesothelioma [30]. The results of the present trial are based on a trial randomizing patients between P/D or observation. This trial was stopped based on slow accrual. Furthermore, only patients with the epithelioid subtype of mesothelioma were selected for surgery. The trend seen in the surgery group between the CD163/CD68 ratio and OS should be confirmed in a larger patient group and we hope that our findings will encourage other researchers who have access to patients undergoing surgery to confirm the data presented in this manuscript. Second, a definitive M1 macrophage marker would enhance the findings of our manuscript for this would give a true insight in the M1/M2 macrophage ratio. NOS2 expression has proven be a useful marker for M1 macrophages in several tumor types [31–33]. However, for mesothelioma, Soini et al. and others [34,35] have demonstrated that NOS2 is highly expressed in healthy pleura as well as in cancerous mesothelioma tissues and mesothelioma cell lines. These findings complicate the use of NOS2 in pleural diseases as mesothelioma. Whether the unique capacity of mesothelial/mesothelioma tumor cells of synthesizing NOS2 is important to control a variety of infections in the pleural space in particular is unknown.

In conclusion, CD163/CD68 ratio was found to be a prognostic marker in a limited number of epithelioid mesothelioma patients, but not a predictive marker for outcome after surgery. This study emphasizes the importance of the balance between M1 and M2 macrophages in tumor behavior. In spite of not being a predictive factor for surgery in mesothelioma, we consider that the prognostic value may be of great importance in patients with mesothelioma. Repolarization of macrophages may be a new therapeutic target in mesothelioma complementing immunotherapeutic strategies.

Acknowledgments

We would like to thank Lisette de Vogel of the Department of Pathology for the technical assistance with the immunohistochemical techniques.

Author Contributions

Conceived and designed the experiments: RC LL JH JA. Performed the experiments: RC LL. Analyzed the data: RC LL JH RH JA AB HH AM. Contributed reagents/materials/analysis tools: RC JH LL. Wrote the paper: RC LL JH RH JA AB HH AM.

References

1. Vogelzang NJ, Rusthoven JJ, Symanowski J, Denham C, Kaukel E, et al. (2003) Phase III study of pemetrexed in combination with cisplatin versus cisplatin alone in patients with malignant pleural mesothelioma. J Clin Oncol 21: 2636–2644. doi:10.1200/JCO.2003.11.136

2. Van Meerbeeck JP, Gaafar R, Manegold C, Van Klaveren RJ, Van Marck EA, et al. (2005) Randomized phase III study of cisplatin with or without raltitrexed in patients with malignant pleural mesothelioma: an intergroup study of the European Organisation for Research and Treatment of Cancer Lung Cancer Group and the National Cancer Institute of Canada. J Clin Oncol 23: 6881–6889. doi:10.1200/JCO.20005.14.589

3. Flores RM, Pass HI, Seshan VE, Dycoco J, Zakowski M, et al. (2008) Extrapleural pneumonectomy versus pleurectomy/decortication in the surgical management of malignant pleural mesothelioma: results in 663 patients. J Thorac Cardiovasc Surg 135: 620–626, 626.e1–3. doi:10.1016/j.jtcvs.2007.10.054

4. Alexander HR Jr, Bartlett DL, Pingpank JF, Libutti SK, Royal R, et al. (2013) Treatment factors associated with long-term survival after cytoreductive surgery and regional chemotherapy for patients with malignant peritoneal mesothelioma. Surgery 153: 779–786. doi:10.1016/j.surg.2013.01.001

5. Haas AR, Sterman DH (2013) Malignant Pleural Mesothelioma. Clinics in Chest Medicine 34: 99–111. doi:10.1016/j.ccm.2012.12.005

6. Gordon GJ, Dong L, Yeap BY, Richards WG, Glickman JN, et al. (2009) Four-gene expression ratio test for survival in patients undergoing surgery for mesothelioma. Journal of the National Cancer Institute 101: 678–686.

7. Suzuki K, Kadota K, Sima CS, Sadelain M, Rusch VW, et al. (2011) Chronic inflammation in tumor stroma is an independent predictor of prolonged survival in epithelioid malignant pleural mesothelioma patients. Cancer Immunology, Immunotherapy 60: 1721–1728. doi:10.1007/s00262-011-1073-8

8. Yamada N, Oizumi S, Kikuchi E, Shinagawa N, Konishi-Sakakibara J, et al. (2010) CD8+ tumor-infiltrating lymphocytes predict favorable prognosis in malignant pleural mesothelioma after resection. Cancer Immunology, Immunotherapy 59: 1543–1549. doi:10.1007/s00262-010-0881-6

9. Anraku M, Cunningham KS, Yun Z, Tsao M-S, Zhang L, et al. (2008) Impact of tumor-infiltrating T cells on survival in patients with malignant pleural mesothelioma. J Thorac Cardiovasc Surg 135: 823–829. doi:10.1016/j.jtcvs.2007.10.026

10. Cornelissen R, Heuvers ME, Maat AP, Hendriks RW, Hoogsteden HC, et al. (2012) New Roads Open Up for Implementing Immunotherapy in Mesothelioma. Clinical and Developmental Immunology: 1–13. doi:10.1155/2012/927240

11. Burt BM, Rodig SJ, Tilleman TR, Elbardissi AW, Bueno R, et al. (2011) Circulating and tumor-infiltrating myeloid cells predict survival in human pleural mesothelioma. Cancer 117: 5234–5244. doi:10.1002/cncr.26143

12. Lan C, Huang X, Lin S, Huang H, Cai Q, et al. (2012) Expression of M2-Polarized Macrophages is Associated with Poor Prognosis for Advanced Epithelial Ovarian Cancer. Technol Cancer Res Treat.

13. Cui Y-L, Li H-K, Zhou H-Y, Zhang T, Li Q (2013) Correlations of Tumor-associated Macrophage Subtypes with Liver Metastases of Colorectal Cancer. Asian Pac J Cancer Prev 14: 1003–1007.

14. Medrek C, Pontén F, Jirström K, Leandersson K (2012) The presence of tumor associated macrophages in tumor stroma as a prognostic marker for breast cancer patients. BMC cancer 12: 306.

15. Herwig MC, Bergstrom C, Wells JR, Höller T, Grossniklaus HE (2013) M2/M1 ratio of tumor associated macrophages and PPAR-gamma expression in uveal melanomas with class 1 and class 2 molecular profiles. Exp Eye Res 107: 52–58. doi:10.1016/j.exer.2012.11.012

16. Niino D, Komohara Y, Murayama T, Aoki R, Kimura Y, et al. (2010) Ratio of M2 macrophage expression is closely associated with poor prognosis for Angioimmunoblastic T-cell lymphoma (AITL). Pathol Int 60: 278–283. doi:10.1111/j.1440-1827.2010.02514.x

17. Becker M, Müller CB, De Bastiani MA, Klamt F (2013) The prognostic impact of tumor-associated macrophages and intra-tumoral apoptosis in non-small cell lung cancer. Histol Histopathol.

18. Mantovani A, Sica A (2010) Macrophages, innate immunity and cancer: balance, tolerance, and diversity. Curr Opin Immunol 22: 231–237. doi:10.1016/j.coi.2010.01.009

19. Lievense LA, Bezemer K, Aerts JGJV, Hegmans JPJJ (2013) Tumor-associated macrophages in thoracic malignancies. Lung Cancer. doi:10.1016/j.lungcan.2013.02.017

20. Fennell DA (2004) Statistical Validation of the EORTC Prognostic Model for Malignant Pleural Mesothelioma Based on Three Consecutive Phase II Trials. Journal of Clinical Oncology 23: 184–189. doi:10.1200/JCO.2005.07.050

21. Hegmans JPJJ, Hemmes A, Hammad H, Boon L, Hoogsteden HC, et al. (2006) Mesothelioma environment comprises cytokines and T-regulatory cells that suppress immune responses. Eur Respir J 27: 1086–1095. doi:10.1183/09031936.06.00135305

22. Heusinkveld M, van der Burg SH (2011) Identification and manipulation of tumor associated macrophages in human cancers. Journal of Translational Medicine 9: 216. doi:10.1186/1479-5876-9-216

23. Brower V (2012) Macrophages: cancer therapy's double-edged sword. J Natl Cancer Inst 104: 649–652. doi:10.1093/jnci/djs235

24. Schmid MC, Varner JA (2010) Myeloid cells in the tumor microenvironment: modulation of tumor angiogenesis and tumor inflammation. J Oncol 2010: 201026. doi:10.1155/2010/201026

25. Ruffell B, Affara NI, Coussens LM (2012) Differential macrophage programming in the tumor microenvironment. Trends Immunol 33: 119–126. doi:10.1016/j.it.2011.12.001

26. Bremnes RM, Al-Shibli K, Donnem T, Sirera R, Al-Saad S, et al. (2011) The role of tumor-infiltrating immune cells and chronic inflammation at the tumor site on cancer development, progression, and prognosis: emphasis on non-small cell lung cancer. J Thorac Oncol 6: 824–833. doi:10.1097/JTO.0-b013e3182037b76

27. De Kleijn S, Langereis JD, Leentjens J, Kox M, Netea MG, et al. (2013) IFN-γ-stimulated neutrophils suppress lymphocyte proliferation through expression of PD-L1. PLoS ONE 8: e72249. doi:10.1371/journal.pone.0072249

28. Topalian SL, Drake CG, Pardoll DM (2012) Targeting the PD-1/B7-H1(PD-L1) pathway to activate anti-tumor immunity. Current Opinion in Immunology 24: 207–212. doi:10.1016/j.coi.2011.12.009

29. Taube JM, Anders RA, Young GD, Xu H, Sharma R, et al. (2012) Colocalization of Inflammatory Response with B7-H1 Expression in Human Melanocytic Lesions Supports an Adaptive Resistance Mechanism of Immune Escape. Science Translational Medicine 4: 127ra37–127ra37. doi:10.1126/scitranslmed.3003689

30. Scherpereel A, Astoul P, Baas P, Berghmans T, Clayson H, et al. (2009) Guidelines of the European Respiratory Society and the European Society of Thoracic Surgeons for the management of malignant pleural mesothelioma. European Respiratory Journal 35: 479–495. doi:10.1183/09031936.00063109

31. Edin S, Wikberg ML, Dahlin AM, Rutegård J, Öberg Å, et al. (2012) The distribution of macrophages with a M1 or M2 phenotype in relation to prognosis and the molecular characteristics of colorectal cancer. PLoS One 7: e47045.

32. Pantano F, Berti P, Guida FM, Perrone G, Vincenzi B, et al. (2013) The role of macrophages polarization in predicting prognosis of radically resected gastric cancer patients. J Cell Mol Med 17: 1415–1421. doi:10.1111/jcmm.12109

33. Kaimala S, Mohamed YA, Nader N, Issac J, Elkord E, et al. (2014) Salmonella-mediated tumor regression involves targeting of tumor myeloid suppressor cells causing a shift to M1-like phenotype and reduction in suppressive capacity. Cancer Immunol Immunother 63: 587–599. doi:10.1007/s00262-014-1543-x

34. Soini Y, Kahlos K, Puhakka A, Lakari E, Säily M, et al. (2000) Expression of inducible nitric oxide synthase in healthy pleura and in malignant mesothelioma. Br J Cancer 83: 880–886. doi:10.1054/bjoc.2000.1384

35. Tanaka S, Choe N, Hemenway DR, Zhu S, Matalon S, et al. (1998) Asbestos inhalation induces reactive nitrogen species and nitrotyrosine formation in the lungs and pleura of the rat. J Clin Invest 102: 445–454. doi:10.1172/JCI3169

36. Veltman JD, Lambers MEH, van Nimwegen M, Hendriks RW, Hoogsteden HC, et al. (2010) Zoledronic acid impairs myeloid differentiation to tumour-associated macrophages in mesothelioma. Br J Cancer 103: 629–641. doi:10.1038/sj.bjc.6605814

37. Popivanova BK, Kostadinova FI, Furuichi K, Shamekh MM, Kondo T, et al. (2009) Blockade of a chemokine, CCL2, reduces chronic colitis-associated carcinogenesis in mice. Cancer Res 69: 7884–7892. doi:10.1158/0008-5472.CAN-09-1451

38. Rogers TL, Holen I (2011) Tumour macrophages as potential targets of bisphosphonates. J Transl Med 9: 177. doi:10.1186/1479-5876-9-177

39. Tang X, Mo C, Wang Y, Wei D, Xiao H (2013) Anti-tumour strategies aiming to target tumour-associated macrophages. Immunology 138: 93–104. doi:10.1111/imm.12023

40. Biswas SK, Mantovani A (2010) Macrophage plasticity and interaction with lymphocyte subsets: cancer as a paradigm. Nat Immunol 11: 889–896. doi:10.1038/ni.1937

41. Beatty GL, Chiorean EG, Fishman MP, Saboury B, Teitelbaum UR, et al. (2011) CD40 agonists alter tumor stroma and show efficacy against pancreatic carcinoma in mice and humans. Science 331: 1612–1616. doi:10.1126/science.1198443

42. Hagemann T, Lawrence T, McNeish I, Charles KA, Kulbe H, et al. (2008) "Re-educating" tumor-associated macrophages by targeting NF-kappaB. J Exp Med 205: 1261–1268. doi:10.1084/jem.20080108

43. Guiducci C, Vicari AP, Sangaletti S, Trinchieri G, Colombo MP (2005) Redirecting in vivo elicited tumor infiltrating macrophages and dendritic cells towards tumor rejection. Cancer Res 65: 3437–3446. doi:10.1158/0008-5472.CAN-04-4262

44. Fong CHY, Bebien M, Didierlaurent A, Nebauer R, Hussell T, et al. (2008) An antiinflammatory role for IKKbeta through the inhibition of "classical" macrophage activation. J Exp Med 205: 1269–1276. doi:10.1084/jem.20080124

45. Chuang C-M, Monie A, Hung C-F, Wu T-C (2010) Treatment with imiquimod enhances antitumor immunity induced by therapeutic HPV DNA vaccination. J Biomed Sci 17: 32. doi:10.1186/1423-0127-17-32

46. Buhtoiarov IN, Sondel PM, Wigginton JM, Buhtoiarova TN, Yanke EM, et al. (2011) Anti-tumour synergy of cytotoxic chemotherapy and anti-CD40 plus CpG-ODN immunotherapy through repolarization of tumour-associated macrophages. Immunology 132: 226–239. doi:10.1111/j.1365-2567.2010.03357.x

47. Pyonteck SM, Akkari L, Schuhmacher AJ, Bowman RL, Sevenich L, et al. (2013) CSF-1R inhibition alters macrophage polarization and blocks glioma progression. Nat Med. doi:10.1038/nm.3337

48. Fridlender ZG, Kapoor V, Buchlis G, Cheng G, Sun J, et al. (2011) Monocyte chemoattractant protein-1 blockade inhibits lung cancer tumor growth by altering macrophage phenotype and activating CD8+ cells. Am J Respir Cell Mol Biol 44: 230–237. doi:10.1165/rcmb.2010-0080OC

Permissions

The contributors of this book come from diverse backgrounds, making this book a truly international effort. This book will bring forth new frontiers with its revolutionizing research information and detailed analysis of the nascent developments around the world.

We would like to thank all the contributing authors for lending their expertise to make the book truly unique. They have played a crucial role in the development of this book. Without their invaluable contributions this book wouldn't have been possible. They have made vital efforts to compile up to date information on the varied aspects of this subject to make this book a valuable addition to the collection of many professionals and students.

This book was conceptualized with the vision of imparting up-to-date information and advanced data in this field. To ensure the same, a matchless editorial board was set up. Every individual on the board went through rigorous rounds of assessment to prove their worth. After which they invested a large part of their time researching and compiling the most relevant data for our readers.

The editorial board has been involved in producing this book since its inception. They have spent rigorous hours researching and exploring the diverse topics which have resulted in the successful publishing of this book. They have passed on their knowledge of decades through this book. To expedite this challenging task, the publisher supported the team at every step. A small team of assistant editors was also appointed to further simplify the editing procedure and attain best results for the readers.

Apart from the editorial board, the designing team has also invested a significant amount of their time in understanding the subject and creating the most relevant covers. They scrutinized every image to scout for the most suitable representation of the subject and create an appropriate cover for the book.

The publishing team has been an ardent support to the editorial, designing and production team. Their endless efforts to recruit the best for this project, has resulted in the accomplishment of this book. They are a veteran in the field of academics and their pool of knowledge is as vast as their experience in printing. Their expertise and guidance has proved useful at every step. Their uncompromising quality standards have made this book an exceptional effort. Their encouragement from time to time has been an inspiration for everyone.

The publisher and the editorial board hope that this book will prove to be a valuable piece of knowledge for researchers, students, practitioners and scholars across the globe.

Contributors

Shengpeng Wang, Lu Wang, Zhangfeng Zhong, Meiwan Chen and Yitao Wang
State Key Laboratory of Quality Research in Chinese Medicine, Institute of Chinese Medical Sciences, University of Macau, Macau, China

Zhi Shi
Department of Cell Biology and Institute of Biomedicine, College of Life Science and Technology, Jinan University, Guangzhou, Guangdong, China

Can Zhou and Jian jun He
Department of Oncology Surgery, First Affiliated Hospital, School of Medicine of Xi'an Jiaotong University, Xi'an, Shaanxi Province, China

Jing Li, Jin hu Fan, You lin Qiao and Rong Huang
Department of Cancer Epidemiology, Cancer Institute and Hospital, Chinese Academy of Medical Sciences and Peking Union Medical College, Beijing, China

Bin Zhang
Department of Breast Surgery, Liaoning Cancer Hospital, Shen yang, Liaoning Province, China

Hong jian Yang
Department of Breast Surgery, Zhejiang Cancer Hospital, Hangzhou, Zhejiang Province, China

Xiao ming Xie
Department of Breast Oncology, Sun Yat-Sen University Cancer Center, Guangzhou, Guangdong Province, China

Zhong hua Tang
Department of Breast-thyroid Surgery, Xiangya Sencod Hospital, Central South University, Changsha, Hunan Province, China

Hui Li
Department of Breast Surgery, the Second People's Hospital of Sichuan Province, Chengdu, Sichuan Province, China

Jia yuan Li
Department of Epidemiology, West China School of Public Health, Sichuan University, Chengdu, Sichuan Province, China

Shu lian Wang
Department of Radiotherapy, Cancer Institute and Hospital, Chinese Academy of Medical Sciences and Peking Union Medical College, Beijing, China

Pin Zhang
Department of Medical Oncology, Cancer Institute and Hospital, Chinese Academy of Medical Sciences and Peking Union Medical College, Beijing, China

Leonarda Ianzano, Sara Bonomo, Carola Missaglia, Maria Grazia Cerrito, Roberto Giovannoni, Laura Masiero and Marialuisa Lavitrano
Department of Surgery and Traslational Medicine, Medical School, University of Milano-Bicocca, via Cadore 48, Monza, Italy

Emanuela Grassilli
Department of Surgery and Traslational Medicine, Medical School, University of Milano-Bicocca, via Cadore 48, Monza, Italy
BiOnSil srl, via Cadore 48, Monza, Italy

Jana Heitmann
Department of Medicine, Section of Hematology/Oncology, The University of Chicago, Chicago, Illinois, United States of America

Tanguy Y. Seiwert, Ezra E. W. Cohen and Everett E. Vokes
Department of Medicine, Section of Hematology/Oncology, The University of Chicago, Chicago, Illinois, United States of America
The University of Chicago Comprehensive Cancer Center, Chicago, Illinois, United States of America

Kerstin Stenson
Department of Surgery, Section of Head and Neck Surgery, The University of Chicago, Chicago, Illinois, United States of America

XiaoZhe Wang, Vivian Villegas-Bergazzi, Kam Sprott, Stephen Finn, David T. Weaver, Esther O'Regan and Allan D. Farrow
On-Q-ity Inc., Waltham, Massachusetts, United States of America

Ralph R. Weichselbaum
Department of Radiation Oncology, The University of Chicago, Chicago, Illinois, United States of America
The University of Chicago Comprehensive Cancer Center, Chicago, Illinois, United States of America

Mark W. Lingen
Department of Pathology, The University of Chicago, Chicago, Illinois, United States of America
The University of Chicago Comprehensive Cancer Center, Chicago, Illinois, United States of America

Hai-Yuan Xu, Li-Qiang Wang and Min-Bin Chen
Department of Medical Oncology, Kunshan First People's Hospital Affiliated to Jiangsu University, Kunshan, People's Republic of China

Wen-Lin Xu
Department of Central Laboratory, Zhenjiang Fourth People's Hospital Affiliated to Jiangsu University, Zhenjiang, People's Republic of China

Hui-Ling Shen
Department of Medical Oncology, Zhenjiang First People's Hospital Affiliated to Jiangsu University, Zhenjiang, People's Republic of China

Monica Mannelqvist
Centre for Cancer Biomarkers CCBIO, Department of Clinical Medicine, University of Bergen, Norway

Elisabeth Wik, Ingunn M. Stefansson and Lars A. Akslen
Centre for Cancer Biomarkers CCBIO, Department of Clinical Medicine, University of Bergen, Norway
Department of Pathology, The Gade Institute, Haukeland University Hospital, Bergen, Norway

Jeeyun Lee, Joon Oh Park and Young Suk Park
Division of Hematology-Oncology, Department of Medicine, Samsung Medical Center, Sungkyunkwan University School of Medicine, Seoul, Korea

Hee Cheol Kim
Departments of Surgery, Samsung Medical Center, Sungkyunkwan University School of Medicine, Seoul, Korea

Anjali Jain, Phillip Kim, Tani Lee, Anne Kuller, Fred Princen and Sharat Singh
Research and Development, Oncology, Prometheus Laboratories, San Diego, California, United States of America

In-GuDo and Suk Hyeong Kim
Pathology, Samsung Medical Center, Sungkyunkwan University School of Medicine, Seoul, Korea

Heather Spencer Feigelson, Chan Zeng and Carsie Nyirenda
Institute for Health Research, Kaiser Permanente Colorado, Denver, Colorado, United States of America

Pamala A. Pawloski
HealthPartners Institute for Education and Research, Bloomington, Minnesota, United States of America

Adedayo A. Onitilo
Department of Hematology/ Oncology, Marshfield Clinic Weston Center, Weston, Wisconsin, and Marshfield Clinic Research Foundation, Marshfield, Wisconsin, United States of America; Clinical Epidemiology Unit, School of Population Health, University of Queensland, Brisbane, Queensland, Australia

C. Sue Richards and Monique A. Johnson
Molecular and Medical Genetics, Oregon Health and Science University, Portland, Oregon, United States of America

Tia L. Kauffman, Jennifer Webster, Denise Schwarzkopf and Katrina A. B. Goddard
The Center for Health Research Kaiser Permanente Northwest, Portland, Oregon, United States of America

Gwen L. Alexander
Henry Ford Health System, Department of Public Health Sciences, Detroit, Michigan, United States of America

Clara Hwang
Henry Ford Health System, Department of Internal Medicine, Division of Hematology/Oncology, Detroit, Michigan, United States of America

Deanna Cross
Marshfield Clinic Research Foundation, Marshfield, Wisconsin, United States of America

Catherine A. McCarty
Essentia Institute of Rural Health, Duluth, Minnesota, United States of America

Robert L. Davis
Department of Pediatrics, University of Tennessee Health Sciences Center, Memphis, Tennessee, United States of America

Andrew E. Williams, Stacey Honda and Yihe Daida
Center for Health Research, Kaiser Permanente Hawai'i, Honolulu, Hawaii, United States of America

Lawrence H. Kushi
Division of Research, Kaiser Permanente Northern California, Oakland, California, United States of America

Thomas Delate
Kaiser Permanente Colorado, Pharmacy Department, Denver, Colorado, United States of America

Ryan R. Gordon, Mengchu Wu, Chung-Ying Huang, William P. Harris, Hong Gee Sim, Jared M. Lucas, Ilsa Coleman and Roman Gulati
Divisions of Human Biology and Clinical Research, Fred Hutchinson Cancer Research Center, Seattle, Washington, United States of America

Peter S. Nelson
Divisions of Human Biology and Clinical Research, Fred Hutchinson Cancer Research Center, Seattle, Washington, United States of America
Department of Medicine, University of Washington, Seattle, Washington, United States of America
Department of Pathology, University of Washington, Seattle, Washington, United States of America
Department of Urology, University of Washington, Seattle, Washington, United States of America

Tomasz M. Beer
Department of Medicine, Oregon Health and Sciences University, Portland, Oregon, United States of America

Celestia S. Higano
Department of Medicine, University of Washington, Seattle, Washington, United States of America
Department of Urology, University of Washington, Seattle, Washington, United States of America

Lawrence D. True
Department of Pathology, University of Washington, Seattle, Washington, United States of America
Department of Urology, University of Washington, Seattle, Washington, United States of America

Robert Vessella and Paul H. Lange
Department of Urology, University of Washington, Seattle, Washington, United States of America

Mark Garzotto
Department of Urology and Cancer Institute, Oregon Health and Sciences University, Portland, Oregon, United States of America
Section of Urology, Portland VA Medical Center, Portland, Oregon, United States of America

Annika Schlamann, Clemens Seidel, Rolf-Dieter Kortmann and Klaus Müller
Department for Radiation Oncology, University of Leipzig Medical Center, Leipzig, Saxony, Germany

André O. von Bueren
Department of Pediatrics and Adolescent Medicine, Division of Pediatric Hematology and Oncology, University of Göttingen Medical Center, Göttingen, Lower Saxony, Germany

Christian Hagel
Department of Neuropathology, University of Hamburg Eppendorf Medical Center, Hamburg, Germany

Isabella Zwiener
Institute for Medical Biostatistics, Epidemiology and Informatics, University of Mainz Medical Center, Mainz, Rhineland-Palatinate, Germany

Shenduo Li, Margaret Kennedy, Sturgis Payne, Kelly Kennedy, Salvatore V. Pizzo and Robin E. Bachelder
Department of Pathology, Duke University Medical Center, Durham, North Carolina, United States of America

Victoria L. Seewaldt
Department of Medicine, Duke University Medical Center, Durham, North Carolina, United States of America

Helen Mahony, Athanasios Tsalatsanis and Ambuj Kumar
Department of Internal Medicine, Division of Evidence-Based Medicine and Health Outcomes Research, University of South Florida, Tampa, Florida, United States of America

Benjamin Djulbegovic
Department of Internal Medicine, Division of Evidence-Based Medicine and Health Outcomes Research, University of South Florida, Tampa, Florida, United States of America
H. Lee Moffitt Cancer Center and Research Institute, Department of Hematology and Health Outcomes and Behavior, Tampa, Florida, United States of America

Shozo Nishida
Division of Pharmacotherapy, Kinki University Faculty of Pharmacy, Higashi-Osaka, Osaka, Japan

Yasuhiro Kidera
Division of Pharmacotherapy, Kinki University Faculty of Pharmacy, Higashi-Osaka, Osaka, Japan
Department of Pharmacy, Kinki University Faculty of Medicine, Osaka-Sayama, Osaka, Japan

Kimiko Fujiwara, Morihiro Nomura and Yuzuru Yamazoe
Department of Pharmacy, Kinki University Faculty of Medicine, Osaka-Sayama, Osaka, Japan

Hisato Kawakami, Tsutomu Sakiyama, Kunio Okamoto, Kaoru Tanaka, Masayuki Takeda, Hiroyasu Kaneda, Shin-ichi Nishina, Junji Tsurutani, Takao Tamura and Kazuhiko Nakagawa
Department of Medical Oncology, Kinki University Faculty of Medicine, Osaka-Sayama, Osaka, Japan

Yasutaka Chiba
Division of Biostatistics, Clinical Research Center, Kinki University Faculty of Medicine, Osaka-Sayama, Osaka, Japan

Jianfang Chen, Yonghai Peng, Feng Pan, Jianjun Li, Lan Zou, Yanling Zhang and Houjie Liang
Department of Oncology and Southwest Cancer Center, Southwest Hospital, Third Military Medical University, Chongqing, China

Zhenyu Ding
Department of Oncology, General Hospital of Shenyang Military Region, Shenyang, Liaoning, China

Michal Munster, Ella Fremder, Valeria Miller, Neta Ben-Tsedek, Shiri Davidi and Yuval Shaked
Department of Molecular pharmacology, Rappaport Faculty of Medicine, Technion, Haifa, Israel

Stefan J. Scherer
Hoffmann La Roche, Basel, Switzerland

Binafsha M. Syed, Andrew R. Green, Christopher C. Nolan, Ian O. Ellis and Kwok-Leung Cheung
School of Medicine, University of Nottingham, Nottingham, United Kingdom

David A. L. Morgan
Department of Oncology, Nottingham University Hospitals, Nottingham, United Kingdom

Peng Zhang, Mian Xi, Lei Zhao, Qiao-Qiao Li, Li-Ru He, Shi-Liang Liu and Meng-Zhong Liu
Sun Yat-sen University Cancer Center, State Key Laboratory of Oncology in South China, Collaborative Innovation Center for Cancer Medicine, Department of Radiation Oncology, Cancer Center, Sun Yat-sen University, Guangzhou, People's Republic of China

Jing-Xian Shen
Sun Yat-sen University Cancer Center, State Key Laboratory of Oncology in South China, Collaborative Innovation Center for Cancer Medicine, Imaging Diagnosis and Interventional Center, Cancer Center, Sun Yat-sen University, Guangzhou, People's Republic of China

Jie Ge, Zihua Chen and Zhikang Chen
Department of Gastrointestinal Surgery, Xiangya Hospital, Central South University, Changsha, Hunan, P. R. China

Jin Huang, Jinxiang Chen and Weijie Yuan
Department of Oncology, Xiangya Hospital, Central South University, Changsha, Hunan, P. R. China

Zhenghao Deng
Department of Pathology, Xiangya Hospital, Central South University, Changsha, Hunan, P. R. China

Jun Li, Jian-Wei Wang, Jin-Jie He, Xiu-Yan Yu, Su-Zhan Zhang and Ke-Feng Ding
Department of Surgical Oncology, Second Affiliated Hospital, Zhejiang University School of Medicine, Hangzhou, Zhejiang Province, China
The Key Laboratory of Cancer Prevention and Intervention, China National Ministry of Education, Hangzhou, Zhejiang Province, China

Yue Liu, Yang Gao and Ye-Ting Hu
The Key Laboratory of Cancer Prevention and Intervention, China National Ministry of Education, Hangzhou, Zhejiang Province, China

Han-Guang Hu and Ying Yuan
The Key Laboratory of Cancer Prevention and Intervention, China National Ministry of Education, Hangzhou, Zhejiang Province, China
Department of Medical Oncology, Second Affiliated Hospital, Zhejiang University School of Medicine, Hangzhou, Zhejiang Province, China

Keya Shah, Kelly Lien, Henry Lam and Yoo-Joung Ko
Sunnybrook Odette Cancer Centre, University of Toronto, Toronto, ON, Canada

Kelvin Chan
Sunnybrook Odette Cancer Centre, University of Toronto, Toronto, ON, Canada
Division of Biostatistics, Dalla Lana School of Public Health, University of Toronto,Toronto, ON, Canada

Doug Coyle
University of Ottawa, Ottawa, ON, Canada

Wenjun Zhao, Lirong Wei, Dongming Tan, Guangsong Su, Yanwen Zheng and Chao He
Cyrus Tang Hematology Center, Jiangsu Institute of Hematology, the First Affiliated Hospital, Soochow University, Suzhou, Jiangsu Province, PR China

Bin Yin
Cyrus Tang Hematology Center, Jiangsu Institute of Hematology, the First Affiliated Hospital, Soochow University, Suzhou, Jiangsu Province, PR China
Thrombosis and Hemostasis Key Lab of the Ministry of Health, Soochow University, Suzhou, Jiangsu Province, PR China
Collaborative Innovation Center of Hematology, Soochow University, Suzhou, Jiangsu Province, PR China

Zhengwei J. Mao
Division of Hematopathology, Department of Laboratory Medicine and Pathology, University of Minnesota Medical Center-Fairview, Minneapolis, Minnesota, United States of America

Timothy P. Singleton
Department of Laboratory Medicine and Pathology, University of Minnesota, Minneapolis, Minnesota, United States of America

Junjie Peng, Debing Shi, Xinxiang Li, Hongbin Wu and Sanjun Cai
Department of Colorectal Surgery, Fudan University Shanghai Cancer Center, Shanghai, China
Department of Oncology, Shanghai Medical College, Fudan University, Shanghai, China

Ying Ding
Department of Biostatistics, University of Pittsburgh, Pittsburgh, Pennsylvania, United States of America

Shanshan Tu
Department of Statistics, University of Pittsburgh, Pittsburgh, Pennsylvania, United States of America

Liang Sun
School of Science and Technology, Georgia Gwinnett College, Atlanta, Georgia, United States of America

Hong Qin, Feng Pan, Jianjun Li, Xiaoli Zhang, Houjie Liang and Zhihua Ruan
Department of Oncology, Southwest Hospital, the Third Military Medical University, Chongqing, PR China

Xu Liu, Ying-jie Jia and Jian-chun Yu
First Teaching Hospital of Tianjin University of Traditional Chinese Medicine, Tianjin, China

Rui-xian Han and Pan Pan
First Teaching Hospital of Tianjin University of Traditional Chinese Medicine, Tianjin, China
Tianjin University of Traditional Chinese Medicine, Tianjin, China

Cui Chen, Qiang-sheng Dai, Hui-wen Weng, He-ping Li and Sheng Ye
Department of Oncology, The First Affiliated Hospital, Sun Yat-Sen University, Guangzhou, China

Peng Sun
Department of Medical Oncology, Sun Yat-sen University Cancer Center, Guangzhou, China

Collaborative Innovation Center for Cancer Medicine, State Key Laboratory of Oncology in South China, Guangzhou, China

Maryam Hafsah Selamat
Department of Postgraduate Studies, University of Malaya, Kuala Lumpur, Malaysia

Siew Yim Loh
Department of Rehabilitation Medicine, Faculty of Medicine, University of Malaya, Kuala Lumpur, Malaysia

Lynette Mackenzie
Discipline of Occupational Therapy, Faculty of Health Sciences, University of Sydney, Sydney, Australia

Janette Vardy
Concord Cancer Centre, Concord Repatriation and General Hospital, Concord, Sydney, Australia
Sydney Medical School, The University of Sydney, Sydney, Australia

Alakesh Bera, Kolaparthi VenkataSubbaRao and Ping Hill
Department of Medicine, Division of Hematology and Oncology, University of Texas Health Science Center at San Antonio, San Antonio, Texas, United States of America

James W. Freeman
Cancer Therapy and Research Center, Experimental and Developmental Therapeutics Program, San Antonio, Texas, United States of America
Research and Development, Audie Murphy Veterans Administration Hospital, San Antonio, Texas, United States of America

Muthu Saravanan Manoharan
Research and Development, Audie Murphy Veterans Administration Hospital, San Antonio, Texas, United States of America

Zhiqi Chen, Ismat Khatri and Anna Podnos
University Health Network, Toronto General Hospital, Toronto, Canada

Reginald M. Gorczynski
University Health Network, Toronto General Hospital, Toronto, Canada
Department of Immunology, Faculty of Medicine, University of Toronto, and Institute of Medical Science, University of Toronto, Toronto, Ontario, Canada

Nuray Erin
Department of Medical Pharmacology, Akdeniz University, School of Medicine, Antalya, Turkey

Ying Huang, Xue-Ming Sun, Xiao-Wu Deng, Fei Han and Tai-Xiang Lu
Department of Radiation Oncology, Sun Yat-Sen University Cancer Center, State Key Laboratory of Oncology in South China, Collaborative Innovation Center of Cancer Medicine, Guangzhou, PR China

Yun-Ming Tian
Department of Radiation Oncology, Sun Yat-Sen University Cancer Center, State Key Laboratory of Oncology in South China, Collaborative Innovation Center of Cancer Medicine, Guangzhou, PR China
Department of Medical Oncology, Sun Yat-Sen University Cancer Center, State Key Laboratory of Oncology in South China, Collaborative Innovation Center of Cancer Medicine, Guangzhou, PR China

Lei Zeng
Department of Radiation Oncology, Sun Yat-Sen University Cancer Center, State Key Laboratory of Oncology in South China, Collaborative Innovation Center of Cancer Medicine, Guangzhou, PR China
Department of Medical Oncology, Sun Yat-Sen University Cancer Center, State Key Laboratory of Oncology in South China, Collaborative Innovation Center of Cancer Medicine, Guangzhou, PR China

Department of Radiation Oncology, Jiangxi Cancer Hospital, Nanchang, PR China

Feng-Hua Wang
Department of Medical Oncology, Sun Yat-Sen University Cancer Center, State Key Laboratory of Oncology in South China, Collaborative Innovation Center of Cancer Medicine, Guangzhou, PR China

Robin Cornelissen, Lysanne A. Lievense, Rudi W. Hendriks, Henk C. Hoogsteden, Joost P. Hegmans and Joachim G. Aerts
Department of Pulmonary Medicine, Erasmus MC Cancer Institute, Rotterdam, The Netherlands

Alexander P. Maat and Ad J. Bogers
Department of Cardio-Thoracic Surgery, Erasmus MC Cancer Institute, Rotterdam, The Netherlands

Index